Prognosis in Neurology

Prognosis in Neurology

Edited by

James M. Gilchrist, M.D.

Associate Professor of Neurology, Brown University
School of Medicine, Providence, Rhode Island;
Director, EMG Laboratory and Director,
Adult Muscular Dystrophy Association Clinic,
Rhode Island Hospital, Providence

With 94 Contributing Authors

Butterworth–Heinemann
Boston   Oxford   Johannesburg   Melbourne   New Delhi   Singapore

Butterworth–Heinemann supports the efforts of American Forests and the Global ReLeaf program in its campaign for the betterment of trees, forests, and our environment.

Library of Congress Cataloging-in-Publication Data

Prognosis in neurology / [edited by] James M. Gilchrist.
      p. cm.
   Includes bibliographical references and index.
   ISBN 0-7506-9888-8
   1. Nervous system--Diseases--Prognosis.   I. Gilchrist, James M.
   [DNLM: 1. Nervous System Diseases--diagnosis.   2. Prognosis. WL
   141 P964 1998]
  RC346.P77   1998
  616.8--dc21
  DNLM/DLC
  for Library of Congress   97-52638
                                        CIP

British Library Cataloguing-in-Publication Data

A catalogue record for this book is available from the British Library.

The publisher offers special discounts on bulk orders of this book.
For information, please contact:

Manager of Special Sales
Butterworth–Heinemann
225 Wildwood Avenue
Woburn, MA 01801-2041
Tel: 781-904-2500
Fax: 781-904-2620

For information on all Butterworth–Heinemann publications available,
contact our World Wide Web home page at: http://www.bh.com

10 9 8 7 6 5 4 3 2 1

Printed in the United States of America

To my parents, Jim and Ann;
to my wife, Maria; and
to my children, Cullen, Greer, James, and Aidan

It appears to me a most excellent thing for the physician to cultivate Prognosis; for by forseeing and foretelling, in the presence of the sick, the present, the past, and the future, and explaining the omissions which patients have been guilty of, he will be the more readily believed to be acquainted with the circumstances of the sick; so that men will have confidence to intrust themselves to such a physician. And he will manage the cure best who has foreseen what is to happen from the present state of matters.

—Hippocrates, *On the Prognostics, I*

Patients and their families will forgive you for wrong diagnoses, but will rarely forgive you for wrong prognoses.

—Albert R. Lamb, *Journal of Chronic Diseases* 1963;16:441

Contents

Contributing Authors

Israel F. Abroms, M.D.
Professor of Pediatrics and Neurology, University of Massachusetts Medical School, Worcester

Lloyd M. Alderson, M.D., D.Sc.
Assistant Professor of Neurology and Neuroscience, Brown University School of Medicine and Rhode Island Hospital, Providence

Paul E. Barkhaus, M.D.
Associate Professor of Neurology, Medical College of Wisconsin, Milwaukee; Director, Neuromuscular Diseases, Clement J. Zablocki Veterans Affairs Medical Center, Milwaukee

Valerie Biousse, M.D.
Chef de Clinique–Assistant, Neurology Department, Lariboisiere Hospital, Paris

Jane G. Boggs, M.D.
Assistant Professor of Neurology and Co-Director, Division of Neurophysiology, Virginia Commonwealth University Medical College of Virginia School of Medicine, Richmond

Mark B. Bromberg, M.D., Ph.D.
Associate Professor of Neurology, University of Utah School of Medicine, Salt Lake City

Mark T. Brown, M.D.
Assistant Professor of Neurology, Duke University School of Medicine, Durham, North Carolina

William D. Brown, M.D.
Assistant Professor of Pediatrics and Neurology, Brown University School of Medicine, Providence, Rhode Island; Attending Physician, Departments of Neurology and Pediatrics, Rhode Island Hospital, Providence

William W. Campbell, M.D., M.S.H.A.
Professor of Neurology and Chair, Division of Adult Neurology, Virginia Commonwealth University Medical College of Virginia School of Medicine, Richmond

David J. Capobianco, M.D.
Assistant Professor of Neurology, Mayo Graduate School of Medicine, Rochester, Minnesota; Consultant in Neurology, Mayo Clinic Jacksonville, Jacksonville, Florida

Percy Chan, B.S.
Research Assistant, Department of Clinical Neurosciences, Brown University School of Medicine and Department of Neurosurgery, Rhode Island Hospital, Providence

William P. Cheshire, M.D.
Assistant Professor of Neurology, Mayo Graduate School of Medicine, Rochester, Minnesota; Consultant in Neurology, Mayo Clinic Jacksonville, Jacksonville, Florida

David B. Clifford, M.D.
Professor of Neurology, Washington University School of Medicine, Washington University Medical Center, St. Louis, Missouri

Cynthia L. Comella, M.D.
Associate Professor of Neurological Science, Rush Medical College of Rush University, Chicago;

Associate Attending Neurologist, Rush-Presbyterian-St. Luke's Medical Center, Chicago

Patricia K. Coyle, M.D.
Professor of Neurology, SUNY at Stony Brook School of Medicine Health Sciences Center, Stony Brook, New York; Director, Multiple Sclerosis Comprehensive Care Center, University Hospital Medical Center, Stony Brook

Jacqueline Crawford, M.D.
Senior Instructor of Neurology, Oregon Health Sciences University School of Medicine, Portland

Allen C. Crocker, M.D.
Associate Professor of Pediatrics, Harvard Medical School, Boston; Associate Professor of Maternal and Child Health, Harvard School of Public Health, Boston; Program Director, Institute for Community Inclusion, Children's Hospital, Boston

Oscar H. Del Brutto, M.D.
Chief of Neurology, Luis Vernaza Hospital, Guayaquil, Ecuador

Robert J. DeLorenzo, M.D., Ph.D., M.P.H.
George B. Bliley III Professor of Neurology; Chairman of Neurology; Professor, Departments of Pharmacology and Toxicology, Biochemistry and Molecular Biophysics; and Director, Molecular Neuroscience Facility, Virginia Commonwealth University Medical College of Virginia School of Medicine, Richmond

John F. Ditunno, Jr., M.D.
Professor of Rehabilitation Medicine, Jefferson Medical College of Thomas Jefferson University, Philadelphia; Project Director, Regional Spinal Cord Injury Center of Delaware Valley, Thomas Jefferson University Hospital, Philadelphia

Curtis Doberstein, M.D.
Assistant Professor of Clinical Neuroscience, Brown University School of Medicine, Providence, Rhode Island; Director, Cerebrovascular Surgery, Rhode Island Hospital, Providence

David W. Dodick, M.D., F.R.C.P.C., F.A.C.P.
Assistant Professor of Neurology, Mayo Graduate School of Medicine, Rochester, Minnesota; Senior Associate Consultant, Mayo Clinic

Gerald Exil, M.D.
Assistant Professor of Neurology and Pediatrics, Brown University School of Medicine, Providence, Rhode Island; Pediatric Neurologist, Rhode Island Hospital, Providence

Daniel M. Feinberg, M.D.
Clinical Fellow in Neurology, Harvard Medical School, Boston; Fellow in Clinical Neurophysiology, Brigham and Women's Hospital, Boston

Christopher S. Formal, M.D.
Assistant Professor of Rehabilitation Medicine, Jefferson Medical College of Thomas Jefferson University, Philadelphia; Staff Physiatrist, Magee Rehabilitation Hospital, Philadelphia

Marc H. Friedberg, M.D., Ph.D.
Neurosurgical Resident, New England Medical Center, Boston

Joseph H. Friedman, M.D.
Professor of Clinical Neurosciences, Brown University School of Medicine, Providence, Rhode Island; Chief of Neurology, Memorial Hospital of Rhode Island, Pawtucket

Gerhard M. Friehs, M.D.
Assistant Professor of Neurosurgery, Brown University School of Medicine and Rhode Island Hospital, Providence

Karen L. Furie, M.D., M.P.H.
Instructor in Neurology, Harvard Medical School, Boston; Assistant in Neurology, Massachusetts General Hospital, Boston

Generoso G. Gascon, M.D.
Professor of Neurology and Pediatrics, Brown University School of Medicine, Providence, Rhode Island; Director, Division of Pediatric Neurology, Rhode Island Hospital/Hasbro Children's Hospital, Providence

James M. Gilchrist, M.D.
Associate Professor of Neurology, Brown University School of Medicine, Providence, Rhode Island; Director, EMG Laboratory, and Director, Adult Muscular Dystrophy Association Clinic, Rhode Island Hospital, Providence

William D. Graf, M.D.
Assistant Professor of Pediatrics and Neurology, University of Washington School of Medicine, Seattle; Attending Physician, Departments of Pediatrics and Neurology, Children's Hospital and Regional Medical Center, Seattle

Neill R. Graff-Radford, M.B.B.Ch., M.R.C.P.
Professor of Neurology, Mayo Clinic Jacksonville, Jacksonville, Florida

Paul E. Greene, M.D.
Assistant Professor of Neurology, Columbia University College of Physicians and Surgeons, New York; Assistant Attending Neurologist, Columbia-Presbyterian Medical Center, New York

Maria Guglielmo, M.D.
Senior Neurosurgical Resident, Brown University School of Medicine and Rhode Island Hospital, Providence

Vladimir Hachinski, B.A., M.D., F.R.C.P.C., M.Sc.(D.M.E.), D.M.Sc.
Richard and Beryl Ivey Professor and Chair of Neurology, University of Western Ontario Faculty of Medicine, London, Ontario; Chief of Clinical Neurological Sciences, London Health Sciences Center-University Campus, London, Ontario

John J. Halperin, M.D.
Professor of Neurology, New York University School of Medicine, Manhasset; Chair of Neurology, North Shore University Hospital, Manhasset

Julie E. Hammack, M.D.
Assistant Professor of Neurology, Mayo Clinic, Rochester, Minnesota

Parissa Jannati, M.D.
Clinical Instructor in Neurology, University of California, Los Angeles, UCLA School of Medicine and the Los Angeles County Harbor/UCLA Medical Center

Gary Johnson, M.D.
Clinical Assistant Professor of Clinical Neuroscience, Brown University School of Medicine, Providence, Rhode Island; Assistant Neurologist, Rhode Island Hospital, Providence

Burk Jubelt, M.D.
Professor and Chair, Department of Neurology, Professor of Microbiology/Immunology and Neuroscience, State University of New York Health Science Center at Syracuse College of Medicine; Attending Neurologist, University Hospital, SUNY Health Science Center at Syracuse

Peter W. Kaplan, M.B., F.R.C.P.
Associate Professor of Neurology, Johns Hopkins University School of Medicine, Baltimore; Chair of Neurology, The Johns Hopkins Bayview Medical Center, Baltimore

George Karpati, M.D., F.R.C.P.C.
Izaak W. Killam Chair of Neurology, Neuromuscular Research Group, Montreal Neurological Institute, McGill University Faculty of Medicine; Senior Neurologist, Montreal Neurological Hospital, Montreal

Douglas I. Katz, M.D.
Assistant Professor of Neurology, Boston University School of Medicine; Director, Neurorehabilitation Programs, HealthSouth Braintree Hospital Rehabilitation Network, Braintree, Massachusetts

Laurence J. Kinsella, M.D., F.A.C.P.
Assistant Professor of Neurology, Case Western Reserve University School of Medicine, Cleveland; Chief, Division of Neurology, Mt. Sinai Medical Center, Cleveland

William C. Koller, M.D., Ph.D.
Professor and Chair of Neurology, University of Kansas School of Medicine and University of Kansas Medical Center, Kansas City

Rhonda G. Kost, M.D.
Staff Investigator, Aaron Diamond AIDS Research Center, New York; Assistant Professor and Associate Physician, Rockefeller University Hospital, New York

Naomi R. Kramer, M.D.
Assistant Professor of Medicine, Brown University School of Medicine, Providence, Rhode Island; Associate Director, Sleep Disorders Center, Rhode Island Hospital, Providence

Eugene C. Lai, M.D., Ph.D.
Assistant Professor of Neurology and Cell Biology, Baylor College of Medicine, Houston; Active Staff, Neurology Service, The Methodist Hospital, Houston

Frank Lieberman, M.D.
Assistant Professor of Neurology and Co-Director of Neuro-Oncology, Mount Sinai School of Medicine of the City University of New York

Alan H. Lockwood, M.D.
Professor of Neurology and Nuclear Medicine, University at Buffalo School of Medicine and Biomedical Sciences and Center for PET, Veterans Affairs Western New York Healthcare System, Buffalo

Eric L. Logigian, M.D.
Associate Professor of Neurology, Harvard Medical School, Boston; Director, Clinical Neurophysiology Laboratory, Brigham and Women's Hospital, Boston

Sydney Louis, M.D.
Professor of Neurology, Brown University School of Medicine, Providence, Rhode Island; Attending Neurologist, Rhode Island Hospital, Providence

Karen S. Marder, M.D., M.P.H.
Associate Professor of Clinical Neurology and Associate Attending, Columbia University College of Physicians and Surgeons, New York

E. Wayne Massey, M.D.
Director of Neurorehabilitation, Duke University Medical Center, Durham, North Carolina

Grace A. Medeiros, M.D.
Clinical Instructor in Neurology, Brown University School of Medicine, Providence, Rhode Island; Senior Fellow in Clinical Neurophysiology, Rhode Island Hospital, Providence

Richard P. Millman, M.D.
Professor of Medicine, Brown University School of Medicine, Providence, Rhode Island; Director, Sleep Disorders Center of Lifespan Hospitals, Providence

Patricia M. Moore, M.D.
Associate Professor of Neurology, Wayne State University School of Medicine, Detroit

Joel C. Morgenlander, M.D.
Assistant Professor of Medicine (Neurology) and Director, Neurology Residency Training Program, Duke University Medical Center, Durham, North Carolina

Richard Munson, M.D.
Clinical Stroke Fellow, University of Western Ontario Faculty of Medicine, London, Ontario

Ruth Nass, M.D.
Professor of Clinical Neurology, New York University School of Medicine, New York

David A. Neumeyer, M.D.
Instructor in Medicine, Harvard Medical School, Boston; Sleep Fellow, Rhode Island Hospital, Providence

Nancy J. Newman, M.D.
Cyrus H. Stoner Professor of Ophthalmology, Associate Professor of Ophthalmology and Neurology, and Instructor in Neurosurgery, Emory University School of Medicine, Atlanta; Director of Neuro-Ophthalmology Unit, Emory Eye Center, Atlanta; Lecturer in Ophthalmology, Harvard Medical School, Boston

Errol R. Norwitz, M.D., Ph.D.
Instructor in Maternal-Fetal Medicine, Department of Obstetrics and Gynecology, Brigham and Women's Hospital, Harvard Medical School, Boston

Brian R. Ott, M.D.
Associate Professor of Neurology, Brown University School of Medicine, Providence, Rhode Island; Associate Chief of Neurology, Memorial Hospital of Rhode Island, Pawtucket

Pinar T. Ozand, M.D., Ph.D.
Director, Inborn Errors of Metabolism Research Laboratory, King Faisal Specialist Hospital and Research Centre, Riyadh, Saudi Arabia

Eric J. Pappert, M.D.
Assistant Professor of Neurological Sciences, Movement Disorders Section, Rush-Presbyterian-St. Luke's Medical Center, Chicago

Roy A. Patchell, M.D.
Chief of Neuro-Oncology, University of Kentucky College of Medicine, Lexington

John M. Pellock, M.D.
Chairman, Division of Child Neurology; Professor of Neurology, Pediatrics, Pharmacy, and Pharmaceutics; and Director, Comprehensive Epilepsy Institute, Virginia Commonwealth University Medical College of Virginia School of Medicine, Richmond

David C. Preston, M.D.
Assistant Professor of Neurology, Harvard Medical School, Boston; Director, Neuromuscular Service, Brigham and Women's Hospital, Boston

John T. Repke, M.D.
The Chris J. and Marie A. Olson Professor of Obstetrics and Gynecology and Chairman, Department of Obstetrics and Gynecology, University of Nebraska College of Medicine and Medical Center, Omaha

Loren A. Rolak, M.D.
Director, Marshfield Multiple Sclerosis Center, Department of Neuroscience, Marshfield Clinic, Marshfield, Wisconsin

Michael Ronthal, M.B.B.Ch.
Associate Professor of Neurology, Harvard Medical School, Boston; Deputy Chief of Neurology, Beth Israel Deaconess Medical Center, Boston

Stacie L. Ropka, M.S.
Senior Research Support Specialist, Department of Neurology, State University of New York Health Science Center at Syracuse College of Medicine

Beth A. Rosen, M.D.
Assistant Professor of Pediatrics and Neurology, University of Massachusetts Medical School and Medical Center, Worcester

Marvin P. Rozear, M.D.
Associate Professor of Medicine (Neurology), Duke University Medical Center, Durham, North Carolina

Allan E. Rubenstein, M.D.
Clinical Associate Professor of Neurology and Director, Mount Sinai Neurofibromatosis Center,
Mount Sinai School of Medicine of the City University of New York

Barry S. Russman, M.D.
Professor of Pediatrics and Neurology, Oregon Health Sciences University School of Medicine, Portland; Pediatric Neurologist, Shriner's Hospital for Children, Portland

George M. Sachs, M.D., Ph.D.
Assistant Professor of Neurology, Brown University School of Medicine, Providence, Rhode Island; Assistant Director, EMG Laboratory, Rhode Island Hospital, Providence

Donald B. Sanders, M.D.
Professor of Medicine, Division of Neurology, Duke University Medical Center, Durham, North Carolina

Harvey B. Sarnat, M.D.
Professor of Neurology, Pediatrics, and Pathology (Neuropathology), University of Washington School of Medicine, Children's Hospital, and Regional Medical Center, Seattle

Jeffrey L. Saver, M.D.
Assistant Professor of Clinical Neurology, University of California, Los Angeles, UCLA School of Medicine; Neurology Director, UCLA Stroke and Medical Center, Los Angeles

Thomas F. Scott, M.D.
Associate Professor of Neurology, Allegheny University Hospitals, Allegheny General Hospital, Pittsburgh

Jeremy M. Shefner, M.D., Ph.D.
Associate Professor of Neurology and Director, Clinical Neurophysiology Laboratory, State University of New York Health Science Center at Syracuse College of Medicine

O. Carter Snead III, M.D., F.R.C.P.C.
Professor of Pediatrics, Neurology, and Pharmacology, University of Toronto Faculty of Medicine; Bloorview Children's Hospital Foundation Chair in Pediatric Neuroscience; and Head, Division of Neurology and The Epilepsy Research Program, The Hospital for Sick Children, Toronto

Yuen So, M.D., Ph.D.
Associate Professor of Neurology, Oregon Health Sciences University School of Medicine, Portland

S.H. Subramony, M.D.
Professor and Vice Chairman of Neurology, University of Mississippi School of Medicine and Medical Center, Jackson

Charlene A. Tate, M.D.
Clinical Assistant Professor of Neurology, Brown University School of Medicine and Rhode Island Hospital, Providence

Alan R. Towne, M.D.
Associate Professor of Neurology and Director, Division of Neurophysiology, Virginia Commonwealth University Medical College of Virginia School of Medicine, Richmond

Stanley Tuhrim, M.D.
Associate Professor of Neurology, Mount Sinai School of Medicine of the City University of New York; Director, Division of Cerebrovascular and Critical Care Neurology, Mount Sinai Medical Center, New York

Kenneth L. Tyler, M.D.
Professor and Vice Chairman of Neurology and Professor of Medicine, Microbiology, and Immunology, University of Colorado Health Sciences Center, Denver; Chief of Neurology Service, Denver Veterans Affairs Medical Center

Beverly C. Walters, M.D., M.Sc., F.R.C.S.C., F.A.C.S.
Associate Professor of Neurosurgery, Brown University School of Medicine, Providence, Rhode Island; Chief, Neurosurgery Service, Miriam Hospital, Providence

James R. White, M.D.
Senior Resident in Neurology, Brown University School of Medicine and Rhode Island Hospital, Providence

Eelco F.M. Wijdicks, M.D., Ph.D.
Professor of Neurology, Mayo Medical School, Rochester, Minnesota; Medical Director, Neurosurgical-Neurological ICU, Mayo Clinic, Rochester

Janet L. Wilterdink, M.D.
Assistant Professor of Neurology and Neurologist, Brown University School of Medicine and Rhode Island Hospital, Providence

Preface

Medicine is practiced very differently now than it was 100 years ago, a change brought about by the scientific method. Modern medicine is built on scientific evidence, and the result has been wonderful advances in knowledge and successes in diagnosis and treatment. But there is a third task for the physician, and it has been sadly neglected of late. That task is prognosis. Before the great life-saving discoveries of the 1900s, a physician's ability was judged less by ability to treat, as that was often limited, and more on ability to foretell the course and events of an illness, often on the basis of only a bedside examination. The physician who could accurately predict which patients would live, which would die, which would suffer, and which would thrive was a physician of much talent. In the headlong scramble to banish death and suffering from the human experience, we have left the ability to prognosticate far behind. As I very much doubt we will be successful in attaining immortality, I think it time to reassess the importance of prognosis.

This is not to say that modern medicine has failed to provide significant improvements in our understanding of the natural history and ultimate ending for many diseases, but there has been little effort to make sense of this information or to process it in a useable fashion. Prognostic data is often dealt with perfunctorily and buried within articles and chapters more concerned with diagnosis and therapy. Yet, many patients' first question after the examination is "What is going to happen to me?" And it is that question to which this book is directed.

Prognosis is a particularly pertinent purpose in neurology. Although neuroscience has seen stupendous advances in chemistry, physiology, pathology, diagnosis, and therapy, the relative inability of the nervous system to regenerate and recover, its sequestration, and its complexity make the nervous system less amenable to therapeutic strategies that are successful in other organ systems. The neurologist is commonly consulted not only to diagnose but to prognosticate. This book is meant to assist in this regard and to serve as a readily accessible guide to prognosis for the clinical neurologist and general internist. It consists of short chapters organized by disease and assumes the correct diagnosis has been made and therapeutic options are known. Other texts of a similar nature are available to guide diagnosis and therapy, and those topics have been purposefully excluded to allow an undiluted discussion of prognosis.

J.M.G.

Part I
Disorders of Consciousness

Chapter 1

Hypoglycemia and Other Metabolic Encephalopathies

Alan H. Lockwood

Metabolic encephalopathies, including hypoglycemia, are a group of disorders caused by a disruption of the normal physiologic state due to the presence of an excess or deficiency of a critical metabolite (e.g., glucose) or a toxin (either produced by the body or present as the result of environmental exposure). The evaluation, treatment, and prognosis of these disorders depend on an understanding of the possible pathophysiologic disruptions of each compound or toxin. As the number of metabolites and toxins that are potential causes of encephalopathy is enormous, this brief discussion focuses on hypoglycemia as a prototype of these disorders.

Natural History

The natural history of the metabolic encephalopathies varies substantially, depending on their cause and severity. Regardless of cause, for example, many episodes of hypoglycemia resolve spontaneously without treatment, whereas other episodes may be fatal. Similarly, the degree of self-awareness of illness and disability also varies. Though some variance in awareness arises as a result of idiosyncratic factors, the fact that metabolic encephalopathies characteristically produce derangements in consciousness and cognitive functions of the brain is a major contributing factor. The relatively recent recognition of the hypoglycemia-unaware syndrome typifies this problem.

Hypoglycemia may originate among outpatients and in hospitalized patients. Several studies have suggested that hypoglycemia is a common occurrence. Stepka et al. evaluated 236 case records of patients with hypoglycemia severe enough to require hospitalization. An error in diet was the most frequent cause in their population and was responsible for approximately half the admissions. Somewhat surprisingly, these authors reported excessive physical activity as the next most common cause (responsible for 55 cases). Errors in doses of hypoglycemic drugs accounted for only 22 cases. Alcohol abuse caused 13 cases. Using a method that evaluated all blood glucose measurements performed by the clinical chemistry laboratory, Stagnaro-Green and colleagues found a 1.9% incidence of hypoglycemia in hospitalized patients.

In an earlier study, Fischer and colleagues found 137 episodes of severe hypoglycemia (defined as serum glucose of less than 50 mg per deciliter) in 94 patients in a 6-month period in a tertiary care hospital. Decreased caloric intake was common and usually was due to the severity of the illness or to disruption of eating patterns owing to hospital routine. Hypoglycemia complicated the treatment of hypokalemia in eight patients and occurred in six patients after treatment of hyperglycemia associated with the use of total parenteral nutrition. Chronic renal insufficiency was present in almost half the cases of hypoglycemia: Only 20 of these 46 patients were diabetics. Thus, renal failure, even in the absence of diabetes mellitus, is an important factor predisposing to the development of hypoglycemia. Other identified causes included liver disease, infection, shock, pregnancy, neoplasia, and burns.

Death is common among hypoglycemic patients. In the Fischer series, hypoglycemia was not the immediate cause of death in any of their indexed cases, but the in-hospital mortality was 27%. The risk of death was highest in patients with the most severe hypoglycemia and the largest number of associated risk factors. Stagnaro-Green and colleagues reported a similar mortality rate of 22.2%. They found the highest mortality rates among black and Hispanic patients (30% and 46%, respectively) and a mortality rate of 6% among white patients.

Hypoglycemia is a relatively uncommon cause of sudden unexpected death. Klatt and coworkers found 123 cases of death due to hypoglycemia (plasma glucose <40 mg per deciliter) among 54,850 autopsies performed by a medical examiner's office in southern California. Alcohol abuse and drugs were associated with 33% and 21% of the cases, respectively. Other associated conditions included cancer, chronic passive congestion of the liver, debilitating neurologic disease, endocrine disorders, and a variety of miscellaneous conditions. The mechanisms implicated were related to the combined effects of liver disease and impaired carbohydrate metabolism, drug or hormonal effects, or inanition due to decreased food intake.

Although diabetes and the use of hypoglycemic agents are risk factors for the development of hypoglycemia, the type of insulin used does not appear to affect the probability of developing hypoglycemia. Both human insulin and insulins derived from animal sources appear to lead to inadvertent hypoglycemia with equal frequency.

Factors Affecting Prognosis

The presence or absence of secondary structural cerebral injury and the presence of permanent or irreversible injury to another organ are the most important factors in determining the ultimate prognosis of metabolic encephalopathy. Patients who experience structural injury to the brain will exhibit variable degrees of recovery dependent on the severity of the brain injury. The metabolic disorder also may predispose to the development of additional neurologic problems. For example, patients with hypoglycemia and secondary epileptic seizures risk seizure-related complications that may compound the effects of hypoglycemia (hypoxia in addition to hypoglycemia). In the absence of a structural injury, most patients should recover completely, once the cause of encephalopathy has been reversed.

Evaluation for Prognosis

The prognosis for patients with hypoglycemia depends on the severity of the metabolic disruption and the presence of other complicating factors, as indicated in Natural History. Levy and associates evaluated 500 adult patients with coma due to causes other than trauma to determine the physical findings that were the most reliable predictors of outcome. Outcome was defined as the best level of function documented in the year following the episode of coma, based on the rationale that subsequent declines were potentially avoidable or unrelated to the episode of coma. The most important objective in these authors' analysis was the avoidance of an incorrect prediction of poor prognosis (e.g., death, persistent vegetative state) among patients who eventually recovered a measure of independent function. In an examination of cause of coma, the group with metabolic etiologies fared best, with 31% experiencing a good recovery. Death or the vegetative state was the result in 54%. For the entire group, these percentages were 12% and 73%, respectively. Regardless of etiology, neurologic examination performed 6 hours after the onset of coma provided reliable information concerning outcome. Of the 120 patients without corneal, pupillary, or oculovestibular reflexes, 97% died or remained in the vegetative state, and only 1% experienced a good recovery. If any two of those reflexes were present and the patient vocalized by moaning, 41% had a good recovery, whereas 59% eventually died or remained in the vegetative state. Thus, as might be expected, indicators of structural damage to the brain stem were associated with the worst outcomes.

Therapies Affecting Prognosis

The intravenous administration of glucose is the primary treatment for hypoglycemia. As hypoglycemia is relatively common and the risk for permanent neurologic injury is high in patients with untreated or delayed treatment, it is appropriate routinely to administer glucose to unconscious patients. This generalization should be considered strongly, even among hospitalized nondiabetic patients. Low risk is associated with the administration of glucose to a patient who already may be hyperglycemic, whereas the potential benefits of prompt treatment are high.

Short- and Long-Term Prognosis

As most episodes of hypoglycemia resolve completely with minimal treatment, full recovery with no sequelae is the rule. The long-term prognosis for patients who experience hypoglycemia is determined by the severity of the episode and by the nature and severity of predisposing causes, such as renal failure, cancer, or alcohol abuse. In the absence of predisposing factors, hypoglycemia rarely causes death, accounting for approximately 0.2% of all cases referred to a California medical examiner. Although hypoglycemia rarely is the immediate cause of death, some 25% of hypoglycemic patients die. For unknown reasons, black and Hispanic patients experience higher mortality (30% and 46%, respectively) than do whites (6%).

Additional Reading

Fischer KF, Lees JA, Newman JH. Hypoglycemia in hospitalized patients. Causes and outcomes. N Engl J Med 1986;315:1245–1250.

Jick SS, Derby LE, Gross KM, Jick H. Hospitalizations because of hypoglycemia in users of animal and human insulins: II. Experience in the United States. Pharmacotherapy 1990;10:398–399.

Klatt EC, Beatie C, Noguchi TT. Evaluation of death from hypoglycemia. Am J Forensic Med Pathol 1988;9:122–125.

Levy, DE, Bates, D, Caronna, JJ, et al. Prognosis in nontraumatic coma. Ann Intern Med 1981;94:293–301.

Lingenfelser T, Renn W, Sommerwerck U, et al. Compromised hormonal counterregulation, symptom awareness, and neurophysiologic function after recurrent short-term episodes of insulin-induced hypoglycemia in IDDM patients. Diabetes 1993;42:610–618.

Stagnaro-Green A, Barton MK, Linekin PL, et al. Mortality in hospitalized patients with hypoglycemia and severe hyperglycemia. Mt Sinai J Med 1995;62:422–426.

Stepka M, Rogala H, Czyzyk A. Hypoglycemia: a major problem in the management of diabetes in the elderly. Aging 1993;5:117–121.

Chapter 2
Anoxic-Ischemic Encephalopathy

Eelco F.M. Wijdicks

Hypoxic-ischemic encephalopathy remains a major cause of persistent disability in hospitals. One-year survival of comatose patients resuscitated from cardiac arrest is between 10 and 25%. However, some patients who survive the systemic complications that triggered the hypoxic-ischemic insult may have a good chance to recover to a premorbid state. Therefore, any prediction of neurologic outcome in patients after successful resuscitation should be considered "best possible outcome"—if the patient survives.

Natural History

The mechanism of anoxic-ischemic encephalopathy is complex, but the most likely pathway is through excitotoxic damage from excitatory amino acids, a derangement in calcium homeostasis, and further neuronal damage from oxygen-derived free radicals. Irrespective of the duration of resuscitation, the most susceptible neurons are located in the hippocampus, cerebellum, putamen, caudate, and thalamus. In most circumstances, cardiac arrest is the main trigger for anoxia, which often is observed in association with acute myocardial infarction or a malignant cardiac arrhythmia. Hypovolemic shock is associated less commonly with a persistent hypoxemic-ischemic insult, but it may occur in patients in need of multiple blood or plasma transfusions or of pharmacologic support of blood pressure. Approximately 50% of all patients die after cardiac arrest. Of the patients who survive, approximately two-thirds die within 6 months and, of the

remaining one-third, a small proportion die in the ensuing year from cardiac failure or sudden death associated with cardiac arrhythmias. In elderly patients and in patients who remain comatose after successful resuscitation, the natural history is less favorable, although accurate neurologic data from the elderly group are not available.

Deterioration to lower levels of consciousness in the first postoperative days is unusual. However, well-documented cases have reported extensive bihemispheric demyelination without pathologic evidence of edema in some patients, with further progression to coma and death. These patients initially were asymptomatic and had sudden deterioration up to 14 days after the ictus. Early ambulation preceded this devastating event, but a metabolic derangement, such as hypoglycemia, hypernatremia, marked hypoxemia, or labile blood pressure, may have contributed. This finding may suggest that after the initial anoxic insult, the white matter is vulnerable to sudden metabolic changes or to sudden changes in blood pressure.

Factors Affecting Prognosis

Several general rules apply to the factors affecting prognosis. Outcome is quite favorable when an intubated patient fends off a painful stimulus immediately after cardiopulmonary resuscitation. On the contrary, lack of a motor response to pain in the first hours does not necessarily imply neurologic impairment is inevitable. The chance of good recovery is expectedly low, but up to 22% of patients recover to a functional state. Patients who awaken on the day of cardiac arrest gradually progress from a dazed state to alertness within 12 hours. Resuscitation of long duration, defined as multiple defibrillations and intravenous administration of epinephrine, usually increases the probability of severe brain damage, resulting in abnormal extensor and flexor responses or flaccidity in the arms and legs. The immediate finding of a localizing response is the best evidence that the duration of anoxia has been brief. Focal neurologic signs are uncommon but may arise from involvement in arterial border zones; they occur more frequently in patients with severe carotid occlusions. Infarction of these borderline zones produces bibrachial paralysis ("man in the barrel") but is uncommon. Many clinical series have highlighted the dire consequences of abnormal brain stem reflexes. However, brain stem reflexes have not been examined systematically in large resuscitation series, or data acquisition has been incomplete. Clinicians must be extremely careful in using abnormal eye movements and pupillary light response as signs of low probability of salvaging the patient, particularly during or immediately after resuscitation efforts. As a rule, the pupil diameter widens, and light response is abolished within a few minutes after cardiac standstill. Frequent systemic use of atropine and epinephrine may cause dilated pupils, but the pupils do not lose their light response.

Several factors have been identified and can be used as indicators of poor outcome within the first postresuscitation day. Myoclonus status epilepticus strongly indicates severe anoxic cortical damage and should be considered an agonal phenomenon. Myoclonus often involves the limbs and face. The rapid and brief jerks in the facial musculature can suggest painful grimacing. The myoclonus can be elicited by hand-clap or pressure to the nail beds or by insertion of central venous catheters but most often is detected after tracheal suctioning. Upward jerking of the eye globes may occur as well, often simultaneously with facial jerks and opening of the eyelids. This type of myoclonus should be differentiated from action myoclonus (so-called *Lance-Adams syndrome*). This syndrome becomes evident only after awakening and, more frequently, after respiratory arrest. Another important early sign of poor outcome is sustained upward gaze (i.e., the eyes turn upward and cannot be brought to a different position). The pathologic substrate of this unusual eye finding is generalized laminar cortical necrosis, often with involvement of bithalamic structures.

A fixed-pupil response to light has been established as an important clinical sign. In the landmark study by Levy and coworkers, it was identified as the only clinical feature that immediately distinguished between the probability of a reasonable outcome or persistent vegetative state and death (Fig. 2-1).

If these early prognostic features are absent, the neurologic examination should be repeated 3 days after the initial event, when any major change in the motor response should be seen. Good recovery can be expected only if, after 72 hours from the time of cardiac arrest, the patient rapidly withdraws the arms to pain, localizes pain, or follows simple, one-step commands. The chance of awakening decreases remarkably in the first week (50% in the first day, 20% in the third day, and 10% at the end of the first week). Awakening after more than 3 days of coma from anoxic ischemic insult very frequently is associated with severe disability (being dependent on others for care).

Evaluation for Prognosis

Several studies may be helpful in delineating prognosis. The yield of the computed tomography scan in postanoxic coma is low, but findings of brain swelling, bilateral watershed infarction, bilateral thalamic hypodensities, and multiple cerebellar infarcts often indicate a poor outcome. These findings are significantly more common in patients with myoclonus status epilepticus. The value of electroencephalographic (EEG) recording is unresolved. Many EEG patterns in postanoxic coma have been described, but only some are strong indicators of poor outcome. More commonly, widespread delta waves are found—sometimes with clear asymmetries between the activities of both hemispheres—and some patients have prominent, superimposed, isolated sharp waves and spikes. Another EEG phenomenon, alpha-pattern coma, is seen in the first days after cardiac arrest and later is replaced by slow delta-wave patterns. Generally, outcome is accepted as poor in patients with alpha-pattern coma, but others have pointed out that prognosis with alpha-pattern coma is not worse. Other postanoxic EEG

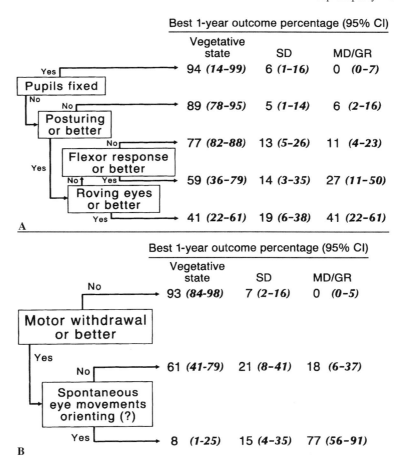

Figure 2-1. Outcome probabilities in postanoxic ischemic coma. A. Initial examination. B. Three days after cardiopulmonary resuscitation. (CI = confidence interval; MD = moderate disability; GR = good recovery; SD = severe disability.) (Modified from DE Levy, JJ Caronna, BH Singer, et al. Predicting outcome from hypoxic-ischemic coma. JAMA 1985;253: 1420–1426. By permission of the American Medical Association.)

patterns, such as spindle coma (activity resembling sleep), are not predictive. Only a burst-suppression pattern has been identified as a predictor of poor prognosis.

A more promising method is to use somatosensory evoked potentials. When a median nerve is stimulated, the lack of scalp potentials indicates an inability to improve beyond a persistent vegetative state. Widespread anoxic-ischemic damage of cortex, thalamus, and cerebellum has been found at autopsy in patients without these cortical scalp responses. It is important that patients should not have had anesthetic agents, which may significantly mute the scalp response. Another laboratory test, analysis of gamma enolase (also known as *neuron-specific enolase*), may be useful but not very practical in the first days of decision making. Enolase can be measured in the cerebrospinal fluid within 24 hours of cardiac arrest, and high values (threshold level unknown) have been associated with contin-

ued unconsciousness and death. The positive predictive value has been 100%, and the negative predictive value has been 89%.

Therapies Affecting Prognosis

No specific treatment has been shown to be effective. Previous reports of randomized trials have included the use of barbiturates and calcium channel blockers, but the results have been disappointing thus far. Apparently, glucocorticosteroid administration in the first 8 hours after cardiac arrest is unsuccessful. Several general guidelines are important. Because many patients have underlying myocardial infarction with arrhythmias and hypotension, blood pressure must be corrected aggressively by plasma volume expansion, with a goal of mild hypertension (mean arterial pressure of 120/140 mm Hg). Maintaining normoglycemia is important, but the significance of hyperglycemia-induced postanoxic brain damage needs to be investigated further.

Intracranial pressure monitoring after cardiopulmonary resuscitation is of no use. Some brain swelling may occur, but it seldom increases intracranial pressure. Nonetheless, frequent suctioning for pulmonary secretions and treatment of agitation in patients fighting the ventilator will help prevent further increase in intracranial pressure. Excessive oxygen may contribute to increased damage from free radicals, and hypocapnia may reduce cerebral blood flow; therefore, arterial oxygen and carbon dioxide tensions should be kept within normal limits.

Short-Term Prognosis

Immediate awakening after cardiac resuscitation (incidence of 20% in a large series) predicts good outcome, and cognitive deficits are unusual. However, many patients have underlying cardiac disease that limits their performance, and a significant number still may die suddenly in the first year. Patients who remain comatose after resuscitation have a high chance of in-hospital death, often from withdrawal of support or recurrent cardiac arrhythmias. Patients who do not withdraw their upper extremities to pain and remain comatose after 24 hours have a very small but significant chance of recovery to independent function if they survive the hospital stay. For a chance of good recovery, recovery should be fairly rapid.

Patients with severe disability after postanoxic coma often are in a tragic state. Rarely, cognitive function may be relatively spared, but action myoclonus may determine disability. These patients, who have been comatose for some time but finally awaken, are unable to stand or walk without support.

Not infrequently, patients have a significant memory deficit, which sometimes can be demonstrated on magnetic resonance imaging as significant bilateral hippocampal damage.

Long-Term Prognosis

The dimension of long-term prognosis has not been assessed thoroughly. Hypoxic-ischemic encephalopathy improves over time, but change to a different outcome category (e.g., severe disability to independent recovery) is highly improbable after 1 year. In fact, the number of patients surviving after 1 year is small (approximately 20%). The cause of death usually is recurrent cardiac arrhythmias or systemic complications associated with persistent vegetative state. Virtually no studies have addressed the possible detrimental effects of cognitive deficits on social relationships or functioning in daily work.

Additional Reading

Levy DE, Caronna JJ, Singer BH, et al. Predicting outcome from hypoxic-ischemic coma. JAMA 1985;253:1420–1426.

Mullie A, Verstringe P, Buylaert W, et al. Predictive value of Glasgow coma score for awakening after out-of-hospital cardiac arrest: Cerebral Resuscitation Study Group of the Belgian Society for Intensive Care. Lancet 1988;1:137–140.

Rothstein TL, Thomas EM, Sumi SM. Predicting outcome in hypoxic-ischemic coma. A prospective clinical and electrophysiologic study. Electroencephalogr Clin Neurophysiol 1991;79:101–107.

Volpe BT, Holtzman JD, Hirst W. Further characterization of patients with amnesia after cardiac arrest: preserved recognition memory. Neurology 1986;36:408–411.

Wijdicks EFM, Parisi JE, Sharbrough FW. Prognostic value of myoclonus status in comatose survivors of cardiac arrest. Ann Neurol 1994;35:239–243.

Chapter 3

Sleep Disorders

David A. Neumeyer, Naomi R. Kramer,
and Richard P. Millman

Sleep medicine is a growing field in neurology. Theory once held that anyone who dozed off had narcolepsy. Now, researchers realize that narcolepsy is fairly uncommon as compared to other causes of hypersomnolence, including insufficient sleep and sleep fragmentation from conditions such as obstructive sleep apnea. This chapter reviews what is known about the prognosis of obstructive sleep apnea (OSA) and narcolepsy.

Obstructive Sleep Apnea

OSA has entered into the forefront of both the medical and lay press. OSA is a common disease involving repetitive collapse of the pharynx during sleep and is manifested by excessive sleepiness, frequent obstructive apneas, and snoring (Table 3-1). Conservative estimates of the prevalence of OSA (per the Wisconsin Sleep Cohort Study) indicate that the disease is present in approximately 2% of women and 4% of men in the 30- to 60-year age group, similar to the prevalence of asthma and diabetes in this age range. Most sleep physicians consider the diagnostic criteria for OSA to include a compatible history along with the presence of at least five apneas and hypopneas per hour of sleep, termed the *respiratory disturbance index* (RDI) as measured by polysomnography. An obstructive apnea is a cessation of airflow lasting at least 10 seconds, with persistent respiratory effort. During an obstructive hypopnea, a partial decrease in airflow occurs, associated with an arousal from sleep

or oxygen desaturation. Although OSA can be treated by several different methods, no ideal regime is available. The pathophysiologic understanding of OSA remains limited.

Natural History

The natural history of OSA is not well characterized, although several key articles have approached this subject. He et al. retrospectively reviewed the mortality of OSA in 385 male patients. In a subgroup of patients with an apnea index (AI) of more than 20 events per hour, the 5- and 8-year mortalities were increased significantly as compared to patients with less severe disease (Fig. 3-1).

Partinen and colleagues retrospectively compared the mortality of 71 patients with OSA, as defined by an AI of greater than 5, treated with a tracheostomy versus 127 patients treated conservatively with weight loss. At 5-year follow-up, the only deaths occurred in the weight-loss group. Eight of the 14 deaths were thought to be vascular (cardiac or cerebrovascular) and potentially related to the sleep apnea.

The understanding of the hemodynamic consequences of OSA are somewhat controversial. Some have thought that heart rate falls during an obstructive event, owing to increased vagal tone, as the patient struggles to breathe against a closed glottis; then, with arousal, tachycardia can occur. Recent studies have suggested heart rate actually rises in many patients during apneas. Severe bradycardia

Table 3-1. Symptoms of Obstructive Sleep Apnea

Loud snoring
Snorting and gasping during sleep
Observed apneas
Choking arousals
Fragmented sleep
Excessive daytime sleepiness
Memory problems
Cognitive difficulties
Personality changes
Depression
Impotence

has been estimated to occur in 10% of patients, and ventricular tachyarrhythmias may occur with severe hypoxemia.

Typically, blood pressure will decrease by 10 to 20% during non–rapid eye movement sleep in normals. Patients with OSA tend not to demonstrate this dip. The mechanism for nocturnal hypertension is not yet defined clearly, but it may be related to increased catecholamine release secondary to a combination of hypoxemia and hypercapnia. Daytime hypertension has been associated with OSA in several studies; however, many of these reports did not control for confounding variables (i.e., adjusting for obesity). A study by Hla and coworkers, using data from the Wisconsin Sleep Cohort Study, was able to document a relationship between OSA and hypertension in patients with an RDI of 5 or greater. The increases in blood pressure seen in patients at night may lead to sustained daytime hypertension.

The relationship between pulmonary hypertension and OSA is less clear. Pulmonary artery pressures typically increase during obstructive apneas and hypopneas in response to alveolar hypoxia, and they fall with the resumption of ventilation. Previous reports concluded that OSA was indeed an independent risk factor for the development of sustained pulmonary hypertension; however, many of these patients had coexisting lung diseases. Sajkov and associates evaluated 27 patients with OSA but without underlying pulmonary disorders by Doppler echocardiography: Of these patients, 11 had mild elevations of their pulmonary pressures. A small percentage of patients with sleep apnea develop cor pulmonale in association with daytime hypoxemia and hypercapnia. This condition has been called the *pickwickian syndrome* or the *obesity-hypoventilation syndrome*, and these patients may be at risk of sudden death.

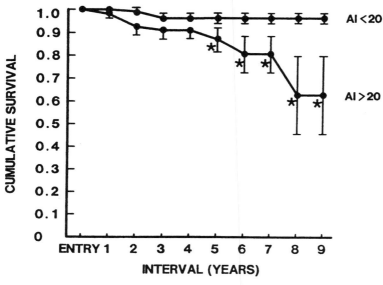

EFFECT OF AI ON MORTALITY
(UNTREATED, ALL AGES)

Figure 3-1. Probability of cumulative survival for all untreated patients with an apnea index (AI) less than 20 (top line) or exceeding 20 (bottom line). *The difference between the curves at that interval is significant at a *p* <0.05. (Reprinted with permission from J He, MH Kryger, FJ Zorick, et al. Mortality and apnea index in obstructive sleep apnea. Experience in 385 male patients. Chest 1988;94:9–14.)

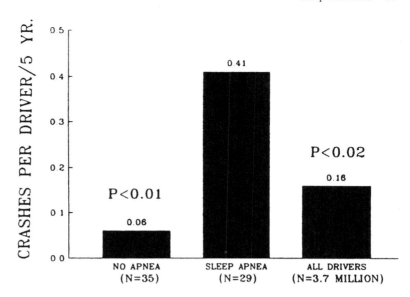

Figure 3-2. Automobile accident rates (accidents per driver per 5-year period) in 29 subjects with obstructive sleep apnea (Sleep Apnea), 35 subjects without sleep apnea (No Apnea), and the 3.7 million licensed drivers in Virginia (All Drivers). The sleep apnea group had significantly more accidents than did either control group. (Reprinted with permission from LJ Findley, ME Unverzagt, PM Suratt. Automobile accidents involving patients with obstructive sleep apnea. Am Rev Respir Dis 1988;138:337–340.)

One of the major consequences of sleep fragmentation from OSA is excessive daytime sleepiness. In the United States, automobile accidents are the third leading cause of death. Excessive daytime sleepiness has been linked with adverse driving outcomes. Numerous studies have related OSA with automobile mortality. In 1988, Findley and coworkers studied 64 subjects, of whom 29 had an RDI of greater than 5. By reviewing the registry of motor vehicle accident reports, these authors demonstrated that patients with OSA experienced considerably increased risk of a motor vehicle accident as compared to those without OSA (Fig. 3-2). This finding seems to correlate with the presence of severe sleep apnea. A similar increased rate of accidents was reported by Stoohs and colleagues in commercial truck drivers.

Other sequelae of chronic sleep deprivation (not necessarily limited to OSA) are depression, increased job-related accidents, personality changes, loss of sexual appetite, and cognitive dysfunction that includes memory disturbances. These changes can affect quality of life.

Factors Affecting Prognosis

The prognosis of sleep apnea appears to be related to disease severity. Thus, any factor that increases the obstruction of the upper airway can worsen the degree of sleep apnea and adversely affect morbidity and mortality. Several known risk factors for OSA include obesity, age, alcohol and tobacco use, nasal obstruction, and sleep deprivation. Alcohol, benzodiazepines, and narcotics, for example, have been shown to worsen snoring and potentiate sleep apnea. These agents directly enhance pharyngeal muscle relaxation during sleep. In addition, apneic periods may be prolonged owing to an increased arousal threshold.

Evaluation for Prognosis

All-night polysomnography has remained the gold standard for the diagnosis of OSA, although the use of portable sleep studies is gaining in popularity. A nighttime sleep evaluation is important in determining disease severity and in following response to specific treatments.

Therapies Affecting Prognosis

OSA, unlike narcolepsy, actually can be cured. Weight loss in some patients may be curative. A successful response to weight loss depends on whether structural abnormalities exist in the jaw or pharynx, contributing to the severity of the sleep apnea.

Surgery also may be curative. In the past, the gold standard for cure of the disorder was a tracheostomy. Uvulopalatopharyngoplasty (UPPP)

Table 3-2. Symptoms of Narcolepsy

Daytime sleepiness
Cataplexy
Sleep paralysis
Hypnagogic hallucinations
Automatic behavior
Disrupted sleep
Cognitive problems
Depression

now is the most common surgical procedure. It removes much of the soft, redundant tissue of the velopharynx, including the uvula, part of the soft palate, and the tonsillar pillars. A recent review of the surgical literature reported by Sher and coworkers revealed that UPPP leads to a partial or complete response in only 41% of patients.

The addition of a mandibular osteotomy with a genioglossal advancement procedure—to pull the tongue forward—has been shown to increase the complete response rate to 61%. The success rate increases to 71 to 78% if the baseline RDI is less than 60 and drops to 41% in the presence of severe sleep apnea. Patients who fail this combined approach can attain a 95% cure rate with the addition of a procedure that advances both the mandible and the maxilla.

An alternative approach simply is to control the sleep apnea. Control can be achieved with nightly use of nasal continuous positive airway pressure (CPAP) or an adjustable oral appliance. In the retrospective study by He and colleagues, treatment with either tracheostomy or CPAP greatly improved survival. In fact, in this study, no patients treated with tracheostomy or nasal CPAP died. Surgery using a UPPP did not alter mortality in those patients with an AI greater than 20. The authors suggested that the low success rate of UPPP, in part, explained the lack of survival benefits.

Short-Term Prognosis

As patients typically present to a sleep physician after having been afflicted with OSA for many years, the short-term prognosis generally is very good. Patients treated with nasal CPAP may notice an alleviation of daytime hypersomnolence. This improvement is important if the patient has such severe sleepiness as to cause fatal motor vehicle or work-related accidents.

Long-Term Prognosis

Few data are available regarding the long-term prognosis of OSA. On the basis of early studies, untreated OSA in the moderate or severe state likely is associated with an increased mortality. Few studies use the current definition of OSA (incorporating hypopneas along with apneas) that address the issue of long-term prognosis. As it is difficult to ferret out the coexisting risk factors among patients with OSA and controls, many of the reported complications associated with OSA may, in fact, be related to comorbid conditions. Further investigation into this and other aspects of OSA is necessary so a comprehensive understanding of disease prognosis can be made.

Narcolepsy

Narcolepsy is a disorder characterized by excessive daytime sleepiness associated with cataplexy, sleep paralysis, and hypnagogic hallucinations (Table 3-2). These symptoms are manifestations of rapid eye movement (REM) sleep fragments. This constellation of symptoms has been termed the *narcolepsy tetrad*. Usually, the syndrome initially presents with irresistible daytime sleepiness with or without other features of the tetrad. Like sleepiness seen in normal subjects after sleep deprivation, sleepiness in narcolepsy is most common when the patient is in a quiet, nonstimulating environment. However, distinguishing features of the sleepiness of narcolepsy include the following: (1) it cannot be alleviated completely by more sleep; (2) it is more profound than normal sleepiness and may occur in unusual situations, such as when patients are talking, standing, walking, or operating heavy machinery; and (3) patients may be unaware of when they are going to fall asleep because they become accustomed to a state of chronic sleepiness. They may thus experience so-called *sleep attacks*.

As with sleep apnea, automatic behavior may occur with narcolepsy. In these situations, the patient may conduct complex activities, such as driving a car or writing messages, but may not remember completing this activity. In addition, the actions taken during these few minutes may be illogical, such as writing nonsensical sentences or writing off the edge of a piece of note paper. It is clear that such symptoms could significantly affect individual work performance and family life.

Cataplexy is an abrupt loss of muscle tone comparable to the atonia seen normally during REM sleep. It is associated with full consciousness and thereby is distinguished from syncope. Usually, it is precipitated by such strong emotions as anger, sadness, or laughter. The severity of episodes may range from complete loss of muscle tone, which results in the patient's fall, to milder forms, such as simple drooping of the head and facial muscles or weakness at the knees. The duration usually is very brief. Cataplexy is thought to be diagnostic of narcolepsy if it is associated with excessive sleepiness.

Natural History

The natural history of narcolepsy is striking in that the degree of sleepiness does not tend to progress as the patient ages. The most common age of onset is in the late teenage years or second decade. Other features of the tetrad may develop at varying points during the course of the illness. Cataplexy may occur in association with the onset of hypersomnolence but, in 10 to 15% of patients, it may not present until 10 or more years later. It rarely precedes the hypersomnolence. Hypnagogic hallucinations and sleep paralysis also may start in conjunction with the sleepiness or at a later date. These latter features may be transient or improve in approximately one-third of patients. In contrast, disrupted nocturnal sleep is usually mild at presentation, but may become more prominent with age. In addition to these unexplained arousals, patients with narcolepsy are also more likely to develop sleep apnea and periodic limb movements.

The sequelae of narcolepsy are most evident in the psychosocial arena and may affect mortality indirectly. Broughton and coworkers found that approximately 66% of patients with narcolepsy reported falling asleep while driving. In addition, patients may experience cataplexy and sleep paralysis while driving. Patients with narcolepsy also have increased incidence of problems at work. Broughton and coworkers found that among patients with narcolepsy who were experiencing difficulties at work, their problems were related either to sleep attacks or to impaired concentration and memory, most likely owing to sleepiness.

Kales and colleagues found that 84% of their patients believed interpersonal relations were affected adversely by their illness. Fifty-six percent of patients deliberately decreased their contact with people to avoid revealing symptoms of their illness. Twenty percent believed their separation or divorce was due to their illness.

Patients with narcolepsy have been reported also to have psychiatric problems. Depression may occur in as much as 30% of the patient population. Although both diseases potentially involve changes in central neurotransmitters, no clear overlapping defect is established. It is most likely that depression is a reaction to psychosocial problems or chronic illness.

Sometimes, patients with narcolepsy are labeled as lazy or are considered drunk or bizarre. This perception often is related to their profound sleepiness as well as to their unusual experiences of hypnagogic hallucinations and cataplexy. On rare occasions, patients with narcolepsy and prominent hallucinations incorrectly have been labeled schizophrenic.

Factors Affecting Prognosis

It is unclear what events may affect the natural history of this disease. The degree of excessive daytime sleepiness and the manifestation of other features of the tetrad varies from patient to patient. Factors that clearly affect prognosis more likely revolve around making the correct diagnosis and the institution of appropriate therapies.

Evaluation for Prognosis

Evaluation of a patient with narcolepsy includes a standard sleep history incorporating questions regarding sleepiness, the presence or absence of the tetrad, sleep cycle information, symptoms of other sleep disorders, and the use of substances that could exacerbate or ameliorate sleepiness. This process establishes the baseline characteristics of the narcolepsy: No method exists for determining the clinical prognosis for any patient.

Therapies Affecting Prognosis

Narcolepsy cannot be cured; it can only be controlled. Therapy affects prognosis only by reducing hypersomnolence and cataplexy. Patient education is a critical part of therapy for narcolepsy. It is important to emphasize that patients take control of their sleep cycle, so that they obtain adequate nocturnal sleep and control daytime sleepiness. Naps may hold sleepiness at bay for 1 to 2 hours and can be scheduled strategically during the day. However, most patients also require stimulants to maintain adequate alertness. Typically, this alertness can be obtained from using the longer-acting stimulants in the morning and a shorter-acting form in the afternoon. Although it is important to maintain alertness for a patient to drive home from work, stimulants in the evening may disrupt nocturnal sleep and should be used with caution. By appropriate use of stimulants and naps, the risks associated with excessive sleepiness may be reduced (though not eliminated). Cataplexy may be very disabling for some patients and may be controlled with tricyclic antidepressants. Serotonin reuptake inhibitors also may be helpful. Sedating tricyclic antidepressants may be used at night to decrease nocturnal awakenings.

Short-Term Prognosis

With drug therapy and naps, patients may quickly notice an improvement in their daytime hypersomnolence and cataplexy.

Long-Term Prognosis

A paucity of data limits documentation of the long-term prognosis of narcolepsy. The morbidity associated with narcolepsy most likely is determined by the adequacy of treatment and the education of patients and their families. Although no cure for narcolepsy exists, controlling sleepiness and cataplexy to the maximum degree possible is essential. As noted, however, sleepiness cannot be abolished completely. It is essential that patients be aware of the possible complications of sleepiness, including highway accidents and accidents at work. Similarly, educating patients' families in the nature of the disease and its impact on work and relationships may enable them to be more supportive. An informed employer may have a much more productive employee if the employee is allowed to take a scheduled nap at lunch time. As with any chronic illness, quality of life may be improved both by treatment and by creating a supportive environment to maximize the person's potential.

Additional Reading

Obstructive Sleep Apnea

Findley LJ, Unverzagt ME, Suratt PM. Automobile accidents involving patients with obstructive sleep apnea. Am Rev Respir Dis 1988;138:337–340.

He J, Kryger MH, Zorick FJ, et al. Mortality and apnea index in obstructive sleep apnea. Experience in 385 male patients. Chest 1988;94:9–14.

Hla KM, Young TB, Bidwell T, et al. Sleep apnea and hypertension. A population-based study. Ann Intern Med 1994;120:382–388.

Partinen M, Jamieson A, Guilleminault C. Long-term outcome for obstructive sleep apnea patients. Mortality. Chest 1988;94:1200–1204.

Sajkov D, Cowie RJ, Thornton AT, et al. Pulmonary hypertension and hypoxemia in obstructive sleep apnea. Am J Respir Crit Care Med 1994;149:416–422.

Sher AE, Schectman KB, Piccirillo JF. The efficacy of surgical modifications of the upper airway in adults with obstructive sleep apnea syndrome. Sleep 1996;19:156–177.

Stoohs RA, Guilleminault C, Itoi A, Dement W. Traffic accidents in commercial long-haul truck drivers: the influence of sleep-disordered breathing and obesity. Sleep 1994;17:619–623.

Weiss JW, Remsburg S, Garpestad E, et al. Hemodynamic consequences of obstructive sleep apnea. Sleep 1996; 19:388–397.

Young T, Palta M, Dempsey J, et al. The occurrence of sleep-disordered breathing among middle-aged adults. N Engl J Med 1993;328:1230–1235.

Narcolepsy

Aldrich MS. Narcolepsy. Neurology 1992;42(S6):34–43.

Broughton R, Ghanem Q, Hishikawa Y, et al. Life effects of narcolepsy in 180 patients from North America, Asia and Europe compared to matched controls. Can J Neurol Sci 1981;8:299–304.

Guilleminault C. Narcolepsy Syndrome. In MH Kryger, T Roth, WC Dement (eds), Principles and Practices of Sleep Medicine (2nd ed). Philadelphia: Saunders, 1994;549–561.

Kales A, Soldatos CR, Bixler EO, et al. Narcolepsy-cataplexy: II. Psychosocial consequences and associated psychopathology. Arch Neurol 1982;39:169–171.

Krishnan RR, Volow MR, Miller PP, Carwile ST. Narcolepsy: preliminary retrospective study of psychiatric and psychosocial aspects. Am J Psychiatry 1984;141:428–431.

Mitler MM, Aldrich MS, Koob GF, Zarcone VP. Narcolepsy and its treatment with stimulants. Sleep 1994;17:352–371.

Richardson JW, Fredrickson PA, Lin SC. Narcolepsy update. Mayo Clin Proc 1990;65:991–998.

Chapter 4

Childhood Attention-Deficit Hyperactivity Disorder

Ruth Nass

Although attention-deficit hyperactivity disorder (ADHD) had been thought to disappear in adolescence, current data indicate that related difficulties may persist through adolescence and into adulthood in one-third to one-half of ADHD children. It is not clear, however, whether childhood ADHD manifests as a continuation of symptoms into adulthood or as a precursor of certain adult psychopathology. Assuming a prevalence of childhood ADHD of 6 to 10% and using one-third of 6% as a minimum figure and two-thirds of 10% as a maximum figure, the prevalence of ADHD may be as high as 2 to 7% of adults. Considered from another vantage, approximately one-fourth of the first-degree relatives (usually the father) of a child presenting with ADHD also will have had ADHD.

Natural History

The frequency of ADHD in a given cohort declines from childhood to adolescence and further from adolescence to adulthood. Long-term follow-up of preschoolers with hyperactivity documents adolescent ADHD in 10% and a psychiatric diagnosis in 50%. Prospective and longitudinal studies document normal to fairly normal outcome in only 30 to 40% of adults who had ADHD in childhood. Significant social-emotional difficulties in adulthood occur in 40 to 50% and serious psychiatric or antisocial disabilities in as many as 10%.

Types of Persisting Problems in Adolescence and Adults

Cognitive Dysfunction

Persisting problems on cognitive tasks measuring attentional and executive functions (initiating, sustaining, shifting, and inhibiting) have been documented in many (but by no means all) adolescents and adults with a history of childhood ADHD.

Academic Performance

At follow-up in early and middle adolescence, many children with ADHD have both academic and behavior problems at school. In late adolescence, both the Montreal and New York ADHD groups were receiving lower grades, failing courses more frequently, and ultimately completing fewer years of school as compared with controls. They also were expelled from school more frequently.

Social Functioning

ADHD teenagers have problems with emotional maturity and self-esteem. Often, they are described as irritable, incorrigible, demanding, and unable to see other points of view. Many are loners, lacking strong friendships. In interpersonal relations, inattentiveness and distractibility often get in the way of intimacy.

Table 4-1. Psychiatric Status of Adults with Attention-Deficit Hyperactivity Disorder (ADHD)

	% Controls (N = 41)	% ADHD (N = 61)
Normal	33*	11
Sexual problems	2.4	20*
Neurotic	51	79*
Psychotic	2.4	8.2
Somatic symptoms	16	27
Suicide attempts	0	6*
Aggression	2	12*

*Statistically significant differences.
Source: Modified from G Weiss, L Hechtman. Hyperactive Children Grown Up (2nd ed). New York: Guilford Press, 1993.

Occupational Status

At age 20, employer ratings of occupational functioning did not differ between ADHD subjects and controls in the Montreal cohort study. These formerly hyperactive children seemed to have chosen professions in which continued restlessness and inattention did not interfere significantly with work performance. However, in longer-term follow-up, the ADHD subjects showed less perseverance, less independence, and poorer relations with supervisors. In another study, prospective follow-up of ADHD young adults compared with their brothers revealed a significant increase in unemployment among the former and failure to achieve the same social class.

Psychiatric Outcome

In general, three outcome groups of adults with a history of childhood ADHD have been identified (Table 4-1): those who fare well and are not particularly different from a control population; those who continue to have problems with attention and impulsivity (the majority of childhood ADHD grown-ups); and those with significant psychiatric or antisocial pathology (a small minority of ADHD grown-ups).

Residual Attention-Deficit Hyperactivity Disorder Symptoms

Although hyperactivity tends to dissipate in adolescence (some studies, however, still find frequencies of hyperactivity as high as 40%), residual impulsiv-

ity, distractibility, inattentiveness, and restlessness are common. An increased risk of accidental death has been documented; motor vehicle accidents are a frequent occurrence. In the Montreal cohort, the frequency of the full ADHD syndrome decreased during adulthood from 31% among young adults to 8% among "older" adults.

Substance Use and Abuse

Substance abuse is more common in ADHD probands than in controls: general substance abuse, 32% versus 7%; alcoholism, 12% versus 5%; drug abuse, 28% versus 3%. Conversely, 14 to 33% of adults with substance abuse meet criteria for a diagnosis of ADHD.

Conduct Problems and Antisocial Behavior

Conduct disorders and oppositional defiant behavior disorders are common comorbid diagnoses with ADHD during childhood. In adolescence and young adulthood, delinquency and arrests (even when social class is considered) are more common in those with childhood ADHD than in controls (58% versus 11%). Prospective follow-up of ADHD young adults compared with their brothers revealed a significant increase in lying, thefts, and time in jail. ADHD adults are 10 times more likely than controls to have antisocial personality disorder. However, de novo antisocial behavior does not occur; there is usually a childhood history of conduct problems. Conduct disorder as a condition comorbid with ADHD is a significant risk for adult antisocial personality disorder. Indeed, some have suggested that delinquency and antisocial personality disorder seen in ADHD follow-up studies relate to the comorbid conduct disorder rather than to ADHD. ADHD girls tend to have little antisocial history.

Specific Psychiatric Diagnoses

Many (but by no means all) studies document an increased frequency of affective disorders (Table 4-2). Comorbidity of ADHD and depression is reported in 0 to 57% of ADHD patients. Suicide attempts are reported with greater frequency than that found among controls (see Table 4-1). The combination of ADHD and bipolar disorder is a risk factor for successful completion of suicide attempts in adolescence. Manic episodes may be provoked rarely by treatment with stimulants, tricyclic antidepressants, and serotonin reuptake inhibitors. Phobias, particularly social phobias, may be more common in the ADHD adult. Although obsessive compulsive disorder is not especially common in the ADHD adult, traits of obsessive compulsive personality disorder are common, specifically perfectionism and preoccupations. Anxiety disorders probably occur with increased frequency in ADHD adults. Notably, the two major prospective studies (New York and Montreal) did not find that childhood ADHD was a risk factor for depressive, bipolar disorder or schizophrenia in adulthood.

Factors Affecting Prognosis

Characteristics of childhood ADHD predictive of poorer long-term outcome include early age at presentation, malicious aggressiveness (as opposed to impulsive aggressiveness), severe ADHD disorder, comorbid neurologic and behavior disorders, and lower IQ. Lack of aggressiveness in childhood (pure hyperactivity) is not totally protective of an antisocial adolescent-adult outcome. The effect of social class on outcome is controversial. Lower socioeconomic status may be related to poorer academic and work functioning and, thus, may affect outcome secondarily. Though family stability appears directly related to outcome, there may be confounding between disrupted families and comorbid conduct disorders. Clearly, the etiology of ADHD affects outcome (Table 4-3). Those causes that are associated with comorbid conditions and compromised intellect or are associated with psychiatric disorders are likely to have a negative impact on outcome. The data, however, correlating electroencephalographic abnormalities in childhood ADHD with poor psychiatric outcome are at best equivocal.

Evaluation for Prognosis

In addition to making a diagnosis of ADHD, workup for comorbid neurologic and psychiatric diagnoses is important to prognosis (see Table 4-2). Family history of ADHD is an obvious risk factor for ADHD but has not been linked with persistence into adulthood. Comorbid diagnoses worsen prog-

Table 4-2. Attention-Deficit Hyperactivity Disorder (ADHD) and Its Comorbidities

Comorbid Disorder	Age Range (years)	Number of Patients	Findings
Antisocial disorder (ASD)	4–25	8,000	Overlap with ASD: 23–64% referred, 47–57% nonreferred ADHD with conduct disorder more severe than ADHD alone
Mood disorder	4–33	3,300	Overlap with mood disorder: 25–75% referred, 15–19% nonreferred
Anxiety disorder	4–23	1,300	Overlap with anxiety disorder: 27–30% referred, 8–26% nonreferred

Source: Modified from S Milberger, J Biederman, SV Faraone, et al. Attention deficit hyperactivity disorder and comorbid disorders: issues of overlapping symptoms. Am J Psychiatry 1995;152:1793–1799.

Table 4-3. Etiology of Attention-Deficit Hyperactivity Disorder

Demographic, genetic
Preperinatal: prematurity, birth asphyxia, maternal anemia, drugs (cocaine, alcohol, smoking)
Sequelae of illness: Reye's syndrome, meningitis or encephalitis, cardiac disease, autoimmune disorder, anemia, epilepsy, otitis
Toxins: lead
Sequelae of metabolic disorders
Sequelae of head injury
Drugs, medications: theophylline, anticonvulsants

Source: Modified from R Nass. Attention deficit disorder: facts and myths. Int Pediatr 1995;10:236–241.

nosis; as many as 20% of ADHD patients have one or more comorbid diagnoses.

Therapies Affecting Prognosis

Few studies report stimulant treatment effects on outcome. Data from the Montreal longitudinal study suggested that although stimulants do not eliminate educational, work, and adult life difficulties, stimulant-treated ADHD children may experience less social ostracism and ultimately have better feelings about themselves and toward others. To the extent that stimulants decrease aggressiveness and aggressiveness is associated with poorer outcome, stimulant treatment also may improve outcome. Psychotherapy, counseling, and remedial help in school have not been documented to predict or affect outcome. However, those receiving such treatment tend toward the more severe end of the disorder spectrum, making interpretation of any findings difficult.

Short-Term Prognosis

In about 15% of preschool children there is a definite concern about ADHD; in 40%, it is considered possible; and in 5%, concerns persist into the elementary school years. During the preschool period, the individual makeup of these three subgroups fluctuates considerably. Aggressiveness increases the risk of persistence. In elementary school, many hyperactive preschoolers have academic difficulties (especially reading), along with continued disruptive and inattentive behavior.

Long-Term Prognosis

Many children and adolescents do not outgrow ADHD. Adult outcome probably reflects the combined interaction of personality characteristics; social, familial, and environmental factors (including mental health of family members); IQ; and socioeconomic status. Persistent ADHD symptoms and aggressive behaviors, such as conduct disorder, bode particularly poorly for long-term prognosis.

ADHD may manifest in different ways in the adult as compared to the child. Comorbid psychiatric conditions are relatively common in the adult with residual ADHD.

Additional Reading

Barkley R, Fischer M, Edelbrock C, Smallish L. The adolescent outcome of hyperactive children diagnosed by research criteria: I. An 8-year prospective follow-up study. J Am Acad Child Adolesc Psychiatry 1990;29:546–557.

Biederman J, Faraone S, Spencer T, Wilens T. Patterns of psychiatric comorbidity, cognition, and psychosocial functioning in adults with ADHD. Am J Psychiatry 1993;150:1792–1798.

Borland BL, Heckman HK. Hyperactive boys and their brothers: a 25 year follow-up. Arch Gen Psychiatry 1976;33:669–676.

Denckla M. ADHD–residual type. J Child Neurol 1991;6 (suppl):S42–S48.

Hechtman L (ed). Do They Outgrow It? Washington, DC: American Psychiatric Press, 1996;39–76.

Herrero ME, Hechtman L, Weiss G. Antisocial disorders in hyperactive subjects from childhood to adulthood: predictive factors and characterization of subgroups. Am J Orthopsychiatry 1994;64:510–521.

Mannuzza S, Klein R, Bessler A, et al. Adult outcome of hyperactive boys: educational achievement, occupational rank, and psychiatric status. Arch Gen Psychiatry 1993;50:565–576.

McGee R, Partridge F, Williams S, Silva A. A twelve year follow-up of preschool hyperactive children. J Am Acad Child Adolesc Psychiatry 1991;30:224–232.

Mendelson W, Johnson N, Stewart M. Hyperactive children as teenagers. J Nerv Ment Dis 1971;153:273–285.

Ratey JJ, Greenberg MS, Bemporad JR, Lindem KJ. Unrecognized ADHD in adult presenting for outpatient psychotherapy. Child Adolesc Psychopharmacol 1992;4:267–275.

Weiss G, Hechtman L. Hyperactive Children Grown Up (2nd ed). New York: Guilford Press, 1993.

Wender P. ADHD in Adults. New York: Oxford Press, 1995.

Chapter 5

Developmental Language Disorders

Ruth Nass

A developmental language disorder (DLD) is diagnosed when a child with adequate intelligence and intact hearing fails to develop normal language. Most children have good receptive language by age 2, along with a 50- to 100-plus-word vocabulary and some two-word phrases. Children who are between 18 months and 3 years and have both expressive and receptive delays are more likely to be diagnosed eventually with a DLD than are those with only expressive delays; these children often catch up. Failure to develop appropriate expressive language by age 3 should be considered pathologic.

Natural History

In general, parents can be told that the majority of children with DLD—with the exception of a significant number of those with verbal auditory agnosia or severe verbal dyspraxia—will learn to speak well or reasonably well by school age. However, even when apparently resolved, a history of a DLD is a risk factor for later academic and reading disability and for emotional difficulties.

A number of risk factors for DLD have been identified by the National Collaborative Perinatal Project: prematurity; small for gestational age; and parental mental retardation. The highest correlations at the 8-month examination, with language deficits at ages 3 and 8, were failure to vocalize to social stimuli (pragmatic deficit) and failure to vocalize two syllables. Another important risk factor is family history of DLD, particularly involving phonol-

ogy. In families with DLD, the gender of the transmitting parent affects the gender ratio and percentage of children with a DLD. If the language disorder is transmitted through the mother, the offspring are more likely to be male, and the children are highly likely to be affected. Paternal transmission does not bias toward sons, and children stand a 50:50 chance of being affected by the language disability. As with other cognitive developmental disorders, girls may need a larger gene load to manifest the problem. DLD also is seen frequently in children with sex chromosome abnormalities involving an extra X (i.e., XXX and XXY).

Factors Affecting Prognosis

In general, the most significant prognostic factors in DLD appear to be nonverbal IQ, the number of language components involved, age at identification, and the number of associated cognitive deficits.

Not all children with DLD are deficient in all aspects of language, nor do they demonstrate identical patterns of language deficits. A variety of subtyping systems have been proposed to encompass the developmental language disorders. Table 5-1 provides a listing based on the Child Neurology Society nosology and indicates the aspects of language that are impaired. The syndromes are named for the aspects of language that are deficient. Both prognosis and treatment response of DLDs depend at least in part on the subtype. Of the higher-order language disorders, the semantic-pragmatic syndrome has a

Table 5-1. Developmental Language Disorders

	Receptive-Expressive		Expressive		Higher-Order	
	Verbal Auditory Agnosia	Phonologic-Syntactic	Verbal Dyspraxia	Phonologic Programming	Semantic-Pragmatic	Lexical-Syntactic
Receptive						
Phonology	↓↓	↓	*	*	*	*
Syntax	↓↓	↓	*	*	*	*
Semantics	↓↓	?	*	*	↓↓	↓
Expressive						
Semantics	↓↓	↓	*	*	↓↓	Nl or ↓
Syntax	↓↓	↓↓	?	*	*	↓
Phonology	↓↓	↓	↓↓	↓	*	*
Repetition	↓↓	↓	↓	↓	↑↑	↓
Fluency	↓↓	↓	Nl or ↓	Nl or ↓	Nl, ↑, or ↓	↓
Pragmatics	Nl or ↓	Nl or ↓	*	*	↓↓	↓

Nl = normal; ? = not known; ↓ = impaired; ↑ = enhanced; ↓↓ = very impaired.
*Presumed normal.

better prognosis than does the lexical-syntactic syndrome. The prognosis of the semantic-pragmatic syndrome is better when it occurs in isolation than when it occurs in the higher functioning autistic child or the child with hydrocephalus. Similarly, prognosis for the lexical-syntactic syndrome is better in the nonautistic child. Of the disorders affecting both expressive and receptive language, verbal auditory agnosia probably has the worst prognosis, even more so when associated with autism. This language disorder can occur with or without epilepsy or electroencephalograph abnormalities. Prognosis probably is equally poor in the two groups. The language deficit in the Landau Kleffner syndrome generally is a verbal auditory agnosia. Some one-third of such patients have a good outcome, one-third a fair outcome, and one-third a poor outcome. Prognosis is somewhat better for the phonologic-syntactic syndrome. Again, association with autism has a detrimental effect on outcome. Associated neurologic dysfunction is especially common in this DLD subtype. Of the predominantly expressive DLDs, the best outcome is seen in the phonologic programming disorder in which children have relatively fluent speech and nearly normal utterance length but poor intelligibility. Serviceable speech usually is achieved, however. This disorder may be a severe articulation problem or a milder form of verbal dyspraxia, and many of the children need prolonged speech and language therapy. Children who have verbal dyspraxia and do not have intelligible speech by 6 years are unlikely to acquire normal speech. Neurologic abnormalities, including spastic diplegia, motor delay, tremor, hemiplegia, and chorea, are relatively commonly associated with this DLD subtype.

Evaluation for Prognosis

Genetic factors often play an important causal role in DLD. Thus, family history is of consequence. Type of language disorder and gender may interact with genetics in affecting prognosis (see the section Natural History).

Neurologic assessment usually is unrevealing but can result in a diagnosis that affects prognosis. Language deficits are found, for example, in children with a number of chromosome abnormalities, including Down syndrome, fragile-X syndrome, Klinefelter's syndrome, and Williams syndrome. The language disorders associated with definable neurologic syndromes often occur with other neuropsychological deficits, including mental retardation, other learning disabilities, and motor dysfunction.

Neuropsychological Assessment

Expressive syntax in elementary school is the best predictor of adolescent language skills. Not only do the language difficulties vary in DLD children but the cognitive deficits vary and may include impairments in auditory processing, attention, verbal and nonverbal short-term memory, hierarchic organization, planning, and sequencing. The more extensive a child's overall problems, the more concern there should be for a poor prognosis.

Electroencephalography

Electroencephalographic evaluation (including a sleep record) is important to the evaluation of and prognosis for the DLD child, particularly of those with a significant receptive component, as the finding of epileptiform activity may alter treatment and therefore outcome.

Imaging

Computed tomography and magnetic resonance imaging generally are normal in the child with a DLD. Research studies suggest typical planum temporale asymmetry patterns may be absent. Dynamic imaging (single photon emission computed tomography, positron emission tomography, functional magnetic resonance imaging) may eventually prove to be of prognostic significance.

Therapies Affecting Prognosis

Opinions regarding referral for early intervention differ, with some advocating delaying referrals until age 4 for expressive-only impaired children and others recommending early identification and prompt intervention for all. For most children with DLD, early intervention is key. Evaluation should be undertaken when the family begins to suspect a problem, particularly when family history is positive. Children as young as 2 years can be assessed and provided with an appropriate intervention program.

Carrying out studies of the effectiveness of remediation is notoriously difficult. Replication of such studies is hampered by limited descriptions of the characteristics of the enrolled children with respect to their histories (e.g., otitis media, socioeconomic status) and their language abilities (e.g., severity of expressive impairment, degree of expressive relative to receptive impairment). Studies rarely describe interventions in adequate detail. Thus, the efficacy of remediation and the specific, most useful remediation method remains controversial.

Short-Term Prognosis

In view of the great variability in the timing of acquisition of language among children with no language difficulties, the definitive diagnosis of a DLD can be difficult to make. In the 2- to 3-year-old, transient (versus persistent) language deficits may be distinguishable on the basis of vocabulary size, time that the child can be engaged in quiet activities, age at initial assessment, and age at follow-up (with poorer outcome the older the child). The reported frequency of DLD in preschool children ranges from 1 to 25%, depending on criteria. At school age, the reported frequency of DLD is somewhat lower, at perhaps 5%. Though improvement and disappearance of deficit are suggested by this decline in frequency, the epidemiologic studies on which these figures are based tend to be cross-sectional (rather than longitudinal), and the criteria for diagnosis differ from study to study. In the National Collaborative Perinatal Project, children with receptive and expressive language problems at age 3 were at significantly increased risk for one of the "minimal brain dysfunction" syndromes (hyperkinesis, soft signs, learning disabilities) at age 7 years. Notably, preschool language ability is the best single predictor of later reading ability.

Long-Term Prognosis

The reported rate of recovery of DLD during elementary school ranges from 20 to 35%. Communication problems continue into adulthood in as many as 50 to 70% given a preschool diagnosis of DLD.

A DLD in the preschool years portends less educational achievement, vocational status, and social adjustment. Nonverbal intelligence in the DLD child seems to be the best single nonlanguage predictor of general outcome. Whether intensive early therapy ameliorates the high rate of residual language and academic difficulties to any degree is yet to be determined.

The more severe the language disorder, the greater the learning difficulties. However, even those children with isolated expressive language delays at age 2 to 3 appear to be at increased risk for language-based learning issues during the school years. Prevalence of academic problems ranges from 45 to 90%, with reading disability most frequently reported. In one study, 71% of 11-year-olds with language difficulties at age 7 required special education. As many as 60% of children with reading disabilities have preceding or persisting language disorders.

With respect to long-term emotional ramifications of DLD, kindergarten children with speech and language disorders are more likely than are controls to evidence behavioral disturbances and to be given diagnoses of a psychiatric disorder, particularly attention deficit hyperactivity disorder (30%) and "emotional problems" (13%). The most significant factor differentiating between those with and without a psychiatric diagnosis is the degree of language deficit. The prevalence rate of speech and language disorders among young children referred for psychiatric services runs as high as 65%. Girls (as compared to boys) with DLD may be affected more frequently by emotional problems and be more socially withdrawn. Thus, children presenting with speech and language difficulties are at significant risk for emotional difficulties and behavioral problems and should be screened and followed carefully.

Additional Reading

Aram DM, Ekelman BL, Nation JE. Preschoolers with language disorders: 10 years later. J Speech Hear Res 1984;27:232–244.

Bashir A, Scavuzzo A. Children with language disorders: natural history and academic success. J Learn Disabil 1992;25:53–62.

Beitchman J, Brownlie E. Childhood Speech and Language Disorders. In L Hechtman (ed), Do They Outgrow It? Washington DC: American Psychiatric Press, 1996;225–254.

Lassman F, Fisch R, Vetter D, La Benz E (eds). Early Correlates of Speech: Language and Hearing. Littleton, MA: PSG Publishing, 1980.

Nass R, Rapin I (eds). DLD. Semin Child Neurol (in press).

Nichols N, Chen M. Minimal Brain Dysfunction. Hillsdale, NJ: Lawrence Erlbaum Associates, 1984.

Nippold MA, Schwarz IE. Children with slow expressive language development: What is the forecast for school achievement? Am J Speech Lang Pathol 1996;5:22–25.

Rescorla L, Schwartz E. Outcome of toddlers with specific expressive language delay. Appl Psycholinguist 1990;11:393–407.

Silva P, Williams S, McGee R. A longitudinal study of children with DLD at age three: later reading, intellectual and behavior problems. Dev Med Child Neurol 1987;29:630–640.

Whitehurst GJ, Fischel JE. Practitioner review: early developmental language delay: What, if anything, should the clinician do about it? J Child Psychol Psychiatry 1994;35:613–648.

Chapter 6

Pervasive Developmental Disorders: Autism and Asperger's Disorder

Ruth Nass

Autism and Asperger's disorder (which probably represents the high-functioning end of the autistic spectrum of disorders) occur with a reported frequency of anywhere from 0.4 to 71 cases per 10,000 children.

Natural History

Like other developmental disorders, autism often shows changing symptoms with age. As many as one-third of autistic children undergo a regression between the ages of 1 and 3. On the other hand, some toddlers and preschoolers with classic symptoms of autism (language difficulties, social relatedness problems, insistence on sameness) no longer look autistic by school age. They may seem a bit odd and have peculiarities of language prosody and pragmatics, and their social skills may be tenuous. Nonverbal learning disabilities or attention deficit hyperactivity disorder may become the school-age diagnosis. Most autistic patients, however, retain the classic picture of autism.

Preschool Through School Age

Dramatic and unpredictable changes can occur between the preschool years and school age. Most, but by no means all, autistic patients develop into school-age children in a pattern commensurate with their intelligence. Nonretarded autistic preschoolers are likely to remain relatively high functioning into

the school years, unless language fails to develop. Even mildly retarded preschoolers may improve as they enter the elementary school years. Daily living skills often improve more than do language skills. Perhaps one-half of autistic children remain largely or entirely mute. During the latency period, in contrast to the preschool years, autistic children generally are calmer (less hyperactive), less bizarre, less resistant to change in routines, more receptive to learning, and more accepting of social advances from others and have fewer stereotypies.

Maturation: School Age into Adolescence

In general, follow-up studies suggest that overall improvement occurs in some 40% of autistic children during adolescence. However, deterioration may occur in adolescence in as many as one-third of patients (Table 6-1).

Adolescent Deterioration

Adolescent autistic deterioration affects both cognitive and behavioral functioning. In Brown's series, one-third of autistic patients did not do as well in adolescence, and 6% became so disturbed that they required hospitalization. In the Maudsley hospital series, 8 of 64 (12.5%) autistic patients deteriorated during their teens, perhaps half in association with the onset of epilepsy. In some instances, the decline showed periodic plateauing

Table 6-1. Adolescent Complications of Autism

Complication	Frequency (%)	Examples and Comments
Epilepsy	20–30; f > m	Partial, complex, and generalized
Deterioration	12–40; f > m	Not necessarily related to epilepsy; some recover
Aggravation of symptoms	35–50	Often periodic, not correlated with deterioration; consists of stereotypies, hyperactivity, self-destructive or unmanageable behavior
Problems associated with sexual maturation	35; m > f	Public masturbation
Depression	22–44	Often highest functioning patients

f = female; m = male.

and then further regression. Previously alert-looking children may emerge from their teens looking dull. Increased maternal age, female gender, and a family history of affective disorder may increase the risk of adolescent deterioration. Higher-functioning children tend to deteriorate less frequently than do low-functioning autistics. Sometimes, deterioration in adolescence reflects a definable neurologic etiology (e.g., tuberous sclerosis). Many (but not all) of the subgroup that deteriorates have seizures, which may not begin until after the decline. Significant deterioration warrants an evaluation for a definable neurologic etiology and for epilepsy. Most patients who deteriorate in adolescence do not recoup their preadolescent language, communication, or social functioning.

By contrast, a small minority (usually the higher-functioning group) improve significantly during adolescence, passing through their teens into adulthood with no more than the usual social issues.

Social Skills and Sexuality

Among those autistic patients who improve in adolescence and adulthood, 50% show interest, friendliness, and involvement with other people, but many lack the social skills to proceed from acquaintance to friend. Social relationships tend to be strongest with parents, teachers, and adults, as contrasted to peers. Autistic adolescents tend to be excluded from social cliques. The ability to perform cognitive shifts appears to predict better social outcome in high-functioning autistic adolescents.

In the Maudsley Hospital series, only 1 of 64 autistic adolescents had a heterosexual friendship. Even tentative expressions of yearning can cause trouble for autistic patients. The typical reaction to the emergence of sexuality is celibacy, which may be imposed by social ineptness rather than by the autistic adolescent's choice. The advent of puberty is not always associated with increased social sophistication about sexually related issues. Seemingly deviant sexual behaviors may reflect this. Thus, lower-functioning autistics with limited behavioral repertoires may begin to masturbate in public or expose themselves as a pleasurable activity, which they do not understand is socially unacceptable. Menstruation can create serious stresses, ultimately requiring hormonal suppression.

Additional Psychiatric Problems Developing During Adolescence

Depression is the most common problem and often occurs in higher-functioning patients who become increasingly aware of the differences between themselves and others. Social skills groups and therapy may prove helpful. Sometimes, antidepressants are valuable in combination with directive psychotherapy in those with good language skills. In some autistic patients, the overactivity of the early years is replaced by underactivity, inertia, and apathy in adolescence. Psychomotor retardation can occur in the absence of depression.

As many as 50% of the autistic population experience a dramatic aggravation of negative behavioral symptoms (self-destructiveness, aggressiveness, and hyperactivity) during the peripubertal period. Some one-half of these patients recoup, and one-half deteriorate further. Family history of affective disorder seems to be a risk factor for adolescent behavioral deterioration. True antisocial behavior is rare. Ritualistic and compulsive behaviors tend to improve during adolescence. Fear and nervousness show little change over time.

Maturation: Adulthood

Population-based outcome studies indicate that two-thirds of adults with autism demonstrate poor social adjustment (limited independence in social relations). Approximately one-half of the patients in combined follow-up series require institutionalization. Nonretarded autistics tend to improve more than those who are retarded. Higher-functioning persons with autism and Asperger's disorder have the best outcome. Fair to good outcomes are reported in 15 to 30%. Only 5 to 15%, however, become competitively employed, lead independent lives, marry, and raise families. Psychiatric problems are common even in this group. Somewhere between 5 and 15% of those in whom autism is diagnosed during childhood no longer appear autistic as adults. Probably for some adults the diagnosis had been overlooked in childhood and adolescence, thus increasing the number with autism who ultimately function in the mainstream. A small proportion of all patients with autism develop into "highly original nonpsychiatrically ill grownups."

Of the group that remains severely impaired, most autistic patients were socially aloof in childhood and remain so as adults. Epilepsy is common. Most are profoundly or severely retarded. All skills are at a low level; even simple self-care skills require supervision. Communication is minimal. Posture and gait tend to be odd. The lack of facial expressions and the presence of odd grimaces further mar appearance. Although some are quiet, many of these very impaired autistic patients are aggressive, destructive, or self-injurious; they may wander aimlessly. Stereotypies and resistance to change persist. Strange habits (e.g., smearing feces) and sexual behaviors (e.g., public masturbation) are harder to manage in the adult than in the child. Such difficulties tend to plateau in the fourth decade. Psychiatric complications include mood swings and catatonia. The frequency of dementia is unknown.

Of the group that improves from childhood to adulthood (some one-fourth), most are socially passive or odd. Most of these patients, although only mildly retarded, do not become independent as adults. Usually, language is adequate for day-to-day life, and many progress in school. They may read books in their particular area of interest. Cognitive profiles reveal large interability variability and areas of special expertise. Behavioral problems are uncommon. Persistent stereotypies (particularly when such patients are excited) and the adherence to meaningless routines, such as repetitive monologs on favorite subjects, keep them from independent living. Social naiveté and immaturity may lead to inappropriate advances to other people, which are even less acceptable in the adult than in the adolescent. Psychiatric complications in this group include anxiety states, depression, obsessional states, mania (rare), and undifferentiated psychotic states. Typical schizophrenia, however, is not reported.

The group living independently is estimated at 5 to 15%. However, this figure likely is an underestimate, because many milder cases remain unidentified. Often, a diagnosis is made when family members learn about autism or when such adults present to physicians who evaluate them at outpatient psychiatric services. Generally, this group, despite independent functioning, has a particular nonempathic style, knowing the rules of social intercourse intellectually rather than instinctively (see Temple Grandin's and Donna Williams's firsthand accounts). Intelligence generally is normal. Those who are most successful tend to have a special skill and the motivation to live as normal a life as possible.

Independence is possible only for those who have outgrown the aggressiveness and destructiveness common to autistic children. Subtle social and language problems may persist. Changing fixed daily routines may be extremely difficult. As adults, even the highest-functioning autistics have trouble with reciprocal interactions, in understanding the nuances of social cues, in making friends, and in responding empathetically to others. Often, they make extensive use of elaborate rules for social relations but fail to generalize them in novel situations. Those living alone may become increasingly eccentric. Affective disorders are fairly common; obsessional and catatonic states occur rarely. Unclassified "psychosis" may occur in response to stress but, in this group too, typical schizophrenia is rare.

Asperger's Disorder

Defining the natural history of Asperger's disorder is more difficult. In such patients, diagnoses may be made only in late childhood, adolescence, or even adulthood because, by definition, early language development must be normal. Nonverbal learning

Table 6-2. Adolescent and Adult Outcome in a Group of Children with Significant Social Relatedness Difficulties

Category	Adolescent Rating, N = 100 (% of total)	Adult Rating, N = 61 (% of total)
Normal-neurotic	38 (38)	23 (38)
Brittle-schizoid (considered odd)	30 (30)	21 (34)
Eruptive-schizoid (too narcissistic for friendships)	21 (21)	7 (11)
Schizophrenic (thought disorder)	9 (9)	10 (17)
Passive-retarded mild (IQ: 70–79)	2 (2)	0 (0)

Source: Modified from J Brown. Adolescent development of children with infantile psychosis. Semin Psychiatry 1969;1:79–89.

disabilities or attention deficit hyperactivity disorder may be the apparent presenting complaint. The characteristic overfocus in a particular, sometimes peculiar, interest area may escalate over time but yet, ultimately, be key to a special form of adult success.

Factors Affecting Prognosis

Language Status

Status of language skills at age 5 to 6 is the key prognostic factor for the long-term outcome of autism. Those autistic patients with conversational language do significantly better than do those with no or rudimentary language. Nonetheless, major speech development may occur late and still be associated with a fair overall outcome. As many as 20% of those without language at 5 years ultimately develop some language. IQ and likelihood of language acquisition run parallel.

Asperger's disorder patients, in contrast to the classic autistic child, tend to be relatively high functioning intellectually and do not by definition exhibit delays in language acquisition. The pragmatic and prosodic deficits, however, may remain prominent. They may learn many of the rules for communication (sometimes even sophisticated rules), but such pragmatic deficits as poor turn tak-

ing, making inappropriate comments, perseverating on a single topic of purely individual interest, or failure to maintain appropriate physical and eye contact with a conversational partner may persist indefinitely. Voice modulation may remain an issue; speech may be mechanical or sing-song. Language status has not, however, been shown to correlate with long-term outcome in this subgroup.

Intelligence

IQ score at the time of diagnosis is an important predictor of outcome in autism, especially for those with low IQ (<50). Although retardation is likely in an autistic child whose IQ is below 50 and who has no language at 3 years, such a child has a 50% chance of having the vocabulary of a 2 year old at age 7 and a 50% chance of scoring above the severely retarded IQ range. From preschool through school age, most autistic children's IQs remain unchanged. Brown has reported the long-term follow-up (midadolescence or beyond) of 100 children (76 boys, 24 girls) of normal intelligence identified in preschool as having severe disturbances of interpersonal relationships. (Many, but not all, had other characteristics of autism; some of the children had language delay, others were hyperverbal.) In contrast to outcome studies of patients meeting full criteria for autism (or pervasive developmental disorder), 38% of the 61 patients followed into adulthood were classified as normal or neurotic (Table 6-2), and almost half had regular jobs (albeit below their socioeconomic and intellectual expectations). Poor outcome generally is predictable in the severely intellectually impaired but more variable in those less impaired. Because of changes (both positive and negative) in adolescence, following patients into adulthood is crucial.

An interaction also exists between language acquisition and IQ. For example, although only 4 of the 48 children in one study with preschool nonverbal IQs greater than 70 did not acquire language, these children scored in the retarded IQ range at age 8 to 12 years despite initial high functioning. Those with poor outcome had more impaired adaptive skills as preschoolers than did their IQ-matched autistic counterparts who did acquire language. Success in education during childhood has the expected predictive power for adolescent and adult outcome.

Neurologic Status and Etiology

Epilepsy (partial and generalized) occurs in up to one-third of patients with autism by early adulthood (see Table 6-1). The first year and peripuberty are particularly vulnerable periods. Those who are retarded are at higher risk, but epilepsy occurs in those who are high functioning as well. Girls may be at greater risk than are boys. Epileptiform electroencephalograms and early epilepsy occur more frequently in very young autistic children who undergo an early regression. The occurrence of seizures may play a role in adolescent deterioration in some patients.

The cause of autism is also a predictor of outcome, highlighting the importance of an etiologic diagnosis. For example, those with autism and tuberous sclerosis do not do as well as those with autism and fragile X chromosome.

Therapies Affecting Prognosis

Families receiving earlier diagnoses and adequate educational programs develop better coping skills than do those whose children receive late diagnoses. This finding may help autistic patients to maximize their potential. Lovaas suggested that autistic children receiving more than 40 hours per week of one-to-one, extremely labor-intensive behavioral treatment for longer than 2 years had higher IQs and less restrictive school placement at age 7 than did a control group receiving less intensive therapy. The Lovaas technique may be most effective for the severely impaired young child. Integrated preschool programs (therapeutic nurseries) also appear to improve outcome. However, all such studies suffer from the lack of matched control groups.

Short-Term Prognosis

In the short term, IQ and language status at school age are the crucial factors predicting short-term prognosis. Dramatic changes can occur between toddler age and school age; classically autistic toddlers may sometimes appear more normal at school age.

Long-Term Prognosis

Most patients with autism maintain the autistic phenotype and remain dependent throughout their life spans. Adolescence is a period of fluctuation characterized by a significant risk of cognitive decline and epilepsy. A small subgroup with autism, generally those who were initially high functioning intellectually, lead normal adult lives and may make significant, even unusual, professional contributions.

Additional Reading

Allen DA. Autistic spectrum disorders: clinical presentation in the preschool child. J Child Neurol 1988;3:548–556.

Brown J. Adolescent development of children with infantile psychosis. Semin Psychiatry 1969;1:79–89.

DeMyer MK, Barton S, Alpern GD, et al. The measured intelligence of autistic children: a follow-up study. J Autism Child Schizophr 1974;4:42–60.

Gillberg C (ed). Diagnosis and Treatment of Autism. New York: Plenum, 1989;375–383, 419–432.

Gillberg C. Outcome in autism and autistic-like conditions. J Am Acad Child Adolesc Psychiatry 1991;30:375–382.

Grandin T. Thinking in Pictures. New York: Vantage Press, 1995.

Kanner L, Rodriguez A, Ashenden B. How far can autistic children go in matters of social adaptation? J Autism Child Schizophr 1972;2:9–33.

McEachen J, Smith T, Lovaas O. Longterm outcome for children with autism who received early intensive behavioral treatment. Am J Ment Retard 1993;4:359–372.

Rutter M, Schopler E (eds). Autism. A Reappraisal of Concepts and Treatment. New York: Plenum, 1978;463–506.

Schopler E, Mesibov G (eds). Diagnosis and Assessment in Autism. New York: Plenum, 1988;167–180, 227–238.

Schopler E, Mesibov GB (eds). High-Functioning Individuals with Autism. New York: Plenum, 1991.

Williams D. Nobody Nowhere. New York: Avon Press, 1992.

Chapter 7

Traumatic Brain Injury

Douglas I. Katz

Traumatic brain injury (TBI) occurs in the form of closed-head injury or penetrating head injury. This chapter emphasizes closed-head injury. TBI is the most common of all disabling neurologic disorders, with an incidence of approximately 200 persons in 100,000. The most frequent causes of TBI are motor vehicle accidents, falls, and assaults. The principle mechanisms of injury involve acceleration-deceleration and direct contact forces. Neuropathologic effects are multiple, involving focal and diffuse, primary, and secondary damage. Primary diffuse damage, usually resulting from rapid deceleration, takes the form of diffuse axonal injury (DAI). Possible associated damage to vascular structures may produce petechial white matter, subarachnoid, and intraventricular hemorrhages. Primary focal damage occurs as a result of either contact or deceleratory forces and takes the form of focal cortical contusions, deep cerebral hemorrhages, or extracerebral hemorrhages (subdural and epidural hematomas). A host of possible secondary events may cause further focal and diffuse damage. These include herniation from mass lesions, strokes (usually posterior cerebral artery territory), diffuse hypoxic-ischemic injury, microvascular injury, excitotoxicity, brain swelling, and edema. Late secondary injury may occur as a result of hydrocephalus or chronic subdural collections.

As with other neurologic disorders, the severity and location of brain damage has a significant relationship with recovery and outcome after TBI. However, diagnosis of the type, severity, and location of brain damage after trauma is more difficult for patients with TBI as contrasted to most other neurologic disorders. Several reasons account for this. First, detecting or measuring some of the major pathologic subtypes of TBI directly is difficult (DAI, secondary hypoxic-ischemic injury). Second, the types of pathology associated with TBI are multiple and often occur in combination. Computing the individual and combined effects of these pathologic components on outcome becomes a difficult task. Third, the most consistent clinical effects of TBI are cognitive and behavioral, areas more elusive to clinical neurologic measurement than most physical impairments. Furthermore, some of the cognitive areas typically affected (e.g., executive functions) have the least well-developed measurement instruments.

Natural History

The clinical, natural history of TBI can be defined in the context of focal or diffuse neuropathologic events. The critical pathophysiologic factors are the type, distribution, severity, and location of the combined neuropathologic events after brain injury. The most consistent and defining characteristics of TBI are disorders of cognition and behavior, and these problems are emphasized in the discussion of natural history. Other elemental neurologic problems, such as motor dysfunction, are common. The elemental problems have a higher incidence in patients with more severe injuries, but their occurrence does not correlate with severity as consistently as does cognitive dysfunction. A mixture of motor problems is typical, such as combinations of spastic paresis, incoordination, imbalance, and dysequilibrium.

Diffuse Injury

The natural history of diffuse injury is characterized by a recognizable pattern of stages that occur across the wide spectrum of severity. Severity determines the duration of recovery stages and levels of impairment at each stage of recovery. The first stage of recovery is coma, a state of unconsciousness without spontaneous eye opening. Patients with DAI are unconscious at the outset, without lucid interval. Patients with the most mild diffuse injuries may not be completely unconscious. The depth of coma in the first hours of recovery, as measured by the Glasgow Coma Scale (GCS), is one of the common markers of injury severity and prognosis.

All survivors resume spontaneous eye opening and sleep-wake cycles while still unconscious, a condition termed *vegetative state*. Except for the small percentage of very severely injured patients who remain permanently vegetative, awareness and purposeful behavior resume, often heralded by visual fixation and tracking. The ability to follow commands is the usual convincing marker of restored consciousness. The total duration of loss of consciousness (LOC) is another common marker of injury severity and prognosis.

In patients recovering slowly, cognitive responsiveness may begin erratically and inconsistently, without any reliable interactive communication. Often, patients are mute. This stage may be termed the *minimally conscious state.* When purposeful cognition is unequivocally established, basic attention and new learning remain severely impaired; this clinical condition may be labeled *confusional state*. At this stage, patients often are highly distractible and exhibit poorly regulated behavior. They may escalate rapidly to agitated behavior with stimulation. Less often, patients may remain in a state of underactivated, hypokinetic, withdrawn behavior. Dense anterograde amnesia also defines this stage; patients are disoriented, have little or no moment-to-moment episodic recall, and display little or no ability to learn new information after even a brief delay. This state is termed *post-traumatic amnesia* (PTA). The end of this stage is characterized by a significant improvement in basic attention and behavior regulation and resumption of continuous, day-to-day memory, albeit still somewhat defective. The duration of PTA is another important index of injury severity and prognosis.

The postconfusional stages of recovery are characterized by a gradual improvement in cognitive and behavioral functioning in those with more severe injuries. This phase of recovery may be broken further into stages of *emerging independence*, as patients' cognitive abilities, self-awareness, and insight allow independence in self-care and safe, unsupervised activity at home and a stage of *social competence*, with restoration of the capacity for independent function in the community or at the higher-level demands of school or the workplace.

Progress through these stages is largely a function of injury severity. Patients with mild, diffuse TBI experience restoration of consciousness in seconds to minutes, if fully unconscious at all; they evolve through confusion and PTA in minutes to hours, and the vast majority progress through the postconfusional stages in up to several weeks. Patients with more severe injuries may remain unconscious (coma and vegetative-state stages) days to weeks, confused (minimally conscious and confusional-state stages) weeks to months, and may evolve through the postconfusional stages (emerging independence and social competence) in months to years. Survivors with the most severe injuries may stall at one or another stage (e.g., those who remain permanently vegetative or minimally conscious).

As implied, a relative proportionality in duration appears to exist between subsequent phases of recovery at any given severity, although the relationships between stages can be highly variable. In general, the period of confusion and PTA is severalfold longer than is the period of unconsciousness and, likewise, the period of postconfusional recovery is several times the duration of confusion.

Focal Injury

The natural history of focal injury resembles that of vascular lesions of other causes, particularly hemorrhagic stroke. The acute phase involves edema and other early secondary phenomena that are maximal over the first few days. The resulting effects may include confusion and, perhaps, decreased arousal, if mass effect compromises diencephalic and mesencephalic structures. Otherwise, primary focal pathology is not associated directly with loss of consciousness.

As edema and other secondary effects wane over the first 1 to 2 weeks, more specific localizing effects of focal damage become more apparent. Recovery during this subacute phase is maximal over the first 3 months, but improvement may continue at a slower rate over several months.

The specific clinical effects of focal cortical contusions usually are different from other causes of focal vascular brain injury, reflecting the distinctive, typical localization of traumatic damage in the anterior and inferior frontal and temporal areas. Of course, focal damage may occur anywhere, particularly as a result of focal contact forces. Damage to limbic neocortical and heteromodal areas of the frontal and temporal lobes determine the usual effects of focal TBI on cognitive and behavioral functioning. The residual syndromes of prefrontal lesions include alterations in affect and behavior (e.g., disinhibition or apathy) and dysfunctional higher-level cognition (e.g., executive functions, insight, social awareness). Lesions in anterior and inferior temporal areas also may contribute to affective and behavioral disturbances. Larger lesions extending to medial temporal areas may produce specific impairments in memory encoding and retrieval (amnesia). Other localizing temporal syndromes involve extension of lesions into auditory association areas (e.g., aphasia with left hemisphere lesions) and visual association areas (e.g., visual agnosias, especially with bilateral lesions). The most common aphasia syndromes after focal temporal trauma are anomic and transcortical sensory aphasia.

The clinical effects of focal lesions often are embedded in the evolving effects of diffuse injury or in the clinical syndromes associated with secondary damage following focal injury. The specific localizing effects of focal pathology cannot be characterized adequately until the confusional state resolves. It is noteworthy that for a similar level of clinical impairment, recovery after focal pathology probably evolves over a shorter course, with an earlier plateau than that observed with severe DAI, which may evolve over a substantially longer period.

Factors Affecting Prognosis

The main factors determining prognosis relate to injury severity. For diffuse injury, animal models and human autopsy studies have confirmed a direct relationship between the amount of DAI, the severity of clinical effects, and duration of recovery. For focal pathology, prognosis relates to lesion characteristics. As with other forms of focal brain damage, longer-term dysfunction depends largely on the location, number, size (particularly depth), and secondary effects of the residual focal lesions. Mass effect from focal pathology is an important cause of death or more severe dysfunction after TBI. Bilateral lesions, especially in homologous areas, are associated with more long-lasting and permanent impairments than are unilateral lesions. The extent of secondary injury in its various forms, from edema to excitotoxicity with delayed neuronal injury to microvascular damage to hypoxic-ischemic injury, is among the important pathologic injury factors determining outcome. Late secondary problems, such as hydrocephalus, chronic subdural collections, and seizures, may cause retardation or reversals in the progression of recovery. Other injuries (e.g., fractures, other organ system damage) and secondary medical complications also may influence outcome.

A host of preinjury factors also are important determinants of recovery. Among these, age is probably the most important. Older age is associated with higher mortality and with slower and less complete recoveries. The effects of age become most apparent after age 40 or 50, but the precise influences on natural history and the ages at which these occur need further clarification. Aside from age, other preinjury prognostic factors include pre-existing psychosocial status, previous neurologic disorders, pre-existing disease, and alcohol or other substance abuse. Premorbid personality and constitutional factors are important influences on outcome. Changes in functional capacity after TBI are understood meaningfully only in the context of a person's previous functioning.

A number of factors probably are important after injury. The effects of treatment are discussed in the section Therapies Affecting Prognosis. Psychological adjustment and family and other social supports are important influences on outcome. The proportional influence of the injury probably wanes as the influence of psychosocial, noninjury factors increases as recovery progresses through the later stages.

Evaluation for Prognosis

Evaluation for prognosis varies with time after injury on the basis of the information available to that point and the outcome questions of interest at that time. In the acute phase of recovery, prognostication for severe TBI largely revolves around predictors of survival and broad gradations of disability. At subacute and later phases of recovery, outcome questions are more fine grained, regarding disability, handicap, and neuropsychological impairments in survivors. At any phase, combinations of evaluation measures produce more powerful prediction models (e.g., age, GCS score, and pupillary reactivity).

Among the most important components of evaluation for prognosis during the early acute period is depth of coma. GCS scores at admission, especially the motor subscore, carry significant prognostic information. Conventional categories for severity have been described using GCS ranges: mild, 13 to 15; moderate, 9 to 12; severe, 6 to 8; very severe, 3 to 5. Neuroimaging provides essential acute prognostic information regarding mass effect from a hemorrhagic lesion (epidural, subdural, or parenchymal) or diffuse edema. Clinical evaluation of brain stem function carries significant prognostic weight; pupillary response in the first 24 hours is among the most useful indicators. Several other early evaluation data may add to prognostication. They include intracranial pressure (ICP), measures of cerebral blood flow, arterial jugular oxygen extraction, and cerebrospinal fluid creatine kinase and lactate measures. Evoked potentials, particularly somatosensory, may have early prognostic value. Event-related potentials may be useful later in recovery. The acute and postacute predictive value of functional neuroimaging, such as single photon emission computed tomography or functional magnetic resonance imaging (MRI), is yet to be determined.

For prognosis in the postacute period, evaluation should center on diagnosis of the type and severity of damage. In patients with diffuse injury, the clinical severity measures described in the section Diffuse Injury carry much prognostic information; in order of increasing predictive value, they are admission GCS score, duration of LOC (e.g., time to follow commands), and duration of PTA (e.g., measured by the Galveston Orientation and Amnesia Test). Determining these parameters may be difficult for patients with mild injuries. Often a patient's subjective report of "unconsciousness" is actually their account of PTA (i.e., the resumption of continuous memory). Other prognostic measures indicating greater diffuse injury severity include deep white-matter lesions on computed tomography (CT) or MRI scans and the degree of atrophy on late scans (>2 months).

In patients with focal injury, neuroimaging is the essential evaluation procedure. The residual lesions on follow-up scans should be considered with respect to location, size, depth, number, bilaterality, and secondary mass effect. Corresponding localizing signs on examination and their recovery rate provide correlative prognostic information.

Evaluation should include an account of possible secondary injury. Indicators include clinical signs of herniation (e.g., unreactive pupil), prolonged ICPs greater than 20 mm Hg, systemic hypotension (e.g., systolic blood pressure <80 mm Hg), or hypoxia and severe edema on early CT (e.g., loss of cisternal markings). Late secondary complications (e.g., hydrocephalus, chronic subdural hematoma [SDH], seizures), additional nonneurologic injuries, and medical complications are also important in determining prognosis.

Evaluation of neuropsychological impairments or levels of disability at specific index times after injury also can be useful outcome predictors. Scores on neuropsychological batteries, certain key measures early in the postconfusional period of recovery, and scores on disability measures, such as the functional independence measure at rehabilitation admission, are commonly used prognostic tools.

Therapies Affecting Prognosis

Aggressive, early, management of TBI patients at the scene, in the emergency room, and in the intensive-care unit has improved survival and reduced morbidity. Some of the more important acute management areas supported by efficacy data are early resuscitation efforts to restore blood pressure and oxygenation, ICP monitoring of patients with severe TBI and abnormal CT scans, treatment of ICP greater than 20 mm Hg, and adequate nutritional support for increased metabolic requirements.

A number of treatment techniques under investigation are aimed at limiting early secondary injury. Of the various strategies, including antagonists of excitatory neurotransmitters, free radical scavengers, and calcium channel blockers, the most promising treatment to date in human studies has been moderate hypothermia. Improved outcome at 3 to 12 months has been demonstrated in patients with severe TBI cooled to 33°C in the hours after injury.

The evidence for the effects of rehabilitation on outcome after TBI is not conclusive, but the preponderance of evidence indicates a beneficial influence across the continuum of recovery. Controlled studies are few, and most reports involve improvement of posttreatment over pretreatment measures in a population assumed to have reached stability of biologic recovery. The rare studies comparing different treatment methods fail to support superiority of one method over another. Critical factors in rehabilitative treatment and the interaction of rehabilitation with natural recovery are yet to be determined.

Short-Term Prognosis

For patients with severe injury, the main short-term prognostic question is survival. The mortality rate for severe TBI is fairly high; one-third to one-half die within the first 6 months, most within the first week. Several factors may worsen prognosis for survival; for instance, SDH and low GCS are associated with nearly 75% mortality. Age has a great influence on mortality; in one series, mortality was 80% in those older than 55 years as contrasted to 30 to 50% in patients younger than 55 years.

More than 80% of patients with mild TBI develop symptoms of the postconcussion syndrome within a few days after injury; noteworthy is that more than 33% of uninjured controls have similar symptoms (e.g., headache, fatigue, dizziness). Most patients recover from the neurologic stigmata within 6 weeks to 3 months, but older individuals may recover considerably more slowly. A small percentage (10 to 15%) of patients have persistent postconcussion syndrome beyond a year after injury, owing to multiple interacting physiologic and psychological factors.

Long-Term Prognosis

Long-term outcome after TBI has been measured in various ways, including impairment levels (e.g., neuropsychological test performance), disability levels (reflected in functional independence in specified activities or settings), and handicap (or ability to return to social roles, such as work or school).

Not surprisingly, the prevalence of neuropsychological impairment at 1 year after injury is higher and occurs across a wider range of tasks in patients with more severe injuries. Very few patients with less than 24 hours LOC have significant impairments 1 year after injury as contrasted to controls. With LOC between 1 and 2 weeks, a high prevalence of impairments is seen in attention, memory, and nonverbal timed tasks (e.g., Wechsler Adult Intelligence Scale Performance IQ scores). In those with more than 2 weeks' coma, significant abnormalities are observed across an even wider array of cognitive measures.

Long-term functional outcome also clearly relates to severity of injury. Of patients with severe diffuse injury (GCS ≤8) followed in a large multicenter study from the time of admission to acute hospital, 29% made a good recovery or had moderate disability (indicating at least basic independence at home and in the community), 31% were severely disabled (dependent for all or some of the day), and 40% were dead or in a vegetative state. Of a group of surviving patients followed from rehabilitation admission, 49% of those with LOC between 1 day and 1 week made a good recovery by 1 year, whereas no patient with LOC more than 3 weeks made a good recovery, and 64% were severely disabled. When PTA was considered, 74% of those with PTA of less than 2 weeks made a good recovery, and only 5% were severely disabled. The probability of a good recovery lessened to 59% for 2 to 4 weeks of PTA, 45% for 4 to 8 weeks of PTA, 12% for 8 to 12 weeks of PTA, and 0 for those with PTA of more than 12 weeks.

The prospects of returning to work at the same or a modified level lessens considerably in patients with more severe injury. The time to return to work is substantially longer than for persons with nonbrain injuries. Most patients with mild or moderate injury return to work at between 1 and 6 months, whereas most of those with severe injury return at between 6 and 12 months, and a significant number require up to 2 years. In one large prospective series, 80% of those with GCS scores of 13 to 15 returned to work, contrasted to 56% of those with GCS scores of 9 to 12 and 26% of those with GCS scores of equal to or less than 8, by 1 year after injury. Some two-thirds of patients with LOC between 5 hours and 1 week, less than 50% of those with LOC of 1 to 2 weeks, and less than 20% of those with LOC of more than 2 weeks returned to work. Age older than 50, lower education, unstable job history, and lower premorbid earnings lessen the likelihood of re-employment.

Continuing improvements in functioning have been observed in patients even beyond 1 to 2 years after injury. Studies have reported better functioning in work or leisure activities, lessened cognitive and behavioral symptoms, and improvements in neuropsychological measures of consistency and reaction times. This supports the observation that TBI has a relatively longer course of recovery and greater prognosis for long-term improvement in functional status than do most other neurologic disorders.

Additional Reading

Alexander MP. Traumatic Brain Injury. In DF Benson, D Blumer (eds), Psychiatric Aspects of Neurologic Disease. New York: McGraw-Hill, 1982.

Dikmen SS, Machamer JE, Winn R, Temkin NR. Neuropsychological outcome at 1-year post head injury. Neuropsychology 1995;9:80–90.

Dikmen SS, Temkin NR, Machamer JE, et al. Employment following traumatic head injuries. Arch Neurol 1994;51: 177–186.

Katz DI, Alexander MP. Predicting course of recovery and outcome for patients admitted to rehabilitation. Arch Neurol 1994;51:661–670.

Levin HS, Benton AL, Grossman RG. Neurobehavioral Consequences of Closed Head Injury. New York: Oxford University Press, 1982.

Levin HS, Gary HE, Eisenberg HM, et al. Neurobehavioral outcome 1 year after severe head injury: experience of the Traumatic Coma Data Bank. J Neurosurg 1990;73:699–709.

Marshall LF, Gautille T, Klauber MR, et al. The outcome of severe closed head injury. Neurosurgery 1991;75(suppl): 28–36.

Part II
Epileptic Disorders

Chapter 8

Neonatal Seizures and Infantile Spasms

O. Carter Snead III

Neonatal Seizures

Volpe has described neonatal seizures as clinical events that may be diagnosed on the basis of a variety of paroxysmal behaviors in the newborn, including focal or generalized tonic posturing; focal or generalized clonic movements; focal, multifocal, or generalized myoclonic movements; apnea; or "bicycling" movements of the lower extremities. Another variant of neonatal seizures is "subtle seizures," which are characterized by motor automatisms, such as orolimentary movements, nystagmus, or intermittent eye deviation. In addition, such autonomic events as apnea may occur either as the primary manifestation or as part of the clinical seizure in the newborn. Apneic seizures usually are not associated with the bradycardia seen with primary apnea of the newborn.

Natural History

Neonatal seizures may be brief and self-limited or prolonged and may evolve into various types of epilepsy beyond the neonatal period. The natural history of neonatal seizures is dependent almost exclusively on the etiology of the seizures. The most common causes of neonatal seizures include hypoxic-ischemic encephalopathy, central nervous system (CNS) infection (either congenital or acquired), congenital anomaly of brain, intracranial hemorrhage, and metabolic abnormalities, including hypoglycemia, electrolyte abnormalities, and hypocalcemia. In addition, many types of inborn errors of metabolism may present with neonatal seizures, including a variety of mitochondrial abnormalities and organic acidurias in conjunction with lactic acidosis. Also, urea cycle defects and pyridoxine dependency or deficiency may present with seizures in the neonate.

Factors Affecting Prognosis

Prognostic considerations in neonatal seizures include the possibility of ongoing seizures beyond the acute setting and the effect on neurodevelopmental outcome. Both are dependent on the etiology of the seizures. The most unfavorable prognosis in neonatal seizures occurs when the seizures occur secondary to either a pre- or perinatal hypoxic-ischemic insult to the brain or owing to a congenital abnormality of brain. In addition, the prognosis for outcome in a child with neonatal seizures resulting from a CNS infection (i.e., meningitis or ventriculitis) may be quite guarded. Neonatal seizures that result from some metabolic abnormalities (e.g., uncomplicated hypocalcemia and some cases of symptomatic hypoglycemia that are diagnosed and treated early) carry a relatively benign prognosis. However, those mitochondrial abnormalities and organic acidurias that present with seizures in the nursery carry a uniformly bad prognosis both for neurodevelopment and for the future development of epilepsy.

Another prognostic feature of neonatal seizures is the clinical manifestation of the seizure. Generalized tonic seizures have the worst prognosis, whereas those children who have subtle seizures tend to do better over the long term. Therefore, careful clinical observation of seizures is important.

An additional prognostic feature of neonatal seizures is the interictal electroencephalogram (EEG). Those children who have had neonatal seizures and have a normal EEG on discharge from the nursery usually have a good prognosis. Conversely, those children with neonatal seizures and an abnormal EEG with multiple paroxysmal events, abnormal background, or burst-suppression do not do well in terms of either ongoing seizures or neurodevelopmental outcome.

Evaluation for Prognosis

The interictal EEG after acute treatment of neonatal seizures is a valuable prognostic tool. To minimize confounding postictal changes, the EEG is most helpful when performed 7 to 14 days after the last seizure. In a neonate whose seizures are well controlled and who has neither evidence of a structural lesion of the brain nor a history of a hypoxic-ischemic insult, a normal EEG carries a good prognosis.

Though the treatment ramifications of cerebrospinal fluid evidence of CNS infection are obvious, CNS infection as a cause of neonatal seizures also carries an adverse prognostic implication. Similarly, an immediate determination of glucose with glucose oxidase strips should be performed in addition to drawing of blood for serum glucose, calcium, magnesium, phosphorus, electrolytes, bicarbonate, blood urea nitrogen, ammonia, and bilirubin. Urine ketones and blood gases should be obtained also. Babies who have seizures secondary to these kinds of metabolic abnormalities tend to register a good prognosis, with the possible exception of hypoglycemia. Neonatal seizures secondary to symptomatic hypoglycemia may produce a poor prognosis if the seizures are not treated promptly and correctly.

The most useful prognostic imaging study in the child with neonatal seizures is the computed tomography (CT) scan. Ultrasonography is easier to obtain; however, it does not provide the full anatomic detail of brain and extra-axial spaces seen with the CT scan. The value of the magnetic resonance imaging (MRI) scan is limited in the neonate because of artifacts conferred by the high amount of water in the neonatal brain and by the logistics of obtaining the scan. The CT scan is important because children with

neonatal seizures secondary to structural congenital abnormalities revealed by the scan have a uniformly poor prognosis. Similarly, radiologic demonstration of hypoxic ischemic injury to the brain also carries a very unfavorable prognosis.

Therapies Affecting Prognosis

Prompt treatment of neonatal seizures is advisable, because the increased metabolic rate and increased cerebral blood flow conferred on the brain by ongoing seizure activity may injure the brain or enhance the damage in a brain already injured by hypoxic-ischemic insult or hemorrhage. Correction of metabolic abnormalities, such as hypoglycemia, hypocalcemia, and hypomagnesemia, should be prompt, as delay has a negative effect on prognosis.

If seizures persist in spite of correction of detectable metabolic abnormalities or occur in the absence of such abnormalities, anticonvulsant drug therapy is indicated. The therapeutic efficacy of anticonvulsant drugs used to treat seizures acutely is related to the peak serum level and the rate at which that level is achieved. Giving the correct loading dose initially is crucial, as lower peak levels result if the loading dose is too low, divided, delivered too slowly, or given by a route other than intravenously.

The drug of choice in the treatment of neonatal seizures is phenobarbital. The drug of choice in those babies who fail to respond to phenobarbital is phenytoin. Although it can be quite effective in the treatment of neonatal seizures, phenytoin has great potential for toxicity and should be used with care. If neonatal seizures prove intractable to treatment with phenobarbital or phenytoin, the next drug to try is a benzodiazepine. The two benzodiazepines recommended for the treatment of seizures in neonates are either diazepam or lorazepam. If the seizures prove intractable to phenobarbital, phenytoin, or benzodiazepines, a therapeutic trial of pyridoxine should be undertaken. Although pyridoxine-deficient or -dependent seizures are quite rare, they are a very treatable cause of intractable seizures.

Prognosis

Neonates who have had seizures and have a normal interictal EEG have a 90% chance of normal development by age 4, whereas only 10 to 15% of those with a multifocally abnormal EEG are normal at age 4. More important than the EEG in this kind of prognostication is the nature of the disease that produced the seizures. Of babies with uncomplicated hypocalcemic seizures, 80 to 100% can be expected to have a normal outcome. Of babies with hypoglycemic seizures, some 50% will be normal. Of those babies with neonatal seizures secondary to CNS infection, roughly 30% will be normal. Of those neonates whose seizures are secondary to perinatal hypoxia, 10 to 20% will be normal. Virtually all babies with neonatal seizures secondary to developmental anomalies of the brain will have an abnormal neurodevelopmental outcome.

Similarly, the risk factors for epilepsy after neonatal seizures include the presence of neurologic deficit, the severity and length of the acute neonatal seizures, an abnormal interictal EEG, and etiology of the seizures. Infants whose seizures are due to hypoxic-ischemic encephalopathy and who are neurologically abnormal at the time of discharge from the nursery have a 30% incidence of epilepsy and should be treated with chronic antiepileptic drug therapy, as should babies in whom cerebral dysgenesis is the cause of neonatal seizures.

Infantile Spasms

The first, and still unsurpassed, clinical description of this disorder was made in 1841 by West in a poignant letter to the *Lancet* wherein he described a mysterious malady afflicting his son and characterized by "bobbings of the head" and "bowings and relaxings" in clusters of "from ten to twenty or more times at each attack" and a progressive deterioration of intellect such that "he … never smiles or takes any notice, but looks placid and pitiful." The clinical presentation of infantile spasms, so clearly described by West, now has been studied carefully and has been characterized further by continuous monitoring with EEG-videotelemetry. The spasms may be divided into categories designated as flexor, extensor, and mixed, with the latter being the most common and extensor spasms being the least common. Flexor spasms consist of flexion of the neck, trunk, arms, and legs. Abdominal flexion may be massive, giving rise to the "jack-knife" or "salaam" seizures that are the hallmark of infantile spasms.

Extensor spasms produce abrupt extension of the neck, trunk, and legs. The mixed flexor-extensor spasms are characterized by flexion of the neck, trunk, and arms and extension of the legs. Infantile spasms usually occur in clusters many times daily (but particularly on awakening) and often are associated with a cry. The doubling over and crying seen with massive abdominal flexor spasms may lead to a misdiagnosis of colic. Infantile spasms are classified etiologically as either symptomatic or cryptogenic. Those children with symptomatic spasms are almost always neurologically abnormal at the onset of the spasms and have a clearly demonstrable cause (e.g., tuberous sclerosis). Patients with cryptogenic spasms are neurologically normal at the onset of the spasms and have no demonstrable etiology of the spasms.

The term *hypsarrhythmia* is used to describe the interictal EEG abnormality classically associated with infantile spasms and refers to a high-voltage chaotic slowing, multifocal spikes, and marked asynchrony. The definition was expanded by Hrachovy and coworkers to include areas of focal abnormality, synchrony, asymmetries, and burst-suppression. *West's syndrome* refers to those children who have infantile spasms, a hypsarrhythmic EEG, and mental retardation.

Natural History

The cumulative spontaneous remission rate of infantile spasms over the first 12 months of seizures is approximately 25%. The spasms are quite age-specific, usually occurring within the first 6 months of life, but the incidence drops off rapidly after the age of 12 months. The spasms rarely occur after the age of 4. Infantile spasms are associated with mortality of 10 to 20% and morbidity of 75 to 90%. The morbidity consists of generally moderate to severe mental retardation, epilepsy, hypotonia, and spasticity. Of those who go on to develop epilepsy, some 20% evolve into the particularly malignant epilepsy syndrome of Lennox-Gastaut.

Factors Affecting Prognosis

A dichotomy is found between the prognosis for seizure control in infantile spasms and that for developmental outcome in these children, the prognosis for seizure control being more favorable. In children with infantile spasms, the ultimate prognosis for normal cognition and development is poor for most and depends heavily on the etiology of the spasms, the pre-existing neurologic and developmental status of the child, the presence or absence of other seizure types that coexist with the spasms, the response of the spasms to therapy, and the age of the patient at the onset of infantile spasms.

Evaluation for Prognosis

The most important prognostic factor in infantile spasms is whether the spasms are cryptogenic or symptomatic. Therefore, an immediate and aggressive attempt should be made to determine the diagnostic category into which the patient falls. This quest should begin with a careful developmental history and thorough physical and neurologic examination. Abnormal development or objective evidence of neurologic abnormality on examination is sine qua non evidence for symptomatic spasms and the dismal prognosis that they imply. Children with new-onset infantile spasms always should undergo a careful physical examination of the skin with a Wood's lamp to expose hypopigmented lesions that are characteristic of tuberous sclerosis. Many children who have tuberous sclerosis and present with infantile spasms may have no other stigmata of the disease. This diagnosis is important for prognosis because children with tuberous sclerosis and infantile spasms have a terrible prognosis in terms of neurodevelopmental outcome and intractable epilepsy.

During the course of a diagnostic work-up of the child with infantile spasms, the single most important study to obtain is an MRI of the brain, because this type of seizure may be a presenting symptom in a significant percentage of neuronal migration disorders. Identifying this group is particularly important, because the spasms in some children in this group may be amenable to surgery. Before the advent of sophisticated MRI technology, these children were classified as having cryptogenic spasms, because often the CT scan was normal. Therefore, an MRI always is indicated in the work-up of infantile spasms and should be performed instead of a CT scan. Furthermore, a normal MRI early in life

does not rule out the presence of neuronal migration disorders of the brain, because these may not become apparent until myelination becomes more mature. Thus, if a child presents with infantile spasms and a pre-existing neurologic abnormality, does not do well, and has a normal MRI, the study should be repeated in a year or so. Another reason for an imaging study before initiation of therapy for infantile spasms is that it serves as a baseline, as either of the most frequently used therapeutic modalities for this disorder—adrenocorticotropic hormone (ACTH) or prednisone—often result in ventricular enlargement.

In addition to careful imaging with MR, a search for a metabolic cause of infantile spasms should be made because the inborn errors of metabolism that lead to symptomatic infantile spasms also uniformly carry a bad prognosis. Inborn errors of amino acids, organic acids, urea cycle defects, lysosomal storage disorders, and mitochondrial abnormalities should be sought in any child who presents with infantile spasms. This caution is particularly true in those children with onset of infantile spasms in the first month or two of life.

Therapies Affecting Prognosis

The desired goals of treatment of a child with infantile spasms are seizure control and an improved intellectual outcome. Though certain therapeutic modalities can achieve seizure control in infantile spasms, the effect of treatment on neurodevelopmental outcome is controversial and uncertain; however, evidence supports the possibility that a positive response to treatment may be associated with a better cognitive outcome, particularly in the cryptogenic group of patients.

Infantile spasms almost always are intractable to treatment with standard anticonvulsant drugs, with the exception of benzodiazepines, valproic acid, and vigabatrin. Either ACTH or oral steroid therapy will result in a significant reduction of seizures in 50 to 65% of patients. An inverse relation probably exists between response to treatment and age, with younger patients responding better. It is not clear whether a short treatment lag time gives a better prognosis. Glaze and colleagues have reported prospective data suggesting that time from diagnosis to treatment makes no difference in ultimate prognosis.

A number of controversial questions concern treatment of infantile spasms and the relation of treatment to ultimate outcome. First, which therapy is the most effective: ACTH, oral steroids, valproic acid, benzodiazepines, vigabatrin, a combination of some or all of these, or some other treatment (e.g., pyridoxine)? Second, in the ultimate outcome, does treating the patient early or late in regard to onset of these spasms make a difference? Third, does treating the spasms at all make any difference in the outcome in a patient with pre-existing mental retardation and an abnormal brain? Fourth, what is the optimal dosage of these drugs? And finally, for how long should the patient be treated once the spasms are brought under control? No definitive answer to any of these questions is found in the literature, and only the first two have been addressed in any detail. Comparing various reports of the efficacy of different treatment regimens and the relation of therapy to outcome is difficult, because no standard treatment regimen has been used. Furthermore, looking at outcome in a mixed group of children with symptomatic and cryptogenic infantile spasms is impossible, because the outcome is determined by the nature of the etiology of the spasms. Any meaningful outcome studies should include either cryptogenic spasms alone or a homogeneous group of symptomatic spasms (e.g., children with neuronal migration disorders).

Although consensus is lacking, I favor an aggressive approach to early treatment—as soon as the diagnosis is made in all patients. The reason for this philosophy of treatment is that in the severely neurologically handicapped child who develops symptomatic infantile spasms, one can never be sure that the retardation and incidence of later debilitating seizures will not be made worse if the spasms are allowed to continue unabated. When this reasoning is applied to the cryptogenic group of patients, the evidence is more compelling.

Prognosis

Few prospective studies are available in regard to short- and long-term prognosis in infantile spasms. Few question that children with cryptogenic infantile spasms have a more favorable short- and long-term prognosis than do children with symptomatic spasms. The rate of response to ACTH in children with cryptogenic spasms probably is on the order of 80 to 95%, whereas that in children with symptomatic spasms is considerably lower at 40 to 60%. Similarly, the rate of relapse or recurrence of spasms is on the order of 50 to 60% in the patients with symptomatic spasms and 15 to 20% in the cryptogenic patients. In addition to outcome regarding seizure control, cognitive outcome also is better in children with cryptogenic spasms. Some 50% of children with cryptogenic infantile spasms will have a normal developmental outcome versus only 15% with symptomatic spasms.

In summary, the child who has infantile spasms and in whom the best prognosis is found is older than 3 years but younger than 12 months, is neurologically normal at the onset of the spasms, and lacks a demonstrable etiology for the spasms (i.e., cryptogenic infantile spasms). The child with a good outcome is one who has no other kind of seizures, does not lose visual following, or does not develop other neurologic deficits during the course of the spasms. Finally, a child who responds completely and early (i.e., within 7 days) to therapy with complete cessation of spasms and normalization of the EEG also would be predicted to have a favorable prognosis both in terms of absence of recurrent seizures and a normal neurodevelopmental outcome.

Additional Reading

Neonatal Seizures

Bergman I, Painter MJ, Hirsch RP, et al. Outcome in neonates with convulsions treated in an intensive care unit. Ann Neurol 1983;14:642–647.

Holden KR, Melits ED, Freeman JM. Neonatal seizures: I. Correlation of prenatal and perinatal events with outcomes. Pediatrics 1982;70:165–176.

Legido A, Clancy RR, Berman PH. Neurologic outcome after electroencephalographically proven neonatal seizures. Pediatrics 1991;88:583–596.

Perlman JM, Volpe JJ. Seizures in the preterm infant: effects on cerebral blood flow velocity, intracranial pressure, and arterial blood pressure. J Pediatr 1983;102:288–293.

Rowe JC, Holmes GL, Hafford J, et al. Prognostic value of the electroencephalogram in term and preterm infants following neonatal seizures. Electroencephalogr Clin Neurophysiol 1985;60:183–196.

Scher MS, Painter MJ. Controversies concerning neonatal seizures. Pediatr Clin North Am 1989;36:281–310.

Volpe JJ. Neonatal seizures: current concepts and revised classification. Pediatrics 1989;84:422–428.

Watanabe K, Hara K, Miyazaki S, et al. Postnatal epilepsy after EEG confirmed neonatal seizures. Am J Dis Child 1982;136:980–984.

Infantile Spasms

Baram TZ, Mitchell WG, Hanson RA, et al. High-dose corticotropin (ACTH) vs. prednisone for infantile spasms: a prospective, randomized, blinded study. Pediatrics 1996;97:375–379.

Cowan LD, Hudson LS. The epidemiology and natural history of infantile spasms. J Child Neurol 1991;6:355–364.

Glaze DG, Hrachovy RA, Frost JD, et al. Prospective study of outcome of infants with infantile spasms treated during controlled studies of ACTH and prednisone. J Pediatr 1988;112:389–396.

Ito M, Okuno T, Fujii T, et al. ACTH therapy in infantile spasms: relationship between dose of ACTH and initial effect or long-term prognosis. Pediatr Neurol 1990;6: 240–244.

Jeavons PM, Bower BD, Dimitrakoudi M. Long-term prognosis of 150 cases of "West syndrome." Epilepsia 1973;14:153–164.

Koo B, Hwang PA, Logan WJ. Infantile spasms: outcome and prognostic factors of cryptogenic and symptomatic groups. Neurology 1993;43:2322–2327.

Lombroso CT. A prospective study of infantile spasms. Clinical and therapeutic correlations. Epilepsia 1983;24:135–158.

Matsumoto A, Watanabe K, Negoro T, et al. Long-term prognosis after infantile spasms: a statistical study of prognostic factors in 200 cases. Dev Med Child Neurol 1981;23:51–65.

Matsumoto A, Watanabe K, Negoro T, et al. Prognostic factors of infantile spasms from the etiological viewpoint. Brain Dev 1981;3:361–364.

Ohtsuka YU, Murashima I, Oka E, Ohtahara S. Treatment and prognosis of West syndrome. J Epilepsy 1994;7:279–284.

Snead OC, Benton JW, Hosey LC, et al. Treatment of infantile spasms with high-dose ACTH: efficacy and plasma levels of ACTH and cortisol. Neurology 1989;39:1027–1030.

Chapter 9
Febrile Seizures

Gerald Exil

Febrile seizure is an age-specific epileptic syndrome characterized by a brief, usually generalized, convulsion in the setting of a febrile illness in an otherwise normal child. This syndrome has been the subject of investigation for many decades, and the natural history and factors influencing prognosis are better understood today.

Natural History

Febrile seizures belong to the category of provoked seizures and, although recurrence is common, must be differentiated from epilepsy, which is defined as recurrent, unprovoked seizures. In 1980, the National Institutes of Health Consensus Development panel on febrile seizures defined febrile seizures as "an event in infancy or childhood, usually occurring between 3 months and 5 years of age, associated with fever but without evidence of intracranial infection or defined causes." According to that definition, children with an underlying toxic metabolic disorder, meningitis, or encephalitis are excluded. Febrile seizure is the most common seizure type in early childhood: 2 to 5% of children aged 5 or younger will develop at least one episode of febrile seizure. After the first febrile convulsion, one-third of children will develop a second febrile seizure; 40 to 50% of the latter group will develop a third seizure.

Simple febrile seizures are associated with a low mortality and morbidity. Verity and colleagues found no intellectual difference in children with febrile seizures as compared with their peers who had no history of febrile seizures.

Factors Affecting Prognosis

Febrile seizures are classified as simple or complex. A simple febrile seizure is a single, brief, generalized convulsion. A complex febrile seizure is characterized by prolonged seizure (>15 minutes) recurrent over a 24-hour period or associated with focalization at the onset of the seizure or during the postictal period. This classification is important from a prognostic standpoint. Simple febrile seizure is a benign entity not associated with permanent neurologic deficit. Complex febrile seizures are more common in children with an underlying neurologic impairment and, in some cases, are associated with later development of epilepsy. As such, complex febrile seizures are an indication for more extensive investigation and more aggressive management.

Risk of Recurrence

More than 90% of all febrile seizures occur between the ages of 6 months and 3 years, with a peak incidence between 9 months and 24 months of age. Although earlier presentation (before 6 months) is not uncommon, a central nervous system infection always should be excluded in this age group. Febrile seizure occurring as late as age 5 to 7 years should raise the suspicion of possible underlying epilepsy. The most predictive factors of recurrence are genetic predisposition and first febrile seizure before 1 year. Genetic predisposition plays a role in the development of febrile seizure but not in later development of epilepsy. An autosomal dominant and a polygenic mode of inheritance have been postulated. The following genetics-related risk factors have been reported: sibling with epilepsy, sibling with febrile seizures, or one parent with history of febrile seizures. The risk increases to 50% if one parent and one sibling have had febrile seizures.

Risk of Epilepsy

The risk of developing epilepsy after a febrile seizure is reported in some studies to be 3%. Certain risk factors have been identified for the later development of epilepsy and include two or more of the following: complex febrile seizures, age less than 1 year at the time of the first febrile seizure, a family history of idiopathic or genetically driven epilepsy, a pre-existent baseline neurologic dysfunction, and first febrile seizure after age 6.

The type of epilepsy after febrile seizure is variable, the most common being generalized tonic-clonic. Mesial temporal sclerosis has been associated with febrile seizures in prospective studies of patients who had complex partial seizures and underwent temporal lobectomy. In particular, prolonged febrile seizures and focal febrile seizures are associated with later development of temporal lobe epilepsy. The mechanism by which febrile seizures cause mesial temporal sclerosis is not understood well. This particular finding on magnetic resonance imaging of children following febrile seizure is not common, implying possible subcellular damage caused by prolonged seizures that is expressed at a later age. Permanent neurologic sequelae after prolonged seizures in children, although rare, has been documented well.

Evaluation for Prognosis

Electroencephalography (EEG) does not have prognostic value in simple febrile seizures and should not be obtained routinely. However, complex febrile seizures are an indication for a more aggressive approach and deserve a more extensive evaluation, including EEG and an imaging study of the brain. Findings that may affect the prognosis include a focal structural abnormality (e.g., stroke), a porencephalic cyst, cerebral dysgenesis, and hypoxic-ischemic injury, among others. An EEG is indicated also in patients with other risk factors, such as underlying neurologic disorder and family history of epilepsy. Recurrence of seizures within the same febrile illness and febrile status epilepticus are indications for a lumbar puncture to rule out an intracranial infection. Febrile seizures in some cases are the initial presentation of a severe metabolic or a progressive neurologic disorder; in that setting, the prognosis is worse and depends on the underlying disease.

Therapies Affecting Prognosis

Short-Term Prognosis

The short-term prognosis is determined by prevention of immediate recurrences. This prevention includes temperature control with antipyretic medications, such as acetaminophen and ibuprofen. Although effective, acetylsalicylate often is avoided, owing to the risk of Reye's syndrome. Tepid sponge bath often is recommended, but it has no proved efficacy. Rectal diazepam is effective in preventing immediate recurrences but should be given only in selected patients. Rectal diazepam does not prevent later development of epilepsy.

Long-Term Prognosis

The long-term prognosis of febrile seizures is excellent even in cases of prolonged seizures in an otherwise normal child with no underlying central nervous system infection. No hard evidence supports the possibility that antiepileptic medications prevent later development of epilepsy. However, such antiepileptic agents as phenobarbital, benzodiazepine, and valproic acid have been reported to prevent recurrences of febrile seizures only in some studies. Mesial temporal sclerosis and temporal lobe epilepsy have been associated with a previous history of complex febrile seizures in some adult studies.

Long-term prophylactic treatment must be selective and should be reserved for children with multiple recurrences of prolonged febrile seizures and for complex febrile seizures in patients with an underlying central nervous system dysfunction. Consideration of long-term prophylaxis must include awareness of risks, benefit, and compliance. Valproic acid must be avoided in young children, owing to associated fetal adverse reactions. Phenobarbital has been associated with behavior disturbances, hyperactivity, and sleep disturbance and may impair cognition. One study by Farwell and coworkers reported the mean IQ to be 7 points lower in patients treated with phenobarbital for 2 years as contrasted to controls.

Additional Reading

Aicardi J. Febrile Convulsions. In J Aicardi (ed), Epilepsy in Children (2nd ed). New York: Raven, 1994;253–275.

Annegers JF, Hauser WA, Elveback LK, Kurland LT. The risk of epilepsy following febrile convulsions. Neurology 1979;29:297–303.

Camfield CS, Camfield PR. Behavior and Cognitive Effect of Phenobarbital in Toddlers. In KB Nelson, JH Ellenberg (eds), Febrile Seizures. New York: Raven, 1981;203–210.

Cendes F, Andermann F, Dubeau F, et al. Early childhood prolonged febrile convulsions, atrophy and sclerosis of the mesial structures, and temporal lobe epilepsy: an MRI volumetric study. Neurology 1993;43:1083–1087.

Farwell J, Lee YJ, Ellenberg JH, Nelson KB. Phenobarbital for febrile seizures. Effects on intelligence and on seizure recurrence. N Engl J Med 1990;322:364–369.

Frantzen E, Lennox-Buchthal M, Nygard A, Stene J. A genetic study of febrile convulsions. Neurology 1970;20:909–917.

Hauser WA, Annegers JF, Anderson VE, Kurland LT. The risk of seizure disorders among relatives of children with febrile convulsions. Neurology 1985;35:1268–1273.

Knudsen FU. Effective short-term diazepam prophylaxis in febrile convulsions. J Pediatr 1985;106:487–490.

Nelson KB, Ellenberg JH. Prognosis in children with febrile seizures. Pediatrics 1978;61:720–727.

Verity CM, Butler NR, Golding J. Febrile convulsions in a national cohort followed up from birth: prevalence and recurrence in the first five years of life. BMJ 1985;116: 329–337.

Chapter 10

Primary Generalized Seizures

Sydney Louis and Charlene A. Tate

Since the 1970s, the prognosis of seizures has improved remarkably from gloomy to quite optimistic. This change is less a consequence of modern treatment than of better data gathering and analysis. Studies conducted up to the 1970s concentrated on institutionalized epileptics, at a time when institutionalization was common. More recent, broader studies of the population have yielded very different results and prognoses. Before current prognoses are detailed, some pertinent definitions are offered.

Definitions

Generalized Versus Primary Generalized Seizures

In 1981, a new international classification of epileptic seizures was based on a phenomenologic description of generalized seizures. This new definition included all generalized seizures plus focal seizures that generalize rapidly and focal seizures from silent areas of the brain that generalize. The result is that the term *generalized seizures*, as used currently, is less pure than the term used before 1981. This term sometimes is used to represent all the various definitions of it; sometimes, it is applied to different entities, and its meaning varies from study to study.

Prognosis for Life

Prognosis, or the ability to predict outcome of disease, must include the likelihood of survival or the risk of death in that condition. Mortality from seizures is a complex issue. Death may result from such complications of the seizures as injury, accident, or suicide. In addition, sudden death can occur in young epileptics.

Prognosis for Development of Epilepsy After the Occurrence of a Single Seizure

Epilepsy (or *seizure disorder*) is defined as the occurrence of more than one spontaneous (not obviously provoked) seizure. It generally is conceded that the occurrence of a single random seizure between birth and death is far more frequent than the likelihood of the recurrent seizures of epilepsy. The occurrence of a single seizure raises the question of the frequency with which epilepsy subsequently will develop.

Prognosis for Remission of Established Epilepsy

When the diagnosis of epilepsy has been made, meaning that two or more unprovoked seizures have occurred, determination of the prognosis for remission can be approached in one of two ways. In the first instance, involving patients in whom the diagnosis of epilepsy has been established and treatment has begun, *remission* is used to mean the disappearance, or lack of continuation, of seizures as a consequence of either treatment or spontaneous remission. In the second instance, involving the selected group of patients who have become seizure-free on medication for periods of 2 to 4 years and in whom medication has gradually been withdrawn, *remission* can be defined as the nonrecurrence of seizures.

Natural History

The natural history of several subtypes of generalized seizure disorders will be enumerated, as their prognoses are unique and well established.

(Primary) Generalized Absence Seizures

(Primary) generalized absence seizures generally start in childhood, commonly at approximately age 4, and usually disappear between 12 and 20 years of age. Data indicate that at puberty, this disorder remits in 40 to 60% of patients. In the remainder, it usually is succeeded by generalized tonic-clonic seizures. This disorder is easily controlled with medications and usually is not associated with brain disease or mental deficiency.

(Primary) Generalized Tonic-Clonic Seizures

(Primary) generalized tonic-clonic seizures are generalized seizures most often commencing in children, teenagers, or young adults (in their 20s) and not usually associated with brain disease or mental deficiency. The seizures generally are easily controlled with medication in 70 to 80% of patients and tend to remit (nonrecurrence off medication) in approximately 40% of patients.

Juvenile Myoclonic Epilepsy

Juvenile myoclonic epilepsy is a condition in which absence attacks, generalized tonic-clonic seizures, and myoclonic jerks begin in the teen years. This syndrome appears to have a genetic origin: A gene on chromosome 6 has been identified as having a possible causative association with this disorder. Most practitioners believe that this disorder is relatively easily controlled with medication (specifically, valproate), but the condition usually does not remit and tends to be prolonged, even lifelong.

Myoclonic Epilepsies

A variety of myoclonic epilepsies begin in childhood or the teen years and are characterized by myoclonus, tonic-clonic seizures, mental deterioration, and a poor outcome. Several different disorders within this category tend to carry poor prognoses for life, seizure control, and mentation.

Factors Affecting Prognosis

Factors that usually are associated with a favorable prognosis are young age at onset of seizure activity, a negative family history, a normal neurologic examination, a normal electroencephalogram (EEG), single versus multiple seizure types, and idiopathic versus remote symptomatic seizures. Examination findings, such as the skin lesions of tuberous sclerosis, neurofibromatosis, or the Sturge-Weber syndrome, may help to determine prognosis.

Evaluation for Prognosis

To allow determination of the prognosis in a patient with generalized seizures, the evaluation must include a careful history of the seizure disorder, a careful family and patient history, a detailed neurologic and general examination (including evaluation of skin), and electrical tests (most especially the EEG). None of these assessments individually determines prognosis, but a complex combination of them helps in prognostication.

Therapies Affecting Prognosis

The two major therapies that modify prognosis are anticonvulsant drugs and surgery. The drugs used in epilepsy (anticonvulsants) attempt to suppress convulsive and nonconvulsive seizures. The drugs' alternate mechanism of use is a possible antiepileptic quality that prevents occurrence or development of the epileptic process after injury, thus increasing the probability of remission. The anticonvulsant effect of drugs has been a confounding variable when measuring remission after seizure disorder has been diagnosed. Whether the drugs also exhibit an antiepileptic function has not been determined, yet most indications are that the drugs do not prevent the development of epileptic foci. For example, after a head injury, phenytoin has failed to prevent development of epilepsy. The complex issue of whether seizures beget more seizures and cause the epileptic process to worsen is too broad and controversial a topic to address in this discussion of prognosis.

Several types of surgery are used to treat epilepsy: (1) The temporal lobe of one side can be removed; (2) the corpus callosum may be sectioned; (3) epileptic foci outside the temporal lobe may be excised or undercut; or (4) a defective hemisphere can be removed (hemispherectomy). Numerous studies of temporal lobectomy allow derivation of prognostic information. Figures for total freedom from seizures range from 30 to 72%. The percentage of patients with no seizures or improved seizure frequency (a decrease of 50% or more) after temporal lobectomy ranges from 61 to 95%. More recent statistics from small studies have suggested that 50 to 60% of patients are free from seizures and another 20% experience improvement in seizure frequency after temporal lobectomy.

The prognosis for remission after hemispherectomy or removal of nontemporal cortex is less satisfactory than after temporal lobe surgery, though the number of patients so treated is much smaller and the data are less firm. After corpus callosal resection, seizure frequency is not diminished and may even be increased, but the seizures do not tend to generalize and, therefore, are less life-threatening.

Remission of Epilepsy

Remission of epilepsy (cessation of seizures on or off medication) is noted, in various studies, to occur in 41 to 76% of patients. Several factors influence cessation of seizures (Table 10-1). Generalized tonic-clonic seizures have a favorable effect on prognosis in some studies, though generalized spike and wave on the EEG increases the probability of recurrence (by 3.47 times) as compared to absence of this pattern on the EEG. According to one study, the younger the patient at age of onset of seizure activity, the better is the probability of remission (67% remission at 2 to 3 years of age; 49% at 4 to 7 years; 46% at 8 to 10 years; and 33% at 11 to 14 years). Multiple seizure types in a single patient

Table 10-1. Recurrence After a First Seizure

	Likelihood of second seizure at year			
	1	3	5	7
Overall percentage	14	29	34	39
Original idiopathic seizure	10	24	29	
No FH in siblings	9		26	
Nonspecific or normal EEG	9		26	
Prior seizure with acute illness	10		39	
Generalized spike and wave on EEG	15		58	
FH positive in sibling	29		46	
Original remote symptomatic seizure	26	41	48	
No prior seizure with acute illness	17	41	48	
Single seizure	21	34	43	
No Todd's palsy	22	31	39	
Multiple seizures, status epilepticus	37		56	
With Todd's palsy	41		75	
Prior seizure with acute illness	60		80	

FH = family history; EEG = electroencephalogram.
Source: Adapted from WA Hauser, SS Rich, JF Annegers, E Anderson. Seizure recurrence after a first unprovoked seizure: an extended follow-up. Neurology 1990;40:1163–1170.

carry a worse remission rate than any single seizure type (49% versus 72%). Remission is much more likely in a patient with a normal neurologic examination than in a patient with mental retardation or neural damage (77% versus 38%). Finally, in some studies, an idiopathic seizure disorder has a better chance of remitting than do seizures that follow symptomatic disease.

Relapse After Seizure Control

The results of studies that evaluated patients who responded satisfactorily to drug therapy (i.e., no further seizures on medication) but then relapsed when their medication was tapered are inconsistent. Comparison of these studies is difficult, as entrance criteria vary. For example, in some studies relapse is considered to have occurred if a seizure is experienced during the withdrawal phase. In most other studies, relapse is considered to have occurred when the patient experiences seizures after the drug has been eliminated completely. This and other discrepancies complicate comparison of such studies.

Nonetheless, the probability of relapse in patients whose seizures were, for a time, controlled by medication, is 20 to 34% for all ages (adults, 26 to 63%; children, 11 to 36%). Among the factors that may increase relapse rate are EEG abnormalities (including abnormalities during drug withdrawal or before drug withdrawal), abnormal neurologic examination, and mental retardation. Frequent seizures before remission are another poor prognostic sign. In most studies, etiology of the seizure disorder, seizure type, age at medication withdrawal, race, gender, family history of seizures, and rate of drug withdrawal do not seem to influence relapse rates.

Sudden Death

Uncontrolled studies show an unexpectedly high mortality in young epileptics, especially men between 20 and 40 years old. Sudden death involves patients in whom seizures are poorly controlled, compliance is poor, and alcohol is abused. It may especially involve patients who have had many seizures but can affect any patient. Incidences ranging from 1 per 250 to 1 per 1,000 have been found in medical examiner studies. The mechanisms postulated have included arrhythmias, central hypoventilation, pulmonary edema, asphyxiation, or aspiration in association with nocturnal seizures. Another recent explanation involves the Romano-Ward syndrome, in which a prolonged cardiac output interval corrected for heart rate develops, resulting in syncope that can masquerade as epilepsy. Sudden death in epileptics is completely unpredictable, except in the Romano-Ward patients, in whom diagnosis is possible on the basis of electrocardiographic abnormalities.

Short-Term Prognosis

The short-term prognosis for occurrence of a second seizure after a single idiopathic generalized seizure is 14% at 1 year but is made more probable if the family history is positive or if generalized spike and wave activity is seen on the EEG. The prognosis for occurrence of a second seizure after one remote symptomatic seizure is higher (26% at 1

year) and is more likely if the patient is affected with Todd's palsy, prior seizure with acute illness, or multiple seizures or status epilepticus.

Long-Term Prognosis

The long-term prognosis for control of seizures with treatment is excellent in most generalized seizure types, the exception being the myoclonic subtypes. The prognosis for successfully withdrawing medication in generalized epilepsy patients is variable, ranging from 26 to 63%. Successful withdrawal of medication is unlikely in juvenile myoclonic epilepsy and in the other myoclonic types of epilepsy, whereas it is much more likely in the absence and tonic-clonic subtypes of generalized seizures. In general, the likelihood of relapsing seizures is greater in those with an abnormal neurologic examination, an abnormal EEG, mental retardation, or frequent seizures before remission.

The sudden death syndrome is more common in young male epileptics whose seizures are poorly controlled, who are noncompliant, and who use alcohol. This behavior affects the prognosis by decreasing life expectancy.

Additional Reading

Berg AT, Shinnar S. Relapse following discontinuation of antiepileptic drugs: a meta-analysis. Neurology 1994;44: 601–608.

Bouma PAD, Westendorp JGJ, van Dijk JG, et al. The outcome of absence epilepsy: a meta-analysis. Neurology 1996;47:802–808.

Hauser WA, Hesdorffer DC. Epilepsy: Frequency, Causes and Consequences. New York: Demos, 1990.

Hauser WA, Rich SS, Annegers JF, Anderson E. Seizure recurrence after a first unprovoked seizure: an extended follow-up. Neurology 1990;40:1163–1170.

Leestma JE, Walczak T, Hughes JR, et al. A prospective study on sudden unexpected death in epilepsy. Ann Neurol 1989;26:195–203.

Mattson RH, Cramer JA, Collins JF, and the Department of Veterans Affairs Epilepsy Cooperative Studies No. 118 and No. 264 Group. Prognosis for total control of complex partial and secondarily generalized tonic clonic seizures. Neurology 1996;47:68–76.

Mitchell WG. Long-term prognosis for children with epilepsy. Curr Probl Pediatr 1995;25:113–120.

Chapter 11

Partial and Secondary Seizures

Alan R. Towne

A seizure is an event that results in an altered state of brain function. In 1870, Hughlings Jackson described a seizure as a "symptom … an occasional, an excessive and a disorderly discharge of nervous tissue." In distinction, epilepsy is a chronic disorder with recurrent symptomatology or seizures. Epilepsy has been described by the World Health Organization as "a chronic brain disorder of various etiologies characterized by recurrent seizures due to excessive discharge of cerebral neurons." Seizures can be classified into two types; partial (or focal) and generalized. Partial seizures develop from an abnormal focus in part of one hemisphere, whereas generalized seizures are characterized by activation of neurons throughout both hemispheres. Partial seizures at times may progress and become secondarily generalized. The ability to differentiate between the different seizure types is important because the various types respond differently to medication and surgery.

Natural History

Seizures occur in a bimodal distribution, with an initial peak in incidence during the first year of life and another peak after the age of 60 years. The incidence of epilepsy is higher in patients older than 75 years and in children younger than 10. It occurs in all age groups and races, with an almost equal distribution among men and women. The incidence of epilepsy is defined as the number of new cases of epilepsy occurring during a specific period in a given population. The cumulative incidence of epilepsy to age 80 ranges from 1 to 3%; partial seizures represent 32 to 52% of incident epilepsy, and generalized seizures account for 39 to 59%. Approximately 60% of patients experience multiple seizures before their first medical contact for this disorder.

A major question addressed to physicians is whether development of seizures affects the mortality and longevity of the patient. However, few well-developed studies have been performed to answer this question. Early epidemiologic studies evaluating individuals with seizures were inconsistent, and it was often difficult to determine accurately whether a person with epilepsy died from seizures or from the underlying cause. A study of insurance company actuarial figures indicates that epilepsy is a minor cause of death, with just fewer than 2,000 deaths ascribed to epilepsy in the United States per year. These figures may be biased as policyholders may have a better survivorship than the general population. Nonetheless, generally studies conclude that mortality is increased in patients with epilepsy.

Factors Affecting Prognosis

The risk of recurrence after a first seizure differs depending on whether the seizure is partial or generalized. Most studies indicate that partial seizures are more likely to recur than are generalized seizures. In a study of recurrence after a first unprovoked seizure in 168 children residing in Halifax,

Nova Scotia, 79% of patients with partial seizures experienced a recurrence, as opposed to 44% of patients with generalized seizures. In another study performed in the Bronx, New York, 283 children, aged 28 days to 19 years, were studied. Using univariate analysis, the recurrence rate was 50% for partial seizures and 30% for generalized seizures. In a large retrospective study that looked at all age groups, Annegers evaluated 424 patients: Of the patients with partial seizures, 31% experienced a recurrence, as compared to 20% of those patients with generalized seizures. As a result of these studies, Hauser concluded that when the neurologic examination, electroencephalographic pattern, and antiepileptic drug regimen remain constant, individuals with a first partial seizure are almost twice as likely to experience recurrence as compared to patients with a first generalized seizure.

Approximately 75% of patients in whom epilepsy is diagnosed will be seizure-free for 5 or more years, and one-half of those will enter remission in the first year after the diagnosis is made. Studies examining seizure remission have been plagued with differences in case ascertainment, the definition of remission (seizure-free interval ranging from 2 to 5 years), and the length of follow-up. Despite these problems, most studies indicate patients with partial seizures are less likely to achieve remission than are patients with generalized seizures. A study of 457 cases of unprovoked epilepsy in Rochester, Minnesota, found that patients with generalized-onset seizures were more likely to become seizure-free for 5 years off medication than were those with complex partial seizures. In another study of children aged 5 to 14 years, 50% of patients with partial seizures attained remission, as compared to 65% of patients with generalized seizures. Among the approximately 75% of patients with epilepsy who achieve remission, antiepileptic medications can eventually be withdrawn in 40 to 90% without seizure recurrence.

Evaluation for Prognosis

The electroencephalogram (EEG) is an essential test in determining the seizure type and can aid in determining prognosis. The presence of epileptiform activity is not necessarily associated with an increased risk of epilepsy. Conversely, up to 20% of patients with epilepsy do not demonstrate epileptiform activity even after multiple EEGs. The majority of patients with partial epilepsy demonstrate complex partial seizures, the most frequent site of onset arising in the anterior temporal region. In these patients, the localizing value of extracranial EEG has ranged from approximately 40 to 90% in published series. In those patients who experience simple partial seizures, the results of surface-recorded EEG monitoring may be unremarkable. In studies that use simultaneous intracranial and extracranial recordings, approximately 80% of patients had no definite extracranial EEG alteration. Lobar onset of a seizure is the most common alteration seen via scalp electrodes in patients with complex partial seizures of anterior temporal lobe origin. The frontal lobe is the second most common site of seizure onset in patients with partial epilepsy, but the interictal EEG is not as sensitive in patients with frontal lobe epilepsy as it is in patients with temporal lobe seizures. Other types of partial seizures that might be diagnosed by EEG criteria include occipital lobe epilepsy and benign childhood epilepsy with central temporal spikes. The prognosis in patients with these disorders is excellent, and the seizures usually do not persist into adulthood.

Neuroimaging is an important component in the evaluation of patients with epilepsy. In most cases, magnetic resonance imaging (MRI) has supplanted computed tomography (CT) as the test of choice. The dramatically improved resolution of MRI permits easy visualization of small, potentially epileptogenic lesions, including mesial temporal sclerosis, and can demonstrate hippocampal asymmetry.

Therapies Affecting Prognosis

Although the search for effective antiepileptic medications began 2,000 years ago, not until the mid–nineteenth century did Locock find bromides that were effective in certain types of seizures. Phenobarbital was introduced in 1912 as the first synthetic chemical agent for the management of seizures. The modern era of pharmacotherapy was heralded by Merritt and Putnam with their discovery in 1938 of the anticonvulsant properties of diphenylhydantoin. This drug was effective for both generalized and partial seizures. Until that time, recurrent seizures and epilepsy were a lifelong condition for which there was little likelihood of control or remission.

The clinical data indicate that antiepileptic drugs (AEDs) are not effective in altering the long-term prognosis for seizure remission. However, AEDs are clearly effective in suppressing seizure activity. The Veterans Affairs (VA) Medical Centers cooperative trials have compared the efficacy of several drugs in adults with newly diagnosed partial or secondarily generalized seizures. The initial trial compared phenytoin, carbamazepine, phenobarbital, and primidone. The VA cooperative study failed to show significant differences between the AEDs' effectiveness in controlling partial-onset seizures. Phenobarbital and primidone produced more frequent adverse events. Carbamazepine was superior to phenytoin in completely controlling partial seizures within 1 year after treatment was initiated (43% versus 26%). Because the first VA cooperative trial did not include valproate, a second study was performed comparing that drug with carbamazepine. Carbamazepine was somewhat more effective in those patients with complex partial seizures only but, in patients with generalized seizures as well, valproate was more effective in obtaining seizure control. Subsequent studies in the United States and Europe have provided similar findings. It appears that carbamazepine, phenytoin, and valproic acid are equivalent as initial medication for partial and secondarily generalized seizures.

A number of new drugs, including felbamate, gabapentin, and topiramate, are available for the treatment of partial seizures. Large-scale, randomized trials, such as the VA cooperative studies, are needed to investigate fully the efficacy of these drugs. However, some information is available concerning their use. In one double-blind comparison trial, lamotrigine was found to have efficacy similar to that of carbamazepine and was better tolerated. The efficacy of felbamate has been demonstrated in refractory patients with complex partial seizures. Drug interactions with this AED are prominent, and its use has been limited because of fatal aplastic anemia and hepatotoxicity. Gabapentin has been effective in partial seizures and is generally well tolerated, demonstrating no hepatic enzyme induction and little effect on plasma levels of other AEDs. Topiramate has been very effective in partial seizures and has one of the highest responder rates when compared to the other new antiepileptic drugs.

Whenever possible, monotherapy should be the goal: In approximately 70% of cases, seizures will be well controlled on a single drug. If a patient's seizures are not controlled on initial therapy, then a second drug should be tried. In the VA cooperative study, an alternative agent succeeded in 46% of patients whose first drug had failed because of adverse events or insufficient seizure control. In the 30% of cases in which single-drug treatment does not control seizures, then combination therapy may be needed.

Although 60 to 80% of patients achieve adequate seizure control with treatment involving existing drugs, the remaining patients will have unsatisfactory control despite multiple AEDs at maximum doses. Referral to a specialized center for possible seizure surgery should be considered in these cases. At most centers, the criteria for surgical referral include disabling seizures that are resistant to high therapeutic levels of AEDs, a well-defined region of seizure onset, and an epileptogenic zone originating in tissue that can be removed without causing disability. The most commonly performed surgical procedure for epilepsy is temporal lobectomy. In a survey by Engel of more than 3,000 patients after temporal lobectomy who were followed up for at least 1 year, 68% were seizure-free, 24% had worthwhile improvement, and 8% showed no improvement. Resection of extra temporal foci results in less favorable improvement and, in the absence of a focal lesion, seizure-free outcomes are relatively rare. Complications of seizure surgery remain low, with small visual field deficits occurring in up to 75% of patients who undergo classic temporal lobectomy and hemiparesis occurring in approximately 3% of patients. Mortality after temporal lobectomy has been estimated to be between 0 and 0.8%.

Short-Term Prognosis

As compared to patients with generalized-onset seizures, patients with partial seizures experience a higher recurrence rate. The probability of recurrence after a first partial seizure is 10 to 79%, with complex partial seizures accounting for the higher percentages. Most second seizures occur within 1 year of the first seizure. In patients with simple or complex partial seizures, an abnormal EEG or an abnormal neurologic examination indicates a greater than 90% chance of recurrence.

Long-Term Prognosis

Numerous studies make clear that most patients' seizures will be controlled with appropriate AED therapy. Approximately 75% of patients with epilepsy will achieve remission within 5 years of diagnosis. However, those patients who have not entered remission after 5 years are less likely to obtain complete seizure cessation. In addition, even those patients who achieve remission can relapse. Patients with complex partial seizures are more likely to relapse (32%) than are those patients with generalized-onset tonic-clonic or absence seizures.

Seizure outcome is only one measure of prognosis. The mortality of patients with epilepsy must be taken into account. The higher-than-expected risk of death may be due in part to the condition underlying the epilepsy rather than to the epilepsy itself. Recent studies indicate the overall mortality for patients with epilepsy is two to three times that of the general population and, for those patients with partial epilepsies, the mortality rate may reach four times that expected in normal controls.

Additional Reading

Annegers JF, Hauser WA, Elveback LR. Remission of seizures and relapse in patients with epilepsy. Epilepsia 1979;20:729–737.

Cockerell OC, Johnson AL, Sander JWAS, Shorvon SD. Prognosis of epilepsy review and further analysis of the first nine years of the British national general practice study of epilepsy, a prospective population-based study. Epilepsia 1997;38:31–46.

DeLorenzo RJ, Towne AR. Epilepsy. In SH Appel (ed), Current Neurology (Vol 9). Chicago: Year Book, 1989;27–76.

Engel J, Van Ness, PC, Rasmussen TB, Ojemann LJ. Outcome with Respect to Epileptic Seizures. In J Engle (ed), Surgical Treatment of the Epilepsies. New York: Raven Press, 1993;615.

Hauser WA, Annegers JF, Roca WA. Descriptive epidemiology of epilepsy: contributions of population-based studies from Rochester, Minnesota. Mayo Clin Proc 1996;71:576–586.

Hauser WA, Hesdorffer DC. Epilepsy, Frequency, Causes and Consequences. New York: Demos, 1990.

ILAE Commission Report. The epidemiology of the epilepsies: future directions. Epilepsia 1997;38:614–618.

Mattson RH, Cramer JA, Collins JF, The Department of Veterans Affairs Epilepsy Cooperative Study No. 264 Group. A comparison of valproate with carbamazepine for the treatment of partial and secondarily generalized tonic-clonic seizures in adults. N Engl J Med 1992;327:765–771.

Merritt HH, Putnam JJ. A new series of anticonvulsant drugs tested by experiments in animals. Arch Neurol Psychiatry 1938;39:1003–1015.

Chapter 12

Status Epilepticus

Jane G. Boggs, Alan R. Towne, Robert J. DeLorenzo, and John M. Pellock

Status epilepticus (SE) is widely recognized as both a medical and a neurologic emergency. The literature has reported mortality figures ranging from 3 to 52% in various populations. This wide variance can be accounted for largely by differences in age, duration of SE, and etiologies. Defining the prognosis for mortality from SE thus depends on the complex interplay of these primary factors. DeLorenzo and colleagues have determined that the overall mortality within 30 days of SE is remarkably consistent at between 20 and 30%.

The neurologic and medical morbidity in the 70 to 80% of SE patients who experience long-term survival depends not only on age, etiology, and duration of the ictus but also on the medical sequelae, iatrogenic complications, and factors affecting general health in epilepsy patients. In this chapter, we review the prognosis for morbidity and mortality after SE.

Natural History

The natural history of SE depends not only on treatment and other factors affecting prognosis but also on how SE is defined. Historically, SE has been considered as an epileptic seizure that is so frequently repeated or so prolonged as to create a fixed and lasting condition. Clinical application of this definition, especially in clinical research, is difficult because the terms of the definition are so general. A more applicable definition is offered by the Epilepsy Foundation of America's Working Group

on Status Epilepticus, which characterizes this diagnosis more precisely as "more than 30 minutes of (1) continuous seizure activity or (2) two or more sequential seizures without full recovery of consciousness between seizures."

Although exact frequency and morphologic criteria for the electroencephalographic characteristics of a seizure are based largely on the electroencephalographer's opinion of the evolution of the event in the context of the electroencephalographic background and reactivity, recent controversy has developed regarding whether periodic epileptiform discharges (PEDs) should consistently be considered a form of SE. Animal studies have documented a progression of electroencephalographic patterns in the natural course of untreated SE, beginning with recurrent convulsions that merge into continuous seizure activity, advance to the development of brief periods of suppression, and finally evolve into PEDs and even burst-suppression. Although similar patterns can be identified in human patients who are treated for SE, it is ethically impossible to withhold treatment and record an electroencephalogram (EEG) continuously to observe this proposed progression to PEDs.

Although early epidemiologic studies indicated an incidence of SE of approximately 60,000 per year in the United States, prospective, population-based data have projected an estimated yearly incidence of 140,000. The Greater Richmond Metropolitan Status Epilepticus Project (GRMASE) has validated 1,000 cases of SE, with a median duration of 92 minutes. Distribution of cases of SE is bimodal, with the greatest number of cases occurring in young children and in the elderly. Although generalized and partial convulsive SE comprise the largest proportion of recognized cases, nonconvulsive SE probably occurs more frequently than is detected, owing to the great variability and subtlety of its presentation.

Factors Affecting Prognosis

Although mortality is highest within the first 30 days after SE, it is unusual for patients to die during SE. No specific factors have been associated with death during SE as opposed to after SE. Mortality from SE increases asymptotically to approximately 30 days but, after this, is no more likely due to SE than to other medical factors. Some investigators have defined mortality in SE patients to include only those patients who die before termination of SE, thus suggesting very low mortality rates. As SE and its treatment can precipitate numerous additive complications and result in a cascade of multiple organ dysfunction, the time immediately subsequent to SE should logically be considered in mortality statistics for this disorder.

Age at onset of seizure activity has long been recognized as a primary determinant of mortality for many medical disorders, including SE. Infants and children to age 16 have an overall mortality of only 3% in the GRMASE. Shinnar and colleagues found that one-third of SE cases in children between 4 and 60 months of age were related to acute febrile illness, with mortality of nearly zero; nonfebrile SE in children has only slightly higher mortality. Series involving high proportions of pediatric cases can thus be expected to have lower overall mortality rates than those involving large numbers of adults. Pediatric patients also have a markedly higher recurrence rate than do adults—that is, a certain encephalopathic group survives to have SE repeatedly rather than dying after a single episode. SE mortality in adults who have had multiple recurrences is lower than the mortality in adults with an isolated episode, suggesting that some adults may share characteristics for a "good" prognosis that predispose them to recurrence rather than death.

As specific definition of neonatal SE remains controversial, determination of mortality statistics in premature and full-term neonates with SE is difficult. Population-based data from the GRMASE suggest that both incidence and mortality of neonatal SE may be higher than in infants older than 1 month.

The age distribution of SE incidence is bimodal, with peaks in very young and very old patients. Mortality, however, steadily and exponentially increases with advancing age. The highest mortality of SE is in the oldest patients, who typically also have multiple medical illnesses. Thus, mortality attributed to SE in the elderly likely is not a factor simply of age but also of reduced physiologic resilience. SE is effectively a convulsive or electrical "stress test," which can easily result in decompensation of underlying medical conditions. It is not uncommon for previously asymptomatic, undiagnosed atherosclerotic cardiovascular disease to be expressed as ischemia or infarction during and immediately after SE. A retrospective review of cardiac enzymes and electrocardiograms obtained during SE found that 10% of patients who underwent such studies met criteria for myocardial infarction during SE.

The elderly similarly are more susceptible to etiologies of SE that are associated with the highest mortality. Hypoxia and especially anoxia occurs more than five times more commonly in adult patients older than 65 years. Overall mortality of anoxia related to SE is 71% in adults but is 92% in patients older than 65. Patients who experience SE resulting from cardiopulmonary arrest rarely survive, but this is expected, as relatively few patients who experience cardiopulmonary arrest, with or without SE, survive. However, mortality among elderly patients with "milder" etiologies (e.g., ethanol-related status epilepticus) is closer to that of younger patients.

Causes of SE that carry intermediate prognoses for mortality in adults include cerebrovascular disease, metabolic derangements, drug overdose, tumor, and trauma. Categorizing causes broadly into acute symptomatic and remote etiologies not surprisingly demonstrates that acute etiologies are associated with higher mortality. Presumably, the combined physiologic stress of SE and the acute causative illness, as well as the acute treatments for both, are additive if not synergistic. Of course, in many patients, multiple etiologies of SE may be present, rendering more complicated the direct association between mortality and a single etiology.

One of the causes of SE that is associated with the highest survival in all age groups is a subtherapeutic anticonvulsant drug level. Studies have not clearly substantiated whether patients with pre-existing epilepsy have a lower risk of death after SE than those in whom SE is the presenting symptom of epilepsy.

Duration of SE is the third primary determinant of mortality. As duration increases to approximately 3 hours, mortality increases exponentially, after which only small increments in mortality are seen. Duration is the only potentially modifiable primary determinant of mortality in SE: Earlier presentation, earlier diagnosis, and a shorter interval to initiation and completion of treatment obviously can shorten the overall SE duration, thereby reducing mortality. In SE treatment, difficulty obtaining intravenous access and slow or prolonged infusions also can significantly delay control of SE. Whether the choice of initial parenteral agent or whether rapid initiation of treatment with *any* agent is more important in SE management has not yet been determined.

Other factors indirectly related to the three primary determinants of age, duration, and etiology contribute to mortality after SE. Although there is no standard definition of electroencephalographic patterns constituting SE in patients with ambiguous clinical signs, slower patterns, such as PEDs, are traditionally not regarded as pathognomonic for SE. In the recently completed Veterans Administration Cooperative Study, "Treatment of Generalized Convulsive Status Epilepticus," stuporous or obtunded patients whose EEGs demonstrated PEDs were considered to be in "subtle SE." Mortality of subtle SE was found to be 64%, whereas the mortality of overt SE was 26.5%. This is consistent with the observation of GRMASE that nonconvulsive SE has a higher mortality than does convulsive SE, as the former is more commonly associated with hypoxic or anoxic etiologies.

Incompetent autonomic nervous system function also can increase mortality after SE. The initial physiologic response to acute seizures is typically tachycardia and hypertension along with other signs of sympathetic activity. Failure to develop sinus tachycardia during seizures that last more than 2 minutes indicates an incomplete and atypical sympathetic response and is significantly associated with higher mortality. Patients who die after SE typically exhibit evidence of autonomic decompensa-tion by slow decrease of both heart rate and systemic blood pressure or inappropriate dissociation of heart rate and blood pressure; both responses can result in critically decreased cardiac output and cerebral perfusion. As death from any condition ultimately results in complete cardiovascular failure, not surprisingly the majority of SE patients, as well as patients with witnessed cardiac death, experience ventricular fibrillation as their terminal rhythm. The infrequency of witnessed cardiac arrhythmias during and immediately after SE suggests that patients who eventually die have a latent arrhythmogenicity of the heart. Conditions prone to abrupt, lethal, cardiac arrhythmia (e.g., catecholamine and cocaine cardiomyopathy, "athlete's heart," "voodoo death") have been associated with cardiac myofibrillar necrosis and contraction band formation. Similar histologic findings have been documented in higher-than-expected numbers of autopsied hearts after SE.

Numerous medical complications have been described in SE and are summarized in Table 12-1. The coexistence of some medical diseases and SE can have synergistic effects on outcome. Patients who have a stroke combined with SE have a higher mortality than would be anticipated from the additive individual mortality rates of these diagnoses.

Experimental models of SE have documented neuronal loss and loss of mediation by gamma-aminobutyric acid (GABA) in the CA1 region of the hippocampus, as well as decreased $GABA_A$ receptors in rat forebrain. These basic scientific findings have suggested that long-term impairment of central nervous system function may result from both electrical and convulsive aspects of SE. Elevation of serum neuron-specific enolase, an enzymatic marker of central nervous system cell damage, has been noted after both convulsive and nonconvulsive SE.

Clinically, cognitive outcome after SE has been variable, but slight deterioration of intellectual function after SE is likely. In a retrospective study of SE, up to 30% of children were reported to have some neurologic morbidity, but a prospective study found the true rate to be 15 to 20%. The proportion of these changes that is transient is undetermined. Separation of the long-term cognitive effects of SE from those of the underlying etiology, medical sequelae, and effects of antiepileptic drugs (AEDs) is a difficult problem but has important implications for treatment. Neuropsychiatric testing of

Table 12-1. Acute Medical Complications
of Status Epilepticus

Cardiovascular
    Cardiac ischemia
    Conduction abnormalities, congestive heart failure
    Hypotension
    Cardiac arrest
Respiratory
    Hypoventilation
    Apnea
    Intubation, ventilator dependence
    Neurogenic pulmonary edema
Gastrointestinal, nutritional
    Mucosal ulceration
    Hepatic dysfunction
    Ileus
    Enteral feeding tubes
    Parenteral nutrition
Renal, electrolytes
    Acute renal failure
    Uremia
Infections
    Aspiration pneumonia
    Intravenous line infections
    Urinary tract infections

---

patients treated chronically with different individual AEDs has failed to document significantly different levels of cognitive impairment except in patients maintained on barbiturates. Similarly, barbiturates have been implicated as contributing to developmental delay in infants born to mothers taking barbiturates during pregnancy and lactation. Whether use of barbiturates in emergency treatment protocols for SE worsens cognitive outcome is unknown.

Therapies Affecting Prognosis

The results of the Veterans Administration Cooperative Study "Treatment of Generalized Convulsive Status Epilepticus" indicate lorazepam, diazepam, phenobarbital, and phenytoin all had similar efficacy when administered promptly. The only statistically significant difference was between lorazepam and phenytoin, with the latter agent being less effective. The most important, modifiable, prognostic factor in termination of SE is the overall interval from the start of SE to completion of medication infusion.

Medications used in the management of SE can cause additional complications. In most centers, treatment is initiated with parenteral benzodiazepines, which, if followed by barbiturates, can result rapidly in respiratory failure. For this reason, most SE protocols recommend that barbiturates be deferred until after both benzodiazepines and phenytoin have failed. Fosphenytoin, which can be infused more rapidly than intravenous phenytoin and with significantly less local irritation and less hypotension, potentially will facilitate rapid treatment of SE. Cases of SE that are refractory to benzodiazepines and phenytoin or fosphenytoin can frequently be managed by continuous infusion of a barbiturate or other anesthetic agent to induce burst-suppression on EEG. Such infusions frequently result in significant hypotension and may require additional use of parenteral pressors, which may precipitate ischemic complications.

Short-Term Prognosis

SE is well established as a medical emergency with significant mortality. The degree to which SE itself, its etiology, and its modulating factors of age and treatment affect short-term prognosis remains a complex problem. The overall risk of death in the subacute period (within 30 days) after SE is 22%. The ability to stratify risk factors to define mortality in particular patient groups is possible only by analyzing and comparing the results of large, prospective, population-based studies.

Long-Term Prognosis

Definition of long-term morbidity is the aspect of prognosis that is most difficult. Medical sequelae are common, but relating them directly to SE can be difficult. Extrapolating from animal research and clinical observations, it is known that long-term cognitive and neurologic impairment is a likely complication of prolonged seizures, but many confounding variables interfere with the determination of whether neurologic function will be altered by the amount and type of seizure activity, its etiology, or its management. In addition, symptoms of cognitive and neurologic impairment may not be apparent for years after SE. In cases of SE that occur early in life, the effect on both maturation of the nervous system and social development must be considered.

Additional Reading

DeLorenzo RJ, Hauser WA, Towne AR, et al. A prospective, population-based epidemiologic study of status epilepticus in Richmond, Virginia. Neurology 1996;46:1029–1035.

Dodrill CB, Wilensky AJ. Intellectual impairments as an outcome of status epilepticus. Neurology 1990;40(suppl 2):23–27.

Hauser WA. Status epilepticus: epidemiologic considerations. Neurology 1990;40(suppl 2):9–12.

Kapur J, Lothman EW, DeLorenzo RJ. Loss of $GABA_A$ receptors during partial status epilepticus. Neurology 1994;44:2407–2408.

Lothman E. The biochemical basis and pathophysiology of status epilepticus. Neurology 1990;40(suppl 2):13–23.

Lowenstein DH, Alldredege BK. Status epilepticus at an urban public hospital in the 1980s. Neurology 1993;43:483–488.

Shinnar S, Pellock JM, Berg AT. An inception cohort of children with febrile status epilepticus: cohort characteristics and early outcome. Epilepsia 1995;36(suppl 4):31.

Towne AR, Pellock JM, Ko D, DeLorenzo RJ. Determinants of mortality in status epilepticus. Epilepsia 1994;35:27–34.

Treiman DM, Meyers PD, Collins JF, et al. Design of a large prospective double-blind trial to compare intravenous treatments of generalized convulsive status epilepticus. Epilepsia 1990;31:635.

Chapter 13

Eclampsia

Errol R. Norwitz, John T. Repke, and Peter W. Kaplan

Eclampsia is the occurrence of one or more generalized convulsions or coma in the setting of preeclampsia and in the absence of other neurologic conditions. Preeclampsia is a multisystem disorder of pregnancy and the puerperium that complicates approximately 6 to 8% of all pregnancies. It is characterized by new-onset hypertension (sitting blood pressure [BP] ≥140/90), proteinuria (≥2+ in a random urine sample or ≥300 mg in a 24-hour collection), and nondependent edema after 20 weeks' gestation. Eclampsia was at one time believed to be the end result of preeclampsia—hence the nomenclature. However, it is now known that seizures are but one clinical manifestation of "severe" preeclampsia. Other manifestations include the HELLP syndrome (*h*emolysis, *e*levated *l*iver enzymes, and *l*ow *p*latelets), disseminated intravascular coagulopathy, acute renal failure, hepatocellular damage, intrauterine growth restriction, congestive cardiac failure, and pulmonary edema.

In the United States and other developed countries, the incidence of eclampsia is relatively stable at approximately 4 to 5 per 10,000 live births. In developing countries, however, the reported incidence varies widely from 6 to 7 to as high as 100 cases per 10,000 live births. Occurrence rates are highest among nonwhite, nulliparous women from lower socioeconomic backgrounds. Peak incidence is in the teenage years and early twenties, but there is also an increased incidence in women older than 35 years.

Despite recent advances in detection and management, preeclampsia and eclampsia together remain the second most common cause of maternal death in the United States (after embolism), accounting for 15% of all maternal deaths and probably accounting for 50,000 maternal deaths per year worldwide.

Natural History

Almost half of all cases of eclampsia occur preterm, and more than one-fifth occur before 31 weeks' gestation. Of those cases occurring at term, the majority (approximately 75%) occur either intrapartum or within 48 hours of delivery. Traditionally, convulsions that occurred more than 48 hours after delivery were not considered to be eclampsia. However, it is now clear that late postpartum eclampsia (i.e., seizures developing more than 48 hours but fewer than 4 weeks postpartum) exists and may account for up to 16% of all cases of eclampsia. Eclampsia before 20 weeks' gestation is extremely rare and should raise the possibility of an underlying molar pregnancy or neurologic disease that predisposes the patient to seizures.

Antepartum cases of eclampsia are often dramatic, with multiple seizures and maternal complication rates of up to 71%. Complications include disseminated intravascular coagulopathy, acute renal failure, hepatocellular injury, liver rupture, intracerebral hemorrhage, cardiorespiratory arrest, bronchial aspiration, acute pulmonary edema, and postpartum hemorrhage. In a retrospective analysis of 990 cases of eclampsia, López-Llera reported an overall maternal mortality rate of 13.9% (138 of 990). The highest maternal mortality rate (22.2%

[12 of 54]) was seen in that subgroup of women with early eclampsia (i.e., ≤28 weeks' gestation). The overall perinatal mortality for eclampsia is on the order of 9 to 23%. As expected, perinatal mortality is closely related to gestational age and may be as high as 93% (50 of 54) in pregnant women with eclampsia before 28 weeks' gestation. Fetal deaths are related to abruptio placentae, premature delivery, and intrauterine asphyxia.

Eclamptic seizures are almost always brief, seldom lasting longer than 3 to 4 minutes. Patients who do not improve rapidly after seizures and hypertension are controlled or those who develop localizing neurologic signs should be evaluated further. Preeclampsia or eclampsia always resolves after delivery, although this may require a few days or even weeks. Diuresis (>4 liters per day) is believed to be the most accurate clinical indicator of resolution.

The relationship between hypertension, symptoms and signs of cortical irritability (headache, visual disturbances, nausea, vomiting, fever, hyperreflexia), and seizures remains unclear and unpredictable. Nonetheless, most women have one or more antecedent symptoms before an eclamptic seizure. In a retrospective analysis of 383 cases of eclampsia in the United Kingdom, Douglas and Redman reported that 59% of eclamptic patients (227 of 383) experienced a prodromal headache, visual disturbance (scotomas, amaurosis, blurred vision, diplopia, homonymous hemianopsia), or epigastric pain. In 38% of cases (146 of 383), however, eclampsia was the first manifestation of pregnancy-related hypertensive disease.

Although it correlates well with the incidence of cerebrovascular accident, the magnitude of BP elevation does not appear to be predictive of eclampsia. Indeed, 20 to 38% of eclamptic patients have a maximal BP of less than 140/90 before their seizure. Similarly, 15 to 22% of patients have no proteinuria before their seizure.

Factors Affecting Prognosis

Factors affecting the prognosis for a woman who has experienced an eclamptic seizure and, if she is pregnant, the prognosis for her fetus, are detailed in Tables 13-1 and 13-2, respectively. In this chapter, *short-term prognosis* refers to events related to the seizure itself as well as to subsequent management while the patient is hospitalized. *Long-term prognosis* refers to events that occur after the patient's discharge from the hospital.

Short-Term Prognosis

Without treatment, approximately 10% of eclamptic women will have repeated seizures. Although there is agreement that patients with eclampsia require anticonvulsant therapy to prevent further seizures and possible cerebrovascular accident, the choice of agent has been controversial. Obstetricians have long favored magnesium as the drug of choice for the prevention and treatment of eclamptic seizures, whereas neurologists have favored more established anticonvulsants such as phenytoin or diazepam. This dispute appears to have been resolved by a number of clinical studies. In 1995, the Eclampsia Trial Collaborative Group reported on a prospective trial in which 905 eclamptic women were randomized to receive either magnesium or diazepam, and 775 eclamptic women were randomized to receive either magnesium or phenytoin. Primary measures of outcome were recurrence of seizures and maternal death. Women allocated magnesium had a 52% lower incidence of recurrent convulsions as compared with those allocated diazepam (13.2% [60 of 453] versus 27.9% [126 of 452], respectively). There was no significant difference in maternal or perinatal mortality or morbidity between the two groups. Similarly, women allocated magnesium had a 67% lower risk of recurrent seizures than did those on phenytoin (5.7% [22 of 388] versus 17.1% [66 of 387], respectively). In this arm of the study, the women who received magnesium were 8% less likely to be admitted to an intensive care facility, 8% less likely to require ventilatory support, and 5% less likely to develop pneumonia as compared with women who were given phenytoin. The differences in maternal mortality and in perinatal outcome were not significant.

Transient fetal bradycardia is a common finding after an eclamptic seizure and does not necessitate immediate delivery. Every attempt should be made to stabilize the mother and resuscitate the fetus in utero before a decision is made about delivery.

Cerebral hemorrhage accounts for 15 to 20% of deaths from eclampsia and often is associated with

Table 13-1. Factors Affecting Maternal Prognosis in Eclampsia

Factor	Effect on Short-Term Prognosis[a]	Effect on Long-Term Prognosis[b]
Proteinuria (≥5 g/24 hrs)	No effect	No effect
Associated with HELLP syndrome	↑ MMR (3–28%)	↑ Chronic HTN (33%)
	↑ Eclampsia (50%)	↑ Recurrent preeclampsia (37%)
	↑ Renal failure (8–66%)	↑ Recurrent HELLP syndrome (3–5%)
	↑ DIC (30–38%)	
	↑ Abruptio placentae (20%)	
Severity of BP elevation	↑ Stroke	—
Duration of seizure	No effect	No effect
Associated with ARF	↑ MMR (34%)	↑ Dialysis (10–20%) if associated with HTN
Gestational age ≤28 weeks	—	↑ Recurrence (20–50%)
		↑ Chronic HTN (18%)
History of preeclampsia	—	↑ Chronic HTN (15–25%)
		↑ Recurrent preeclampsia (19–47%)
		↑ Recurrent eclampsia (2–21%)
		↑ Abruptio placentae (2–3%)
African-American race	↑ MMR	↑ Chronic HTN
	↓ HELLP syndrome	
Associated with diabetes	—	↑ Chronic HTN
Associated with abruptio placentae	↑ MMR (24%) especially in older, multiparous women	—
Multiparity	↑ MMR	—
	↑ HELLP syndrome	
Associated intracranial hemorrhage or coma	—	↑ Recurrence (37%)
		↑ Neurologic sequelae

HELLP syndrome = hemolysis, elevated liver enzymes, low platelets; MMR = maternal mortality rate; HTN = hypertension; DIC = disseminated intravascular coagulopathy; BP = blood pressure; ARF = acute renal failure; ↓ = decreased incidence; ↑ = increased incidence.

[a]*Short-term* refers to the seizure itself and to subsequent management while the patient is hospitalized.

[b]*Long-term* refers to the outcome after the patient's discharge from the hospital.

Table 13-2. Factors Affecting Fetal Prognosis in Eclampsia

Factor	Effect on Short-Term Prognosis[a]	Effect on Long-Term Prognosis[b]
Proteinuria (≥5 g/24 hrs)	No effect	No effect
Associated with HELLP syndrome	↑ PNMR (23–40%)	No effect
Severity of BP elevation	↑ PNMR	—
Duration of seizure	No effect	No effect
Associated with ARF	↑ Premature delivery (72%)	—
Gestational age ≤28 weeks	↑ PNMR	—
History of preeclampsia	↑ PNMR (2–4%)	—
Associated with abruptio placentae	↑ PNMR (41–45%)	—
Associated with IUGR	↑ PNMR	—
African-American race	↑ PNMR	—
Maternal age ≥35 yrs	↑ PNMR due to chronic HTN	—
Associated with chronic HTN	↑↑ PNMR	—
Decreased EDF on Doppler ultrasonography	?↑ PNMR	—

HELLP syndrome = hemolysis, elevated liver enzymes, low platelets; PNMR = perinatal mortality rate; BP = blood pressure; ARF = acute renal failure; IUGR = intrauterine growth restriction; HTN = hypertension; EDF = end-diastolic flow; ↑ = increased incidence; ↑↑ = markedly increased incidence; ?↑ = increased incidence possible.

[a]*Short-term* refers to the seizure itself and to subsequent management while the patient is hospitalized.

[b]*Long-term* refers to the outcome after the patient's discharge from the hospital.

significant elevation in BP (≥170/120). For this reason, aggressive BP control is recommended in all patients. However, BP control alone does not appear to affect the natural course of the disease and does not prevent recurrent seizures.

Long-Term Prognosis

Long-term prognosis for the mother depends largely on the degree of injury sustained as a result of the disease. Hepatocellular damage, renal dysfunction, coagulopathy, and hypertension all resolve after delivery. However, cerebrovascular accident (stroke) may result in permanent neurologic sequelae.

Stroke is responsible for approximately 5% of the estimated 420 to 450 pregnancy-related maternal deaths in the United States each year. Whether the risk of stroke is increased during pregnancy remains controversial. Earlier studies, which were mostly hospital-based and not controlled, suggested pregnancy increased the risk of cerebral infarction by nearly 13-fold. More recent case-controlled studies, on the other hand, have estimated that the incidence of stroke is 4.3 to 20 per 100,000 deliveries, similar to that reported for nonpregnant women of childbearing age. However, the risk for both cerebral infarction and intracerebral hemorrhage does appear to be increased in the immediate postpartum period (relative risk of 8.7 and 28.3, respectively). Eclampsia has been identified as a risk factor for stroke during both pregnancy and the puerperium and may be responsible for up to 47% of all pregnancy-related cerebral infarctions. Although some patients have persistent neurologic deficit and neuroradiologic abnormalities after an eclamptic seizure (which suggests brain infarction), the vast majority of patients return to their clinical baseline within a few days or weeks and suffer no long-term neurologic sequelae (which argues against the existence of true cerebral ischemic necrosis). These stroke-like focal defects that follow an eclamptic seizure have been purported to be the result of critical ischemia due to vasospasm, an inflammatory process, or intimal proliferation. Alternatively, preeclampsia or eclampsia may cause intraparenchymal hemorrhage, especially in patients with underlying cerebrovascular anomalies. Approximately 3.5% of arteriovenous malformations will bleed during pregnancy. Although contentious, the literature suggests that the incidence of bleeding complications does not increase during normal pregnancy. Whether this is true also of pregnancies complicated by preeclampsia or eclampsia is not clear. It is clear, however, that a bleed during pregnancy carries a far more guarded prognosis than does a bleed in a patient who is not pregnant, with the mortality rate increasing from 10% to approximately 28%.

In terms of risk of recurrence, patients with a history of preeclampsia or eclampsia are at increased risk (12 to 68%; average, 33.7%) for developing preeclampsia in some form in a subsequent pregnancy. In a prospective study, Sibai and colleagues compared the subsequent pregnancies of 406 women with a history of preeclampsia or eclampsia in their first pregnancy with subsequent pregnancies in 409 controls (matched for age, race, gestational age at delivery, obstetric complications, and month of delivery) who were normotensive in their first pregnancy. Follow-up was a minimum of 2 years (range, 2 to 24 years). The preeclamptic and eclamptic group had a higher incidence of preeclampsia in their second pregnancies (46.8% [190 of 406] versus 7.6% [31 of 409]) as well as in subsequent pregnancies (20.9% [85 of 406] versus 7.7% [43 of 557]) when compared with the normotensive group. In that subgroup of women with severe preeclampsia or eclampsia at ≤30 weeks' gestation, the recurrence rate in the next pregnancy was 76% as compared with 38% in women who developed their disease at ≥37 weeks' gestation. The reported incidence of recurrent eclampsia ranges widely from 0 to 21% (average, 10.3%). Prediction of which patients are at risk for recurrent eclampsia as opposed to other manifestations of severe preeclampsia is not possible.

Aside from the risk of recurrence, pregnancies in women with a history of preeclampsia or eclampsia have an increased incidence of other obstetric complications. These include an increased incidence of abruptio placentae (2.5 to 6.5% versus 0.8% in patients with no history of preeclampsia or eclampsia), preterm delivery (15 to 21% versus 7 to 8%), intrauterine growth restriction (12 to 23% versus 10%), and a higher perinatal mortality (4.6 to 16.5% versus 1 to 3%). Once again, a history of preeclampsia or eclampsia remote from term (i.e., <28 weeks' gestation) increases the likelihood of such complications. The risk appears to be the same whether the patient had severe preeclampsia or eclampsia.

Therapies Affecting Prognosis

Short-Term Prognosis

The only effective treatment for preeclampsia or eclampsia is expeditiously to empty the uterus of all products of conception. Immediate delivery does not necessarily imply cesarean section, although the chance of effecting a vaginal delivery in a patient with severe preeclampsia who is remote from term and who has an unfavorable cervix is only on the order of 14 to 20%. More recently, there has been a trend toward expectant management of severe preeclampsia at less than 32 weeks' gestation. However, even in such studies, eclampsia was considered a contraindication to expectant management.

If the fetus is delivered intact from the unfavorable intrauterine environment, without evidence of asphyxia or birth injury, the prognosis for mother and child is good. Long-term outcome for the child depends largely on gestational age at delivery and problems related to prematurity.

Long-Term Prognosis

Low-dose aspirin (60 to 100 mg per day) reportedly reduces the incidence of preeclampsia among women at high risk for this complication. However, whether aspirin is of value in healthy nulliparous women is not clear. Furthermore, in one study, low-dose aspirin therapy was associated with an increased risk of placental abruption. Dietary supplementation with calcium (≥2,000 mg elemental calcium per day) has also been shown to decrease the incidence of preeclampsia in patients at high risk (typical odds ratio, 0.34; 95% confidence interval, 0.22 to 0.54). The effect of these agents on the incidence of eclampsia is not known.

Magnesium, aside from preventing recurrent convulsions in patients who have already had an eclamptic seizure, has also been shown to prevent the primary seizure in patients with severe preeclampsia. Furthermore, magnesium appears to be superior to other medications in this regard. In a nonblinded, prospective study of 2,138 preeclamptic women, Lucas and coworkers reported seizures in 10 of the 1,089 women randomly assigned to prophylactic phenytoin therapy as compared with none of the 1,049 women given magnesium. There were no differences in maternal or neonatal outcomes.

Conclusions

Eclampsia is an obstetric emergency occurring in 4 to 5 per 10,000 live births. Both the fetus and the mother are at immediate risk for death or lifelong neurologic disability. The ultimate goals of management should be safety of the mother first and then delivery of a live newborn in optimal condition. Delivery is the only effective treatment. With prompt and effective management and in the absence of cerebrovascular hemorrhage, maternal prognosis is good. Fetal prognosis depends largely on gestational age at delivery.

Additional Reading

Chesley LC, Annitto JE, Cosgrove RA. The remote prognosis of eclamptic women. Am J Obstet Gynecol 1976;124: 446–459.

Douglas KA, Redman CWG. Eclampsia in the United Kingdom. BMJ 1994;309:1395–1400.

Eclampsia Trial Collaborative Group. Which anticonvulsant for women with eclampsia? Evidence from the Collaborative Eclampsia Trial. Lancet 1995;345:1455–1463.

Lamy C, Sharshar T, Mas J-L. Prognosis of cerebrovascular pathology associated with pregnancy and the postpartum period. Rev Neurol (Paris) 1996;152:422–440.

López-Llera M. Main clinical types and subtypes of eclampsia. Am J Obstet Gynecol 1992;166:4–9.

Lucas MJ, Leveno KJ, Cunningham FG. A comparison of magnesium sulphate with phenytoin for the prevention of eclampsia. N Engl J Med 1995;333:201–205.

Pritchard JA, Cunningham FG, Pritchard SA. The Parkland Memorial Hospital protocol for treatment of eclampsia: evaluation of 245 cases. Am J Obstet Gynecol 1984; 148:951–963.

Sibai BM, el-Nazer A, Gonzalez-Ruiz A. Severe preeclampsia-eclampsia in young primigravid women: subsequent pregnancy outcome and remote prognosis. Am J Obstet Gynecol 1986;155:1011–1016.

Sibai BM, Sarinoglu C, Mercer BM. Eclampsia: VII. Pregnancy outcome after eclampsia and long-term prognosis. Am J Obstet Gynecol 1992;166:1757–1761.

Sibai BM, Spinnato JA, Watson DL, et al. Eclampsia: IV. Neurologic findings and future outcome. Am J Obstet Gynecol 1985;152:184–192.

Sibai BM. Eclampsia: VI. Maternal-perinatal outcome in 254 consecutive cases. Am J Obstet Gynecol 1990;163: 1049–1054.

Part III

Vascular Disease

Chapter 14

Carotid Stenosis and Transient Ischemic Attacks

Janet L. Wilterdink

Identification of a patient with a transient ischemic attack (TIA) or carotid stenosis identifies an individual at significant risk for subsequent stroke and provides an opportunity for intervention that may prevent a potentially devastating cerebral infarction in the future. TIAs have been defined as a temporary focal neurologic deficit due to focal cerebral ischemia. Though the established duration has traditionally been defined as 24 hours or less, most agree this is excessive; most TIAs are brief, lasting minutes; longer events are likely minor cerebral infarctions. Stenosis of the carotid artery occurs in patients with traditional atherosclerosis risk factors and provides a substrate for embolism to the cerebral circulation.

Natural History

As is true for stroke in general, the pathophysiology of TIAs is diverse. Expectedly, different etiologies carry different prognoses for subsequent stroke, and so studies that lump together TIAs from all causes are not very helpful. In the aggregate, however, the risk of stroke after TIA is in the range of 35% over the next 5 years, or 5 to 6% annually. The risk of stroke after TIA is intermediate between that of transient retinal ischemia, which carries a 2 to 3% annual stroke risk, and cerebral infarction, which carries a 6 to 10% annual recurrent stroke risk.

Carotid stenosis is an important risk factor for stroke, causing between 40 and 60% of infarctions within the internal carotid artery distribution. The randomized controlled clinical trials of carotid endarterectomy for carotid stenosis have demonstrated a 32.3% 2-year risk of stroke and death for patients with symptomatic high-grade stenosis and a 31.9% 5-year risk of stroke and death for patients with asymptomatic high-grade stenosis.

Factors Affecting Prognosis

Careful studies of prognostic factors in TIA patients are lacking. In a study of TIA patients in which cause was not specified, male gender, a history of hypertension, and age older than 60 carried an unfavorable prognosis for subsequent survival but not for cerebral infarction. A history of cardiac disease or peripheral arterial disease also increased the risk of future mortality.

As alluded to in the preceding section, defining the underlying pathogenesis of TIA is helpful in defining prognosis as well as treatment. Cardiac conditions that may lead to embolism, TIA, and stroke are diverse (Table 14-1) and probably carry different prognoses for subsequent stroke. For example, patients with stroke associated with a patent foramen ovale have a low rate of stroke recurrence (1.9% annually), whereas patients with TIA or stroke and nonvalvular atrial fibrillation have a higher (17%) annual rate of recurrence. Assessing the risk of stroke after TIA in patients with other cardiac conditions is limited, as most patients are treated primarily (i.e., before their TIA) with anticoagulants, and virtually all are treated after their TIA.

Table 14-1. Cardiac Conditions Causing Embolism, Transient Ischemic Attack, and Stroke

Major risk
  Nonvalvular atrial fibrillation
  Acute myocardial infarction
  Ventricular aneurysm
  Cardiomyopathy
  Rheumatic heart disease
  Prosthetic valvular disease
  Intracardiac thrombus
  Atrial myxoma
Minor or unclear risk
  Mitral valve prolapse
  Annular or valvular calcifications
  Aortic plaque
  Spontaneous echo contrast
  Patent foramen ovale
  Atrial septal aneurysm

The Warfarin-Aspirin Symptomatic Intracranial Disease Study demonstrated that intracranial arterial stenosis, most common in the carotid siphon, middle cerebral artery main stem, and vertebral and basilar arteries, carries a high stroke risk—10.4 per 100 patient-years. TIAs are a less common manifestation of small-artery occlusive (lacunar) disease. This may imply a less favorable prognosis for subsequent stroke than is associated with other TIA etiologies, but data are lacking. Whereas TIAs attributed to occlusive vertebrobasilar disease often are believed to herald impending infarction, precise data on the prognosis of TIAs attributed to this cause are lacking. Though they did not specify etiology, Muuronen and Kaste found similar stroke rates in patients with vertebrobasilar ischemic symptoms and in those with carotid ischemic symptoms.

Prognosis after TIAs attributed to carotid stenosis was better defined by the symptomatic carotid stenosis surgery trials. The North American Symptomatic Carotid Endarterectomy Trial (NASCET) demonstrated that TIAs associated with high-grade (>70%) carotid stenosis (i.e., symptomatic carotid stenosis) carry a very high risk of subsequent ipsilateral stroke—26% over the next 2 years. Whereas carotid stenosis also carries a higher risk of stroke in asymptomatic individuals, the risk is substantially lower than in symptomatic patients; the Asymptomatic Carotid

Artery Study (ACAS) demonstrated an 11% 5-year risk of subsequent ipsilateral stroke.

Subgroup analysis in the surgical trials demonstrated other factors that influence prognosis in patients with carotid stenosis. In NASCET, single events carried a less severe prognosis—19% 2-year risk of ipsilateral stroke, as compared to a 41% 2-year risk after recurrent events. NASCET also identified nine risk factors: age older than 70 years, male gender, systolic blood pressure in excess of 160, diastolic blood pressure in excess of 90, carotid stenosis greater than 80%, prior history of stroke, recent symptoms (within preceding 31 days), plaque ulceration, and a history of any one traditional atherosclerosis risk factor. The presence of seven or more of these risk factors in patients with symptomatic high-grade stenosis carried a higher risk of ipsilateral stroke—39% over 2 years, as compared to 17% in patients who had five or fewer of these risk factors. ACAS, but not NASCET, suggested that women with carotid stenosis carried a lower 5-year risk of stroke (8.7%) as compared with men (12.1%).

Evaluation for Prognosis

Perhaps the major imperative in the evaluation of a patient with TIA is to define the presence or absence of significant carotid disease. Three modalities are currently in wide use for carotid imaging: cerebral angiography, carotid duplex ultrasonography (CDUS), and magnetic resonance angiography (MRA). Cerebral angiography remains the gold standard, because it alone has been correlated to prognosis and benefit from carotid endarterectomy in clinical trials. However, it is invasive, expensive, and risky (approximately 1% risk of stroke and death). Therefore, most patients undergo MRA or CDUS as a screening procedure before angiography. Studies indicate that these two modalities have a similar sensitivity (73 to 100%) and specificity (76 to 92%) for predicting angiographic stenosis. Other investigators are studying the use of combined MRA and CDUS without angiography in evaluating patients for potential high-grade carotid stenosis. Patel and coworkers found that combined MRA and CDUS studies, when concordant, had sufficient sensitivity and specificity (100% and 91%, respectively) as to make angiography unnecessary. Though this conclusion remains controversial, future analyses of this type will be important in improving the safety of evaluating patients for carotid stenosis and for their overall prognosis.

Whereas carotid imaging is performed primarily to identify carotid disease amenable to surgery (i.e., >70% stenosis), other features may further define prognosis for future stroke. NASCET demonstrated that even among patients with high-grade stenosis, the precise degree of stenosis is important, with ipsilateral 2-year stroke rates of 20% for 70 to 79% stenosis, 28% for 80 to 89% stenosis, and 35% for 90 to 99% stenosis. The presence of intraluminal thrombus, plaque ulceration, or contralateral or tandem artery disease on imaging studies has been found by some investigators to be associated with higher risks of stroke.

Echocardiography is used to identify structural cardioembolic disease in patients with TIA (see Table 14-1). An important caveat is that the prevalence of echocardiographic abnormalities increases significantly if cardiac disease is clinically suspected by history, examination, or electrocardiogram. In TIA patients with no evidence of cardiac disease, the prevalence of major echocardiographic abnormalities is very low (<10%). Transesophageal echocardiography increases by as much as 30% the identification of potential cardioembolic disease over transthoracic echocardiography but does so primarily for minor abnormalities for which the precise risk of stroke or appropriate therapy is not defined.

Patients with TIA frequently undergo computed tomography (CT). A small percentage of TIA patients with normal examinations and nonpersistent symptoms will have CT evidence of infarction. Studies suggest that such patients may be at higher risk for future stroke and death than are those with normal CT scans. The presence of ischemic lesions in patients with apparently asymptomatic carotid disease also might imply a higher-risk patient.

Therapies Affecting Prognosis

Atherosclerosis risk factor management is very important in reducing stroke risk in patients with TIA and carotid stenosis. This has been most convincingly demonstrated for hypertension and smoking. Hypertension is the single most impor-

tant treatable risk factor for stroke, with a population attributable fraction (an estimate of the percentage of excess stroke attributable to hypertension) of 60%. Meta-analysis of treatment trials of blood pressure reduction demonstrated a reduction in stroke incidence: An average blood pressure reduction of 5.8 mm Hg produced a reduction in stroke incidence of 42% over a 2- to 5-year follow-up period. Aggressive treatment of hypertension has been credited with the observed decline of stroke incidence and mortality since the 1970s. Cigarette smoking is associated with an approximately 50% increased risk for all stroke subtypes and has a strong dose-response relationship for ischemic stroke. Smoking cessation decreases stroke risk. In both the Framingham Heart Study and the Nurses' Health Study, the risk of stroke in former cigarette smokers dropped within 1 to 2 years of smoking cessation. After 5 years, the risk of stroke was similar to that for persons who had never smoked.

Antiplatelet agents interfere with activation and aggregation of platelets on the wall of a diseased artery, an important pathophysiologic step in the development of the arterial thrombi that subsequently cause cerebral infarction. In 1994, the Antiplatelet Trialists' Collaboration published a meta-analysis of 145 randomized clinical trials, involving more than 100,000 patients, which compared antiplatelet therapy to placebo in the prevention of stroke, myocardial infarction (MI), and vascular death among high-risk patients. The vast majority of these patients were treated with aspirin. Among the 10,000 cerebrovascular patients included in this study, antiplatelet therapy had similar efficacy in secondary stroke prevention and prevention of MI and vascular death, with a composite risk reduction of 22%. Different genders and age groups and those patients with and without diabetes or hypertension benefited equally from antiplatelet therapy.

The efficacy of ticlopidine (a newer antiplatelet agent) in cerebrovascular disease has been studied in two trials. The Canadian American Ticlopidine Study found a substantial reduction in stroke, MI, and vascular death in patients treated with ticlopidine as compared with placebo, with an overall relative risk reduction of 30%. The Ticlopidine Aspirin Stroke Study found, in patients with recent TIA or mild stroke, a relative risk reduction in stroke of 21% for ticlopidine as compared with placebo. This small improvement in risk is offset by potentially life-threatening complications of ticlopidine, including neutropenia, which occurs in fewer than 3% of patients and reaches serious levels in fewer than 1%. Ticlopidine is reserved as a second-line agent for most patients with TIA, being reserved for those who fail on aspirin treatment or who cannot take aspirin.

Warfarin therapy is reserved mainly for primary and secondary prevention of stroke from cardioembolic disease, the most common cause of which is nonvalvular atrial fibrillation. Most studies that have demonstrated a benefit for warfarin in this setting have focused on primary prevention. The European Atrial Fibrillation Trial, however, studied patients with TIA and minor stroke in the setting of nonvalvular atrial fibrillation. The trial study group demonstrated a benefit of anticoagulation over aspirin, with a reduction in the incidence of stroke from 12 to 4% annually. Anticoagulation is used also for patients with TIA who are found to have other major risk factors for cardioembolic disease (see Table 14-1). The relative benefit of warfarin versus aspirin for minor cardiac abnormalities is undefined.

The Warfarin-Aspirin Symptomatic Intracranial Disease Study suggested that warfarin might also be the treatment of choice for secondary prevention of stroke due to intracranial atherosclerosis, with a relative risk reduction over aspirin of 0.46. The use of warfarin versus aspirin in the prevention of atherothrombotic stroke is currently being investigated.

Carotid endarterectomy improved outcome in several well-performed, randomized, controlled clinical trials of patients with high-grade carotid stenosis. The benefit from surgery, however, is substantially different in patients with symptomatic versus asymptomatic disease. NASCET demonstrated a reduction from 26 to 9% in the 2-year ipsilateral stroke rate in patients with symptomatic carotid stenosis of more than 70%, which is an absolute risk reduction of 17% and a relative risk reduction of 65%. In contrast, ACAS demonstrated a smaller, though still significant, effect on future stroke risk, reducing the 5-year ipsilateral stroke rate from 11 to 5.1%, which is an absolute risk reduction of 5.9% and a relative risk reduction of 55%. NASCET continues analysis of surgical therapy for symptomatic patients

with 30 to 69% stenosis, despite the fact that the European Carotid Surgery Trial has demonstrated no benefit from surgery, as regards future stroke risk, in patients with less than 70% symptomatic stenosis.

Short-Term Prognosis

The risk of stroke after TIA is highest in the weeks and months immediately following the event and then decreases with time. With appropriate evaluation and treatment, however, the short-term risk of future stroke in patients with TIA or carotid stenosis can be very favorable.

Long-Term Prognosis

An underappreciated fact is that patients with cerebrovascular disease, particularly those with carotid stenosis, have a high incidence of cardiovascular disease. In fact, patients with carotid disease are more likely to die of cardiac causes than from cerebrovascular disease. In ACAS, 50% of deaths at 5 years were attributable to cardiovascular disease, as compared with 11% of all deaths from cerebrovascular disease. Further study of cardiovascular evaluation and treatment of patients with cerebrovascular disease is needed.

Additional Reading

Antiplatelet Trialists' Collaboration. Collaborative overview of randomized trials of antiplatelet therapy: I. Prevention of death, myocardial infarction, and stroke by prolonged antiplatelet therapy in various categories of patients. BMJ 1994;308:81–106.

Chimowitz, MI, Kokkinos J, Strong J, et al. The Warfarin-Aspirin Symptomatic Intracranial Disease Study. Neurology 1995;45:1488–1493.

Collins R, Peto R, MacMahon S, et al. Blood pressure, stroke, and coronary heart disease: 2. Short-term reductions in blood pressure: overview of randomized drug trials in their epidemiological context. Lancet 1990;335:827–838.

Easton JD, Wilterdink JL. Carotid endarterectomy: trials and tribulations. Ann Neurol 1994;35:5–17.

European Atrial Fibrillation Trial Study Group. Secondary prevention in non-rheumatic atrial fibrillation after transient ischaemic attack or minor stroke. Lancet 1993;342:1255–1262.

Executive Committee for the Asymptomatic Carotid Athero-sclerosis Study. Endarterectomy for asymptomatic carotid artery stenosis. JAMA 1995;273:1328–1331

Hass WK, Easton JD, Adams HP, et al. A randomized trial comparing ticlopidine hydrochloride with aspirin for the prevention of stroke in high-risk patients. N Engl J Med 1989;321:501–507.

Kawachi I, Colditz GA, Stampfer MJ, et al. Smoking cessa-tion and decreased risk of stroke in women. JAMA 1993;269:232–236.

Muuronen A, Kaste M. Outcome of 314 patients with tran-sient ischemic attacks. Stroke 1982;13:24–31.

Patel MR, Kuntz KM, Klufas RA, et al. Preoperative assess-ment of the carotid bifurcation: can magnetic resonance angiography and duplex ultrasonography replace contrast arteriography? Stroke 1995;26:1753.

Chapter 15

Cervicocerebral Arterial Dissections

Jeffrey L. Saver and Parissa Jannati

Cervicocerebral arterial dissections are an important cause of ischemic stroke. Dissections account for 1 to 2% of all cerebral infarcts and as many as one-fifth of those in the age group 30 and younger. In a population-based study among adults, the average annual incidence of extracranial internal carotid artery (ICA) dissections was 3.5 per 100,000. Dissection may occur in any cervicocerebral vessel, but the cervical vasculature is most susceptible. Extracranial ICA dissections account for 66% of reported cases, extracranial vertebral artery dissections for 18%, intracranial internal carotid and middle cerebral artery dissections for 6%, intracranial vertebral artery dissections for 5%, and basilar artery dissections for 4%.

The most common presentation is unilateral neck pain, face pain, and headache accompanied by focal cerebral ischemic symptoms. In cervical ICA dissections, an ipsilateral Horner's syndrome often is present, as the expanding wall compresses sympathetic fibers running on the external surface of the artery. Tinnitus, subjective pulsatile bruit, and ocular or lower cranial nerve palsies are less common accompanying features.

A history of minor trauma or intense physical activity precedes "spontaneous" cervicocerebral dissections in 20 to 25% of reported cases, demonstrating that arterial tears are occasioned by a continuous spectrum of predisposing mechanical insults and cannot be divided strictly into categories of *spontaneous* and *traumatic*. However, overtly traumatic dissections caused by major blunt or penetrating injury do have a distinctive natural history,

strongly influenced by the nature and extent of the overall traumatic insult. This chapter focuses on spontaneous cervicocerebral dissections, defined as those incurred during normal daily activities or related to only minimal preceding stress or trauma. In spontaneous dissections, underlying arteriopathies are not infrequent and include fibromuscular dysplasia in 15% of cases in addition to Ehlers-Danlos syndrome, Marfan syndrome, and cystic medial necrosis. Most dissections, however, occur in apparently healthy arteries in apparently healthy individuals.

Natural History

The true natural history of cervicocerebral dissections is unknown, as no large reported case series has avoided antiplatelet or anticoagulant therapy. Conversely, however, no controlled clinical trial has ever demonstrated that antithrombotic therapy alters the natural history in any way. As the impact (if any) of antiplatelet and anticoagulant agents on the course likely is small, outcomes observed in series of patients treated with diverse medical therapies likely approximate the disease's true natural history. These observations have changed dramatically since 1975. Early case series were dominated by cases from autopsies and suggested a grave, frequently fatal, prognosis. Subsequently, advances in noninvasive imaging, including cervical and transcranial ultrasonography, computed tomography (CT), magnetic resonance imaging (MRI), and magnetic resonance angiography (MRA), have permitted identification of ever more mildly affected patients. Some case series provide a decidedly more roseate and accurate picture of the course of cervicocerebral dissections.

In clinical settings, six questions regarding the prognosis commonly demand attention:

1. Will the patient presenting with only pain or other local symptoms develop cerebral ischemia?
2. Will the patient with an initial transient ischemic attack (TIA) or stroke develop early infarct progression or recurrence?
3. What is the likelihood and timing of radiologic vessel recanalization?
4. What is the long-term risk of stroke recurrence in a patient with an initial stroke?
5. What is the risk of recurrent dissection?
6. What is the long-term functional outcome?

This chapter addresses these questions in detail for the most common variety of cervicocerebral arterial dissections, dissections of the cervical ICA and cervical vertebral artery, for which a robust database exists. Dissections at other locations are considered briefly in Factors Affecting Prognosis.

Among patients with identifiable minor precipitating trauma, the interval between the minor injury and local or cerebral ischemic symptoms tends to be brief. In one series, time from trauma to first symptom ranged from 0 to 15 days, with a mean of 2.3 days, and the time from trauma to TIA or completed stroke ranged from 0 to 31 days, with a mean of 4.8 days.

The Patient with Only Local Symptoms

Some one-fourth of cervical ICA patients present with local complaints alone and three-fourths with TIA or cerebral infarction. The largest study examining development of ischemia among patients with inaugural local symptoms reported on 53 patients with initial isolated head or neck pain, Horner's syndrome, or tinnitus. Subsequently, no cerebral ischemic events developed in 26% of the patients, TIAs only appeared in 30%, TIAs followed by cerebral infarction occurred in 13%, and cerebral infarction without preceding TIA transpired in 30%. Most ischemic events occurred within the first week of local symptoms. The mean time to first TIA was 10.5 days. The mean time to cerebral infarction after inaugural local signs or TIA was 6 days, with a range from a few minutes to 31 days. More than 80% of completed strokes occurred in the first 7 days.

Early Worsening: The Patient with Transient Ischemic Attack or Infarction

Data on early stroke progression or recurrence are surprisingly scarce. In the foregoing series, cervical ICA dissection patients with TIAs developed completed cerebral infarctions in 30% of cases, a mean of 4 days after the TIA. In contrast, our clinical impression is that among patients presenting with cerebral infarction, stroke progression, or early recurrence (recurrence within 2 weeks of first stroke) is uncommon, likely occurring in less than 15% of cases.

Likelihood and Timing of Radiologic Recanalization

Vessels stenosed by a dissection show a remarkable propensity to spontaneous improvement in lumen caliber, without surgical intervention or stenting. Approximately 85% of stenoses improve or return to normal at follow-up angiography. Similarly, dissections are one of the few causes of complete angiographic ICA occlusion that permit spontaneous recanalization. Recanalization occurs in approximately 50% of occlusions. Serial ultrasonographic studies demonstrate that the median time to resolution of vessel narrowing is 6 to 7 weeks, most arteries recover by 3 months, and vessels that fail to reconstitute a normal lumen by 6 months are highly unlikely to improve thereafter.

Pseudoaneurysm formation is uncommon in cervical ICA dissection, affecting less than 6% of patients in a multicenter European study. Across all series reporting follow-up angiography, aneurysms resolve or improve spontaneously, without surgical intervention, in approximately 45% of cases.

Late Stroke Recurrence

Late infarcts—those occurring more than 2 weeks after diagnosis of dissection—are infrequent in cervical artery dissection. Among more than 500 reported cases of extracranial carotid or vertebral dissection with extended follow-up (mean, 3.4 years), fewer than 1.6% experienced late cerebral infarction. This finding yields a crude annualized stroke risk of 0.5%, but most infarcts actually occurred in the first year after dissection. The rate is likely higher for patients with persisting ICA occlusion than for those with recanalization.

Late Dissection Recurrence

The risk of recurrent dissection in the initially dissected artery is low; the risk of subsequent dissection in another cervicocerebral vessel is slightly higher. In a Mayo clinic series of 200 patients with cervical internal carotid or vertebral artery dissections, the recurrence rate was 2% in the first month and 1% per year thereafter over 7 years of follow-up. In a collaborative European study of 105 patients, the rate of recurrent dissection also approximated 1% per year over 10 years. Across all large, long-term series, second cervicocerebral dissections occurred in 5% of 303 patients with initial ICA dissections and in 6% of 114 patients with initial vertebral artery dissections. The mean time to recurrence was 4.1 years, with a range of 2 days to 8.6 years. Factors predisposing to recurrent dissection were underlying frank arteriopathy, either Ehlers-Danlos syndrome or fibromuscular dysplasia, and positive family history of dissection.

Long-Term Functional Outcome

In those patients who have experienced a cerebral infarct, the severity of the stroke is the major determinant of outcome in patients with cervical arterial dissection. Reflecting their generally younger age, dissection patients tend to show greater functional recovery from acute neurologic deficits than do most older patients with cerebral infarcts. At 3 months after onset among patients with cervical ICA dissection, 50% are neurologically normal, 21% have mild residual deficits, 25% have moderate to severe persisting deficits, and 4% have died. Among patients with cervical vertebral artery dissection, 83% are neurologically normal or have only mild deficits, 11% have moderate to severe deficits, and 6% have died.

Factors Affecting Prognosis

The site of the affected vessel strongly influences prognosis. In contrast to extracranial dissections, the course of intracranial dissections generally is more severe. Intracranial carotid system dissections typically affect the terminal ICA or middle cerebral artery. Major stroke is the rule, often progressing over several days. Seizures or syncope can be the initial symptom, and one-half of patients have early alteration of consciousness. Subarachnoid hemorrhage occurs in one-fifth of cases. Among 59 reported cases, fatal outcome was observed in 72%, and moderate to severe neurologic deficits were present in 50% of the survivors. However, specific, noninvasive imaging and angiographic features for identifying intracranial internal carotid system dissections are lacking. The resulting reliance on pathologic findings for diagnosis likely results in underrecognition of nonfatal cases and overestimation of the gravity of the prognosis.

Intracranial vertebral artery dissections are distinguished by a high frequency of subarachnoid hemorrhage (SAH). SAH is the presenting feature in more than one-half of cases; brain stem, cerebellar, or hemispheric infarction in one-third; and both SAH and infarction in one-tenth. More rarely, dissenting aneurysms acting as mass lesions produce cranial nerve or brain stem compression. In patients presenting with SAH, rebleeding occurs in one-fourth if endovascular or surgical intervention is not undertaken.

The typical course of basilar dissection is abrupt onset of severe brain stem ischemia leading rapidly to coma. Death was the outcome in more than 60% of reported cases.

Multivessel dissections are more likely to produce severe ischemic deficits than are single-vessel dissections. Some 15% of all cervical ICA dissections are bilateral, and at least one-half of these occur in patients with fibromuscular dysplasia.

Patients with underlying arteriopathies appear to have increased risk of recurrent dissection. Vasculopathies associated with cervicocerebral dissection include fibromuscular dysplasia, Marfan syndrome, Ehlers-Danlos syndrome type IV, polycystic kidney disease, pseudoxanthoma elasticum, osteogenesis imperfecta, alpha$_1$-antitrypsin deficiency, migraine, and cystic medial necrosis. Family history of cervicocerebral, aortic, or renal dissection is also a risk factor for dissection recurrence. Second dissection appeared in 50% of the 10 patients with familial disease in a Mayo series.

Evaluation for Prognosis

Standard physical examination, brain imaging, and vessel imaging provide a wealth of prognostic information. Among patients with completed infarcts, the extent of the initial deficit plus the MRI or CT depiction of infarct site and volume allow estimation of the potential for long-term functional recovery.

MRA and conventional angiography allow assessment of degree of vessel compromise. The greater the vessel narrowing, the more likely cerebral ischemia will develop. In one study, 35% of patients with mild-to-moderate cervical ICA stenosis developed TIA or infarct versus 89% of patients with near-occlusion or occlusion.

In occasional patients, measurement of cerebrovascular reserve with acetazolamide (Diamox)-single photon emission computed tomography, acetazolamide-xenon CT scan, or CO_2 or acetazolamide transcranial Doppler studies may aid in determining the risk of hemodynamic ischemia. Similarly, preliminary reports suggest that transcranial Doppler embolus detection studies may help in judging risk of symptomatic artery-to-artery embolization.

Follow-up MRA or conventional angiographic imaging 3 months after onset is useful in determining long-term prognosis. Patients with persisting occlusion or severe residual stenosis are at higher risk of late ischemia.

Therapies Affecting Prognosis

No prospective, randomized, controlled clinical trial of any intervention for cervicocerebral dissections has been reported. Treatment is guided by current understanding of disease pathogenesis and informed opinion rather than by definitive data. For cervical arterial dissections, anticoagulation usually is undertaken for the first 3 months, to discourage distal embolization and thrombus propagation at the dissection site. Anticoagulation does not appear to increase the risk of recurrent dissection. In patients with strong contraindications to anticoagulation, antiplatelet therapy is a reasonable alternative. The first week after onset appears to be the time of greatest risk, so immediate anticoagulation with unfractionated heparin or a low-molecular-weight heparin followed by warfarin is advocated in patients with small infarcts or no infarcts and after a 5- to 9-day delay in large infarcts.

The role of thrombolytic therapy in dissection patients presenting within 3 hours of onset of ischemic symptoms is undefined. The theoretic risks of provoking extension of the dissecting hemorrhage—or SAH if the dissection already has an intracranial component—argues for extreme caution in use of systemic thrombolytics. Intra-arterial thrombolysis through selective catheterization directly onto a distal thrombus beyond the dissection site may have a lower risk of dissection exacerbation while affording beneficial reperfusion.

Long-term therapy is guided by 3-month vessel imaging. If the vessel has recanalized with only minimal luminal irregularities or if a smooth occlusion persists, anticoagulation is discontinued, and antiplatelet therapy is begun. If severe luminal stenosis and irregularity persist, anticoagulation is continued, and imaging is repeated at 6 months. When 3-month imaging demonstrates a dissecting aneurysm, anticoagulation is continued, and serial imaging is pursued. Surgery or endovascular aneurysm therapy is reserved for those patients with further ischemia despite medical therapy or progressive cranial nerve compression.

Short-Term Prognosis

The first 2 weeks (and especially the first few days) after onset of a cervicocerebral dissection are the period of greatest risk. Often, the diagnosis is overlooked until cerebral ischemia develops but, if infarction can be prevented or minimized in this epoch, the course generally will be benign.

Long-Term Prognosis

Late strokes after cervicocerebral dissection are remarkably uncommon. Perhaps 10% of patients will have a second cervicocerebral dissection over the next 10 years, more frequently in patients with identifiable underlying arteriopathies or familial disease. The eventual functional outcome is good to excellent in 70% of cervical ICA and in 80% of cervical vertebral artery dissections.

Additional Reading

Bassetti C, Bogousslavsky J, Eskenasy-Cottier AC, et al. Spontaneous intracranial dissection in the anterior circulation. Cerebrovasc Dis 1994;4:170–174.

Bassetti C, Carruzzo A, Sturzenegger M, Tuncdogan E. Recurrence of cervical artery dissection: a prospective study of 81 patients. Stroke 1996;27:1804–1807.

Biousse V, D'Anglejan-Chatillon J, Touboul P-J, et al. Time course of symptoms in extracranial carotid artery dissections. Stroke 1995;26:235–239.

Desfontaines P, Despland P-A. Dissection of the internal carotid artery: aetiology, symptomatology, clinical and neurosonological follow-up, and treatment in 60 consecutive cases. Acta Neurol Belg 1995;95:226–234.

Leys D, Moulin T, Stojkovic T, et al. Follow-up of patients with history of cervical artery dissection. Cerebrovasc Dis 1995;5:43–49.

Saver JL, Easton JD. Dissections and Trauma of Cervicocerebral Arteries. In HJM Barnett, JP Mohr, BM Stein, FM Yatsu (eds), Stroke: Pathophysiology, Diagnosis, and Management (3rd ed). New York: Saunders (in press).

Schievink WI, Mokri B, O'Fallon WM. Recurrent spontaneous cervical-artery dissection. N Engl J Med 1994;330: 393–397.

Schievink WI, Mokri B, Piepgras DG, Kuiper JD. Recurrent spontaneous arterial dissections: risk in familial versus nonfamilial disease. Stroke 1996;27:622–624.

Steinke W, Rautenberg W, Schwartz A, Hennerici M. Noninvasive monitoring of internal carotid artery dissection. Stroke 1994;25:998–1005.

Sturzenegger M, Mattle HP, Rivoir A, Baumgartner RW. Ultrasound findings in carotid dissection: analysis of 43 patients. Neurology 1995;45:691–698.

Chapter 16

Brain Infarction

Karen L. Furie and Marc H. Friedberg

Natural History

Ischemic stroke is the third leading cause of death in the United States and a major cause of disability in millions of Americans. The majority of ischemic strokes are embolic, either cardioembolic or due to cryptogenic (unknown source) emboli. Cryptogenic strokes may be due to an unidentified cardiac source or, on the basis of recent reports, aortic atheromas of more than 4 mm. Atherothrombotic disease of the extracranial carotid arteries and vertebrobasilar system is associated with established vascular risk factors: hypertension, diabetes mellitus, smoking, and hypercholesterolemia. Lacunar strokes are believed to be due primarily to lipohyalinosis of the small perforating vessels; however, they can be caused by small emboli. Other factors, such as alcohol consumption, diet, inborn errors of metabolism, and clotting disorders, also contribute to stroke in the general population. The genetic basis of cerebrovascular disease has become a major focus of basic and clinical research, and considerably more knowledge of genetic determinants of stroke risk should be known in the near future. Currently, though certain polymorphisms appear to predispose to stroke, environmental factors seem more important in precipitating clinical events.

Primary and secondary stroke prevention requires the identification of a stroke risk or mechanism and the initiation of proper therapy. Atherosclerotic disease, both intra- and extracranial, should be managed with modification of vascular risk factors. Clinical trials have shown a benefit to carotid endarterectomy in patients with high-grade symptomatic (>70%) or asymptomatic (>60%) carotid stenosis. Ongoing studies are assessing the use of angioplasty and stenting in these populations. Several trials have demonstrated the efficacy of warfarin in reducing the stroke risk in patients with atrial fibrillation. However, for the majority of strokes as yet no clearly superior medical therapy is available. Another ongoing study seeks to assess warfarin and aspirin in reducing the risk of recurrent stroke. Although other antiplatelet agents (ticlopidine, clopidogrel, dipyridamole [Persantine]) have been shown to be beneficial in preventing stroke, they have not supplanted aspirin as the mainstay of preventive therapy.

Factors Affecting Prognosis

Recovery

Large hemispheric infarcts carry a poorer prognosis than do smaller, deep infarcts. They are more likely to develop hemorrhagic transformation, but that condition rarely serves as an independent predictor of poor outcome. The location of an initial stroke can affect functional outcome. Unexpectedly, lesions of the basal ganglia alone seem to have a poorer prognosis than do those isolated to the cerebral cortex or those involving both the cortex and basal ganglia.

Of the lacunar syndromes, patients with pure motor hemiparesis and sensorimotor deficits have a worse functional outcome than do patients with ataxic hemiparesis or a pure sensory deficit. In one study of functional outcome in patients with lacunar stroke, 24% were dependent for activities of daily living at 3 years.

In a population of stroke rehabilitation patients, predictors for returning to independence after a stroke include symptoms of less than 60 days' duration before beginning rehabilitation therapy; living independently or being employed before the stroke; and a higher functional independence measure at the time of admission.

Mortality

Thirty-day case fatality rates as high as 20% have been reported after an ischemic stroke, although these findings vary significantly on the basis of age, gender, and nationality. Stroke patients have a higher mortality rate than do their age-matched stroke-free peers, mainly as a result of cardiac disease. After a first stroke, those surviving the first 30 days will have survival rates of 87, 79, 73, and 72% at 1, 2, 3, and 4 years, respectively. Factors associated with higher mortality include older age, a history of myocardial infarction, the number of stroke deficits, cardiac arrhythmia, and diabetes mellitus.

Lacunar disease carries a 4-year survival rate of approximately 80% and a recurrent stroke rate of 85%. Higher mortality is associated with diabetes, the degree of neurologic dysfunction and functional disability at 7 days, cigarette smoking, and age. Dementia is an independent predictor of long-term survival, with demented patients more likely to die from recurrent stroke.

Recurrence

The rate of recurrent stroke is highest in the period immediately after a stroke. National Institute of Neurological and Communicative Disorders and Stroke and Oxfordshire data indicated a 3.3% rate of recurrent stroke in the first month and 1- and 5-year cumulative incidence rates of 6 to 14% and 20 to 37%, respectively. The Copenhagen Stroke Study evaluated patients who presented with an acute stroke; 23% of these patients had experienced a previous stroke. Recurrence was associated with male gender, hypertension, atrial fibrillation, and a history of transient ischemic attack. Mortality was significantly higher in patients with recurrent stroke. Stroke severity, measured by functional status, was worse in patients whose recurrent stroke was contralateral to the initial infarct.

Recurrent stroke risk varies on the basis of the mechanism of stroke. For patients with atrial fibrillation, the rate of untreated stroke is approximately 15% per year. High-grade carotid stenosis conveys an 18% risk of stroke after 1 year, even with best medical therapy.

Evaluation for Prognosis

One study compared three stroke rating scales: the National Institutes of Health Stroke Scale (NIHSS), the Canadian Neurological Scale, and the Middle Cerebral Artery Neurological Score. The NIHSS provided the best prognostic information, with sensitivity to poor outcome of 71% and specificity of 90%. In predicting the 3-month outcome, the NIHSS, using a cut-point of 13, added significantly to the predictive value of all other scores, though no other score added useful information to the NIHSS.

Radiologic assessment of ischemic strokes may help to predict outcome. Infarct volumes on magnetic resonance imaging T2-weighted images of middle cerebral artery territory strokes of less than 80 cc correlated with a better 30-day outcome, according to the Scandinavian Stroke Scale.

Therapies Affecting Prognosis

Acute stroke therapies may impact on short- and long-term outcome. The use of intravenous tissue plasminogen activator within 3 hours of an acute stroke was associated with improved function at 90 days, using the NIHSS, Barthel index, modified ranking scale, and Glasgow Outcome Scale. A criticism of this study, however, was that it was not empowered to look at outcome differences based on stroke subtypes. In addition, 6% of the patients who received tissue plasminogen activator experienced a symptomatic intracerebral hemorrhage, almost half of them fatal.

Medical therapy also may reduce the risk of death or recurrent stroke. In the primary prevention of stroke in patients with atrial fibrillation, warfarin reduces the risk of recurrent stroke by approximately 70% as contrasted to 36% with aspirin. Using end points of stroke, systemic embolism, or death, the risk reductions are 48% for sodium warfarin (Coumadin) and 28% for aspirin. For noncardioembolic strokes, aspirin reduces the risk of stroke by approximately 20%. Ticlopidine may provide a marginal advantage over aspirin for reduction of stroke risk, but that advantage must be weighed against the higher risks (particularly neutropenia) associated with its use.

Stroke recovery may be enhanced by such new neuroprotective agents as lubeluzole, fosphenytoin, and citicoline, all of which currently are under investigation. Fibroblast growth factor is being studied as a therapy in acute stroke on the basis of its ability to facilitate prolonged cell survival and postischemic recovery.

Hyperthermia in the first 7 days after a stroke has been shown to be an independent predictor of poor outcome. Not clear is whether the fever source may be a key feature in determining the causal link with the observed increase in mortality. Hypothermia has been demonstrated to reduce neuronal damage in animals, but inducing it clinically in humans as a safe method of reducing ischemic injury has been difficult.

Patients in stroke rehabilitation units, as compared to general medical wards, have a shorter length of stay and improved functional outcome as measured by the Barthel index. Ninety-five percent of patients reach maximal recovery within 12 weeks of their stroke. Younger patients (younger than 75) have shorter lengths of stay and better Barthel scores at discharge. On average, neurologic recovery precedes functional improvement by 2 weeks. No improvement is reported, even in those with very severe strokes, after 5 months. Medications that may retard recovery after stroke include sedative-hypnotics, phenothiazines, and anticonvulsants.

Quality of life analyses have found that stroke survivors enjoy a quality of life similar to others in the community. Depression, which has a prevalence of 16 to 30%, has been a major determinant of quality of life after stroke in several studies. Identification and treatment of depression can significantly improve the mood and function of stroke survivors.

Short-Term Prognosis

Overall, the rate of stroke mortality has declined since the 1970s. This reduction seems to be due to increased survival rather than to a lower incidence of stroke, as the prevalence of patients with stroke has increased. Therefore, recent improvements in acute stroke management seem to have led to better short-term survival. This change cannot be attributed to any one practice or therapy. In general, fatal cardiovascular disease has decreased over the same time period, likely owing to modification of risk factors and to early identification of milder disease as a result of increased health awareness in the general population.

Long-Term Prognosis

Patients who have had an ischemic stroke have a rate of recurrent stroke or death in the first 30 days as high as 20%. Those who survive the first 30 days have a 15% risk of stroke or death in the first year. Acute medical therapies, such as intravenous tissue plasminogen activator and neuroprotective agents, may improve the functional outcome of stroke. For certain subgroups of stroke patients, such as those with atrial fibrillation or high-grade carotid stenosis, certain effective interventions can reduce the risk of recurrent stroke. For the majority of strokes, however, modification of risk factors and treatment with either an antiplatelet or antithrombotic therapy remains the standard of care.

Additional Reading

Burn J, Dennis M, Bamford J, et al. Long-term risk of recurrent stroke after first-ever stroke—Oxfordshire. Stroke 1994;25:333–337.

Jorgensen HS, Nakayama H, Raaschou HO, et al. Outcome and time course of recovery in stroke: II. Time course of recovery. The Copenhagen Stroke Study. Arch Phys Med Rehabil 1995;76:406–412.

Kalra L. The influence of stroke unit rehabilitation on functional recovery from stroke. Stroke 1994;25:821–825.

Kalra L. Does age affect benefits of stroke unit rehabilitation? Stroke 1994;25:346–351.

Lai SM, Alter M, Friday G, Sobel E. Prognosis for survival after an initial stroke. Stroke 1995;26:2011–2015.

Muir KW, Weir CJ, Murray GD, et al. Comparison of neurological scales and scoring systems for acute stroke prognosis. Stroke 1996;27:1817–1820.

Sacco RL, Ellenberg JH, Mohr JP, et al. Infarcts of undetermined cause: the NINCDS Stroke Data Bank. Ann Neurol 1989;25:382–390.

Samuelsson M, Soderfeldt B, Olsson GB. Functional outcome in patients with lacunar infarction. Stroke 1996; 27:842–846.

Saunders DE, Clifton AG, Brown MM. Measurement of infarct size using MRI predicts prognosis in middle cerebral artery infarction. Stroke 1995;26:2272–2276.

Ween JE, Alexander MP, D'Esposito M, Roberts M. Factors predictive of poor outcome in a rehabilitation setting. Neurology 1996;47:388–392.

Wilkinson PR, Wolfe CDA, Warburton FG, et al. A long-term follow-up of stroke patients. Stroke 1997;28: 507–512.

Chapter 17

Spinal Cord Infarction

William P. Cheshire and E. Wayne Massey

Spinal cord infarction is an uncommon condition resulting from interruption of the spinal cord's vascular supply. Disease in, or surgery of, the aorta is the most frequent cause of this malady, whether from atherosclerosis, dissection, aneurysm, or trauma. Other causes, similar to the differential diagnosis of cerebral infarction, include global hypoxic ischemia, arteriovenous malformation, hypercoagulability, embolism, epidural hematoma, arteritis, and decompression sickness. Rarely, spinal infarction follows trauma to radicular arteries from retroperitoneal procedures or intervertebral foraminal stenosis. Incidence is greatest among older individuals and affects men twice as often as women.

Though the level of infarction may affect any segment of the spinal cord, the majority involve the lower thoracic cord, which receives its principal blood supply from the artery of Adamkiewicz joining the anterior spinal artery variably from T5 to L2, most commonly on the left (from T9 to T12). Thoracic and cervical radicular arteries also contribute to the anterior spinal artery, which originates from the vertebral arteries and culminates in extensive anastomoses surrounding the spinal cord in conjunction with the paired posterior spinal arteries.

Intrasegmentally, the prevailing configuration of infarction is known as the *anterior spinal artery syndrome*. This condition affects the anterior two-thirds of the cord, sparing the posterior columns that receive perfusion from the posterior spinal arteries. The Brown-Séquard syndrome involves only the lateral half of the spinal cord and yields dissociated deficits of ipsilateral paralysis (with or

without ipsilateral posterior column dysfunction) and contralateral loss of pain and temperature sensibility. Posterior spinal artery and spinal venous infarction are rare and presentation is more varied. Decompression syndrome is believed to be venous infarction secondary to nitrogen bubbles.

Natural History

The clinical course of spinal cord infarction is monophasic, with abrupt onset followed by a variable degree of neurologic recovery over days to weeks. Patients present with the acute onset of flaccidity, weakness (most commonly paraplegia or paraparesis), areflexia, decreased pain and temperature sensibility below the level of the lesion, atonic urinary bladder, and paralytic ileus. Transient pain in the back or in a radicular distribution may occur at the level of the lesion.

The chronic state develops within weeks. Flaccidity and areflexia are followed by spasticity, hyperreflexia, ankle or knee clonus, and Babinski's responses. Occasionally, co-involvement of the lower motoneuron masks these upper motoneuron deficits. Prickling, burning, or constricting paresthesia or painful dysesthesia below the level of the lesion can resist therapy.

Autonomic dysfunction may be transient or permanent. The urinary bladder, atonic once acutely severed from the sympathetic nervous system, will develop detrusor hyperreflexia and sphincter dyssynergia chronically. Erectile impotency can occur. Lesions superior to the origin of the greater splanchnic nerve at T4 to T9 can cause orthostatic hypotension. Impaired vasomotor and sudomotor tone may compromise thermoregulation. Spinal dysautonomia refers to the excessive sympathetic response of tachycardia, hypertension, and diaphoresis that chronically disinhibited neurons of the intermediolateral cell column (T1 to L2) may mount in response to mildly noxious stimuli, such as bladder distension.

Factors Affecting Prognosis

Survival depends largely on the potential for the disease causing the spinal cord infarction not to lead otherwise to cardiac or peripheral vascular failure. The infarction itself indirectly influences morbidity, as paralysis places the patient at risk for decubitus ulceration and deep venous thrombosis with pulmonary embolism, and neurogenic bladder dysfunction predisposes to urinary tract infection, hydronephrosis, and urosepsis. Respiratory compromise from bilateral interruption of diaphragmatic innervation at C3 to C5 is rare in spinal cord infarction but has been seen in vertebral artery dissection.

The extent of neurologic recovery depends on the amount and distribution of neuronal loss and on determining what portion of the initial deficit is due to reversible ischemia or edema. Unlike cerebral stroke, in which adjacent neurons may be capable of assuming some lost function, the spinal cord's compact arrangement limits the possibilities of recovery through neuronal plasticity.

Chronic pain and clinical depression are most common in patients who fail to regain ambulation. This combination of conditions produces significant ongoing disability. Prognosis for functional recovery is more favorable in cryptogenic cases in which no underlying disease is discovered.

Evaluation for Prognosis

The most important prognostic indicator is serial neurologic examination. An improving course portends a more favorable outcome, and return to ambulation is much more likely if hip abductor and knee extensor strength initially is preserved. Subsequent improvement is unlikely if none occurs within 1 month.

Beyond the bedside evaluation, assessment of prognosis requires diagnostic spinal imaging, as the natural history depends on the pathophysiology. Magnetic resonance imaging (MRI) is a sensitive means of detecting structural lesions, such as arteriovenous malformation or compressive hematoma, to which the infarction may be secondary. MRI will help to distinguish spinal cord infarction from multiple sclerosis or other causes of transverse myelitis and from tumors. In spinal infarction, MRI acutely may demonstrate increased cord signal, edema, or enhancement but does not help with prognosis, as profound or irreversible deficits can accompany a normal study. Sometimes, a small arteriovenous malformation can be missed by MRI but be detected by prone and supine myelography or by MRI with high-dose gadolinium. If the patient is too ill to undergo MRI, plain radiography can help to exclude metastatic vertebral erosion or infectious discitis, and computed tomography scan, or even spiral computed tomography scan, can help to exclude epidural or subdural hematoma or hematomyelia.

Cerebrospinal fluid analysis can be helpful in the diagnosis of arteritis or meningovascular syphilis but should not be undertaken in the presence of a possible spinal block from a mass lesion.

Electromyography can determine whether involvement extends to spinal nerve roots or anterior horn cells. Somatosensory evoked potentials contribute little to prognosis, as they monitor only the posterior columns, which usually are spared in spinal cord infarction. The postvoid residual bladder volume is a useful and essential screen for neurogenic bladder in the patient who is not dependent on an indwelling catheter. Blood pressure should be measured supine and standing or upright to detect orthostatic hypotension.

Therapies Affecting Prognosis

The literature remains mute on the question of acute thrombolytic therapy for the infrequent diagnosis of spinal cord infarction. However, isolated cases of documented anterior spinal artery embolism suggest a valid rationale for the judicious use of heparin in appropriate clinical circumstances. As in cerebral stroke, intravenous hydration and avoidance of even modest degrees of relative hypotension may prevent subsequent infarction of an ischemic penumbra. No evidence exists in support of steroids as helpful. Any benefit from chronic antiplatelet therapy or tissue plasminogen activator is also unproved. Enoxaparin still is unproved in this situation.

Short-Term Prognosis

Of patients receiving a diagnosis of spinal cord infarction, approximately 20% will regain the ability to walk, another 20% will reach a lesser degree of neurologic improvement, 40% will not improve significantly, and the remaining 20% will not survive their underlying illness. In most cases, neurologic improvement reaches a plateau within 4 weeks.

Long-Term Prognosis

The long-term outlook after spinal cord infarction has not been well studied. The risk of subsequent vascular events, whether spinal or cerebral stroke,

myocardial infarction, or peripheral vascular occlusion, depend primarily on the status of underlying atherosclerotic risk factors. Some individuals with self-limited, corrected, or undiscovered conditions causing their spinal cord infarction have survived for many years without further incident.

Additional Reading

Cheshire WP, Santos CC, Massey EW, Howard JF Jr. Spinal cord infarction: etiology and outcome. Neurology 1996;47:321–330.

Foo D, Rossier AB. Anterior spinal artery syndrome and its natural history. Paraplegia 1983;21:1–10.

Kim SW, Kim RC, Choi BH, Gordon SK. Non-traumatic ischaemic myelopathy: a review of 25 cases. Paraplegia 1988;26:262–272.

Sandson TA, Friedman JH. Spinal cord infarction: report of 8 cases and review of the literature. Medicine 1989;68:282–292.

Satran R. Spinal cord infarction. Stroke 1988;19:529–532.

Chapter 18
Subarachnoid Hemorrhage

Janet L. Wilterdink

Subarachnoid hemorrhage (SAH) is one of the most dreaded acute medical conditions because of its high rate of early mortality and long-term morbidity. Because 80% of all nontraumatic SAHs are due to aneurysmal rupture, this chapter focuses on aneurysmal SAH.

Natural History

Understanding of the natural history of cerebral aneurysm rupture is limited, as most reported series do not include patients who die before or shortly after arrival to the hospital. Also, surgical intervention has become routine in the management of aneurysmal subarachnoid hemorrhage since the mid-1960s. Studies previous to that are potentially limited because computed tomography (CT) scans, now a mainstay in the diagnosis of SAH, were not in wide use.

Population data suggest that approximately 10 to 15% of patients with SAH die before arriving at hospital. An additional 10 to 15% die within the first 24 hours. For those who survive the first day, the outlook remains guarded. Another 20 to 30% will die in hospital, and half of the long-term survivors will have substantial neurologic deficits and disability. Only 20 to 30% of patients make a good functional recovery after SAH.

Most of the death and disability occurring among those who survive the initial hemorrhage occurs as a consequence of rebleeding and cerebral ischemia. The risk of rebleeding is highest immediately after the initial hemorrhage and occurs in

some one-third of patients within the first month. The risk of rebleeding tapers over time; approximately one-half of patients rebleed in 6 months, after which the risk stabilizes at perhaps 3% per year. Recurrent hemorrhage carries a dire prognosis: From 42 to 75% will die. Death and disability not attributable to the original or subsequent hemorrhage is largely due to cerebral ischemia and infarction, much of which is believed to occur as a consequence of vasospasm. Cerebral ischemic deficits occur in 25 to 75% of all patients.

Factors Affecting Prognosis

Prognosis after SAH is determined by a complex interaction among the severity of the hemorrhage at presentation, specific demographic characteristics of the patient, and the development of complications. These are not independent variables. Table 18-1 lists the causes of death and disability observed in the International Cooperative Study on the Timing of Aneurysm Surgery (ICSTAS). Notably, this study observed 3,521 patients who were admitted to hospital within 3 days of their SAH; thus it excluded many patients with very early mortality.

Demographic Factors

Virtually all models of prognosis after SAH include age as an independent variable. SAH mortality in

Table 18-1. Causes of Death and Disability Among 3,521 Patients in the International Cooperative Study on the Timing of Aneurysm Surgery

Cause	Death (%)	Disability (%)
Direct effect of bleed	7.0	3.6
Vasospasm	7.2	6.3
Rebleeding	6.7	0.8
Hydrocephalus	0.3	1.4
Intracerebral hemorrhage	1.0	1.0
Surgical complication	1.7	2.3
Medical treatment complication	0.7	0.1
Other	1.3	1.0
Unknown	0.0	0.1
Total	**26**	**16.3**

Source: Adapted from NF Kassell, JC Torner, EC Haley, et al. The International Cooperative Study on the Timing of Aneurysm Surgery. J Neurosurg 1990;73:18–47.

Table 18-2. Outcome at 6 Months by Age

Age (yrs)	Good Recovery (%)	Disabled (%)	Dead (%)	Total
18–29	86	7	7	261
30–39	70	13	17	476
40–49	64	15	22	833
50–59	56	17	27	1,043
60–69	44	20	36	681
70–87	26	26	49	227
Total	**58**	**16**	**26**	**3,521**

Source: Adapted from NF Kassell, JC Torner, EC Haley, et al. The International Cooperative Study on the Timing of Aneurysm Surgery. J Neurosurg 1990;73:18–47.

individuals surviving the first hospital day increased from 7% in patients ages 18 to 29 to 49% for those older than 70 (Table 18-2). Older patients are more likely to have a larger amount of blood on initial CT scan, hydrocephalus, and associated intraventricular hemorrhage. The incidence of rebleeding and symptomatic vasospasm also was higher in older patients. The increased incidence of premorbid medical disease in these patients may play a role. Data also suggest that women have a more serious prognosis than do men, with higher mortality rates, decreased incidence of independent status on discharge, and higher rates of symptomatic vasospasm.

Clinical Features at Presentation

The neurologic status of the patient at presentation is another consistent predictor of outcome. Clinical grade in various series is defined by Glasgow Coma Scale or, simply, level of consciousness. In the ICSTAS, of those in coma at onset, 72% died as contrasted to only 13% of alert individuals (Table 18-3). Separate from clinical grade, a history of loss of consciousness at the ictus was predictive of poorer prognosis in some series. A history of sentinel hemorrhage also worsened the overall prognosis.

Other variables less consistently studied or reported to have an impact on prognosis after SAH include a high diastolic and systolic blood pressure on admission or a history of long-standing hypertension. An elevated blood glucose also has been associated with a poor outcome. A poor baseline general medical condition has the expected negative effect on survival and morbidity after SAH.

Complications

Most complications occur within the first 2 weeks after SAH. Patients who survive this period without major complication are likely to do quite well. Rebleeding is the most dreaded complication and

Table 18-3. Outcome at 6 Months by Consciousness Level on Admission

Consciousness Level	Good Recovery	Disabled	Dead	Total
Alert	1,279 (74%)	218 (13%)	225 (13%)	1,722
Drowsy, stuporous	713 (48%)	306 (21%)	465 (31%)	1,484
Comatose	35 (11%)	53 (17%)	227 (72%)	315
Total	**2,027 (58%)**	**577 (16%)**	**917 (26%)**	**3,521**

Source: Adapted from NF Kassell, JC Torner, EC Haley, et al. The International Cooperative Study on the Timing of Aneurysm Surgery. J Neurosurg 1990;73:18–47.

is associated with a very high mortality, up to 75%. It appears to occur more commonly in those who lose consciousness at the ictus and in those who have intraventricular blood on initial CT. Although uncontrolled hypertension would appear to be a likely risk factor, a relationship between rebleeding and noninduced hypertension is not established definitively. Older patients and women also may be at higher risk of recurrent hemorrhage.

Cerebral ischemia may occur as a consequence of vasospasm and accounts for one-third to one-half of death and disability secondary to SAH. Cerebral ischemia usually occurs some time after the ictus of SAH; the peak incidence is between 4 and 14 days. Vasospasm occurs in 30 to 40% of patients and is a risk factor for the development of cerebral ischemic deficits. Symptomatic vasospasm occurs in 20%. Cerebral ischemia appears to occur in the absence of vasospasm, however, and may represent effects of the initial hemorrhage, thromboses, or embolism. Vasospasm and infarction are more likely to occur in patients with high blood volume in the subarachnoid space, especially when in close proximity to the basal cerebral blood vessels. Hyponatremia, hypovolemia, hypertension (induced or spontaneous), and a premorbid history of hypertension are risk factors for vasospasm and cerebral ischemia.

The incidence of acute hydrocephalus (within the first month) varies according to diagnostic criteria and may be seen radiographically in up to two-thirds of patients. Clinical deterioration from hydrocephalus is less common and occurred in 22% of 660 patients followed by Vermeij and colleagues. In multivariate analysis, neurologic deterioration attributed to hydrocephalus was predicted by tranexamic acid treatment, volume of cisternal blood on initial CT, intraventricular blood, and hydrocephalus on initial CT. Other studies suggest that age and aneurysm site (posterior circulation aneurysms) also may be predictive of hydrocephalus. Hydrocephalus occurring in the first 3 days worsens ultimate prognosis for recovery. In the series by van Gijn and coworkers, 20 of 34 such patients died. Acute hydrocephalus may be a risk factor for vasospasm.

Medical complications of SAH include disordered sodium balance (syndrome of inappropriate diuretic hormone or diabetes insipidus), which is associated with higher risk of vasospasm, cerebral infarction, hydrocephalus, and seizure. Neurogenic pulmonary edema, cardiac arrhythmia (ventricular

and supraventricular), cardiac failure, hepatic or kidney failure, thrombocytopenia, infection (pneumonia or ventriculitis), deep venous thrombosis, and gastrointestinal hemorrhage also occur. Age, gender, and race do not predict, but clinical grade and a large amount of blood on CT scan do predict, the incidence of medical complications.

Medical complications have an impact on outcome. In one study, 83% of patients who died had a severe medical complication, whereas only 30% of those surviving had a severe medical complication. Medical complications occurred in the majority but were severe and life-threatening in 40%. Overall, the number of deaths attributed to medical complications was 4.4% of the study total or 23% of all deaths. Pulmonary complications (adult respiratory distress syndrome, embolus, and aspiration) contributed to half of the medical deaths; the rest were caused by cardiac arrhythmia, central nervous system infection, sepsis, and gastrointestinal complications.

Evaluation for Prognosis

Primary Radiographic Features

The initial CT scan not only provides the diagnosis in 75 to 85% of patients with SAH, it provides important prognostic information. Absence of blood on CT scan or blood isolated to the perimesencephalic space is more likely to have a very favorable overall prognosis. A large blood volume, whether defined by diffuse deposition or a thick layer of blood, predicts a high risk of vasospasm, cerebral ischemia, and poor prognosis, with a twofold to threefold increase in mortality. Associated intracerebral, intracerebellar, intraventricular, or subdural hematoma also increases mortality (Table 18-4).

Cerebral angiography determines the cause of bleeding in patients with SAH. Although magnetic resonance angiography may identify the aneurysm in patients with SAH, it is less sensitive than is conventional angiography, less reliable in identifying multiple aneurysms, and does not provide anatomic detail sufficient for planning surgery. Absence of aneurysm on a well-performed angiogram is an excellent predictor of good outcome. Aneurysm site also is a determining factor of prognosis. Mortality in hospitalized patients was lowest for internal carotid and middle cerebral artery aneurysms (24%

Table 18-4. Mortality Rates and Risk Ratios After Subarachnoid Hemorrhage Based on Computed Tomographic Findings

	Mortality Rate (%)	Mortality Risk Ratio
Detrimental findings		
Intracranial blood (any site)	28	4.3
Intraventricular blood	46	2.2
Intracerebral blood	44	2.0
Diffuse subarachnoid blood (any site)	23	1.7
Hydrocephalus	37	1.6
Local, thick collection of subarachnoid blood	32	1.4
Favorable findings		
Local, thin collection of subarachnoid blood	10	0.4
Normal	6	0.2

Source: Adapted from HP Adams, NF Kassell, JC Torner. Usefulness of computed tomography in predicting outcome after aneurysmal subarachnoid hemorrhage: a preliminary report of the cooperative aneurysm study. Neurology 1985;35:1264.

and 21%, respectively) and was highest for anterior cerebral and vertebrobasilar artery aneurysms (30% and 31%, respectively). The size of the aneurysm also is important; in one series, patient mortality was 41% for aneurysms of more than 24 mm, as contrasted to 28% for those between 12 and 24 mm and 25% for those of less than 12 mm (Table 18-5).

Secondary Radiographic Features

Follow-up imaging studies are important to identify the cause of clinical deterioration in patients with SAH. CT scan is sensitive for determining rebleeding and hydrocephalus; however, findings of cerebral ischemia generally are delayed after clinical onset of symptoms. Magnetic resonance imaging may be more sensitive than is CT scan for presence and extent of ischemic injury, but clinical deterioration still precedes radiographic abnormality.

Follow-up angiography evaluates success of surgical clipping and is important in the diagnosis of vasospasm in the patient whose clinical deterioration is thought to be secondary to cerebral ischemia. The incidence of angiographic vasospasm is between 30 and 40% but has been reported as high

Table 18-5. Outcome at 6 Months by Aneurysm Size

Aneurysm Size	Good Recovery (%)	Disabled (%)	Dead (%)	Total (no.)
<12 mm	60	15	25	2,748
12–24 mm	52	19	29	703
>24 mm	39	20	41	70
Total	**58**	**16**	**26**	**3,521**

Source: Adapted from NF Kassell, JC Torner, EC Haley, et al. The International Cooperative Study on the Timing of Aneurysm Surgery. J Neurosurg 1990;73:18–47.

as 70%. Though probably not the sole pathologic mechanism underlying cerebral ischemic complications in SAH, the relationship between vasospasm severity and delayed focal neurologic deficits has been described well. The presence of vasospasm on angiography is predictive of morbidity and mortality. The presence and site of vasospasm may be predicted by the site of largest blood volume on CT scan. Vasospasm is more likely in women and in those who have poorer clinical grades on admission.

Transcranial Doppler ultrasonography has become an increasingly popular modality for detecting vasospasm in SAH patients. Studies have indicated good correlation between increasing flow velocities in the middle cerebral artery and the degree of arterial narrowing, with a sensitivity of 60% and specificities approaching 90%.

Therapies Affecting Prognosis

Surgical Therapy

Aneurysmal clipping, first introduced in the 1950s and 1960s, now is a mainstay in the treatment of aneurysmal SAH to reduce the risk of rebleeding. In the 1970s, microsurgical techniques were introduced, and the benefit from surgery became more apparent. The ICSTAS reported that, of 2,922 patients undergoing aneurysm surgery, 69% had good recovery and 14% died. However, patients selected to undergo surgery had better neurologic status on admission. Age, aneurysm size (but not location), and clinical grade on admission predicted surgical outcome.

Controversy remains, however, as to the timing of surgery. Though operative outcome is improved with surgery performed later (2 weeks) than that accomplished earlier, delayed surgery leads to increased mortality and morbidity, owing to the rebleeding in the interim. The ICSTAS was a non-randomized clinical trial that studied the effect of timing of surgery on outcome. Early surgery resulted in less than one-half the rate of rebleeding (6% versus 13%) and lower risks of delayed ischemic deficits (27% versus 32%). This finding must be balanced, however, against the increased operative mortality (17% on day 1) contrasted to 7% operative mortality that occurs with delayed surgery. Overall, no benefit or detriment was found for planned early surgery versus late surgery. More recent series using newer surgical and anesthetic techniques suggest even more favorable outcomes with early surgery, and this trend now is well established for patients with good clinical grade on presentation. Clinical grade and patient's age contribute to operative risk and to their overall prognosis and may influence surgical decisions. The ICSTAS also demonstrated wide center-to-center variability in outcome not explained by differences in clinical grade or other prognostic factors for death and disability. The variability was concluded to be, in part, the result of differences in medical management.

Inoperable aneurysms present a more serious prognosis than do those that are operable, making difficult the assessment of the benefit of other techniques aimed at reducing recurrent aneurysm rupture rates, such as coiling. Other invasive procedures include the use of angioplasty for the treatment of vasospasm; this surgical approach has a complication rate of at least 17%, and its overall efficacy is unclear.

Ventriculostomy and cerebrospinal fluid drainage are the most common methods of treating acute hydrocephalus associated with clinical deterioration but may lead to rebleeding or ventriculitis, especially if continued for more than 3 days. The role of prophylactic antibiotics in this setting is not clear.

Medical Therapy

The goal of antifibrinolytic therapy (ε-aminocaproic acid, tranexamic acid) is to decrease the rate of rebleeding preoperatively. However, this therapy appears to do so at the expense of an increased risk of ischemic complications and does not improve outcome clearly.

Nimodipine, though not reducing the incidence of vasospasm, appears to improve prognosis. A meta-analysis of randomized trials of nimodipine in SAH demonstrated increased odds of good outcome: (Glasgow Outcome Scale = 1) odds ratio = 1.86; good or fair outcome (Glasgow Outcome Scale ≥2) odds ratio = 1.67; decreased odds of death and disability due to vasospasm, odds ratio = 0.46; and CT scan infarction rate, odds ratio = 0.58. No significant difference was found in overall mortality.

Hypervolemic hypertensive therapy combines volume expansion and augmentation of cardiac index with dobutamine and induced systemic hypertension. This approach decreases the incidence and severity of delayed ischemia. Dangers of this therapy include rebleeding of unsecured aneurysms, pulmonary edema, and aggravation of cerebral edema. This therapy requires early aneurysm clipping.

Though in the past hyponatremia was attributed to syndrome of inappropriate diuretic hormone and was treated with fluid restriction, recent data suggest that it is more likely representative of sodium and volume loss and is treated better with intravenous fluids, thus decreasing the incidence of cerebral ischemia.

Short-Term Prognosis

The 10 to 20% death rate occurring in SAH patients before reaching the hospital is unlikely to be changed by modern medical therapy, although a recent population-based study in Washington suggested a rate less common than in previous reports (<5%). Similarly, reductions in mortality rates in the first few hospital days are unlikely to be large. In the ICSTAS, the mortality among hospitalized SAH patients was 26% at 6 months, somewhat less than earlier studies had reported. A somewhat higher mortality, 32%, was reported in the Washington population-based study.

Long-Term Prognosis

Detailed neuropsychological testing of patients surviving SAH has demonstrated conflicting results.

Some researchers reported a high incidence of neuropsychiatric deficits early (6 weeks) that largely resolved when testing was repeated 3 to 6 months later. Others reported significant cognitive impairment in a large percentage (more than half) of these patients more than 1 year after SAH. Twenty percent of survivors are unable to return to premorbid functioning. Older patients are more likely than are younger to experience significant emotional and cognitive dysfunction. Though anterior communicating artery aneurysms traditionally were believed to have a higher association with neuropsychological sequelae, this belief has not been borne out clearly in studies.

Delayed hydrocephalus resulting from impaired resorption of cerebrospinal fluid by the arachnoid villi may occur months to years after SAH. The incidence is low, less than 10% over a 15-year period. Epilepsy also may occur as a delayed complication in a small number (10 to 15%) of SAH survivors; the first seizure generally occurs within the first 18 months.

Additional Reading

Adams HP, Kassell NF, Torner JC. Usefulness of computed tomography in predicting outcome after aneurysmal subarachnoid hemorrhage: a preliminary report of the cooperative aneurysm study. Neurology 1985;35:1263–1267.

Barker FG, Ogilvy CS. Efficacy of prophylactic nimodipine for delayed ischemic deficit after subarachnoid hemorrhage: a meta-analysis. J Neurosurg 1996;90:405–414.

Hutter BO, Gilsbach JM, Kreitschmann I. Quality of life and cognitive deficits after subarachnoid haemorrhage. Br J Neurosurg 1995;9:465–475.

Kassell NF, Torner JC, Haley EC, et al. The International Cooperative Study on the Timing of Aneurysm Surgery. J Neurosurg 1990;73:18–47.

Lanzino G, Kassell NF, Germanson TP, et al. Age and outcome after aneurysmal subarachnoid hemorrhage: why do older patients fare worse? J Neurosurg 1996;85:410–418.

Longstreth WT, Nelson LM, Koepsell TD, van Belle G. Clinical course of spontaneous subarachnoid hemorrhage: a population-based study in King County, Washington. Neurology 1994;43:712–718.

Ohman J, Servo A, Heiskanen O. Risk factors for cerebral infarction in good-grade patients after aneurysmal subarachnoid hemorrhage and surgery: a prospective study. J Neurosurg 1991;74:14–20.

Solenski NJ, Haley EC, Kassell NF, et al. Medical complications of aneurysmal subarachnoid hemorrhage: a report of the multicenter, cooperative aneurysm study. Crit Care Med 1995;23:1007–1017.

van Gijn J, Hijdra A, Wijdicks EFM, et al. Acute hydrocephalus after aneurysmal subarachnoid hemorrhage. J Neurosurg 1985;63:355–362.

Vermeij FH, Hasan D, Vermeulen M, et al. Predictive factors for deterioration from hydrocephalus after subarachnoid hemorrhage. Neurology 1994;44:1851–1855.

Chapter 19

Cerebrovascular Malformations

Curtis Doberstein, Maria Guglielmo, and Percy Chan

Cerebrovascular malformations are a heterogeneous group of lesions with varying natural histories and treatment requirements. In general, such malformations can be categorized variously as arteriovenous malformations, cavernous malformations, venous angiomas, or telangiectases, depending on their pathologic features. Arteriovenous and cavernous malformations are the lesions encountered most commonly in clinical practice. They typically present in young adults and children with intracerebral hemorrhage, headaches, or seizures. Once identified, certain cerebrovascular malformations can follow an aggressive course; thus, they warrant prompt intervention, underscoring the need to understand the pathophysiology and natural history of each of these different vascular anomalies. Given the diversity in clinical presentation, prognosis, and options for therapeutic intervention with respect to each type of vascular malformation, these lesions are reviewed separately (Table 19-1).

Arteriovenous Malformations

Cerebral arteriovenous malformations (AVMs) are congenital lesions composed of three major components: the nidus (the core of abnormal blood vessels), feeding arteries, and draining veins. In general, the nidus is a compact tangle of dysplastic blood vessels interwoven with nonfunctional brain tissue separated from normal brain parenchyma by a rim of gliotic tissue (Fig. 19-1). Direct communication is apparent between AVM feeding arteries and draining veins, owing to a lack of the normally interpositioned arteriolar and capillary networks. The absence of these high-resistance networks, which regulate blood flow, creates a system in which high-pressure arterial blood shunts directly into the cerebral venous system. Because the arteries and veins subserving the nidus also can be an integral component of adjacent functional brain tissue, unique physiologic alterations in the surrounding vasculature can occur (e.g., "cerebrovascular steal"). In addition, owing to the hemodynamic change imposed by the increased volume of blood flow imposed by the AVM, aneurysms can form on arteries that feed the nidus and are found in 10% of AVM cases.

Arteriovenous malformations typically present with symptoms during early adulthood, although they can become symptomatic in children and the elderly. Cerebral hemorrhage is the most common presentation and occurs in approximately 50% of cases. Seizures, headaches, and progressive neurologic deficits not related to hemorrhage are the presenting features in most other cases. The widespread use of computed tomography (CT) scans and magnetic resonance imaging (MRI) also has resulted in diagnoses of an increasing number of asymptomatic AVMs.

Natural History

Cerebral hemorrhage is the most common and serious sequela of an AVM and remains the over-

Table 19-1. Natural History of Vascular Malformations

Type	Definition	Hemorrhage Risk (%)	Treatments
AVM	Congenital, direct connections between dysplastic cerebral arteries and veins	2–4/yr	Microsurgical resection Stereotactic radiosurgery Endovascular embolization
Dural AVM	Acquired dura-based arteriovenous shunt	1.6/yr	Endovascular embolization Microsurgical resection
Cavernous angioma	Dilated vascular channels without normal intervening brain tissue	1–5/yr	Microsurgical resection
Venous malformation	Dilated vein or cluster of veins	Rare	Usually none

AVM = arteriovenous malformation.

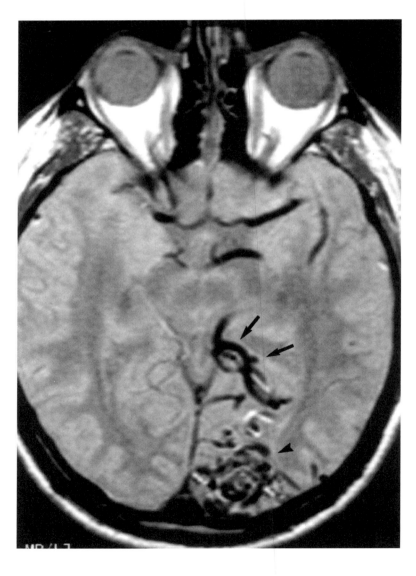

Figure 19-1. Magnetic resonance imaging of a left occipital arteriovenous malformation (arrowhead). Note feeding arteries (arrows).

whelming concern with respect to its natural history. The mortality associated with an AVM-induced hemorrhage is approximately 15%, with serious neurologic morbidity occurring in another 30% of cases. The risk of bleeding in a previously unruptured AVM is believed to be 3 to 4% per year, with an annual risk of death approximating 1%. In lesions presenting with hemorrhage, however, the rate of rebleeding is higher during the first year after the event. The risk of rebleeding in cases that previously have bled is 6 to 10% during the first year, but this risk then declines and resembles that of unruptured lesions: 3 to 4% per year.

Factors Affecting Prognosis

Numerous anatomic and angiographic factors have been investigated to ascertain whether they alter the risk of experiencing a cerebral hemorrhage secondary to an AVM. Patients who have an aneurysm arising from an AVM feeding artery have an increased risk of subsequent hemorrhage. In addition, the presence of an aneurysm within the AVM nidus strongly correlates with hemorrhage. However, these aneurysms often are difficult to visualize in the dense tangle of abnormal blood vessels composing the nidus. Although AVM location does not appear to alter its natural history with respect to bleeding, the risk related to lesion size remains controversial. Several small series seem to indicate that smaller malformations have higher hemorrhage rates, although a consistent relationship between AVM size and hemorrhage has not been proved. The role of deep venous drainage, magnitude of arteriovenous shunting, and presence of draining vein stenosis require further study but currently are not thought to alter significantly the natural history of brain AVMs.

It has been thought that pregnancy increases the risk of AVM-related cerebral hemorrhage. However, the two most comprehensive studies regarding this subject have shown conflicting results. In their analysis of 451 pregnant women harboring AVMs, Horton and coworkers found a hemorrhage rate of 3.5% and concluded that pregnancy was not a significant risk factor for bleeding. In contrast, Ondra and associates analyzed 166 Finnish AVM patients and found that 14% of all hemorrhages occurred during the third trimester of pregnancy. These authors concluded that pregnancy poses an increased risk of AVM-related intracerebral bleeding. In both studies, no hemorrhages occurred during labor, cesarean section, or abortion.

Evaluation for Prognosis

Diagnostic studies required for the diagnosis and treatment of brain AVMs include MRI scanning and cerebral angiography, and these studies may aid also in prognostication. For example, the presence of an associated intranidal or feeding artery aneurysm may increase the likelihood of hemorrhage. Location, size, and venous drainage may influence the risks of intervention (Fig. 19-2).

Therapies Affecting Prognosis

The decision to proceed with treatment is based on the natural history of the disorder combined with the patient's general health and the location and size of the malformation. Generally, seizures are controlled well with anticonvulsant therapy, and headaches often respond to standard analgesics. Once the decision is made to intervene with definitive treatment, therapies can be initiated on an elective basis. In rare circumstances, an associated intracerebral hemorrhage may require surgical evacuation on an emergent basis, and the AVM can be dealt with accordingly.

Microsurgical resection of cerebral AVMs remains the best therapy for most malformations and results in the complete obliteration of the structural abnormality (Fig. 19-3). In addition, surgical extirpation provides an immediate cure with respect to bleeding originating from abnormal AVM blood vessels. Modern microsurgical and neuroanesthetic techniques have reduced the risk associated with the removal of these malformations. The risk of surgery is variable and depends on patient characteristics, the location and anatomy of the AVM, and the experience of the surgeon. In general, operable lesions carry a 5 to 15% risk of neurologic morbidity.

Stereotactic radiotherapy and endovascular embolization also can play an important role in the treatment of cerebral AVMs. Interventional neuroradiologic treatment typically involves the selective catheterization of arteries feeding the malformation, followed by the administration of particles (e.g., Ivalon, Avitene, or coils) or specialized glue poly-

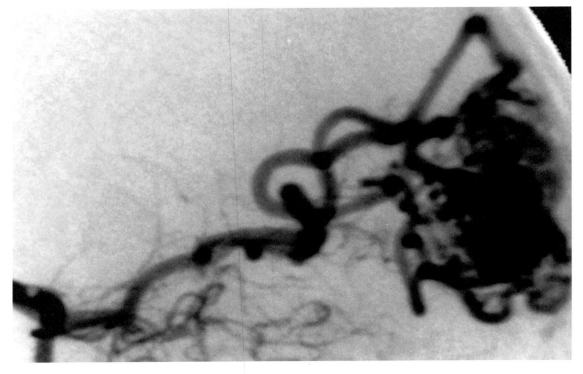

Figure 19-2. Preoperative lateral vertebrobasilar angiogram shows occipital arteriovenous malformation shown in Fig. 19-1.

mers. This approach can result in obliteration of portions of the malformation but rarely results in a cure. Embolization usually is used as a surgical adjunct, reducing blood loss during surgery and facilitating microsurgical resection. Stereotactic radiotherapy is becoming a major treatment modality for cerebral AVMs, particularly for lesions deemed inappropriate for surgical resection. Malformations best suited for radiotherapy are less than 3 cm in size, and approximately 85% of these lesions will eventually obliterate over a 2- to 3-year period. Larger lesions have less chance of obliteration after radiotherapy. It should be noted also that during the interval between radiotherapy and complete obliteration of the AVM, cerebral hemorrhage remains a risk.

Short- and Long-Term Prognosis

The mortality associated with the acute rupture of a cerebral AVM is usually within the first 30 days after presentation. However, mortality associated with rupture of an AVM is less than 15%. In patients surviving the initial hemorrhage, the prognosis after treatment generally is good. Microsurgical resection can result in immediate cure and, although obliterating the lesion radiosurgically requires approximately 18 months to 2 years, cure can be seen in 80 to 85% of AVMs of less than 3 cm. The prognosis for untreated malformations is guarded, given an annual risk of death of approximately 1% from the time of detection.

Dural Arteriovenous Malformations

Dural arteriovenous malformations (DAVMs) are a subset of AVMs, exhibit unique characteristics, and account for approximately 10 to 15% of all cerebral AVMs. They are thought to be acquired (rather than congenital) lesions resulting from previous venous sinus thrombosis. Arteriovenous shunts normally

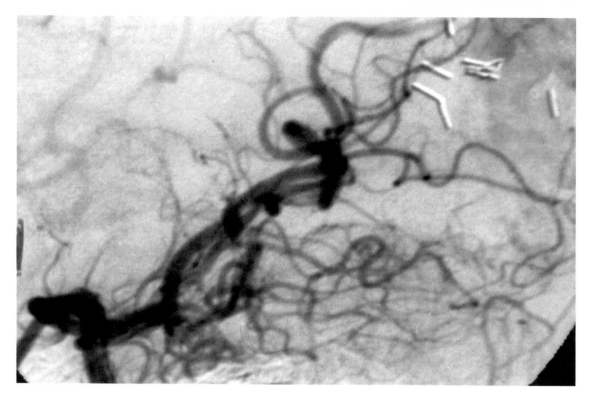

Figure 19-3. Postoperative angiogram, lateral view, demonstrates complete obliteration of the arteriovenous malformation (see Figs. 19-1 and 19-2) by a combination of endovascular embolization and microsurgery.

are present in the dura, and arise from the primary anastomotic arteries, which form a layer on the periosteal dural surface. Factors that alter the arteriovenous pressure gradient, such as venous thrombosis and direct trauma to the dura, are thought to produce an increase in the size and number of these existing physiologic shunts. The higher incidence of DAVMs in women and during pregnancy has been speculated to have a hormonal etiology. A subset of DAVMs of the cavernous sinus, termed *carotid-cavernous fistulas* (CCFs), can occur either spontaneously or after trauma.

Natural History

As with other vascular malformations, significant mortality and morbidity associated with DAVMs occur primarily from episodes of hemorrhage, which may be subarachnoid, intraparenchymal, or subdural. Other presentations include focal neuro-logic symptoms not related to hemorrhage and arterial steal phenomenon but frequently related to focal venous hypertension. The most common symptom associated with these lesions is pulsatile tinnitus, especially in DAVMs of the transverse and sigmoid sinuses. Neuro-ophthalmic manifestations of DAVMs typically occur with CCFs and include papilledema or both isolated and combined palsies of cranial nerves III, IV, V, and VI.

Factors Affecting Prognosis

Leptomeningeal retrograde venous drainage appears to be the greatest factor predisposing DAVMs to hemorrhage. Awad's analysis of 377 patients with DAVMs demonstrated that fistulas of the tentorial incisura follow the most aggressive course and those at the transverse-sigmoid or cavernous sinus follow the most benign. In another study, of 54 conservatively managed patients with average follow-up of

6.6 years, five hemorrhages were seen, yielding a yearly 1.6% risk of hemorrhage. This study also noted a tendency for lesions with leptomeningeal drainage to hemorrhage, although it did not reach significance. A significantly increased risk of hemorrhage was seen with an associated venous varix on a draining vein.

DAVMs of the transverse and sigmoid sinuses, the most common subtype, are less likely to have retrograde leptomeningeal venous drainage and, therefore, are more likely to follow a benign course. In contrast, almost all tentorial-incisural DAVMs drain into pial perimesencephalic and cerebellar veins and are the most aggressive subtype.

The natural history of CCFs varies depending on whether the lesion is post-traumatic or spontaneous. Traumatic CCFs generally progress very rapidly, with severe exophthalmos and decreasing vision that may lead to permanent blindness. Fistulas that extend into the sphenoid or ethmoid sinuses may cause massive nasal hemorrhage. Classically, spontaneous CCFs are described as resulting from a ruptured intracavernous aneurysm, but often no evidence of an aneurysm is found. Their natural history is not understood as well as the more common traumatic CCFs, and a large number spontaneously thrombose.

Evaluation for Prognosis

CT with and without contrast can demonstrate thrombosed sinuses, dilated veins, or varices and is the test of choice when an acute hemorrhage is suspected. Usually, visualizing the DAVM itself is difficult. MRI has limitations similar to those of CT scan but is more sensitive in diagnosing an associated thrombosed sinus if present. Angiography, including selective injection of the external carotid artery, remains the test of choice for diagnosing a DAVM and best delineates the anatomic location and venous drainage pattern that are the most important factors in prognosis.

Therapies Affecting Prognosis

Treatment generally is considered in patients who present with intracranial bleeding or a progressive neurologic deficit, including progressive loss of vision (usually from CCFs) and tinnitus that becomes progressively intolerable and interferes with normal activities. Endovascular therapy with coils or detachable balloons or glue polymers is the procedure of choice for most lesions, especially for CCFs and transverse-sigmoid lesions. Surgical approaches are preferred for anterior cranial fossa lesions, and combined therapies have been employed. Stereotactic radiosurgery also has shown some success in smaller lesions.

Short- and Long-Term Prognosis

Short-term prognosis for patients with DAVMs is related to mode of presentation. The mortality and morbidity of lesions presenting with hemorrhage is related to the extent and location of bleeding, although the risk of death or significant neurologic morbidity is low. After treatment, the prognosis is very favorable for patients with lesions presenting with symptoms other than hemorrhage. Untreated lesions must be observed carefully, particularly if they are tentorial and anterior fossa DAVMs, which typically have pial venous drainage and are more likely to hemorrhage.

Cavernous Malformations

Cavernous malformations (CMs), also known as *angiomas* or *cavernomas*, are well-circumscribed anomalies composed of dilated sinusoidal vascular channels that do not subserve normal brain tissue. They are located most commonly in the supratentorial white matter but can occur also in the cerebellum or brain stem. Multiple lesions are common and are present in approximately 20% of affected patients. Although generally sporadic, familial forms of CMs occur in some 6% of cases. The clinical manifestations of CMs differ from those of AVMs. Seizures are the most common presenting problem and occur in approximately 50% of symptomatic cases. Symptoms related to mass effect (e.g., headache or nausea) or focal neurologic deficits also are common. Cerebral hemorrhage is the initial presentation in approximately one-third of patients. Radiographic evidence of hemorrhage surrounding the lesion, however, is extremely common, even in asymptomatic lesions. An increasing number of incidental CMs are being recognized on cerebral CT scan and MRI studies.

Figure 19-4. Preoperative T1-weighted axial magnetic resonance imaging scan of a cavernous angioma (arrow) with classic "popcorn" appearance of mixed-age blood products.

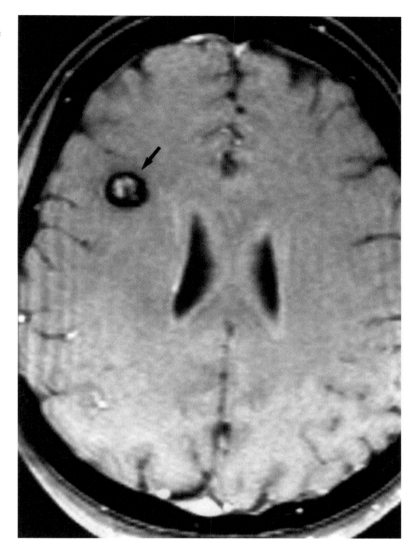

Natural History

The natural history of CMs has been characterized poorly. The general belief holds that previously unruptured CMs have an annual hemorrhage rate between 0.5 and 1%. However, in patients with previous symptomatic hemorrhage, the annual bleeding rate increases to approximately 4.5%.

Factors Affecting Prognosis

The risk of hemorrhage has not been related significantly to patient gender or age or lesion location.

The familial form of the disease may carry a slightly higher risk of hemorrhage and previous hemorrhage increases the likelihood of future bleeding. The effect of pregnancy remains speculative, although pregnant women accounted for the majority of hemorrhages in one series.

Evaluation for Prognosis

The routine use of MRI has led to the identification of a greater number of CMs (Fig. 19-4). These lesions usually appear as well-defined, circumscribed abnormalities surrounded by a rim of decreased sig-

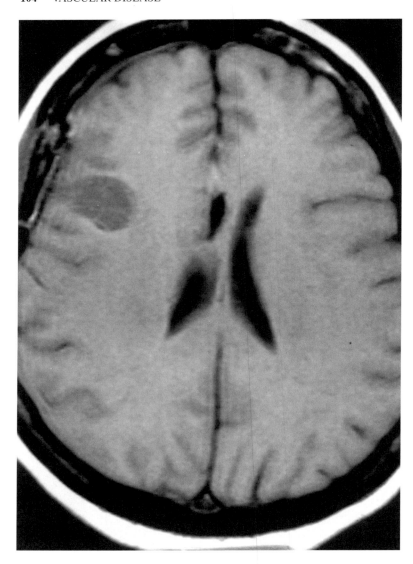

Figure 19-5. Postoperative T1-weighted axial magnetic resonance imaging scan demonstrates complete removal of cavernous angioma (see Fig. 19-4) using stereotactic microsurgical techniques.

nal intensity. The hypodense rim is secondary to the presence of hemosiderin, and the demonstration of blood by-products in various stages of evolution is common. Occasionally, venous angiomas are found to coexist with cerebral CMs. The appearance of CMs on CT scan imaging typically is characterized by a focal area of increased attenuation. Areas of calcification are not uncommon and can be seen in 15 to 20% of lesions. In addition, contrast administration results in faint enhancement. CMs are angiographically occult because of their low blood flow. Radiographic studies, although useful for diagnosis, do not provide clues to prognosis.

Therapies Affecting Prognosis

The majority of incidental lesions do not require treatment; however, microsurgical resection remains the main therapy for symptomatic CMs (Fig. 19-5). Surgically, these lesions have a papillary shape often likened to a mulberry. Modern neurosurgical techniques, such as the operating microscope and stereotactic localization, have reduced the morbidity associated with operative intervention. The role of radiosurgery is controversial, given that obliteration of the lesion cannot be confirmed radiographically and long-term follow-up studies are inconclusive.

Short- and Long-Term Prognosis

Most hemorrhages from CMs are asymptomatic, and significant morbidity and mortality are low. Familial lesions appear to yield a somewhat poorer prognosis; thus, a more aggressive therapeutic approach to symptomatic familial lesions is justified. In lesions that have caused either symptomatic hemorrhage or medically intractable seizures, long-term results after resection appear to be very favorable.

Capillary Telangiectasia

Telangiectasias are composed of small capillaries that have normal brain tissue interposed between them. Commonly, they involve the brain stem and deep brain regions and typically are identified as incidental findings at autopsy or during cerebral angiography. These lesions are not visualized well on CT scan or MRI and are asymptomatic.

Natural History

The natural history of cerebral capillary telangiectasias generally is benign. However, in rare instances, they can hemorrhage. No surgical intervention or medical therapy is required for treatment of these lesions.

Short- and Long-Term Prognosis

Capillary telangiectasias almost never cause significant hemorrhage. As a result, they yield an excellent prognosis.

Venous Angioma

Venous angiomas, or malformations, are composed of groups of histologically normal-appearing veins separated by intact brain parenchyma. A venous varix is a solitary vein or a smaller cluster of dilated veins and is a subtype of venous malformation. Venous malformations are thought to be functionally important and to represent an anomalous configuration of normal cerebral venous drainage. These malformations are diagnosed as incidental findings on CT scan, MRI, and angiographic studies.

Natural History

In general, venous anomalies have a benign natural history but, on rare occasions, they can bleed and result in cerebral hemorrhage. Given the fact that they do not behave in an aggressive fashion and that they are thought to represent potentially functionally important venous drainage, no treatment is warranted. Venous infarction can result when these abnormalities are resected or interrupted.

Short- and Long-Term Prognosis

Venous angiomas almost never cause significant hemorrhage. For this reason, they yield an excellent prognosis.

Additional Reading

Awad IA, Little JR, Akrawi WP. Intracranial dural arteriovenous malformations: factors predisposing to an aggressive neurological course. J Neurosurg 1990;72:839–850.

Brown RD, Wiebers DO, Nichols DA. Intracranial dural arteriovenous fistulae: angiographic predictors of intracranial hemorrhage and clinical outcome in nonsurgical patients. J Neurosurg 1994;81:531–538.

Horton JC, Chambers WA, Lyons SL, Adams RD. Pregnancy and the risk of hemorrhage from cerebral arteriovenous malformations. Neurosurgery 1990;27:871–872.

Kondziolka D, Lunsford LD, Kestle JK. The natural history of cerebral cavernous malformation. J Neurosurg 1995;83:820–824.

Mullan S. Fistulas and Vascular Malformations of the Dura and Dural Sinuses. In MJ Apuzzo (ed), Brain Surgery: Complication Avoidance and Management. New York: Churchill Livingstone, 1993.

Ondra SL, Troupp H, George ED, Schwab K. The natural history of symptomatic arteriovenous malformations of the brain: a 24-year follow-up assessment. J Neurosurg 1990;73:387–391.

Rigamonti P, Hsu FPK, Monsein LH. Cavernous Malformations and Related Lesions. In RH Wilkins, SS Rengachary (eds), Neurosurgery. New York: McGraw-Hill 1992;2503–2508.

Chapter 20

Intracerebral Hemorrhage

Stanley Tuhrim

Intracerebral hemorrhage (ICH) occurs when arterial blood extravasates into the brain parenchyma. Usually, this event results from rupture of small, penetrating arteries deep in the brain and that have been damaged by hypertension or age (amyloid angiopathy). ICH may occur also secondary to trauma, drug use (especially cocaine), a coagulation defect, a vascular malformation (e.g., angioma, arteriovenous malformation), or tumor. In these situations, the immediate prognosis may not differ from that of primary hemorrhage, but the longer-term prognosis depends on the severity of the underlying pathology.

ICH can be classified also according to the location in which it occurs. Approximately 30% of intracerebral hemorrhages occur in the putamen, 25% in the thalamus, 5% in the caudate, and 25% in the lobes of the hemispheres. The remaining 15% of ICHs occur infratentorially, with two-thirds originating in the cerebellum and the remainder in the pons.

Natural History

Mortality is the least equivocal of the outcome measures used in studies of stroke prognosis and usually is expressed as the 30-day case fatality rate, as few deaths attributable to stroke occur after the first month. For ICH, the reported mortality rate ranges from 30 to 50%. Death after ICH usually occurs within 1 week of onset. Transtentorial herniation is the most frequent cause of death in supratentorial lesions, whereas direct destruction of the brain stem usually is responsible in infratentorial lesions.

Since 1950, the incidence of ICH has dropped in parallel with the decline in cerebral infarction. This decrease is due largely to the advent of aggressive treatment of hypertension, the primary modifiable risk factor for stroke. This drop has more than offset the increase in ICH due to anticoagulant-related hemorrhages, which were not seen before the advent of the widespread use of this therapy in the mid 1950s. For example, in a population-based study of residents of Rochester, MN, the age-adjusted incidence of nontraumatic ICH fell from 15.7 per 100,000 in the years 1945 to 1952 to 9.3 from 1961 to 1968 and to 6.0 from 1969 to 1976. This progressive decline appeared to reverse by 1980, when the rate returned to 9 per 100,000. However, this apparent reversal can be attributed to a second major medical development: the advent of computed tomography (CT). Previously, ICH was diagnosed either at autopsy or on the basis of clinical criteria that implied profound neurologic compromise. Routine scanning of acute stroke patients allowed correct classification of smaller hemorrhages with milder symptoms that otherwise would have been diagnosed mistakenly as infarctions. This advance had the dual effect of increasing the apparent incidence of ICH and decreasing the case fatality rate, as most patients with these smaller hemorrhages survived.

Accurate identification of ICH during life has provided an opportunity to correlate clinical findings with outcome. These studies take one of two general approaches. In one, outcome for specific lesion sites (e.g., thalamus or cerebellum) are described as a function of various presenting characteristics in relatively small series of patients. Another approach uses more heterogeneous but larger groups of patients (e.g., supratentorial hemorrhage), applying sophisticated statistical techniques that allow inferences to be drawn about the joint effects of the identified factors. Because this approach examines aggregate data and attempts to generalize about broad categories of patients, no inferences can be drawn about clinical signs found in a small subgroup of patients. The sections that follow review the information provided by these complementary approaches. Outcome correlates for specific lesion sites are considered first, followed by a discussion of the analyses of aggregate data.

Factors Affecting Prognosis

Clinical Signs Related to Specific Lesion Sites

Putamenal Hemorrhage

The clinical spectrum of putamenal hemorrhage is extremely broad, ranging from very small, asymptomatic lesions to very large, invariably fatal ones. The overall mortality for putamenal hemorrhage is comparable to ICH in general.

The clinical signs associated with a poor chance for survival include pupillary abnormalities, disturbance in extraocular movements, and bilateral Babinski's signs, whereas lack of impairment of higher cortical functions and at least partial sparing of motor function are associated with survival. Large hemorrhage size and presence of intraventricular blood on CT scan are associated also with a high mortality rate. Extension of the hemorrhage to the level of the lateral ventricle implies destruction of the posterior limb of the internal capsule, making recovery of motor function improbable. Lesions involving only the anterior limb of the internal capsule fare much better than those that involve the posterior limb.

Caudate Hemorrhage

Although the caudate is supplied by deep penetrating branches of the large superficial cerebral vessels similar to those supplying the putamen and thalamus, hemorrhage rarely originates there. Caudate hemorrhage may mimic subarachnoid hemorrhage with meningismus, vomiting, headache, and changes in level of consciousness and behavior. Intraventricular blood always is present and frequently is accompanied by hydrocephalus. Hemiparesis and conjugate gaze paresis also may be present, indicating compression of the internal capsule. Patients so afflicted rarely die and usually recover completely. The almost uniformly good outcome in these patients, despite the invariant feature of intraventricular hemorrhage, contrasts sharply with putamenal hemorrhage, wherein such extension frequently is associated with death.

Thalamic Hemorrhage

Though the overall survival prognosis in thalamic hemorrhage appears comparable to that of putamenal hemorrhage, little consensus exists regarding prognostic factors. The clinical findings associated with thalamic hemorrhage have been described well but, other than level of consciousness, are related inconsistently to survival. An exception to this finding is the syndrome of posterior thalamic hemorrhage consisting of ipsilateral ptosis and miosis, contralateral sensory neglect and sensorimotor hemiparesis, defective pursuit toward the lesion, and hypometric saccades away from the lesion. These lesions limited to the posterior thalamus rarely result in significant permanent deficit. Similarly, the aphasia seen with left-sided thalamic hemorrhage usually is transient. Hemorrhage size appears to be the single best predictor of outcome in thalamic hemorrhage. Although reports differ as to the largest hematoma size consistent with survival, when the diameter exceeds 3 cm, patients rarely survive. Ventricular extension occurs in more than 50% of cases and carries a variable prognosis, but hydrocephalus, usually occurring as a result of intraventricular hemorrhage, is associated with a high mortality rate (>50%).

Lobar Hemorrhage

Lobar hemorrhages differ from other supratentorial hemorrhages in that a history of hypertension is found less frequently, occurring in one-third to one-half of cases. Those with no history of hypertension have a substantially better prognosis. The reported mortality rates for lobar hemorrhage range from 9 to 32%, lower than those for other lesion sites. Level of consciousness, hemorrhage size, intraventricular extension, and degree of midline shift have been identified as important prognostic variables.

Pontine Hemorrhage

The majority of pontine hemorrhages involve the paramedian area bilaterally, generally rupture into the ventricular system, and are fatal. Frequently, survivors are devastated neurologically. However, the advent of CT scanning has resulted in the demonstration of small hemorrhages limited to the pontine tegmentum or to a small portion of the basis pontis. These lesions produce signs and symptoms similar to those of lacunar infarctions in that region and carry a similarly good prognosis. These lesions are more likely associated with vascular malformations than are the more severe, medial lesions.

Cerebellar Hemorrhage

The clinical course of cerebellar hemorrhage is highly variable, but certain prognostic signs have been identified. Patients who are alert and either remain so or undergo surgery before becoming comatose fare far better than those who become stuporous or comatose, regardless of whether they undergo operation. If evacuation is performed after the patient becomes stuporous, the mortality rate is 75%, whereas the survival rate for those undergoing surgery before they reach this point is 75%. Clinical findings at presentation other than level of consciousness have not been reliable predictors of worsening or outcome, but CT scan findings may be more helpful. Hemorrhage diameter of greater than 3 cm, obstructive hydrocephalus, and intraventricular hemorrhage are associated with a decreased level of consciousness and a poor outcome. Overall, the survival rate for cerebellar hemorrhage may be higher than that for other ICH locations. In the National Institute of Neurological Disorders and Stroke (NINDS) Data Bank series, more than 80% of cerebellar hemorrhages survived for at least 30 days. The patients who survive usually make excellent recoveries.

General Prognostic Features

For patients with supratentorial ICH, prognosis studies that have performed multivariate analyses, despite minor variations in patient selection, variables assessed, and statistical methods, demonstrate consistent results. Hemorrhage size, intraventricular extension of blood, and Glasgow Coma Scale (GCS) score (or level of consciousness) emerge as consistent independent predictors of survival. Although the consistency of these findings provides a measure of assurance of their accuracy, ideally a multivariate model developed by analyzing data from one cohort should be validated externally by testing its ability to predict outcome in an independent data set.

Tuhrim and coworkers attempted to validate a logistic regression model developed with data from the pilot phase of the NINDS study on data from an independent group of patients collected in the main phase of that project. The initial model contained three factors: hemorrhage size, GCS score, and pulse pressure (defined as systolic-diastolic blood pressure) and correctly predicted life or death outcome at 30 days for 92% of the patients in the original data set. Application of this model to all patients with complete information in the NINDS study main phase resulted in 90% correct prediction. For practical purposes, the initial three-factor model provides an accurate means of determining the likelihood of survival for a patient at the time of hospital admission by using the following equation:

$$\text{Mortality probability} = e^{pi}/(1 + e^{pi})$$

where *pi* (predictive index) is defined as

$$-4.0630 + 2.9039 \, (\text{GCS score}) + 0.8777 \, (\text{hemorrhage size}) + 0.9086 \, (\text{pulse pressure})$$

where GCS = 0 ($\geq$9) or 1 (<9); hemorrhage size = 0 (small), 1 (moderate), or 2 (large); and pulse pressure = 0 ($\leq$45), 1 (46 to 65), or 2 (>65).

The use of this equation may be exemplified by considering a patient in the category with the poorest prognosis, having a GCS score of 6, a large hemorrhage, and a pulse pressure greater than 65. The predictive index for this patient is $-4.0630 + 2.9039 \, (1) + 0.8777 \, (2) + 0.9086 \, (2) = 2.4136$, and the estimated probability of dying within 30 days of ICH onset is $e^{2.4136}/(1 + e^{2.4136}) = 0.9179$ or approximately 92%.

Therapies Affecting Prognosis

Anticoagulant Therapy

The use of long-term anticoagulation has contributed to the incidence of ICH. The risk of ICH has been estimated at 8 to 11 times higher for patients older than 50 and on oral anticoagulant therapy. The majority of patients have a prothrombin time or international normalized ratio that is within the target range. The tendency is for anticoagulant-related hemorrhages to occur in the cerebellum, in particular in the vermis.

Forsting and colleagues reported that 20 of 40 patients with anticoagulant-related hemorrhage did not survive, but 18 of 20 survivors recovered completely. Five patients experienced concomitant subdural hematomas, but no patient had multiple ICHs. Radberg and associates found that 28 of a series of 200 patients with ICH had been taking warfarin at the time of the hemorrhage. The overall mortality was 30%, but 57% of patients with the anticoagulant-related hemorrhages died. These hemorrhages also were larger on average.

Anticoagulant-related hemorrhages tend to be larger than others and carry a somewhat poorer prognosis. The same prognostic factors—hemorrhage size, intraventricular hemorrhage, and level of consciousness or GCS score—predict outcome in these patients. These patients do not appear to differ in degree of recovery, frequently returning to a high level of functioning.

Surgical Evacuation

Surgical evacuation of ICH clearly is beneficial if the hemorrhage occurs in the cerebellum and the patient is not yet moribund. Anecdotal reports tell of good outcomes with surgical evacuation of brain stem hemorrhages, but this procedure is not performed widely and is unlikely to benefit patients presenting with marked impairment. Numerous trials of evacuation of supratentorial ICH have failed to show a consistent benefit. However, some have suggested that early evacuation (less than 6 hours from onset) may improve outcome, but this theory remains untested. The large Japanese experience, as related by Kanaya, suggested that outcome in at least some supratentorial ICH may be improved with surgical extirpation, but data from randomized trials are lacking.

Medical Therapy

Numerous protocols for medical management of the ICH patient have been suggested, but no specific protocol has been shown to affect outcome. In general, medical management is directed at controlling elevated intracranial pressure, moderating extremely high blood pressure (albeit in the absence of consensus regarding the ideal target pressure), and treating comorbidities or complications. Although higher blood pressures have been associated with a higher mortality rate, no existing data demonstrate that controlling blood pressure reduces mortality. The use of corticosteroids has been studied in a randomized trial by Poungvarin and coworkers and has been found to be of no benefit.

Short-Term Prognosis

The bulk of the preceding discussion pertains to short-term mortality, as the majority of studies of prognosis in ICH have focused on 30-day survival. In fact, most acute deaths occur in the first 2 weeks, owing mainly to increased intracranial pressure and immediate tissue destruction. Deaths beyond this period generally are attributed to complications arising from severe neurologic impairment, such as aspiration pneumonia and pulmonary embolus.

Long-Term Prognosis

Long-term outcome in ICH has been studied less thoroughly. Daverat found that more than 75% of ICH survivors functioned independently after 6 months. Helweg-Larsen and colleagues followed patients for a median of 4.5 years and found that 8 of 29 had returned to work and 9 had no neurologic deficits, whereas 5 were incapacitated. Tuhrim and coworkers found that the same factors that predicted short-term survival (pulse pressure, GCS score, ICH size) predicted a good outcome, defined as a Barthel's index of activities of daily living greater than 60. More recently, Lampl and associates found that functional outcome after 6 months was related to initial hemorrhage size in lobar and putamenal—but not thalamic—hemorrhages. Patients with temporal lobe hematomas appeared to recover most completely.

In summary, the prognosis for a patient with ICH can be determined largely by a careful neurologic assessment and review of imaging studies at time of hospital admission. Both in-hospital mortality and long-term prognosis for recovery have been linked to the clinical and radiologic appearance at that time, with general prognostic features accurately predicting mortality probability and site-specific findings yielding some important additional information regarding functional return.

Additional Reading

Daverat P, Castel JP, Dartigues JF, Orgogozo JM. Death and functional outcome after spontaneous intracerebral hemorrhage: a prospective study of 166 cases using multivariate analysis. Stroke 1991;22:1–6.

Feldmann E (ed). Intracerebral Hemorrhage. Armonk, NY: Futura, 1994.

Forsting M, Mattle HP, Haber P. Anticoagulant-related intracerebral hemorrhage. Cerebrovasc Dis 1991;1:97–102.

Helweg-Larsen S, Sommer W, Stange P, et al. Prognosis for patients treated conservatively for spontaneous intracerebral hematomas. Stroke 1984;15:1045–1048.

Kanaya H. Results of conservative and surgical treatment in hypertensive intracerebral hemorrhage—co-operative study in Japan. Jpn J Stroke 1990;12:509–524.

Kase CS, Caplan LR. Intracerebral Hemorrhage. Boston, MA: Butterworth–Heinemann, 1994.

Lampl Y, Gilad R, Eshel Y, Sarova-Pinhas I. Neurological and functional outcome in patients with supratentorial hemorrhage. Stroke 1995;26:2249–2253.

Poungvarin N, Bhoopat W, Viriyavejakul A, et al. Effects of dexamethasone in primary supratentorial intracerebral hemorrhage. N Engl J Med 1987;316:1229–1233.

Radberg JA, Olsson JE, Radberg CT. Prognostic parameters in spontaneous intracerebral hematomas with special reference to anticoagulant treatment. Stroke 1991;22:571–576.

Tuhrim S, Dambrosia JM, Price TR, et al. Prediction of intracerebral hemorrhage survival. Ann Neurol 1988;24:258–263.

Chapter 21

Vascular Dementia

Richard Munson and Vladimir Hachinski

Vascular dementia (VD) is a term used to define a collection of disorders that cause an acquired mental impairment resulting from brain injury secondary to blood vessel disease. Defining the prognosis of VD is like defining the prognosis of cancer or infection. To give meaning to a prognosis of VD, one must make clear the type of VD under discussion. This can be accomplished by describing the proposed mechanism of the VD, the proposed etiopathology, and the operational definitions of both the vascular and the dementia components of the disease. A variety of pathologies can cause these proposed mechanisms, including cardiac disease; small-, medium-, and large-vessel angiopathies; atherosclerosis; hypercoagulable states; and others.

Proposed Mechanisms of Vascular Dementia

Multi-Infarct Dementia

The term *multi-infarct dementia* (MID) describes a process whereby the accumulation of multiple ischemic events—whether large or small, cortical or subcortical—leads to cognitive decline. This decline includes the "lacunar state" wherein multiple lacunes can cause a "subcortical dementia syndrome."

Strategic Infarcts

Strategic infarcts are small or large infarcts localized to areas of the brain that can affect multiple cogni-tive processes. Examples of this malady include the angular gyrus syndrome and some thalamic infarcts.

Single Infarcts Leading to Dementia

In a hospitalized cohort of patients with stroke compared to those of a normal control group, Tatemichi and coworkers showed that the risk of dementia per 100 person-years was 8.4 as contrasted to 1.3 in the control group, for a relative risk of 5.5 for dementia occurring with stroke. In a longitudinal study following 158 patients with first-ever ischemic stroke, Treves and colleagues showed a cumulative risk of dementia of 29% at 1 year and 34% at 3 years.

Single Infarcts Interacting with Alzheimer's Disease

Snowdon and coworkers showed in the "Nun study" that the presence of one or more infarcts in nuns with dementia correlated with decreased Mini-Mental State Examination scores. The prevalence of dementia was 88% for those with an infarct and 57% for those without an infarct, for an odds ratio of 11.1. These authors further showed that in nuns with pathologically validated Alzheimer's disease, the presence of one or more infarcts correlated with a reduced number of neurofibrillary tangles found in demented patients. This suggests that having a stroke may worsen the clinical expression of Alzheimer's disease.

Chronic Ischemia

The existence of chronic ischemia in the brain has not been demonstrated conclusively. Various pathologic reports have described an incomplete ischemia involving gliosis and demyelination. Some cases of leukoaraiosis seen on computed tomography (CT) or magnetic resonance imaging may reflect this mechanism. Many would put the proposed Binswanger's disease into this category of VD. Some case reports speak of decreased perfusion associated with severely stenosed carotid arteries and reversal of apparent dementia after carotid endarterectomy or extracranial-intracranial bypass, which may suggest a role for hypoperfusion (or misery perfusion) as a cause of VD.

Diagnostic Criteria

Multiple criteria currently are employed to diagnose VD. A recent review using seven different criteria on 124 patients with VD showed significant differences in the frequencies of diagnosis of VD versus Alzheimer's disease versus mixed dementia. Currently, the most popular criteria are available through the *Diagnostic and Statistical Manual of Mental Disorders*, Fourth Edition; the State of California Alzheimer's Disease Diagnostic and Treatment Centers; the international work group of the American National Institute of Neurological Disorders and Stroke; and the European Association Internationale pour la Recherché et l'Enseignement en Neurosciences. Each of these criteria uses course of the disease, risk factors, behavioral features, neurologic signs, temporal relationship of dementia to stroke, and neuroimaging in varying ways to determine the diagnosis. All these criteria incorporate memory loss and functional impairment in their definition of dementia.

Natural History

The natural history of VD, therefore, depends on the type of VD (as described) and on the criteria for diagnosis. Little is conclusively known at this time. The clinical picture can be one of smooth, progressive deterioration, stepwise deterioration, fluctuations, or remitting disease. Moroney and coworkers followed 115 patients with MID (defined in their study by abrupt onset, fluctuating course, history of strokes, focal neurologic symptoms and signs) for 6 years. One hundred and two patients died, and the mean 6-year survival rate was 11.9% versus 45.2% expected survival rate. This finding demonstrates a survival rate worse than the 21.1% survival rate of those with Alzheimer's disease. The mean duration of MID was 5.2 years, and the mean age at death was 82.4 years. The survival rate was independent of the severity of dementia. The underlying cause of death was dementia in 38.2% of cases and acute cerebrovascular event in 33.3% of cases. Skoog and colleagues looked at 85 year olds and, using criteria for VD proposed by Erkinjuntti, including MID, probable VD or mixed dementia, and hypoperfusion dementia, found a 3-year mortality of 66.7% as contrasted to 42.2% in Alzheimer's disease and 23.1% in those without dementia. Meyer and associates studied 125 patients with MID defined by a modified Hachinski ischemic scale, cognitive testing, brain imaging, and history of sudden onset of stepwise and progressive mental deterioration. These authors found a mean age of 67.1 years and a 5.1% mortality rate.

Tatemichi and coworkers found that dementia after stroke was a predictor in long-term survival. In their study of 251 patients after stroke, they found that 66 (26.3%) were demented at 3 months. The mortality rate was 19.8 deaths per 100 person-years as contrasted to 6.9 deaths per person-years in patients without dementia after stroke.

The variable mortality rates reflect differences in definition of VD, diagnostic criteria, age of the patients, and study designs. These studies do not describe the etiopathology underlying their cases, such as probable cardioembolic versus small-vessel disease. These etiopathologies may confer different risks for the patients. However, the diagnosis of VD by all these methods appears to confer an increased short-term mortality as compared to those of similar age without this diagnosis.

Factors Affecting Prognosis

Most definitions of dementia are derived from patients with Alzheimer's disease. Thus, the definitions require memory loss and a level of cognitive decline that interferes with daily function, meaning that patients are affected severely by the time they receive diagnosis of VD.

Three mechanisms of VD—multi-infarct, strategic infarct, and infarct acting on underlying Alzheimer's disease—result in risk factors for stroke that are presumably the most important factors for prognosis (age, male gender, race, hypertension, cardiac disease, prior cerebrovascular event, cigarette smoking, diabetes, and hyperlipidemia). Moroney and associates looked for factors that may increase the risk of dementia after stroke. They found that patients with hypoxic-ischemic disorders (cardiopulmonary arrest, congestive heart failure, myocardial infarction, cardiac arrhythmia, seizures, syncope, pneumonia, respiratory failure, etc.) had a relative risk of 4.3 of becoming demented compared with those without an hypoxic-ischemic event. Some so-called instances of chronic ischemia may be due to severe extracranial artery stenosis; others may have chronic hypertension as their basis.

The risk associated with the apolipoprotein E-4 allele in patients with VD has not been differentiated clearly from its risk for Alzheimer's disease. However, it may become another factor affecting prognosis in the near future.

Evaluation for Prognosis

Many tests required for the diagnosis of VD are important to understanding the mechanism of the dementia and the underlying pathology. White-matter changes can be seen on CT scanning or magnetic resonance imaging. On CT scan, these changes appear as hypodense areas surrounding the ventricles and at times extending into the centrum semiovale. Pathologic studies have described a variety of substrates for these changes, including demyelination, lacunar infarction, dilated perivascular spaces, and hydrocephalus. To avoid presupposition on the etiology of this finding, the term *leukoaraiosis* was introduced. Although leukoaraiosis can be found in normal patients, moderate to severe leukoaraiosis is more common in patients with VD than in normal controls. The presence of leukoaraiosis has been related also to an increased risk of future stroke in patients with transient ischemic attacks or minor stroke. The CT scan of the brain also can show the number and locations of strokes that the patient may have experienced, giving evidence for the possible underlying etiology of the strokes.

Therapies Affecting Prognosis

Therapies affecting the prognosis of VD are presumably those for the secondary prevention of stroke. Proved therapies for secondary prevention of stroke are carotid endarterectomy for symptomatic carotid artery stenosis measured greater than 70% on angiography using the method of the North American Symptomatic Carotid Endarterectomy Trial; antiplatelet agents (aspirin, ticlopidine); and anticoagulation for atrial fibrillation. Other treatments include aggressive management of such stroke risk factors as hypertension, diabetes mellitus, hyperlipidemia, cigarette smoking, and possibly homocystinemia. Although the benefit of aggressive secondary stroke prevention for an improved course of VD makes clinical sense, it has not been tested in a clinical trial.

In a study with few patients, Meyer and coworkers found improved cognition and clinical course in patients with MID after smoking cessation, 325 mg per day of aspirin, and control of systolic blood pressure to between 135 and 150 mm Hg. Further studies with larger numbers of patients are needed to confirm these observations.

A trial of propentophylline is being conducted to assess its benefit in VD. The impact that thrombolysis or other acute stroke treatment has on the development of VD is not known at this time, although theoretically they could be beneficial. The study by Moroney and associates suggests that aggressive treatment of comorbid illnesses causing hypoxia or ischemia might be beneficial in VD.

Short-Term Prognosis

The short-term prognosis of VD is not known at this time. The major obstacles to determining the prognosis of VD have been described. First, further studies are needed to indicate better the type of VD being studied, including the mechanism and etiopathology of the dementia. Second, as vascular causes of dementia likely are preventable and treatable, identifying patients is necessary early in the course of the disease process, when interventions could be most beneficial. This approach could be accomplished by assessing patients with amounts of cognitive impairment less severe than are required for the current definitions of dementia. For this reason, the term *vascular cognitive impairment* has been suggested to replace VD. Vascular cognitive impairment would encompass a full spectrum of patients from those with high risk but no cognitive deficit to those with mild cognitive impairment to those with full dementia.

Long-Term Prognosis

The long-term prognosis of VD also is not known. Two epidemiologic studies described in Natural History showed poor long-term survival associated with the diagnosis. Owing to the multiple possible mechanisms and pathology of this group of diseases, its natural history is unclear, and the effect on survival or quality of life of the treatments described in Therapies Affecting Prognosis are not known. With studies clearly defining the vascular components of this disease group and perhaps identifying cognitive impairment at an earlier stage, it can be hoped that, in the future, more will be known about the prognosis of this potentially treatable disease.

Additional Reading

Hachinski VC. Preventable senility: a call for action against the vascular dementias. Lancet 1992;340:645–648.

Hachinski VC. Vascular dementia: a radical redefinition. Dementia 1994;5:130–132.

Meyer JS, Rogers RL, Mortel KF. Multi-infarct dementia: demography, risk factors, and therapy. In MD Ginsberg, WD Dietrich (eds), Cerebrovascular Diseases. New York: Raven, 1989;199–206.

Molsa PK, Marttila RJ, Rinne UK. Survival and cause of death in Alzheimer's disease and multi-infarct dementia. Acta Neurol Scand 1986;74:103–107.

Moroney JT, Bagiella E, Desmond DW, et al. Risk factors for incident dementia after stroke. Role of hypoxic and ischemic disorders. Stroke 1996;27:1283–1289.

Skoog I, Nilsson L, Palmertz B, et al. A population-based study of dementia in 85-year-olds. N Engl J Med 1993;328:153–158.

Snowdon DA, Greiner LH, Mortimer JA, et al. Brain infarction and the clinical expression of Alzheimer Disease. The Nun Study. JAMA 1997;277:813–817.

Tatemichi TK, Paik M, Bagiella E, et al. Dementia after stroke is a long term predictor of long term survival. Stroke 1994;25:1915–1919.

Tatemichi TK, Paik M, Bagiella E, et al. Risk of dementia after stroke in a hospitalized cohort: results of a longitudinal study. Neurology 1994;44:1885–1891.

Treves TA, Arnovich BD, Bornstein NM, Korczyn AD. Risk of dementia after a first-ever ischemic stroke: a 3-year longitudinal study. Cerebrovasc Dis 1997;7:48–52.

Verhey FRJ, Lodder J, Rozendaal N, Jolles J. Comparison of seven sets of criteria used for the diagnosis of vascular dementia. Neuroepidemiology 1996;15:166–172.

Chapter 22

Immune-Mediated Vasculopathies of the Central Nervous System

Patricia M. Moore

Immune-mediated neurovascular diseases comprise a wide group of disorders, defined by immune-mediated damage to the vessel wall and attendant tissue ischemia. Because many diseases have a central feature of vasculitis or immune-mediated vasculopathy and tissue injury occurs at various stages in the course of the disease, the disorders are grouped into idiopathic vasculitides, secondary vasculitides, and immune-mediated vasculopathies. Clinically, the most easily recognized are the idiopathic and secondary vasculitides, which share evidence of tissue inflammation and may be distinguished by their distinctive clinical profiles and underlying etiologies. Neurovascular abnormalities also are a component of chronic, systemic inflammation and connective tissue diseases; in many cases, the tissue ischemia may be dispersed temporally from evidence of acute disease. The prognosis depends on the cause of the inflammation and the nature of the vascular injury. Factors influencing the prognosis of disease may be local to the region of the central nervous system (CNS) or peripheral nervous system ischemia or may be systemic. In general, the local features largely determine the extent of recovery. The systemic features, particularly organ failure, are crucial to mortality (Table 22-1).

Natural History

Inflammation in and around blood vessels is integral to numerous physiologic and pathologic processes. The physiologic processes provide rapid response and delivery of cells to regions where the integrity of tissue is threatened. The pathophysiologic mechanisms causing disease are multiple and well defined in only a few disorders. Many observed pathologic processes differ from physiologic inflammation principally in extent, duration, and location.

The combination of physical obstruction of blood flow by immune cells, increased coagulation, and contraction of vessel diameter (in those arteries with smooth muscle cells) seen in pathologic inflammation may precipitate tissue ischemia. The clinical manifestations and outcome then depend on the location and extent of tissue ischemia and on the ability of the specific tissue to regenerate or recover function. Generally, ischemia of the peripheral nervous system heals more quickly and completely than does that of the CNS. Nonetheless, depending on the extent of ischemia, neuropathies heal over months to years. The CNS features of vasculitis vary with the location of ischemia. Clinical episodes may be transient, despite tissue infarction (probably because viable cells rapidly subsume the lost function) or permanent, such as often occurs in infarction of the occipital lobes, cerebellum, or brain stem. The longer-term outcome of the vasculitides depends on the extent of scarring in the blood vessel wall and whether the vascular inflammation is recurrent (Table 22-2). Scarring of the vessel wall by inflammation renders it vulnerable to additional damage from hypertension, hyperlipidemia, and potentially adverse effects of corticosteroid therapy.

The systemic manifestations of inflammation are critical to morbidity and mortality even in those diseases in which local neurologic consequences of vascular inflammation can be quieted or cured. Two

Table 22-1. Factors Determining Prognosis

Local factors
  Location and extent of tissue ischemia associated with
    initial immune event
  Healing of the vessel with normal integrity or by scarring
  Recurrence of vasculitis or immune vascular injury
Systemic factors
  Distribution of vascular injury and the presence of organ
    failure
  Systemic effects from inflammation
  Recurrence of vascular inflammation
  Efficacy and consequences of therapy

prominent aspects are the presence of organ failure—particularly renal, cardiac, and pulmonary—and complications of therapy, notably infections and such side effects as vasoconstriction.

Specific Diseases

Idiopathic Vasculitides

Polyarteritis Nodosa

Polyarteritis nodosa (PAN) affects medium- and small-sized vessels throughout the body and has various clinical manifestations, a spectrum of severity and, probably, numerous causes. Hepatitis B–associated PAN has been separated from other forms of PAN to emphasize that antiviral agents in association with immunosuppressive and anti-inflammatory therapy can improve the outcome.

Systemic Disease.   The 5-year survival of patients with systemic PAN rose from 18% untreated to 55% treated with corticosteroid therapy alone to 79% with combination prednisone and cyclophosphamide therapy. The mortality is greatest in the first year of disease and historically remains associated most closely with organ failure, particularly gastrointestinal tract disease. A prospective study of 326 patients confirmed that organ failure remains the predominant feature determining survival over the 3-year course of the study. Gastrointestinal tract failure is largely irreversible. Although early proteinuria is associated with increased mortality, overt renal failure is reversible in many patients. CNS disease and cardiomyopathy are overall risk factors for death but do not individually increase early mortality. The other feature determining survival and morbidity is the complication rate of immunosuppressive therapy, especially infections.

Table 22-2. Prognosis of Various Immune-Mediated Vasculopathies

Disease	Recovery from Initial Event	Recurrent Inflammation	Vascular Scarring	Organ Failure
Idiopathic vasculitides				
Polyarteritis nodosa	Good	+++	Yes	Yes
Wegener's granulomatosis	Fair	++	Yes	Yes
Churg-Strauss syndrome	Good	+	?	+/–
Temporal arteritis	Fair	+	+/–	No
Isolated angiitis of the CNS	Good	+	+	No
Secondary vasculitides				
Secondary to infection	Fair	+/–	+/–	Yes
Secondary to toxins	Fair	+/–	+/–	No
Secondary to neoplasia	Fair	+/–	+/–	Yes
Vasculopathies associated with immune-mediated injury				
Systemic lupus erythematosus	Fair	Yes	Yes	Yes
Hematologic abnormalities	Good	No	No	Yes
Systemic inflammation	Fair	Yes	Yes	?
Autoantibodies	?	No	No	?

CNS = central nervous system; +++ = very common; ++ = common; + = less common; +/– = possible; ? = unclear.

Neurologic Disease. Peripheral neuropathies are one of the defining features of polyarteritis nodosa. Except for seizures and subarachnoid hemorrhage that may occur early, such CNS abnormalities as stroke usually occur later in the course of disease. The frequent ischemic neuropathies heal well, albeit slowly (months to years) and, when recurrence of the PAN is controlled, the neuropathies are not prominent in the morbidity and mortality of disease. Similarly, seizures seldom are recurrent and are controlled easily with medications. Visual abnormalities develop from vasculitis in regions spanning the orbits, the optic nerve and tracts, the visual cortex, and the cranial nerves and brain regions controlling ocular motility.

Substantial experience by several groups revealed that the later complications of PAN affect survival but, as they are distributed over the life span of patients, a separate analysis of risk is needed. The longer-term morbidity results from degenerative and hypertensive vascular disease affecting the heart, CNS, and kidneys. Not clear is whether the origin of the degeneration is a subclinical vasculitis in the coronary and cerebral vasculature healing with fibrosis and scarring or whether the vasculopathy is primarily degenerative and is exacerbated by hypertension and medications. I anticipate, although it is not yet studied, that the addition of therapeutic agents that minimize platelet aggregation and vasoconstriction to the medical regimen and the use of the lowest clinically effective dosages of corticosteroids will reduce the longer-term complications.

Churg-Strauss Syndrome

Churg-Strauss syndrome (CSS) initially was classified with PAN but is increasingly regarded as a distinct entity, though a recognized overlap exists. Features traditionally marking CSS are asthma, hypereosinophilia, and systemic small-vessel vasculitis that often affects peripheral nerves.

Systemic Disease. The mortality of the disease reflects the distribution of the systemic vasculitis, with visceral organ failure the prominent determining feature. Asthma plays little role in the outcome. Some investigators consider the disease to be less aggressive than is Wegener's granulomatosis or PAN. One study indicated that both the sequelae of

early episodes and the relapse rate are lower in CSS than in the other systemic vasculitides.

Neurologic Disease. Clinically, neuropathies occur in more than 65% of patients and, as in PAN, often are defining features of the disease. The CNS manifestations vary, but the 10 to 15% of patients with subarachnoid hemorrhage, visual loss, or stroke do not influence the mortality figures. Encephalopathies appear more frequently than in the other systemic necrotizing vasculitides, but whether this reflects increased incidence or increased recognition is not known.

Wegener's Granulomatosis

Wegener's granulomatosis is another systemic necrotizing vasculitis. Characteristic features are upper and lower respiratory tract involvement, glomerulonephritis, and systemic vasculitis. The strong association of Wegener's granulomatosis and circulating antineutrophilic cytoplasmic antibodies is an aid in diagnosis, although none of the forms of antineutrophilic cytoplasmic antibodies currently are useful in determining overall relapse rate, type of relapse, morbidity, or longevity. Patients have had a dramatic improvement in survival with the advent of cyclophosphamide therapy.

Previously, Wegener's granulomatosis was fatal over 4 to 6 months in untreated patients and 11 months with prednisone therapy alone. Long-term survivals now are routine in patients treated with prednisone-cyclophosphamide therapy. To reduce the long-term features of diseases and the side effects of medication, recent trials have examined other therapies. Notably, treatment with trimethoprim-sulfamethoxazole may decrease relapse rate, particularly in those patients who are nasal carriers of certain staphylococcal strains.

Systemic Disease. The early mortality results from progressive disease leading to organ failure despite therapy. Because of a relapse rate higher in Wegener's granulomatosis than in PAN or CSS, acute complications of disease extend beyond 1 year.

Neurologic Disease. Overall, neurologic abnormalities have declined since the advent of combination therapy, but peripheral neuropathies and cranial neuropathies remain frequent. The very erosive nature of the early lesions produces prominent tissue destruction; healing of the upper respiratory tract and the cranial neuropathies often is incomplete. After the systemic disease is under control, the onset of neurologic abnormalities is unlikely.

Temporal Arteritis (Giant Cell Arteritis)

Temporal arteritis typically affects persons older than 50 and appears more prevalent among women of Northern European background. Several studies reveal both a seasonal and cyclic variation (over 5 to 7 years) in incidence.

Systemic Disease.   Although temporal arteritis is a systemic arteritis, clinical features (except for malaise and arthralgias) seldom occur below the neck. When systemic features are prominent, the diagnosis is more likely to be PAN or CSS.

Neurologic Disease.   Headaches, tender temporal arteries, and jaw claudication predominate in temporal arteritis, although ischemic optic neuropathies remain the feared complication. Occasionally, intracranial disease referable to the posterior circulation occurs. The natural history, based on several older series, indicates the disease is self-limited, although several exacerbations often occur before symptoms subside. In recent studies, survival was not diminished in patients with temporal arteritis as compared with age-matched cohorts. Corticosteroid therapy alone appears effective in preventing the devastating ischemia to the visual system, but little evidence substantiates that it alters the course. When blindness arises, recovery of vision is infrequent, occurring in less than 15% of patients. The less frequent ophthalmoplegias share a better prognosis, with substantial improvement or resolution in most patients. Given the real and potential complications of corticosteroid therapy, determining the necessary duration of therapy is important, albeit difficult. Given the documented relapses with visual loss after short-term corticosteroid therapy, most specialists in vasculitis continue the medication for at least 1 year.

Isolated Angiitis of the Central Nervous System

Isolated angiitis of the CNS is an idiopathic vasculitis affecting blood vessels of the CNS within the dural reflections. Although the disease was originally described as fatal, treatment with cyclophosphamide dramatically decreases the morbidity and mortality of the disease. Current issues focus more on the definition and prevalence than on therapy for the disease. I use criteria published previously: clinical features consistent with recurrent, multifocal vascular disease; exclusion of an underlying systemic inflammatory process or infection; neuroradiographic studies, usually a cerebral angiogram, supporting diagnosis of vasculopathy; and brain biopsy to establish the presence of vascular inflammation and to exclude infection, neoplasia, or alternate causes of vasculopathy. In my experience, the recent increased frequency of diagnosis well may reflect lax criteria rather than rising incidence.

Systemic Disease.   Systemic features are absent from this disease, which targets the CNS vasculature. Any evidence of systemic disease should initiate a search for alternative diagnoses.

Neurologic Disease.   Neurologic features are protean, although typically headaches, encephalopathy, and multifocal signs suggest the diagnosis. Untreated, recurrent ischemia leads to coma and death, although the time frame is not established clearly. Early studies described the mortality in untreated patients as 9 months to 1 year. More recently, I have observed that untreated disease may smolder over several years, although recurrent disease is the rule. Patients treated with prednisone alone have a high relapse rate, in one study greater than 90%. Therapy with cyclophosphamide, usually in combination with a low dosage of prednisone, results in a cure in many patients. Although the relapse rate cannot be determined accurately given the rarity of the disease, it appears to be below 10%. To some extent, this figure depends on the duration of cyclophosphamide therapy. An early series of patients treated for 6 months after clinical remission of symptoms developed a relapse in 30%. The current protocol of 12 months of therapy corresponds to a relapse rate lower than 10%. The outcome of individual neurologic episodes is fairly good, with many patients returning to normal function. As with other types of vascular injury, the occipital cortex heals poorly, and hemianopsias usually are persistent. The radiculopathy-myelopathy features encountered in some patients do heal, albeit slowly. Episodes of mania or psychoses may recur, and treatment may be difficult, but episodes may subside with therapy.

Secondary Vasculitides

Successful prognostication requires recognition and correct diagnosis of the secondary vasculitides: vasculitis secondary to infections, to toxins, and to neoplasia. These diseases share several features: They occur more frequently than do the idiopathic vasculitides; prompt diagnosis and appropriate therapy greatly improve prognosis; and tissue biopsy often is the sole test in distinguishing secondary from idiopathic disorders. The secondary vasculitides involve the CNS more than the peripheral nervous system, although this tendency may be an artifact of recognition.

The secondary vasculitides are grouped together not because of an absence of differences in prognoses between vasculitis secondary to infections and vasculitis secondary to toxins but because the prognosis is so dependent on the specific underlying etiology that differences between the groups are less critical. In general, as would be anticipated, the more virulent the underlying process, the worse the outcome for the vasculitic components of disease (e.g., vasculitis associated with a bacterial meningitis has a higher mortality and morbidity—strokes, cranial neuropathies—than does vasculitis associated with treponemal infections). With indolent infections, an important variable in prognosis is duration of disease before diagnosis and treatment. In these cases, treatment of the acute inflammation does not diminish the damage from chronic cicatrization of the blood vessel wall. Ischemia from scarring is as devastating as that from acute inflammation.

Vasculitides associated with malignancy occur infrequently. This group emphasizes the need for histology in making a diagnosis. Isolated angiitis of the CNS, CNS vasculitis secondary to a lymphoma, and CNS lymphoma without vasculitis may be clinically and radiographically indistinguishable. The treatment and prognosis depend on accurate diagnosis.

Vascular diseases associated with toxins are well known. However, vascular inflammation occurs in only a small percentage of toxin-mediated vascular injury. The relevance of this finding to the prognosis is substantial, as a great deal of toxin-mediated CNS vascular disease is chronic and hemorrhagic and is unrelieved by prednisone or immunosuppressive therapy.

Vasculopathies Associated with Immune-Mediated Injury

Immune-mediated injuries with which vasculopathies might be associated include systemic lupus erythematosus (SLE), hematologic abnormalities, systemic inflammation, and autoantibodies. Vascular inflammation often is a dramatic manifestation of an illness and directs the patient and physician to early diagnosis and intervention. Inflammation is, however, only part of the spectrum of immune-mediated vascular disease. An examination of the effects of inflammation itself on the vasculature renders apparent that numerous mediators may increase coagulation, alter vasomotor tone, stimulate cell proliferation in the vessel wall, and modify the turnover and transport of essential nutrients within the vascular tree. Although eliciting inflammation in the CNS is more difficult than in the systemic vasculature, the extent of responses of the CNS to injury is only beginning to be understood. The range of diseases that may share immune-mediated vascular damage is large. In some, such as thrombotic thrombocytopenic purpura, the abnormalities are histologically mild and clinically transient. If the underlying disorder is treated, recovery is typical.

At the other end of the spectrum is SLE. Vasculitis of the CNS is rare in SLE, although chronic, degenerative changes or a bland vasculopathy in the vessel wall are frequent. Studies in animal models of autoimmunity indicate that persistent, albeit low-level, circulating immune complexes are associated with a degenerative process rather than with the inflammatory disorder usually associated with induced immune complex disease. The numerous features contributing to the CNS vascular abnormalities are not yet definable, yet they profoundly influence the prognosis of SLE. The vascular disease, when clinically manifest, is not treatable with anti-inflammatory medications, which may cause deterioration of the histologic picture. Further studies and the prevention of vascular disease are more likely to have an impact on prognosis.

Similarly, the role of antiphospholipid antibodies in inflammatory or immune-mediated vasculopathies is yet to be defined. To date, therapies aimed at reducing the titer of antiphospholipid antibodies have not altered the recurrence or sequelae of vascular disease.

Additional Reading

Abu-Shakra M., Smythe H, Lewtas J, et al. Outcome of polyarteritis nodosa and Churg-Strauss syndrome. An analysis of twenty-five patients. Arthritis Rheum 1994;37: 1798–1803.

Cohen P, Guillevin L, Baril L, et al. Persistence of antineutrophil cytoplasmic antibodies (ANCA) in asymptomatic patients with systemic polyarteritis nodosa or Churg-Strauss syndrome: follow-up of 53 patients. Clin Exp Rheum 1995;13:193–198.

Giang DW. Central nervous system vasculitis secondary to infections, toxins, and neoplasms. Semin Neurol 1994; 14:313–319.

Guillevin L, Lhote F, Amouroux J, et al. Antineutrophil cytoplasmic antibodies, abnormal angiograms and pathological findings in polyarteritis nodosa and Churg-Strauss syndrome: indications for the classification of vasculitides of the polyarteritis nodosa group. Br J Rheumatol 1996;35:958–964.

Guillevin L, Lhote F, Gayroud M, et al. Prognostic factors in polyarteritis nodosa and Churg-Straus syndrome. A prospective study in 342 patients. Medicine 1996; 75:17–28.

Moore PM. Diagnosis and management of isolated angiitis of the central nervous system. Neurology 1989;39: 167–173.

Moore PM. Neurological manifestation of vasculitis: update on immunopathogenic mechanisms and clinical features. Ann Neurol 1995;37:S131–S141.

Nishino H, Rubino FA, DeRemee RA, et al. Neurological involvement in Wegener's granulomatosis: an analysis of 324 consecutive patients at the Mayo Clinic. Ann Neurol 1993;33:4–9.

Parisi JE, Moore PM. The role of biopsy in vasculitis of the central nervous system. Semin Neurol 1994;14: 341–348.

Part IV

Degenerative Disorders

Chapter 23

Alzheimer's Disease and Other Cortical Dementias

Brian R. Ott

Alzheimer's Disease

Alzheimer's disease is the leading cause of dementia, accounting for at least 55 to 65% of cases in the elderly. An estimated 4 million persons are affected with Alzheimer's disease in the United States. Prevalence of the disease no doubt will increase as the longevity of the population increases.

The disease is progressive and leads ultimately to a state of total dependence on others for activities of daily living. More than 50% of those admitted to nursing homes have Alzheimer's disease or a related dementia disorder, making it a major socioeconomic and medical burden on the population. Dementia itself is an adverse prognostic indicator for mortality among the institutionalized.

Other cortical diseases causing dementia are considerably less common; therefore, Alzheimer's disease will be the primary focus of this chapter. Knowledge about the prognosis of Alzheimer's disease is essential for the physician to properly advise families about long-range medical and financial planning.

Natural History

Alzheimer's disease is a degenerative disorder that, like other cerebral degenerations, follows a progressive course of clinical deterioration characterized by loss of cognitive and functional abilities and by changes in mood and behavior. The earliest symptoms consist of amnesia and impairment in word finding. Depression and relative retention of insight into deficits may coexist. Personality and social behavior generally are preserved in the beginning.

Eventually, patients develop additional problems of cognition, including aphasia, apraxia, agnosia, and executive and visuospatial impairments. Psychiatric or noncognitive behavior problems develop and include sleep disturbances, apathy, irritability, depression, delusions, hallucinations, wandering, and pacing. Insight and judgment become impaired. Late stages of the disease are accompanied by impaired movement and rigidity, complete loss of communication abilities, and loss of bowel and bladder control. Myoclonus and seizures may occur as late manifestations in some 10 to 20% of cases.

Though this pattern of decline is well recognized, heterogeneity exists in rate of decline and qualitative features of decline among individuals. Efforts have been made by longitudinal research studies to define (1) predictors of rate of cognitive decline, (2) predictors of mortality, and (3) functional impairments or behavioral problems that lead to institutional placement. The absence of a treatment that alters the disease process has allowed researchers to accumulate recent data about the natural history of the disease and the significance of specific prognostic factors.

Factors Affecting Prognosis

The original case described by Alois Alzheimer in 1907 was that of a 51-year-old woman with amnesia, aphasia, and delusions. Subsequently, patients with onset of dementia in the presenium (younger than 65 years) were said to have Alzheimer's disease or presenile dementia, whereas those with onset after the age of 65 were deemed as having senility or senile dementia. Although all patients with a degenerative dementia of the Alzheimer type, regardless of age, now are said to have probable Alzheimer's disease, evidence has accumulated to suggest that age of onset nevertheless may affect prognosis. Early age at onset has been associated with more rapid cognitive decline in several studies; however, conflicting results from others have been reported. Even less convincing evidence suggests a relationship between family history of dementia and rate of progression in Alzheimer's disease.

Psychotic features, such as paranoia and hallucinations, and extrapyramidal signs, such as bradykinesia, have been related to faster decline in self-care activities. Aggression, sleep disturbance, psychosis and extrapyramidal signs, and lower scores on verbal neuropsychological tests have been related to faster decline in cognition.

Men tend to have a lower survival rate than do women with dementia. This observation is explainable at least partially by the lower survival rate of elderly men in general. Other factors that have a less well-defined adverse effect on prognosis include myoclonus, late age at onset, history of alcohol abuse, and hearing impairment.

Evaluation for Prognosis

The rate of cognitive decline in Alzheimer's disease is not linear. Patients with early-stage disease decline at a slower rate than do those in a more advanced stage. Cognitive screening tests, such as the Mini-Mental State Examination, the short or long versions of the Blessed Information-Memory-Concentration test, and the Mattis Dementia Rating Scale, provide reasonable measurements of disease progression. Through results of such measures, initial severity of cognitive impairment and the rate of decline can predict clinical disease progression in Alzheimer's disease. Measures of instrumental daily activity function, though important, tend to reach a floor before late stages of disease.

Magnetic resonance images, computed tomography scans, and electroencephalography generally have not provided clinically useful measures of prognosis. Temporal lobe degeneration (as evidenced by atrophy on radiographic studies) or regional cerebral blood flow on single-photon emission computed tomograms has been related to more severe psychotic features and faster rate of cognitive decline.

Most recently, the presence of the apolipoprotein (apo) E-4 allele has been shown by multiple investigation sites to be a strong risk factor for developing Alzheimer's disease and a risk factor for earlier onset. Despite this association, evidence for the apo E-4 allele as an adverse prognostic factor for disease progression is weak. Recent studies have shown that the apo E genotype does not predict either cognitive or functional decline in patients with established Alzheimer's disease. The apo E-4 allele may be more important as a determinant of disease progression in the preclinical phase. It also may prove useful to predict response to cholinomimetic agents.

Therapies Affecting Prognosis

Epidemiologic studies have not examined psychoactive drug treatments as confounders of the natural history of disease progression. This issue is particularly important in trying to understand the effect of psychosis on progression, as adverse effects of neuroleptic agents for paranoia, hallucinations, or aggression may influence functional as well as cognitive abilities. Despite advances in treatment for many other types of medical problems, the last several decades have seen no evidence of improved survival for dementia patients. Therefore, it seems unlikely that survival will be altered substantially until development of disease-specific treatment that will slow or block the process of neurodegeneration.

The advent of cholinomimetic therapy for cognitive dysfunction in Alzheimer's disease has raised hope that pharmacotherapy may alter the dire prognosis of Alzheimer's disease. In a retrospective analysis done 2 years after completion of a randomized trial of tacrine for Alzheimer's disease, Knopman and coworkers reported that patients receiving higher doses of tacrine were less likely to die and less likely to be placed in a nursing home than were those on lower doses of the drug (i.e., <120 mg per day).

Accumulating evidence suggests that the drop in estrogen levels at menopause accounts for the increased incidence of Alzheimer's disease in women and that estrogen replacement therapy may ameliorate this effect. Estrogen has a number of salutary properties, including enhancement of acetylcholine release and synaptic function and serving as a potential nerve growth factor. Prospective trials are assessing the effect of estrogen on the development of Alzheimer's disease and its effect on disease progression. A number of other compounds also are being tested as potential agents to restore nerve function (e.g., nerve growth factor) or to retard the degeneration process (e.g., anti-inflammatory agents and selegiline).

Short-Term Prognosis

As mentioned, hallucinations and delusions independent of cognitive status may identify a subgroup of patients with rapid functional decline. Psychosis and extrapyramidal signs are associated with more rapid cognitive and functional decline and subsequently with earlier nursing home placement and death.

Up to 75% of persons with Alzheimer's disease ultimately are placed in nursing homes, where they live for an average of 3 years. The survival of outpatients with dementia is better than for those in nursing homes, a finding probably owing to differences in disease severity. In one comparative study, van Dijk and coworkers reported that the 2-year survival rate for outpatients was 75% as contrasted to 50% for nursing home residents.

Long-Term Prognosis

The mean length of time from dementia onset to death ranges from 5 to 8 years. Older individuals die sooner than do younger individuals after onset of disease. Conditions associated with death in those with Alzheimer's disease often are treatable and include infections (particularly pulmonary), trauma, nutritional deficiency, decubitus, aspiration, sensory deficits, Parkinson's disease, and epilepsy.

Factors identified with early mortality in Alzheimer's disease include male gender, severity of impairment on scales of general cognition and activities of daily living, wandering, agitation, vascular disease, and sensory impairment. Severity of language impairment and measures of overall cognitive impairment are predictive of institutionalization and death, particularly among those with early-onset disease. Though shortened survival has been associated with severity of disease, duration of disease is a relatively poor predictor of clinical course.

Other Dementia Disorders

Several longitudinal studies have associated vascular dementia with a prognosis poorer than that for Alzheimer's disease. Wang and Whanger reported mean survival of 6.8 years for early-onset Alzheimer's disease, 5.1 years for late-onset Alzheimer's disease, and 3.8 years for vascular dementia. In a more recent study, Barclay reported a mean survival of 8.1 years for Alzheimer's disease and 6.7 years for vascular dementia (Fig. 23-1).

Dementia after stroke is an adverse predictor of long-term survival. In an 8-year follow-up study of 606 nursing home dementia patients, van Dijk reported that comorbid factors independent of disease severity were strong predictors of mortality. Stroke patients with pulmonary infection had the worst prognosis.

Complicating the interpretation of clinical studies of prognosis in vascular dementia are its common overlap with Alzheimer's disease and the lack of uniform and generally accepted diagnostic criteria. Approximately 10 to 15% of patients with Alzheimer's disease also have stroke. Identification of those in whom there is a significant contribution of vascular pathology to dementia is important, as medical treatment of risk factors and the use of antiplatelet or anticoagulant medications may reduce disease progression.

As mentioned in Factors Affecting Prognosis, the presence of psychosis and extrapyramidal signs connotes a poor prognosis in Alzheimer's disease. One possible explanation for this observation is that these patients constitute a distinct subgroup who have either the Lewy body variant of Alzheimer's disease or diffuse Lewy body disease. Although it is unclear whether such signs are stage-specific, patients with hallucinations and delusions at the onset of their dementia should be suspect for one of these two diagnoses. Other features of diffuse Lewy body disease include fluctuating mental status and marked sensitivity to the extrapyramidal side effects of neuroleptic agents.

Infrequently, dementia patients present with a predominantly frontotemporal degeneration, wherein neurobehavioral characteristics and results of brain imaging studies differ from Alzheimer's disease. Historically, the most well defined of these disorders is Pick's disease. Age of onset is somewhat earlier than in Alzheimer's disease, and the clinical course usually is more prolonged. Most patients develop the disease before age 60 and survive for 6 to 12 years. Prominent changes in behavior, personality, and judgment that occur early in disease may lead to nursing home placement. Apathy, irritability, disinhibition, and sexual indiscretion are particularly problematic management issues.

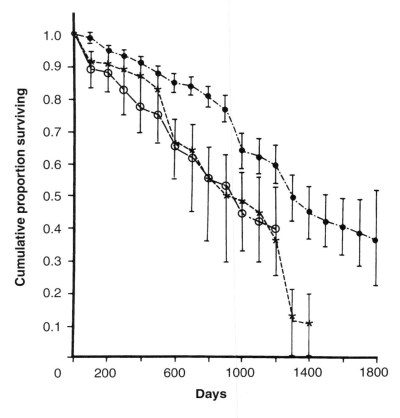

Figure 23-1. Prognosis for survival in dementia of the Alzheimer type (•) and multi-infarct (*) or mixed vascular dementia (○). (Reprinted with permission from LL Barclay, A Zemcov, JP Blass, J Sansone. Survival in Alzheimer's disease and vascular dementias. Neurology 1985;35:837.)

With the development of magnetic resonance imaging and such functional brain imaging studies as positron emission tomography and single-photon emission computed tomography, asymmetric and focal cortical degeneration syndromes are being recognized increasingly. Among the asymmetric degenerations is the syndrome of progressive aphasia. Although half of such patients eventually go on to develop more typical Alzheimer's disease or Pick's disease, a significant proportion remain relatively focal. In the perisylvian area, nonspecific pathologic changes consisting of spongiform change and subcortical gliosis are seen. Recognizing such patients is important, as their prognosis is better than that of patients with probable Alzheimer's disease. Independent functioning may be preserved for many years, with actual dementia being delayed for periods of 3 to 10 years.

Additional Reading

Barclay LL, Zemcov A, Blass JP, Sansone J. Survival in Alzheimer's disease and vascular dementias. Neurology 1985;35:834–840.

Galasko D, Corey-Bloom J, Thal LJ. Monitoring progression in Alzheimer's disease. J Am Geriatr Soc 1991;39:932–941.

Knopman D, Schneider L, Davis K, et al. Long-term tacrine (Cognex) treatment: effects on nursing home placement and mortality. Neurology 1996;47:166–177.

Mortimer JA, Ebbitt B, Jun SP, Finch MD. Predictors of cognitive and functional progression in patients with probable Alzheimer's disease. Neurology 1992;42:1689–1696.

Rossor MN (ed). Unusual Dementias. In Bailliere's Clinical Neurology (Vol 1, No. 3). London: Bailliere Tindall, 1992.

Salmon DP, Thal LJ, Butters N, Heindel WC. Longitudinal evaluation of dementia of the Alzheimer type: a comparison of three standardized mental status examinations. Neurology 1990;40:1225–1230.

Stern Y, Albert M, Brandt J, et al. Utility of extrapyramidal signs and psychosis as predictors of cognitive and functional decline, nursing home admission, and death in Alzheimer's disease: prospective analyses from the Predictors Study. Neurology 1994;44:2300–2307.

van Dijk PT, Dippel DW, Habbema JD. Survival of patients with dementia. J Am Geriatr Soc 1991;39:603–610.

van Dijk PT, Dippel DW, van der Meulen JH, Habbema JD. Comorbidity and its effect on mortality in nursing home patients with dementia. J Nerv Ment Dis 1996;184:180–187.

Wang JA, Whanger A. Brain Impairment and Longevity. In E Palmore, FL Jeffers (eds), Prediction of Life Span. Lexington, MA: Heath, 1971.

Chapter 24

Parkinson's Disease

Joseph H. Friedman

The diagnosis of Parkinson's disease (PD) rests on clinical criteria alone. Laboratory tests may reveal abnormalities besides PD but cannot exclude the diagnosis. Studies looking at accuracy of diagnosis suggest a 20% error rate, with other akinetic rigid syndromes misdiagnosed as PD. The heterogeneity of signs creates this difficulty. Most research criteria for the diagnosis of PD require the presence of three of four cardinal criteria—tremor at rest, rigidity, bradykinesia, and postural instability—and the absence of such atypical features as gaze palsies, corticospinal tract, and cerebellar signs. Accuracy of diagnosis is enhanced by the presence of all four cardinal features: asymmetry at the time of presentation, postural instability developing later than the other signs, dementia (if present) developing as a late manifestation, and beneficial response to L-dopa. Diagnosis can be confirmed only by autopsy.

The median PD age at onset is approximately 60 in the United States and Europe, with some 5% of cases beginning younger than age 40 (young-onset PD). Although rare families develop PD in an autosomal dominant–inherited fashion and familial aggregation of cases is common, most people with PD do not have a family history. The etiology of PD is unknown.

Prognosis in PD refers to the two issues of mortality and disability. Mortality occurs secondary to pneumonia, urinary tract infections, inanition, and complications of falls. Disability occurs as the result of dementia, depression, and motor dysfunction. Such non–drug-induced parkinsonian conditions as progressive supranuclear palsy and striatonigral degeneration, which mimic PD, almost always carry a significantly worse prognosis than does PD in every area of function.

Natural History

Although PD is defined clinically by the presence of four cardinal features, the severity of each sign is highly variable. For example, 20% of patients have no tremor at rest. Thus, some patients may have severe bradykinesia and no tremor, whereas others may have the reverse. Being a very noticeable sign, tremor is the single most common feature bringing patients to medical attention. Gait disturbances, stiffness, slowness, and loss of dexterity are the next most frequent early symptoms. As the disease progresses, the early prominent features tend to remain most prominent. In addition, the rate of disease progression measured from functional (rather than biochemical) markers tends to remain fairly constant.

Using the Hoehn-Yahr staging system (stage I, unilateral parkinsonism; stage II, bilateral; stage III, mild to moderate disability with postural impairment; stage IV, severe disabling disease, able to walk unassisted but markedly incapacitated; stage V, confined to bed or wheelchair unless aided) in the pre–L-dopa era, the median duration of symptoms for those in stage I was 3 years; stage II, 6.0 years; stage III, 7.0 years; stage IV, 9.0 years; and stage V, 14.0 years, with an enormous range at each level. One-third of patients in stage I reportedly had symptoms for more than 5 years.

Once L-dopa became available, natural history studies became ethically unacceptable other than for studying progression in patients not yet requiring L-dopa. One study looking at early, mild, untreated patients with presumed PD not yet requiring symptomatic therapy reported that 60% required the addition of L-dopa within 18 months of entry. The average rate of decline in Unified Parkinson's Disease Rating Scale (UPDRS) scores was 14 points per year. The UPDRS's ranking of 44 items rates the most severe impairment per item at a 4. A moderately severe patient has a score of perhaps 80. Long-term follow-up studies are affected by the usual confounding variables, such as the occurrence of other diseases, particularly Alzheimer's disease, which increases in prevalence with age and may occur concurrently with PD. Cerebrovascular disease also occurs as an independent factor.

A newly recognized disorder, diffuse Lewy body disease (DLBD), further complicates prognosis, as the pathology of PD and DLBD are identical in the brain stem and differ only in the cortex, so that extrapyramidal signs and symptoms are identical. However, the presence of early dementia and behavioral abnormalities makes for a very different clinical course.

Factors Affecting Prognosis

Studies looking at prognostic data have been in relative agreement that the prognosis for patients with "tremor-predominant" PD is better than that for patients with the postural-instability and gait-difficulty (PIGD) variant. However, part of this discrepant outcome is due to the higher error rate of diagnosis. The majority of patients with presumed PD of the PIGD variant are discovered at autopsy not to have PD. Also, as tremor generally is not associated with functional impairment, the PIGD form is more functionally disabling.

Younger age at onset generally predicts a more benign disease progression, possibly explained partly by better compensating mechanisms. As aging itself produces some neurologic changes identical to those of PD, normal aging adds to the functional progression of the disease, independent of the continuing pathologic changes of PD.

The single most important risk factor for death is dysphagia. Usually (but not always) associated with dysarthria, impaired coordination of swallowing muscles leads to frequent aspiration. Dysphagia is particularly severe for nonviscous fluids such as water. Death comes unpredictably and may be delayed by a feeding gastrostomy, depending on the patient's and family's instructions, sometimes for years.

Evaluation for Prognosis

Laboratory data, such as imaging and physiologic studies, are not useful for prognostication.

Therapies Affecting Prognosis

Response to L-dopa is a risk factor that has never been assessed for prognosis. Some 90% of patients in whom PD is clinically diagnosed respond to L-dopa, and many of the 10% of nonresponders are found to have other akinetic rigid syndromes. Rare autopsy-confirmed PD patients, however, have been reported to experience no improvement from L-dopa. The extent of the improvement on L-dopa therapy is highly variable, with some patients improving dramatically and others only minimally. The extent of L-dopa response cannot be predicted, other than that the PIGD subset of patients, reflecting a higher percentage of non-PD parkinsonian syndromes, are less likely to respond. The improvement on L-dopa is important for prognosis, as failure to respond to L-dopa generally predicts a failure to respond to other anti-Parkinson medications.

Psychosis is not a feature of untreated PD but is a common side effect of L-dopa and other anti-PD medications. Psychosis is the single most important risk factor for nursing home placement, exceeding motor impairment. Dementia is the largest risk factor for a psychotic response to L-dopa. Therefore, dementia is a major prognostic feature clearly tied to a worse outcome, as drug treatment for motoric function is limited by mental side effects. It is also a major risk factor for death.

Short-Term Prognosis

The short-term prognosis in PD hinges on the response to L-dopa. In general, patients who fail to

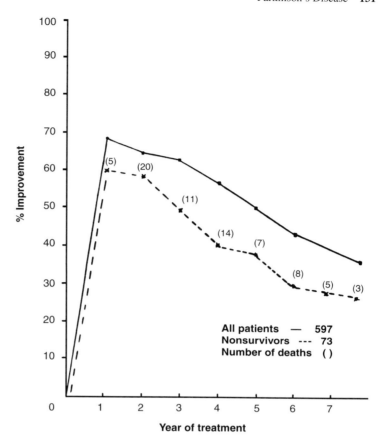

Figure 24-1. Declining improvement over time on L-dopa. (Reprinted with permission from MD Yahr. In W Birkmayer, D Hornykiewicz (eds), Advances in Parkinsonism. Basel: Editones Roche, 1976;444–455.)

respond to this drug rarely respond to the other anti-PD medications in any significant way. Although 50% of patients develop complications of L-dopa therapy within 3 to 5 years of drug initiation, it is unknown whether these complications are due to total drug dose, duration of therapy, or other factors. As a result of this uncertainty, many PD specialists attempt to postpone initiation of L-dopa therapy until "needed" rather than simply at diagnosis. Using this highly individualized approach, 60% of mildly affected, untreated PD patients "required" L-dopa within 2 years of diagnosis. The patients with tremor have perhaps an 80% response rate to L-dopa, and the patients who have postural instability as an early feature have only a 30% response rate, owing in part to diagnostic errors. The degree of response to the drug varies considerably, from a near miraculous recovery to a minimal improvement in speed or tremor. In any patient, the degree

of benefit is unpredictable, but younger patients generally show a better response. Of the cardinal features of PD, tremor generally is the least predictable in its response to medications. Tremor may resolve almost completely on L-dopa or may not improve at all. Tremor may be more responsive to anticholinergics or amantadine, to all, or to none. Anticholinergics work best on tremor and rigidity and not as well on bradykinesia and dexterity—problems much more likely to respond to L-dopa and dopaminergic drugs.

At a mean dose of 300 mg L-dopa per day, mild to moderate PD patients had motor scores on the UPDRS improve from 44 to 20. The score on an activities-of-daily-living scale improved from 80 to 86% (wherein 100% is normal). L-Dopa is thought to have no impact on disease progression, although the theoretic concern remains that the drug may hasten disease progression (Fig. 24-1).

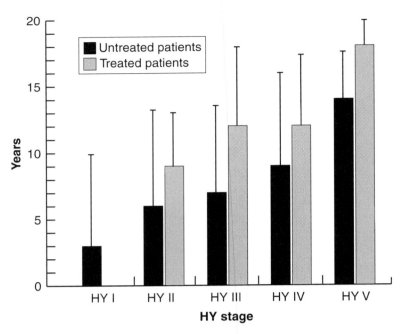

Figure 24-2. Median disease duration to reach Hoehn-Yahr (HY) stage. Comparison of untreated and L-dopa–treated patients. (Reprinted with permission from W Poewe, GK Wenning. The natural history of Parkinson's disease. Neurology 1996;47(suppl 3):S147.)

Once started on L-dopa, 41% of patients develop "wearing off," 30% develop dyskinesias, and 25% develop "freezing" within 2 years. In the large prospective study from which these data were drawn, wearing off was more common in younger patients with more rapidly progressive disability. In another study, motor fluctuations developed in only 20% of patients within 5 years. Using carbidopa and levodopa (Sinemet CR) (long-acting preparation) or standard-release carbidopa–L-dopa revealed no difference.

Long-Term Prognosis

The long-term prognosis for PD is not good but, as in many neurodegenerative conditions, is highly variable. The disease always is considered progressive, and even if the pathologic condition were to be truly static, normal aging would produce its own progression of deficits.

The death rate from PD is probably lower with L-dopa than without it, although the increase in parkinsonian life span since the development of L-dopa is due also to better medical care in general. Pre–L-dopa mortality for PD varied from 1.5 to 2.9 times that of age-matched control rates. More recent studies have shown mortality rates varying from normal to 2.9, depending in part on duration of follow-up, with longer follow-up yielding a greater percentage increase in the death rate. Almost all studies show a mortality rate of 1.2 to 2.5 as compared with age-matched controls.

Disease progression changes with the decline in the substantia nigra cell population and with the response to anti-PD medications. Progression is equal for men and women but is slower in patients in whom disease onset occurs early and in those with prominent tremor. Fifty percent of patients are only mildly disabled at up to 6 years after disease onset, 5% of patients continue to have mild disease after 10 years, and 5% are disabled severely within 3 to 5 years of disease onset. Progression of disability is stable for each patient (i.e., slow progression at onset predicted slow progression later on while a rapid decline early on would not be arrested).

L-Dopa and other PD medications have shifted the curves describing the decline of function to the right (Fig. 24-2). Selegiline, for example, prolongs by 12 months the time until patients require L-dopa. Once L-dopa is added, motor dysfunction and disability improve but rarely increase the Hoehn-Yahr stage by more than 1 month. The addition of other drugs improves disability by decreasing fluctuations and other L-dopa–induced problems rather than simply by enhancing the L-dopa peak response. The recent addition of pallidotomy helps the occasional PD patient with L-dopa–induced dyskinesias and fluctuations but does not slow disease progression.

Dementia occurs in perhaps 30% of PD patients, sometimes owing to the concurrence of Alzheimer's or other illnesses but most often owing to PD itself. The dementia progression is as variable as is the motor dysfunction, but generally the mental decline parallels the physical. Dementia is considerably more likely with advancing age. Drug-induced psychosis occurs in approximately 5 to 8% of drug-treated patients, far more commonly in the demented but not restricted to this subgroup. It is more common also in the elderly.

Additional Reading

Birkmayer W, Knoll J, Riederer P, et al. Increased life expectancy resulting from addition of L-deprenyl to madopar treatment in Parkinson's disease: a long-term study. J Neural Transm 1985;64:113–127.

Clarke CE. Does levodopa therapy delay death in Parkinson's disease? A review of the evidence. Mov Disord 1995;10:250–256.

Goetz CG, Tanner CM, Stebbins GT, Buchman AS. Risk factors for a progression in Parkinson's disease. Neurology 1988;38:1841–1844.

Hoehn MM, Yahr MD. Parkinsonism: onset, progression and mortality. Neurology 1967;17:427–442.

Kurtzke JF, Goldberg ID. Parkinsonism death rates by race, sex and geography. Neurology 1988;38:1558–1561.

Martilla RJ, Rinne UK. Disability and progression in Parkinson's disease. Acta Neurol Scand 1977;56:159–169.

Parkinson's Study Group. Effects of tocopherol and deprenyl on the progression of disability in early Parkinson's disease. N Engl J Med 1993;328:176–183.

Parkinson's Study Group. Impact of deprenyl and tocopherol treatment on Parkinson's disease in DATATOP patients requiring levodopa. Ann Neurol 1996;39:37–45.

Rajput AH, Pahwa R, Pahwa P, Rajput A. Prognostic significance of the onset mode in parkinsonism. Neurology 1993;43:829–830.

Zeretusky WJ, Jankovic J, Pirozzolo FJ. The heterogeneity of Parkinson's disease: clinical and prognostic implications. Neurology 1985;35:522–526.

Chapter 25

Amyotrophic Lateral Sclerosis

Jeremy M. Shefner

Amyotrophic lateral sclerosis (ALS) is a degenerative disease characterized by a variable combination of upper and lower motor neuron loss. Over the course of years, patients become progressively weaker and clumsier in their movements, with death due primarily to pulmonary failure approximately 3 to 5 years after diagnosis. The disease most often begins in the limbs, subsequently spreading throughout the neuraxis. However, in one-half of patients, the initial symptoms are slurred speech or swallowing difficulties, suggesting onset in the bulbar region. Men are affected slightly more frequently than are women. The average age of onset is the late fifth decade, but the distribution is quite broad. The cause of ALS has not been determined completely, though in approximately 10% of patients, a clear family history can be obtained. Some 20% of these patients have a known mutation in the gene for a Cu/Zn-requiring superoxide dismutase. In other patients, no clear genetic basis has been determined, and transport of excitotoxic neurotransmitters and abnormalities in protection from oxidative stress have been found.

Natural History

Although ALS affects the entire neuraxis, patients present initially with quite focal signs and symptoms. Perhaps one-half of all ALS patients will present with unilateral arm weakness. Wrist drop is a characteristic early sign, often noted concurrently with intrinsic hand-muscle wasting. For unclear reasons, flexor compartment forearm muscles usually are affected later in the disease. Because of this asymmetry of forearm involvement, the hand often assumes a clawed posture. The disease spreads regionally, going from the distal to proximal arm, where biceps and deltoid muscles usually are affected before the triceps.

Approximately one-fourth of patients present with lower-extremity symptoms, most commonly a unilateral foot drop. As in the upper extremity, weakness tends to spread regionally, first to more proximal muscles in the same leg and then to the opposite leg, before ascending to involve the arms.

Most of the remaining patients present with symptoms of bulbar dysfunction, alone or in combination with other symptoms. Change in the clarity of speech often is the first bulbar symptom, with difficulty in swallowing also noted early. Swallowing liquids becomes difficult before problems arise with swallowing solids; carbonated and alcoholic liquids are the least likely to be tolerated, thicker liquids being better tolerated.

The signs and symptoms that bring most ALS patients to medical attention are related to lower motor neuron dysfunction. Though they may be appreciated by the examining physician early in the course of ALS, upper motor neuron signs rarely are the cause of symptoms. Occasionally, patients will present with complaints of limb stiffness and slowed movements, but such patients are the exception. Even as the disease progresses and upper motor neuron signs become more flagrant, lower motor neuron loss continues to be the most important factor affecting disability. A rare exception to this rule are those patients with significant emotional lability or pseudobulbar affect. Uncontrollable laughing or crying occasionally can be the presenting symptom, and many patients with prominent upper motor neuron bulbar signs may be prevented from working because of this problem.

Regardless of the site of initial presentation, patients experience a slow, steady progression of symptoms. Patients with limb-onset disease may not experience bulbar symptoms until quite late; in contrast, bulbar-onset patients usually will develop symptoms in the extremities within months of diagnosis. By 2 years after diagnosis, most patients require ambulation aids. The rate of progression often is characterized as "stuttering," with periods of relative stability followed by more rapid change. However, studies quantitatively assessing changes in strength over time have shown that, within any body area, changes are remarkably linear. Thus, patients with slow early rates of decline most often will have a relatively long course, whereas those with a rapid early course will continue to worsen rapidly. The average survival time for all patients is approximately 3 years after diagnosis, but some patients may live more than 10 years, though others die in less than 1 year.

For most ALS patients, death is related to a pulmonary event. Primary respiratory failure can occur in the absence of infection but often is associated with aspiration and consequent pneumonia. Inadequate nutrition also can lead to death, but alterations in diet consistency and gastrostomy, when indicated, usually are sufficient to treat this complication. Less often, venous thrombosis and pulmonary embolus are causes of patient death.

Factors Affecting Prognosis

There are several factors that are important determinants of prognosis in ALS. Genetics certainly plays an important role. In general, distinguishing patients with familial ALS from those with sporadic disease is impossible. On average, age of onset is slightly lower in familial ALS, but rate of progression is highly variable. However, the specific mutation dramatically influences rate of progression. In the United States, the most common identified mutation is a point mutation in the super-

oxide dismutase–1 gene wherein valine is substituted for alanine at position 4 (A4V). Rosen and colleagues showed that patients with this mutation have very aggressive disease, with survival after diagnosis averaging 1.2 years. In contrast, other point mutations in the same gene are associated with a very slowly progressive course in which disease duration averages more than a decade. As more mutations are characterized, more specific information about prognosis will be available. In the meantime, it should be stressed that genetic determinants of prognosis are available only for a very small minority of patients.

Age of disease onset is another factor that affects prognosis. Younger patients tend to have more slowly progressive disease, whereas the course is more rapid in patients older than 65. Eisen and coworkers reported a mean disease duration of more than 8 years for patients with disease onset at younger than age 40, as contrasted to 2.6 years for patients with onset between 61 and 70 years of age. With few exceptions, epidemiologic studies have shown also that the prognosis for patients with onset of symptoms in the bulbar region is significantly worse than that for patients with limb onset. In a study from Norway, mean survival after diagnosis was 26 months for limb-onset patients and 12.1 months for patients with initial bulbar involvement.

Another important factor influencing prognosis is the rate of disease progression. Natural history studies have shown that rate of progression can be estimated if patients are assessed monthly with quantitative strength testing over 3 months. Thus, after a relatively brief period, patients can be given useful information about the rate of progression of their disease. Although progression in the limbs does not predict duration of disease, Ringel and colleagues have shown that rate of change of pulmonary function is extremely predictive of survival time.

Evaluation for Prognosis

Evaluation for prognosis is similar to the evaluation required to make the diagnosis of ALS. Electromyography is useful in defining the distribution of the disease at the time of study. However, repeated electrophysiologic study has not proved useful in following patients. An exception may be the use of a recently described technique called *motor unit estimation* (MUNE). MUNE can be performed in a number of different ways, but its goal is to estimate the number of functioning motor axons innervating a given muscle. Sequential MUNE studies are employed increasingly to assess rate and distribution of disease progression and may be useful in assessing prognosis.

As described in Factors Affecting Prognosis, the major factors that affect prognosis for patients with ALS are epidemiologic, such as age, site of onset, and concurrent disease. Determination of these factors is accomplished during a routine clinical evaluation. In addition, rate of change of pulmonary function clearly affects survival and should be evaluated through monthly measurements of respiratory mechanics, including forced vital capacity. Sequential quantitative assessment of muscle groups in the limbs also is very useful in predicting disease progression in those areas but does not predict overall disease duration.

Therapies Affecting Prognosis

Since the early 1990s, remarkable advances in both specific and supportive therapy of ALS have altered prognosis for ALS patients. With regard to supportive care, nutritional support probably has had the greatest impact. Patients with impaired swallowing function often can maintain adequate nutrition with high-calorie liquid supplements. When this becomes insufficient, percutaneous endoscopic techniques for placing gastrostomy or jejunostomy tubes are tolerated well by debilitated patients. The early use of gastrostomy-jejunostomy has reduced greatly the incidence of malnutrition in the ALS patient population, and at least one recent study has suggested that patients who receive gastrostomies may have a reduced mortality as contrasted to equivalent patients who refused the procedure.

Advances in pulmonary technology also have affected prognosis. An increasing percentage of patients in the United States choose to have a tracheostomy and chronic positive pressure ventilation when respiratory failure is imminent. Sizes of ventilators have diminished, and patients can live at home and remain ambulatory even when ventilator-dependent. For patients choosing this option, life span clearly is prolonged. However, a tremendous investment of money and caretaker time is required to maintain a ventilator-dependent ALS patient at home.

For the majority of ALS patients who do not choose the foregoing option, ventilatory assistance in the form of noninvasive positive pressure ventilators also can improve prognosis. Although only a few studies have been performed, evidence suggests that life span is prolonged in patients using nocturnal bilevel positive pressure support. Air flow is provided by mask, and patients may use nocturnal bilevel positive pressure support only at night or for rest periods during the day.

Other supportive therapy also may improve prognosis. Although it has not been studied adequately, depression is frequent in ALS patients. Appropriate treatment with antidepressant medications can improve quality of life. In addition, studies of patients with other serious diseases (e.g., breast cancer) have shown that treating depression prolongs survival. Data on this question are not available for ALS patients, but at least the possibility exists for altering that prognosis.

Prognosis for patients with ALS can be improved also by specific therapy. In 1996, the first drug shown to prolong survival in ALS was approved for general use by the U.S. Food and Drug Administration. Riluzole (Rilutek) is an oral agent shown modestly to prolong survival. In two placebo-controlled clinical trials, Rilutek was well tolerated and produced an average increase in life span of 3 months. Clearly, this improvement in life span is not dramatic. However, currently at least five other agents in clinical trials are likely to have similar or greater efficacy. Researchers hope that by combining multiple agents with modest efficacy, a more dramatic treatment response will be obtained.

Short-Term Prognosis

Many patients with ALS experience a delay of more than 1 year between the onset of symptoms and the diagnosis of the disease. Despite this period, most patients are ambulatory and without respiratory symptoms at the time of diagnosis. Quality of life can be high during this time and should remain so for the next 12 to 18 months. Patients often continue to work and participate normally in everyday life activities. During this period, depression may be the most important factor to recognize and treat.

Within 2 years after diagnosis, most patients require ambulation assistance in the form of a walker or wheelchair, and patients with bulbar-onset disease will experience communication problems.

Long-Term Prognosis

Despite advances in care, the long-term prognosis for patients with ALS is grim. Approximately 50% of patients will die sometime between 3 and 5 years after diagnosis. Death is preceded by a period during which the patient is completely dependent on family members or caretakers for activities of daily living. For those patients electing chronic ventilatory support, this period can be prolonged indefinitely. Communication with patients who have lost speech and hand function can be extremely difficult. Computer-based communication devices have made this problem somewhat more tractable, but such devices are very expensive, and their use is cumbersome. Nutrition also may be a problem, although many patients have had gastrostomy tubes placed by the time they become totally dependent.

Near the end of life, many ALS patients become extremely limited in their communication abilities, despite maintaining normal intellectual capacity. For this reason, discussions between patients and caregivers regarding terminal care decisions must begin early and continue throughout the course of the patient's illness.

Additional Reading

Bensimon G, Lacomblez L, Meininger V. A controlled trial of riluzole in amyotrophic lateral sclerosis. N Engl J Med 1994;330:585–591.

Brown RH. Superoxide dismutase and familial amyotrophic lateral sclerosis: new insights into mechanisms and treatments. Ann Neurol 1996;39:145–146.

Eisen A, Schulzer M, MacNeil M, et al. Duration of amyotrophic lateral sclerosis is age dependent. Muscle Nerve 1993;16:27–32.

Gurney ME, Cutting FB, Zhai P, et al. Benefit of vitamin E, riluzole, and gabapentin in a transgenic model of familial amyotrophic lateral sclerosis. Ann Neurol 1996;39:147–157.

Lacomblez L, Bensimon, G, Leigh PN, et al. Dose ranging study of riluzole in amyotrophic lateral sclerosis. Lancet 1996;347:1425–1431.

Ringel SP, Murphy JR, Alderson MK, et al. The natural history of amyotrophic lateral sclerosis. Neurology 1993; 43:1316–1322.

Rosen DR, Bowling AC, Patterson D, et al. A frequent ala 4 to val superoxide dismutase–1 mutation is associated with a rapidly progressive familial amyotrophic lateral sclerosis. Hum Mol Genet 1994;3:981–987.

Rosen DR, Siddique T, Patterson D, et al. Mutations in Cu/Zn superoxide dismutase gene are associated with familial amyotrophic lateral sclerosis. Nature 1993;362: 59–62.

Chapter 26
Huntington's Disease

Karen S. Marder

Although chorea is the feature associated most often with the hereditary condition eloquently described by George Huntington in 1872, it is now clear that there is a triad of motor, cognitive, and psychiatric signs described more aptly as Huntington's disease (HD). In 1983, genetic linkage was shown between HD and DNA markers on chromosome 4p. Ten years later, in 1993, the Huntington's Disease Collaborative Research Group reported the discovery of a CAG repeat that is identified in the 5' region of a novel gene on 4p16.3 and is expanded beyond the normal polymorphic range in individuals with HD (see Huntington's Disease Collaborative Research Group in Additional Reading). The discovery of the HD gene and the 348-kD protein it encodes, named *huntingtin*, has generated more questions than answers about the biologic basis of HD and about the relationship between CAG repeat length, age of onset, and clinical progression.

Natural History

In North America and Western Europe, the prevalence of HD is 5 to 10 per 100,000, whereas in African blacks, Japanese, Chinese, and Finnish, the prevalence is 10-fold lower, owing to both a lower CAG repeat length on normal chromosomes and to an altered frequency of DNA haplotypes. The mean onset age is from 36 to 45 years but has been reported as early as age 2 and as late as age 90. Death occurs on average 15 to 20 years after onset (usually dated from the onset of chorea), but duration up to 40 years after diagnosis has been described. In adults, chorea gradually increases and peaks at perhaps 10 years and then either plateaus or declines, whereas dystonia and gait impairment tend to increase with disease duration.

Approximately 6% of patients present with HD before the age of 20. These juvenile cases are characterized by dystonia and rigidity, occasional seizures and myoclonus, and (rarely) chorea. Juvenile HD predominantly is paternally inherited and has more rapid progression than does adult-onset HD. Duration of juvenile HD rarely extends beyond 14 years. In both adult- and juvenile-onset cases, dysphagia, impaired eye movements and fine alternating movements, and gait impairment (but not chorea) are the major correlates of functional impairment. The most frequent cause of death is aspiration pneumonia, but accidents, subdural hematomas, and suicide also are common.

Factors Affecting Prognosis

A number of studies have examined the association between CAG trinucleotide repeat length, age of onset of HD, and disease progression. In normal alleles, the range of CAG repeats may be from 6 to 39, with the vast majority less than 30 and a mean of 18 to 19 CAG repeats. HD alleles show repeat lengths of 36 to 121 CAG repeats, with the majority greater than 40 CAG repeats and a mean of 42 to 46 CAG repeats. A highly significant negative correlation between CAG repeat length and HD onset age has been demonstrated in a number of studies; higher repeat lengths are associated with younger onset age. This negative correlation is strongest for those with a high number of repeats and weaker for those alleles within the 40 to 50 repeat range that constitute the majority of HD alleles. Despite the strong correlation, repeat length appears to account for only 50% of the variance of onset age. Therefore, such other factors as modifying genes or environmental factors may vary the age of onset within individuals and families. Most HD alleles, unlike normal alleles, manifest meiotic instability (in this case, a tendency toward repeat expansion), which is more common in paternal transmission. The tendency for greater expansion in sperm than in eggs explains why juvenile cases of HD tend to be inherited paternally. Meiotic instability also may explain both genetic anticipation (the earlier onset of disease in subsequent generations) and new mutations. Individuals with sporadic HD, known to occur in 1 to 3% of all cases of HD, tend to have parents, often fathers, who have repeat lengths in the 30 to 39 range, who do not manifest HD, but whose children have alleles within the HD range, owing to CAG repeat expansion. Therefore, repeat lengths equal to or less than 29 now can be characterized as normal, lengths of 30 to 35 are considered intermediate, lengths of 36 to 39 are thought of as incomplete penetrance (meaning some people do and some do not manifest disease with this repeat length), and lengths equal to or greater than 40 are characterized as being within the HD range (see Nance in Additional Reading).

Repeat length has been examined also in terms of disease progression. The largest study, by Brandt and colleagues, demonstrated a more rapid decline in neurologic and cognitive function for 21 patients with repeat lengths equal to or greater than 47 repeats compared to 25 patients followed for 2 years with 37 to 46 repeats. Longer repeat lengths have been associated also with greater pathologic severity after adjusting for disease duration. Not all studies have found an association between higher repeat length and disease progression. At least one study specifically has refuted any relationship between progression of psychiatric symptoms and repeat length.

In another study of 42 adults before the availability of CAG repeat length, Myers and coworkers found that younger onset age and lower weight at first examination were associated with more rapid functional decline.

Evaluation for Prognosis

Before the availability of genetic testing, all studies on diagnosis and prognosis of HD were based on the presence of unequivocal signs of a movement disorder on neurologic examination. Several investigators have now focused on defining the earliest signs of HD in asymptomatic carriers. In the largest study of cognitive impairment in at-risk individuals without signs or symptoms of HD, Foroud and associates compared cognitive function in 260 non-HD gene carriers and 120 HD gene carriers. Performance on two tests from the Wechsler Adult Intelligence Scale, Revised (digit symbol and picture arrangement) was significantly worse in carriers, and scores were correlated negatively with the number of CAG repeats in the expanded HD allele. Within the same cohort, through the use of computer-based tasks, asymptomatic gene carriers were found to have slower saccadic velocity and slower movement and visual reaction time. These findings suggest that in presymptomatic individuals with HD, subtle subclinical cognitive and motor changes that are present may reflect changes in basal ganglia function before the onset of clinically apparent disease.

Imaging studies have been used also to determine the existence of anatomic or functional correlates of presymptomatic gene carriers. Gene carriers have been shown to have reductions in basal ganglia volume and, in some, abnormal glucose metabolism on positron emission tomography studies. Using this technology, dopaminergic D1 and D2 receptor binding were lower for presymptomatic gene carriers than for noncarriers. Magnetic resonance spectroscopy has demonstrated increased cortical lactate levels, a measure of impaired mitochondrial energy production, in symptomatic HD patients. This tool now is being used to study presymptomatic carriers.

Determining the point at which disease is manifest in a person carrying the HD gene will have important implications for both short- and long-term prognosis and treatment. Were an effective treatment without significant side effects available, intervening at the earliest stage of the illness would be appropriate. Once a diagnosis of HD is made, however, no specific laboratory tests can establish prognosis.

Therapies Affecting Prognosis

At the present, therapy for HD may be divided into two categories: symptomatic (either blockade of nigrostriatal pathway or replacement therapy) or neuroprotective. Symptomatic treatment of the movement disorder is confined to neuroleptics, atypical neuroleptics, benzodiazepines, and such dopamine-depleting agents as reserpine or tetrabenazine. These agents may improve the chorea, but they tend to worsen the voluntary movements, such as gait and swallowing, and may themselves cause tardive dyskinesia, parkinsonism, acute dystonic reactions, sedation, and depression. Therefore, the movement disorder should not be treated unless it becomes functionally or psychiatrically disabling.

Neuroprotective strategies designed to slow the progression of HD have included a trial of baclofen, which may inhibit corticostriatal release of glutamate and aspartate. A large, double-blind trial of baclofen, 60 mg per day, in 60 patients, showed an actual nonsignificant worsening of total functional capacity in the active arm. A 1-year, double-blind trial of high-dose d-alpha tocopherol (3,000 IU) versus placebo and a multicenter trial of OPC-14117, a free radical scavenger, yielded no improvement in neurologic, neuropsychological, or functional domains.

Psychiatric disorders may occur in anywhere from 35 to 75% of HD patients. In fact, affective symptoms may precede motor manifestations by up to 5 years. Because suicide occurs four to eight times as often as in the general population and tends to occur early in the disease, recognizing risk factors for suicide and treating depression aggressively are important. The single factor most predictive of suicide in a retrospective review of 300 HD patients (9 of whom committed suicide) was being childless, followed by being male, being unmarried, having a family history of suicide, living alone, and being depressed. Because HD patients also are prone to impulsivity and irritability, suicide always should be considered a possibility.

A number of nonpharmacologic interventions definitely can affect prognosis. Gait impairment is a major cause of morbidity due to falls and also is a frequent reason for institutionalization. Physical therapy can be helpful in improving balance, strength, and endurance; reducing muscle tone; and improving perceptual skills. Dysphagia also is a common life-threatening complication of HD. Swallowing therapy to prevent aspiration is extremely effective at all stages of the illness.

HD patients require 4,000 to 6,000 calories per day and, late in the illness, may require a feeding tube to maintain caloric intake. Ideally, a discussion of such an arrangement should include the patient and should occur before a crisis situation. Indications for a feeding tube include 10% weight loss over a 1-month period, inadequate hydration, repeated aspiration, and severe swallowing incompetence. Contraindications include irreversible lack of communication and comprehension, lack of informed consent, or the patient's clearly expressed refusal.

Short-Term Prognosis

A large extended family with Huntington's disease has been examined annually by the United States–Venezuela Cooperative Huntington's Disease Project since 1981. Among 171 gene-positive individuals who were seen between 1981 and 1988 and had not received a diagnosis of HD, abnormalities of saccadic eye movement and slowness of rapid alternating movements were the most common abnormalities on neurologic examination. Over the 7-year period, 30 incident cases of HD were identified. The likelihood of developing HD over a 3-year period was 3% for at-risk individuals with a normal examination at first evaluation, 23% for those with mildly abnormal neurologic examinations, and 60% of those with highly abnormal examinations. Penney and coworkers suggested that this progression of signs from mild saccadic pursuit and fine-motor abnormalities to more definitive abnormalities and eventual chorea represents a "zone of onset" rather than a discrete age of onset.

Many longitudinal studies use the total functional capacity (TFC) score, designed by Shoulson and Fahn, to measure disease progression. Worldwide, a consistent 0.5 to 1.0 decline per year exists in this 13-point scale in longitudinally followed populations. No interventions have altered this finding substantially. In the Venezuela family, the rate of decline on the TFC was 1.4 per year (Fig. 26-1). Decline was linear for symptomatic persons at the two highest stages of the scale and then became variable at scores representing more severely impaired patients. Whether the plateau of the scale in more impaired persons reflects actual disease progression or insensitivity of the scale is unknown.

Long-Term Prognosis

A new era of HD research and clinical care has been entered. Presymptomatic gene carriers may be

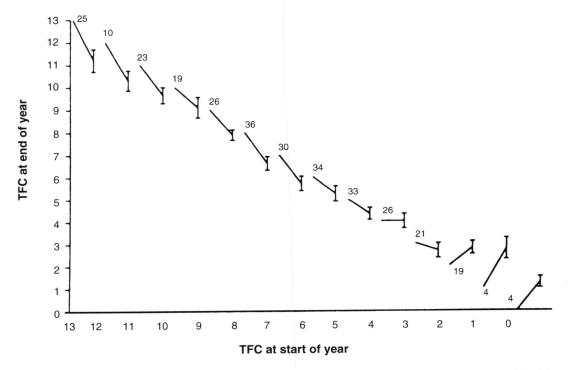

Figure 26-1. Average yearly rate of decline of functional capacities on the Shoulson-Fahn scale for patients with adult-onset Huntington's disease. Total functional capacity (TFC) was derived by calculating the average decline of each group's TFC in the next year and subtracting from the initial TFC (bars = standard error of the mean). The number of persons in each group is given by the first point in each set. The apparent increase in follow-up TFC of those with low initial TFCs is due to exclusion of those who died in the next year. (Reprinted with permission from JB Penney, AB Young, I Shoulson, et al. Huntington's disease in Venezuela: 7 years of follow-up on symptomatic and asymptomatic individuals. Mov Disord 1990;5:96.)

identified easily, but there is no way to tell these people when they will manifest disease. There is no effective treatment, and it is not known whether earlier treatment will lead to improved function. These considerations render all the more imperative that people receive adequate genetic counseling before making a decision to determine their gene status.

Additional Reading

Brandt J, Bylsma FW, Gross R, et al. Trinucleotide repeat length and clinical progression in Huntington's disease. Neurology 1996;46:527–531.

Foroud T, Siemers E, Kleindorfer D, et al. Cognitive scores in carriers of Huntington's disease gene compared to non-carriers. Ann Neurol 1995;37:657–664.

Gusella JF, Wexler NS, Conneally PM, et al. A polymorphic marker genetically linked to Huntington's disease. Nature 1983;306:234–238.

The Huntington's Disease Collaborative Research Group. A novel gene containing a trinucleotide repeat that is expanded and unstable on Huntington's disease chromosomes. Cell 1993;72:971–983.

Myers RH, Sax DS, Koroshetz WJ, et al. Factors associated with slow progression in Huntington's disease. Arch Neurol 1991;48:800–804.

Nance M. Huntington disease—another chapter rewritten. Am J Hum Genet 1996;59:1–6.

Penney JB, Young AB, Shoulson I, et al. Huntington's disease in Venezuela: 7 years of follow-up on symptomatic and asymptomatic individuals. Mov Disord 1990;5:93–100.

Shoulson I, Fahn S. Huntington's disease: clinical care and evaluation. Neurology 1979; 29:1–3.

Chapter 27

Spinal Muscular Atrophy

Barry S. Russman

Spinal muscular atrophy (SMA) is an autosomal recessive disease manifested clinically by weakness and progressive loss of motor function. The disorder typically begins before age 5. Laboratory examinations necessary to make the diagnosis include DNA testing, neurophysiology testing, and muscle biopsy. If the patient's history and physical examination are consistent with the clinical presentation of SMA (fasciculation, finger trembling, etc.), only DNA testing for deletion of the *survival motor neuron* gene is necessary for the diagnosis. Once the diagnosis has been made, the patient is classified into one of three categories. The current classification system, which relates to prognosis, is based on age at onset and maximum function achieved. The age of onset for SMA I is less than 6 months, and these patients never achieve the ability to sit without support. SMA II (juvenile or chronic SMA) patients typically develop weakness after age 6 months (although exceptions occur), and they are able to sit independently when placed. SMA III patients develop weakness after age 18 months (exceptions also occur), and they are able to walk independently at some point in their lives.

Natural History

SMA I (Werdnig-Hoffman disease) presents during the first 6 months of life with lack of motor development, muscle weakness, and poor muscle tone and progresses inexorably to death by age 2. The infants in whom the gravest prognosis is identified have problems sucking or swallowing in the perinatal period or during the first few months of life. The worst prognosis is for patients who exhibit abdominal breathing during the first few months of life. In one series, 50% of the patients were dead by age 7 months and 80% by 1 year (see Thomas in Additional Reading).

SMA II (juvenile or chronic SMA) usually is symptomatic between the ages of 6 and 18 months but may start earlier. Patients at this stage attain independent sitting when placed and may live into adolescence or longer. Some of these patients may gain function for the first few years but ultimately lose function slowly over time. In one series, 75% of SMA II patients still sat after age 7, regardless of age of onset; 50% of this group sat independently after age 14 (see Russman in Additional Reading). Only rarely can such patients get to the sitting position on their own. Fifty percent of SMA patients in whom the maximum function achieved is walking with assistance lose this ability by age 7, unrelated to age of onset; none walks with assistance after age 14. The life expectancy of patients with SMA II is not known. Anecdotal information suggests that patients live into adolescence and the early twenties (see Hausmanowa-Petrusewicz and colleagues, Zerres and Rudnik-Schoneborn in Additional Reading).

SMA III (juvenile SMA or Kugelberg-Welander disease) becomes symptomatic after age 18 months; all patients walk independently at some time. Fifty percent of SMA patients who walk without assistance and whose onset is younger than age 2 lose the ability to walk independently by age 12. Fifty percent of SMA patients who walk and whose onset is between 2 and 6 years lose walking ability by age 44. Eighty-five percent of SMA walkers cannot negotiate stairs without holding onto a rail. They can raise their hands above the head; however, as they lose walking ability, they lose this function as well.

Factors Affecting Prognosis

SMA I patients with severely impaired breathing have the poorest prognosis for life expectancy. A poor suck is a second factor indicating an early demise in this group of patients. The loss of function in SMA II, such as the ability to sit independently, does not correlate necessarily with early demise but rather is an indication of disease progression only. Scoliosis development has not been correlated with progressive disease in SMA II or III. SMA III patients will lose function and forced vital capacity over time; however, life expectancy has not been correlated with these factors, although, by intuition, the development of pulmonary insufficiency should raise concerns.

Evaluation for Prognosis

Little evaluation is necessary to assist in prognostication. The course of disease correlates to some degree with pulmonary function. All SMA patients gradually lose forced vital capacity, which should be monitored as part of routine care, as life expectancy may correlate with this loss.

Therapies Affecting Prognosis

No treatment is known to cure, slow, or reverse the course of SMA. (Studies are under way to determine whether glutamate inhibitors or nerve growth factors might be effective in altering the natural course of disease.) Supportive care can alter the prognosis for life expectancy, for function, and for quality of life. The management of SMA I involves monitoring for respiratory infection. Early discussion with the family about orders not to resuscitate is helpful. As discussed, some children with SMA I (Werdnig-Hoffman disease) do not suck or swallow well, and a feeding gastroscopy may be necessary. Long-term ventilatory support for children with SMA I has not been reported. Inadvertently, a 4-month-old patient in my practice was placed on a ventilator. She is now 13. Although she attends regular public school, she requires extensive medical support there and at home.

Ventilatory support has been recommended and used successfully in SMA II patients. The eventuality of respiratory support should be discussed before it becomes necessary for survival, so that management options can be considered. The development of deformities in patients with SMA II and III is common. SMA I patients rarely require orthopedic intervention because they do not live long enough to develop spinal deformity. However, scoliosis is a major problem in most SMA II patients and 50% of SMA III patients. Before age 10, perhaps half of SMA patients, especially those who are nonambulatory, develop spinal back curvatures of more than 50 degrees. Scoliosis repair is carried out safely if the forced vital capacity is greater than 40%. The use of an orthosis before surgical intervention does not prevent the development of scoliosis but will allow the patient to be upright rather than bedridden. Patients will lose some upper-extremity function after operative intervention. On the other hand, the advantages of a stable trunk and the opportunity to sit unassisted in an upright position far outweigh the disadvantages. Whether scoliosis repair prevents further deterioration of pulmonary function or prolongs life is unclear.

Short- and Long-Term Prognosis

No explanation exists for functional loss in all SMA patients. Several authors have speculated that strength of muscle groups changes very little over the years. Such factors as weight and height gain, contracture development, or disuse in conjunction with deterioration of pulmonary function may be the explanation. Regardless, loss of function occurs in all types of SMA, more precipitous in the more severely affected (SMA I) and more gradual in SMA II and SMA III. Table 27-1 summarizes this deterioration.

Table 27-1. Function Loss Over Time Correlated with Spinal Muscular Atrophy Type

Classification	Mortality Risk	Stop Sitting When Placed	Stop Standing or Walking
SMA I	Death by age 2 in 100%	—	—
SMA II	Live until age 20–40 yrs	By age 15 yrs in 50%; indefinite in 50%	—
SMA III	Indefinite	Indefinite	By age 15 yrs in those with onset before age 2; otherwise, in the fourth decade

SMA = spinal muscular atrophy.

Additional Reading

Hausmanowa-Petrusewicz I, Badurska B, Ryniewicz B. The natural history of proximal chronic childhood spinal muscular atrophy (forms 2 and 3). Acta Cardiomiol 1992; 4:19–33.

Russman BS, Buncher CR, White M, et al. Function changes in spinal muscular atrophy II and III. Neurology 1996; 47:973–977.

Thomas NH, Dubowitz V. The natural history of type I (severe) spinal muscular atrophy. Neuromuscul Disord 1994;4:497–502.

Zerres K, Rudnik-Schoneborn S. Natural history in proximal spinal muscular atrophy. Clinical analysis of 445 patients and suggestions for a modification of existing classifications. Arch Neurol 1995;52:518–523.

Chapter 28

Inherited Ataxias

S.H. Subramony

The inherited ataxias are disorders that cause progressive difficulties with balance and a variety of other motor functions. These diseases are being increasingly understood at a molecular genetic level, and genotypic classification is emerging (Tables 28-1 and 28-2). However, in many families with inherited ataxia, the gene loci and mutations still are unknown. Earlier reports on ataxia patients dealt with clinically and genetically heterogeneous patient populations, and a paucity of data limits discussion of the prognosis and natural history of different diseases. A significant factor in the prognosis of these disorders is the nature of the gene mutations responsible, resulting in variability of clinical features, natural history, and prognosis even within the same genotype. Neither the mechanisms resulting in phenotypic variability nor the specific phenotypic features that result in altered prognoses are understood completely.

This chapter summarizes the available information in different disorders in terms of natural history, factors affecting prognosis, and the long-term outlook. No proved therapeutic interventions can alter the course of the neurologic syndromes in any of these disorders. Patients and families with such diseases have concerns over and above their own prognoses, always giving rise to questions about risks for family members. Some issues regarding genetic counseling are addressed.

Autosomal Recessive Ataxias

Friedreich's Ataxia

Friedreich's ataxia (FRDA) typically has onset within the first two decades of life, but the age of onset can be much wider. Several siblings in a family may be affected but, in many small families, singleton patients are found. The disease is characterized by progressive gait ataxia, early occurrence of areflexia, and proprioceptive deficits and dysarthria. Other signs include oculomotor abnormalities, dysphagia, muscle weakness, wasting, and extensor plantar signs. Systemic features include cardiomyopathy, skeletal deformities, and diabetes.

Natural History

The age of onset for FRDA varies from 2 to 51 years. Considerable variation in age of onset can occur within a family, and onset beyond the age of 21 occurs in up to 17% of cases. Natural history has been looked at mainly for classic FRDA of early onset. The mean age at onset in many series was 11 to 13 years. The mean time to chair-bound status was 9 to 16 years. The rate of disease progression varied considerably, even within a family. The age at death in an early series of cases diagnosed clinically ranged from 5 to 71 years, with a mean of 37 years. This figure may have to be revised, as now later-onset cases

Table 28-1. Autosomal Recessive Ataxias

Ataxia	Prevalence	Gene Locus	Mutation	Protein
Friedreich's ataxia	1.2–4.7 per 100,000	Chromosome 9	GAA repeat expansion	Frataxin
Ataxia telangiectasia	—	Chromosome 11	Deletions and insertions	ATM
Ataxia with vitamin E deficiency	—	Chromosome 8	Deletions, missense-nonsense mutations	Alpha-tocopherol transfer protein
Early-onset ataxia with retained tendon reflexes	—	Likely hetero-geneous	Unknown (many due to FRDA mutation)	Unknown
Ataxia with hypogonadism	—	Unknown	Unknown	Unknown
Ataxia with myoclonus	—	Unknown	Unknown	Unknown
Ataxia with known metabolic errors	—	Variety of gene mutations	Different types	Different types

ATM = gene mutated in ataxia telangiectasia; FRDA = Friedreich's ataxia.

Table 28-2. Autosomal Dominant Ataxias: Prevalence as Percentage of Dominant Ataxias

	Prevalence (%)	Gene Locus	Mutation	Protein
Spinocerebellar ataxia 1	5–40	Chromosome 6p	CAG repeat expansion	Ataxin 1
Spinocerebellar ataxia 2	13	Chromosome 12q	CAG expansion	Ataxin 2
Spinocerebellar ataxia 3	11–21	Chromosome 14q	CAG expansion	Ataxin 3
Spinocerebellar ataxia 4	Unknown	Chromosome 16q	Unknown	Unknown
Spinocerebellar ataxia 5	Unknown	Chromosome 11	Unknown	Unknown
Spinocerebellar ataxia 6	Unknown	Chromosome 19p	CAG expansion	Calcium channel alpha subunit
Spinocerebellar ataxia 7	Unknown	Chromosome 3p	CAG expansion	Unknown
Dominant episodic ataxias	Unknown	Chromosome 12 and 19	Point mutations	K channel; calcium channel alpha subunit
DRPLA	2	Chromosome 12p	CAG expansion	DRPLA protein

DRPLA = dentatorubral-pallidoluysian atrophy.

may be diagnosed with precision. Some 56% of these patients died from cardiac failure; 44% had miscellaneous immediate causes of death, including pneumonia, strokes, and diabetic ketosis.

Many signs occur earlier than do others in the disease; thus, ataxia, loss of position sense, and areflexia are present very early in the disease. Dysarthria, dysphagia, loss of vibration sense, muscle weakness and wasting, and extensor plantar reflexes often appear later. Hearing loss, visual loss, and sphincter problems are late and not universal features.

Factors Affecting Prognosis

The gene mutation involves the homozygous expansion of an intronic, unstable GAA repeat in the gene X 25 on chromosome 9. Disease onset age is related inversely to the degree of expansion, espe-

cially of the smaller allele. Also, an inverse correlation appears between repeat size and the time to a chair-bound status, but the correlation is not as strong. Cardiomyopathy, diabetes, scoliosis, and muscle weakness also may be correlated with the presence of larger expansions. Earlier age of onset is associated with poorer prognosis for disability and life. The occurrence of symptomatic cardiomyopathy and diabetes has an adverse effect on prognosis. Progressive scoliosis can affect prognosis as well and tends to be more common among patients with onset age before 12 years.

Evaluation for Prognosis

Patients with suspected FRDA should have the number of repeats in their X 25 gene estimated for both diagnosis and prognosis to convey the degree of expansion. Clinical evaluation should ensure careful assessment of neurologic features that result in morbidity and mortality, including the degree of impairment of mobility in general, the severity of bulbar deficits (including the degree of dysphagia and alteration in cough mechanisms), and difficulty with bladder control. Systemic features that result in morbidity and mortality should be evaluated periodically. They include clinical and radiologic assessment of spinal curvature, fasting blood sugar, and clinical and (if necessary) laboratory assessment of cardiac function. Many nonambulatory patients will not develop the classic symptoms of cardiac failure; hence, careful evaluation should include questions about orthopnea, accurate cardiopulmonary examination and, if necessary, echocardiography.

Therapies Affecting Prognosis

Interventions directed at cardiomyopathy, cardiac failure, scoliosis correction, and diabetes control will improve morbidity and mortality. Beyond that, no treatments can affect the course of FRDA.

As FRDA is a recessive disease, patients can be reassured that disease transmission to the next generation is unlikely. All children of patients with FRDA will be carriers of the mutated gene. Risk for siblings not yet beyond the age of onset is 1 in 4. Siblings may wish to be tested for possible carrier state through a search for a heterozygous expansion of the GAA repeat. This search will be meaningful if an affected person in the family has homozygous expansion of the repeat. Occasionally, patients with FRDA will have an expanded repeat on one allele and a point mutation on the other, rendering carrier detection more difficult. Of course, a carrier has a chance of transmitting the disease only by having offspring with another carrier. The FRDA gene frequency in the general population has been estimated to be 1 in 110.

Ataxia Telangiectasia

Ataxia telangiectasia (AT) tends to have an onset earlier than that of FRDA, with postural instability and ataxia around 12 to 14 months of age. Ataxia becomes more severe during the second half of the first decade, and children develop a variety of other neurologic signs, including hypotonia, bradykinesia, choreoathetosis, proprioceptive deficits, and areflexia. Other signs include a characteristic oculomotor disorder typified by difficulty with initiating saccades that often necessitates head thrusts and spasmodic blinking to move the eyes to the side. In addition, typical oculocutaneous telangiectasia develops between 3 and 6 years of age and spreads in a symmetric fashion over the conjunctivae, external ears, eyelids, creases of the neck, and cubital and popliteal fossa. Laboratory abnormalities that support the diagnosis include the universal elevation of serum alpha-fetoprotein and decreased levels of serum IgA, IgG, and IgE. Altered radiosensitivity of cultured cells occurs.

Natural History

The natural history of AT is one of relentless progression. Most of the patients are chair-bound by early in the second decade. Few patients live beyond the age of 30. The natural history has changed since the 1970s because of better treatments for sinopulmonary infections and lymphoreticular malignancies, so that death often is postponed to the fourth and fifth decades. With the current possibility of identifying variant phenotypes as being due to mutations in the same gene, AT patients with longer survival are likely.

Approximately 1% of children affected by AT develop a malignancy every year, usually lymphomas or leukemias. In addition, many of the patients exhibit a tendency for sinopulmonary infections. More than 80% of cases in one series had frequent infections of the respiratory tract. This condition is related to abnormal immunologic function. The major causes of death in AT include pulmonary infections (in almost half the patients), problems related to malignancy (in some 25% of cases), and a combination of the two disorders in others.

Factors Affecting Prognosis

The gene mutated in AT (ATM) encodes a putative 350 Kd protein with a PI-4-kinase-like domain. The AT phenotype and, thus, the prognosis in AT are related to the types of mutations present in an affected person. Close to 90% of the mutations inactivate the protein, often by truncating it, resulting in the classic phenotype. Milder phenotypes have been related to some degree of normal splicing from the mutant allele. The large size of the ATM transcript renders a systematic search for mutations laborious.

Both neurologic and systemic factors have an obvious relation to prognosis. More rapid neurologic progression with major impairment of mobility and bulbar deficits leads to earlier death. Prognosis also is determined by the presence and absence of malignancies and infections.

Evaluation for Prognosis

Assessment of the specific mutation to predict the phenotype is not practical at this point. In addition to monitoring for critical neurologic features, these patients need to be evaluated periodically for lymphomas and hematologic malignancies. Assessment of immunoglobulin levels may allow some prediction of frequent respiratory infections, but low Ig levels alone do not account completely for the tendency to such infections. In female patients with AT, prognosis for long-term survival may be better if they develop normal puberty, as early death in females always is associated with hypoplastic ovaries and absence of secondary sexual characteristics.

Genetic Counseling

Many aspects of genetic counseling are similar to those for other recessive disorders, such as FRDA. However, mutation detection is more difficult, and carrier detection may be more laborious. Over and above the genetic aspects of carrier detection, one should be aware also that heterozygote carriers of the ATM gene may be at increased risk for malignancies, especially of the breast.

Early-Onset Cerebellar Ataxia with Retained Tendon Reflexes

Harding pointed out that a number of patients with childhood-onset progressive ataxia differed from FRDA in retaining their reflexes, a disorder she named *early-onset cerebellar ataxia with retained tendon reflexes*. Many such patients are likely to be variant phenotypes of FRDA. The remaining patients with such a syndrome are likely to be clinically and genetically heterogeneous. As a group,

they may have slower progression rates, often becoming chair-bound at a mean of 21 to 33 years after onset.

Autosomal Dominant Ataxias

The dominantly inherited ataxias are clinically confusing disorders that just now are being sorted out at the molecular level. In the older literature, many of these diseases were included under the rubric of *olivopontocerebellar atrophies* or "Marie's Ataxia." All the disorders so far elucidated have been due to unstable CAG repeat expansions, accounting for the phenotypic variability within families; such variability makes a clinical diagnosis of the genotype involved very difficult. In almost all the diseases, a larger expansion is associated with earlier onset, more rapid progression, and (probably) a more widespread involvement of the nervous system, resulting in poorer prognosis. The specific affected gene also has a major impact on prognosis, because some of the disorders have relatively late onset and slower progression. An estimated 40% of the dominant ataxias cannot yet be identified at a genotypic level.

Unlike recessive ataxias, none of the dominant ataxias have any intrinsic systemic features that affect prognosis. Therefore, the prognosis is determined solely by the nature of the neurologic deficits and the rate of progression of the neurologic syndrome. Earlier onset of the disease is associated with more rapid progression and possibly more widespread dysfunction in the nervous system. The occurrence of prominent bulbar deficits, including dysphagia, tongue atrophy, poor palatal movements, and poor cough, is related to poorer prognosis. Both the nature of the specific gene mutation and the degree of unstable expansion probably influence the occurrence of these clinical signs. Prognosis is influenced further by the degree of involvement of the lower motor neuron and the resultant respiratory problems and changes in bladder control. Nutritional problems occur late and result from dysphagia; in addition, many of these patients undergo weight loss unexplained by poor nutritional intake. Thus, assessment for prognosis primarily involves evaluation of bulbar deficits, nutritional status, and sphincter control. In addition, knowledge of the degree of CAG expansion involved and the age of onset allow some speculations regarding the prognosis as well. Death in many patients is related to pulmonary complications, but many patients with late-adult-onset disease will die of unrelated causes.

Spinocerebellar Ataxia 1

Autosomal dominant spinocerebellar ataxia 1 is related to an unstable CAG expansion in the ataxin 1 gene on chromosome 6. The age of onset varies from 6 to more than 70 years. The disease begins with progressive ataxia and dysarthria. Clinical signs observed early in the disease include hyperreflexia, nystagmus, gait ataxia, limb ataxia, and dysarthria. Relentless progression results in loss of ambulation; eye movements become slow and incomplete. Dysphagia and poor cough develop. Often, a mild peripheral polyneuropathy occurs, with loss of ankle reflexes and distal sensory loss.

Natural History

The duration from onset to death has varied from 1 to 38 years in different families: Some families have clusters of relative later-onset cases with slower progression rates; others have early onset with rapid progression. The mean duration of illness ranges from 9 to 16 years and the mean age at death from 37 to 55 years. Some of the signs that appear to change over the course of the disease include nystagmus, which disappears as the saccade velocity becomes slower; the development of gaze palsy; and change from generalized hyperreflexia to distal areflexia. Although bulbar deficits including dysarthria and choking spells during deglutition can occur early, severe bulbar deficits, including markedly abnormal cough, tend to be later features. Other late features include mild amyotrophy and choreic or dystonic movements.

Factors Affecting Prognosis

The unstable CAG expansion in the ataxin 1 gene and the degree of expansion in different patients offer a major explanation for the phenotypic variability and, consequently, the prognosis. Normal alleles contain 6 to 40 repeats, often with CAA interruptions. The expanded range varies from 39 to 81 uninterrupted repeats. All studies have shown an inverse correlation between repeat size and age of onset. However, considerable scatter is found in the age of onset for a given repeat size. Approximately 66% of the variation in onset age can be related to the CAG repeat number. The duration of disease from onset to death and the rate of disability progression also are correlated with number of repeats but less strongly than with age of onset. Thus, though larger repeat sizes result in earlier onset of disease and faster progression, probably other epigenetic and environmental factors play a role in progression and duration of disease. Repeat sizes greater than 50 occur mostly in patients with onset at 20 years or younger, and patients with repeat numbers greater than 52 are disabled significantly by 5 years into the illness. Homozygous expansion of the CAG repeat does not seem to add any further severity, other than that predicted by the larger allele. Whether the gender of the affected parent has any influence on the duration of the illness remains unclear.

Spinocerebellar Ataxia 2

A large group of patients with dominant ataxia from the eastern provinces of Cuba was shown initially not to be linked genetically to the SCA 1 locus on chromosome 6 and eventually were linked to markers on chromosome 12. This disorder, known as *spinocerebellar ataxia 2* (SCA 2), also has been seen in other geographic areas. Clinically, the disease resembles SCA 1. SCA 2 may exhibit greater intrafamilial disease variability than does SCA 1. Progressive ataxia and dysarthria are early and universal. Oculomotor findings can be distinct in some of these families; early and severe slowing of saccades may be seen, and the prevalence of nystagmus is low. Usually, a prominent peripheral neuropathy appears, especially in the upper limbs, and thus hyporeflexia is more common than hyperreflexia. Fasciculations, cramps, and tremor also have been reported in this disease. Spasticity, extrapyramidal rigidity, dementia, and dystonia have been reported in some families as well.

Natural History

The duration of the illness varies from 7 to 18 years. Progression varies considerably, so that some are disabled severely in their forties and others still mildly affected in their sixties. Overall, the natural history of this disease resembles that of SCA 1 but is more variable.

Factors Affecting Prognosis

The gene mutation in SCA 2 is an unstable expansion of a CAG repeat within the responsible gene on chromosome 12q. The normal SCA 2 allele contains 15 to 29 repeats, with 22 or 23 repeats accounting for the majority. The expanded range is 36 to 59. An inverse relation between age of onset and the number of repeats was noted, with most of the juvenile cases having more than 45 repeats. A homozygous expansion may not give rise to any disease more severe than the usual heterozygous expansion.

Anticipation in onset age is observed in SCA 2, and it may exhibit a paternal bias toward greater anticipation. Intergenerational instability is seen in the expanded repeat, but the issue of parental bias in the degree of intergenerational expansion is not settled.

Spinocerebellar Ataxia 3: Machado-Joseph Disease

An autosomal dominant disorder—spinocerebellar ataxia 3 (Machado-Joseph disease [MJD]; SCA 3/MJD)—with cerebellar ataxia and a variety of other clinical features was described originally among the Portuguese Azorean emigrants to the United States in the 1970s. What apparently were rather distinct clinical phenotypes among scattered families in the United States were shown to be due to the same genetic defect after examination of large families in the Azores revealed extraordinary variability of the clinical findings within the same family. A similar disorder was described among other ethnic groups as well. The mutation was identified in 1994 to be an unstable CAG expansion within the responsible gene on chromosome 14. Families with dominant ataxia unrelated to Portuguese ancestry were shown also to have the same mutation, which is one of the most common abnormalities accounting for dominant ataxia. The clinical picture is very similar to that of SCA 1 and 2; however, in many families, the degree of intrafa-

milial variability is somewhat larger than in SCA 1. Most patients have progressive ataxia, upper motor neuron signs, nystagmus, slow saccades, amyotrophy, and the eventual appearance of distal areflexia and (occasionally) generalized areflexia. Occasional patients within the same families exhibit an early akinetic-rigid syndrome often responsive to L-dopa with little ataxia. Still other patients have had fairly typical parkinsonian syndromes, often with onset in middle adult life. Patients with prominent spastic-rigid syndromes are labeled as type I; with progressive ataxia and upper motor neuron signs as type II; and with ataxia, areflexia, and amyotrophy as type III. Many patients will progress from one type into another. Families with limited intrafamilial variability, with disorders often completely indistinguishable from SCA 1, have been labeled as having SCA 3.

Natural History

SCA 3/MJD is a disease of relentless progression, though at a variable rate. The duration of the disease from onset to death has varied from 6 to 29 years as reported in the available literature. The mean duration of the illness in 36 patients from the Azores was 15.6 years. The course in my experience is not dissimilar from that in SCA 1, with loss of ambulation at between 5 and 15 years into the illness. Many patients evolve from an initial syndrome comprising cerebellar ataxia, hyperreflexia, and nystagmus into one that includes severe imbalance, distal or total areflexia, gaze palsies, dysphagia and poor cough, and dystonic and choreic movements. Others evolve from an extrapyramidal syndrome into a predominantly cerebellar syndrome.

Factors Affecting Prognosis

The normal repeat number in the MJD gene varies from 12 to 40. The abnormal range is 64 to 84. An inverse correlation exists between the number of repeats and the age of onset. In general, juvenile onset is associated with repeat numbers in excess of 75. Some 58 to 70% of the variability in onset age is explained by the repeat numbers. "Type I" phenotype seems to be correlated with larger repeat sizes; patients with 64 to 71 repeats often present with a late adult-onset type III phenotype.

Some degree of anticipation in onset age is seen in many families, up to a mean of 12 years, but not all anticipation can be accounted for by intergenerational expansion of the repeat. Often, paternally inherited cases have earlier onset than do maternally inherited cases, and this simply may reflect the bias toward larger expansions with paternal transmission of the expanded allele.

Spinocerebellar Ataxia 4

The spinocerebellar ataxia 4 disorder, which has been linked to markers on chromosome 16, has been described in a single Utah family. The age of onset is typically in the third and fourth decade, with median onset age near 39. Progressive ataxia was associated with prominent signs of a sensory polyneuropathy, with areflexia in the lower limbs in the majority and significant loss of vibration and position senses. In contrast to other dominant ataxias, dysarthria was less common, as were other signs of brain stem disease, including eye movement problems and other lower cranial nerve deficits. This condition resulted in an overall slower progression with a relatively normal life span.

Spinocerebellar Ataxia 5

Spinocerebellar ataxia 5 disease, which is linked to markers on chromosome 11, has been reported in a single family descended from the paternal grandparents of President Abraham Lincoln, though many other previously reported families have similar clinical features. The age of onset ranged from 10 to 68 years but typically occurred in the third to fourth decade. The disorder was more benign than many other dominant ataxias, with slower progression, lack of bulbar signs, and (often) a normal life span.

Spinocerebellar Ataxia 6

Researchers have described a form of dominant ataxia, spinocerebellar ataxia 6, due to a rather modest expansion of a CAG repeat sequence in the gene coding for the alpha subunit of the voltage-gated calcium channel. This disease also seems to

have a relatively late adult onset, occasionally with episodic symptoms and a relatively benign course compatible with a normal life span. The patients mostly have progressive pure cerebellar signs with little in the way of bulbar or upper motor neuron deficits, and pathologically the disease is characterized as cerebello-olivary atrophy.

Spinocerebellar Ataxia 7

The spinocerebellar ataxia 7 form of dominant cerebellar ataxia exhibits associated visual loss related to a maculopathy. The phenotypic variability within families with this disorder can be enormous, with wide variation in onset age and related variation in clinical phenotype and rate of progression. The age of onset is bimodal, with a significant proportion having onset in infancy and childhood and others in middle adult life (30 to 39 years). The disease can begin either with progressive visual loss or imbalance or both, and some persons in the family may exhibit one or the other symptom alone. In some adults, visual signs that can be detected only with sophisticated testing may be the only indication of the disease. Electroretinography and tritan color axis defects are useful methods for detecting such visual dysfunction. With childhood onset, the disorder is characterized by a rapidly progressive neurodegenerative disease that combines visual loss, ataxia, upper motor neuron signs, remarkable intention tremor, and other widespread neurologic signs, including seizures, myoclonus, and dementia. Adult-onset disease is characterized by a combination of ataxia, hyperreflexia, visual loss, and slow saccades. Signs of peripheral nerve disease are unusual.

Natural History

The natural history is one of progression. Childhood onset results in rapid progression, with death occurring within 5 years. In adults, the duration of disease varies from 5 to 41 years, with a mean of 18 years.

Factors Affecting Prognosis

Often, remarkable anticipation is seen in onset age from one generation to the next, especially among paternally inherited cases. This condition may result in children presenting with the disease and perhaps even dying from it before the affected parent becomes symptomatic. The gene mutation is on chromosome 3p; once again, the mutation is a highly unstable CAG repeat expansion.

Dentatorubral-Pallidoluysian Atrophy

Dentatorubral-pallidoluysian atrophy (DRPLA) is a relatively rare disorder in the West and has been described as mostly from Japan. The key to the clinical diagnosis of DRPLA is its extreme clinical variability within the same family. The age of onset varies from 6 months to older than 60 years. With childhood onset, the disease presents with myoclonic epilepsy, progressive dementia, ataxia, and chorea. Presentation in adult life results in a syndrome that combines chorea, ataxia, and dementia, often leading to the erroneous diagnosis of Huntington's disease.

Natural History

This progressive disorder has a variable course that appears to be related primarily to onset age. The time from onset to death has varied from 1 to 30 years in several reports, with earlier-onset cases having rapid progression.

Factors Affecting Prognosis

The mutation responsible for DRPLA is the unstable expansion of a CAG repeat in a gene on chromosome 12p. The normal allele has 7 to 34 repeats. Affected persons carry one allele in the expanded range with 54 to 75 repeats. Age of onset is correlated inversely with the number of repeats; juvenile cases with myoclonic epilepsy have a larger number of repeats, usually more than 62. Homozygous state probably leads to a disease state more severe than the usual heterozygous state.

Considerable anticipation is seen in age of onset. Paternal transmission often results in greater anticipation than maternal transmission. A paternal bias also is seen in the intergenerational instability of the repeat, with paternal transmission resulting in a mean expansion of five repeats (range +1 to +14) and maternal transmission leading to a mean expansion of 2 repeats (range –3 to +4).

Genetic Counseling in Dominant Ataxias

In the dominant ataxias, each offspring of an affected person has a 50% risk of being affected. As the person at risk grows older than the typical age of onset for a given disorder, the risk gradually diminishes but, given the wide scatter of onset age of these diseases, the risk does not vanish completely until very late in life. Thus, many at-risk persons have to make life decisions regarding their own offspring and career before they can be certain whether they will be affected by the disease.

In the many disorders in which the mutation already has been identified, presymptomatic testing is possible. The issues are very similar to those in Huntington's disease. The ethical dilemmas surrounding such decisions are a matter of some debate; in general, such testing should be offered only to adults, probably in the setting of a formal presymptomatic testing program. This approach often involves several sessions, including formal psychological assessments, genetic counseling, and follow-up. Issues regarding job and insurance discrimination, confidentiality of records, and the possible psychological reactions (both positive and negative) to the results of the test need to be discussed as well.

Summary and Conclusions

In a dramatic fashion, molecular genetic studies clearly have advanced the knowledge regarding inherited ataxias. Most of these ataxias, especially the dominantly inherited entities, result from unstable trinucleotide expansions and share a variety of features. An inverse correlation is observed between the age of onset and the number of repeats; also, a less well-defined relation appears to exist between clinical parameters of disease severity and the number of repeats, suggesting factors other than the repeat numbers alone may contribute to disease progression. The unstable nature of the expanded repeats may explain a number of previously baffling aspects of these illnesses, including intrafamilial variability of clinical features and anticipation in age of onset, both of which have a bearing on prognosis. However, the exact mechanisms by which larger expansions lead to earlier ages of onset and somewhat more severe disease remain unclear.

Clearly, anticipation is evident in onset age in most of these diseases, but not all anticipation can be explained by the degree of intergenerational expansion, suggesting some degree of ascertainment bias as an additional factor. Typically, in the dominant ataxias, anticipation and intergenerational expansion of the repeat size are greater with paternal than with maternal transmission.

Additional Reading

Durr A, Brice A, Lepege-Lezin A, et al. Autosomal dominant cerebellar ataxia type I linked to chromosome 12q (SCA II: spinocerebellar ataxia type II). Clin Neurosi 1995;3:12–16.

Durr A, Cossee M, Agid Y, et al. Clinical and genetic abnormalities in patients with Friedreich's ataxia. N Engl J Med 1996;335:1169–1175.

Enevoldson TP, Sanders MD, Harding AE. Autosomal dominant cerebellar ataxia with pigmentary macular dystrophy. A clinical and genetic study of eight families. Brain 1994;117:445–460.

Filla A, De Michelle G, Cavalcanti F, et al. The relationship between trinucleotide (GAA) repeat length and clinical features in Friedreich ataxia. Am J Hum Genet 1996;59:554–560.

Flanigan K, Gardner K, Alderson K, et al. Autosomal dominant spinocerebellar ataxia with sensory axonal neuropathy (SCA 4): clinical description and genetic localization to chromosome 16q22.1. Am J Hum Genet 1996;59:392–399.

Ikeuchi T, Koide R, Onodera O, et al. Dentatorubral-pallidoluysian atrophy (DRPLA). Clin Neurosci 1995;3:23–27.

Ranum LPW, Schut LJ, Lundgren JK, et al. Spinocerebellar ataxia type 5 in a family descended from the grandparents of President Lincoln maps to chromosome 11. Nature Genet 1994;8:280–284.

Sedgwick RP, Boder E. Ataxia Telangiectasia. In JMBV de Jong (ed), Handbook of Clinical Neurology (Vol 16): Hereditary Neuropathies and Spinocerebellar Atrophies. Amsterdam: Elsevier, 1991;347–424.

Sequiros J, Coutinho P. Epidemiology and clinical aspect of Machado-Joseph disease. Adv Neurol 1993;63:139–153.

Zhuchenko O, Bailey J, Bonnen P, et al. Autosomal dominant cerebellar ataxia (SCA6) associated with small polyglutamine expansions in the alpha 1A-voltage-dependent calcium channel. Nat Genet 1997;15:62–69.

Part V
Movement Disorders

Chapter 29

Essential Tremor

William C. Koller

Natural History

Essential tremor probably is the most common of the movement disorders. Tremor is the sole symptom and affects a variety of body parts, including the hands, head, voice, and (less often) the legs and trunk. Essential tremor occurs in families and is transmitted as an autosomal dominant gene. The condition is slowly progressive, can start anytime in life, and can cause significant disability.

Usually, the disease starts late in life, although it can begin in childhood. Initially, the symptoms and the resultant disability are mild, and patients often will not seek medical attention. The exact pattern of disease progression is unclear. Predicting which patients will develop more severe tremor is difficult, as the rate of progression of essential tremor is highly variable. Tremor in some patients may remain dormant (without change) for a long period (e.g., several decades) and then might increase to a new plateau. Patients often present to a doctor with concerns that they may have Parkinson's disease; alternatively, they seek a diagnosis because, after 20 to 30 years of experiencing tremor, they have functional disability. The severity of disability, of course, is related to such individuals' daily activities and to their perceived dysfunction.

Many patients with essential tremor never visit a physician because their tremors are mild and cause only a minimal functional problem. Very little investigation has focused on patients in this category.

Factors Affecting Prognosis

Tremor can be enhanced significantly by stress and emotional events. In contrast, repose often will decrease the tremor. Alcohol ingestion, even in modest amounts, often will reduce tremor dramatically for a short period.

Clearly, disability is determined in part by the occupation and activities of the patient. For those with hand tremor, the extent to which these people use their hands will affect the prognosis. The individual for whom hand manipulations are an essential element of his or her occupation (e.g., surgeon, draftsperson) will likely consider tremor more disabling than the individual whose work does not depend on hand dexterity. Likewise, teachers or real estate salespersons may be rendered nonfunctional by their voice tremor. Embarrassment can be a major problem for patients with essential tremor, particularly those with severe head tremors. Some individuals avoid going to restaurants or other public places, and social isolation may be the result.

Evaluation for Prognosis

The evaluation for essential tremor is based on history and clinical examination. Tremor severity can be estimated by the clinician; however, it is important to note that severity of tremor can fluctuate significantly both over time and by circumstance. For instance, patients often feel increased stress in the doctor's office.

The physician can achieve an adequate understanding of the tremor's effect on an individual's daily functioning by obtaining a precise history of how the tremor interferes with the patient's activities. Patients sometimes underestimate their disability or do not understand clearly how the tremor has adversely affected their activities. Because a patient may have coped with his or her tremors for many years, the patient may not be a good judge of the effect the tremor has on his or her life. The physician might elicit the opinion of friends and family members, which may aid in the assessment of disability and prognosis.

Although essential tremor is a very slowly progressive condition, in some patients the tremor worsens much more quickly. Such patients are much more concerned about the future and about how tremor will alter their activities.

Therapies Affecting Prognosis

Existing pharmacologic and surgical treatments can control tremors in many patients, though pharmacologic treatment of essential tremor often is inadequate. Primidone and the beta-adrenergic blocking drugs, such as propranolol, are the only drugs with proved efficacy. These agents, though reducing hand tremor, appear to have much less effect on tremor of the head and voice. In only 40% of patients who present to a neurologist for treatment of essential tremor will tremor be controlled with the use of these drugs.

It is not possible to predict the point at which patients will respond to pharmacologic therapy. Patients must be given the drugs in gradually increased doses to determine responsiveness. Adverse reactions will limit drug use in some. Tolerance to the effect of drugs has not been studied well, but the drugs do appear to have long-term efficacy in patients who respond.

Botulinum toxin injections can be helpful for patients with essential head or voice tremor. Surgical thalamotomy and deep-brain stimulation (DBS) of the thalamus exist for patients with severe, disabling tremors unresponsive to drugs. These procedures have risks but may provide very effective tremor control. Some estimate that 90% of patients have good results after DBS. Both thalamotomy and DBS of the thalamus appear to possess long-term efficacy in essential tremor; however, further study is needed.

Short-Term Prognosis

At onset, essential tremor usually is mild, is made worse by stress, but otherwise is rarely a major problem, and treatment may not be indicated. Because essential tremor is very slowly progressive in most patients, when disability occurs, pharmacologic or surgical treatment can be employed. If good tremor control results from these therapies, the prognosis is favorable.

Long-Term Prognosis

In some patients with essential tremor, all forms of treatment eventually will fail. The severity of tremor in these individuals may prevent them from performing the most basic activities of daily living. Eating, writing, drinking liquids, and other hand manipulations may be impossible. The prognosis for these patients is poor. Nonetheless, most patients with essential tremor will not experience such a poor quality of life.

Additional Reading

Bain PG, Findley LJ, Thompson PD, et al. A study of hereditary essential tremor. Brain 1994;117:805–824.

Benabid AL, Pollak P, Gervason L, et al. Long-term suppression of tremor by chronic stimulation of the ventral intermediate thalamic nucleus. Lancet 1991;337:403–406.

Eible R, Koller WC. Tremor. Baltimore: Johns Hopkins University Press, 1990.

Fahn S, Tolosa E, Marin C. Clinical Rating Scale for Tremor. In J Jankovic, E Tolosa (eds), Parkinson's Disease and Movement Disorders. Baltimore: Urban & Schwarzenberg, 1988.

Findley LJ, Koller WC. Essential tremor: a review. Neurology 1987;37:1194–1197.

Hubble JP, Busenbark KL, Koller WC. Essential tremor. Clin Neuropharmacol 1989;12:453–482.

Koller WC, Busenbark K, Miner K. The relationship of essential tremor to other movement disorders: report on 678 patients. Essential Tremor Study Group. Ann Neurol 1994;35:717–723.

Koller WC, Hubble J, Busenbark K. Essential Tremor. In DB Calne (ed), Neurodegenerative Disease. Philadelphia: Saunders, 1994;717–742.

Lou JS, Jankovic J. Essential tremor: clinical correlates in 350 patients. Neurology 1991;41:234–238.

Selby G. Stereotaxic Surgery. In WC Koller (ed), Handbook of Parkinson's Disease. New York: Marcel Dekker, 1987;421–436.

Chapter 30

Idiopathic Dystonia

Cynthia L. Comella

Torsion dystonia is an idiopathic disorder defined clinically by the Scientific Advisory Board of the Dystonia Medical Research Foundation as "a syndrome of sustained muscle contractions, frequently causing twisting and repetitive movements, or abnormal postures." The disorder is classified according to three schemes: age of onset, body distribution, and etiology. The prognosis of dystonia varies, depending on the patient's classification in each of these categories. In the vast majority of patients, dystonia is not a life-threatening disorder.

Natural History

Dystonia is recognized as a lifelong disorder that fluctuates in severity and intensity over its course. However, the natural history of dystonia has not been determined in longitudinal studies, and the availability of effective symptomatic medications has rendered future studies of natural history problematic.

The prevalence of dystonia is estimated to be 20 per 100,000 population. The onset of childhood dystonia usually occurs between age 3 to 9 and is roughly equal in female and male children. Adult-onset dystonia often begins between 30 and 50 years and, with the exception of arm dystonia, affects women more than men in an approximate 2 to 1 ratio.

Adult-onset focal dystonia is the most common type of dystonia. Among the focal dystonias, the most frequently involved area is the neck (cervical dystonia), with involuntary turning or twisting of the head. Blepharospasm refers to involvement of the eyes, with increased blinking and forced eye closure. Spasmodic dysphonia is dystonia of the laryngeal muscles, causing a whisper or strangled voice. Oromandibular dystonia involves jaw muscles with forced opening or closing. Generalized dystonia involves several body areas, including at least one leg and trunk and is the rarest form of dystonia, representing only one-ninth of the cases.

Idiopathic dystonia may be inherited as an autosomal dominant disorder with variable penetrance. The DYT1 gene is localized to chromosome 9q34. The DYT1 gene is responsible for most cases of childhood-onset generalized dystonia, especially in Ashkenazi Jews. In contrast, adult-onset focal dystonia has been considered a sporadic disorder. However, recent family studies in cervical dystonia have suggested that focal dystonia also may be autosomal dominant with a low penetrance. The DYT1 gene is not the cause of focal adult-onset dystonia, and the putative gene or genes have yet to be identified.

An intriguing aspect of dystonia is the effect of positional and sensory factors. Dystonic symptoms tend to change with voluntary activity of the involved body area and with the position of that body area. Many patients find certain sensory "tricks," such as touching the chin for cervical dystonia, can improve symptoms dramatically (albeit temporarily). These types of sensory tricks, or *geste antagonists*, have been described in all forms of dystonia. The mechanism of sensory tricks is not known.

Despite the chronicity of dystonia, it is not considered a progressive, neurodegenerative disease.

Table 30-1. Prognosis for Spread of Dystonia, Depending on Site of Initial Presentation

Initial Body Area Involved	Onset Age	Percentage with Spread to Other Body Areas	Percentage Developing Generalized Dystonia
Lower limb (crural dystonia)	8.4	94	89
Neck (cervical dystonia)	44	25	6
Eyes (blepharospasm)	54	37	6
Larynx (spasmodic dysphonia)	NG	14	0
Arm (brachial dystonia)	NG	41	27

NG = not given.
Source: Adapted from P Greene, UJ Kang, S Fahn. Spread of symptoms in idiopathic dystonia. Mov Disord 1995;10:143–152.

No evidence suggests ongoing deterioration of brain structure or function, as is the case in other chronic neurologic disorders, such as Parkinson's disease or amyotrophic lateral sclerosis. However, the symptoms of dystonia can result in major disability, with significant impact on the capacity of many patients to lead a normal life.

The natural history of dystonia is, in part, predicted by the age of onset, the area of the body first affected, and the occurrence and duration of spontaneous remission. The likelihood of dystonia spreading from one body region to another was analyzed by Greene and associates in 115 patients with onset less than 22 years and in 472 patients with older-age-onset dystonia. In the young-onset group, the most frequent body area involved was the leg. The mean age of symptom onset was 4 years. The first symptoms were foot inversion, especially in running. Later, the intensity of the symptoms increased such that foot involvement would occur with less activity and then began to occur even at rest. Ninety-four percent of the children with presentation in the leg went on to develop dystonia in other body areas, and 71% developed generalized dystonia. The spread from focal foot dystonia to generalized dystonia occurred approximately 5 years after disease onset. Older children (≥10 years) had an increased frequency of symptom onset in the arm and neck region. Of the older children, 33% later developed generalized dystonia. Adult-onset dystonia, defined as dystonia beginning after the age of 21 years, usually involves upper face, vocal cords, neck, or arms. In Greene's study, 36% of the blepharospasm patients had spread of dystonia to other facial muscles, but only 21% had spread beyond cranial structures. Adults with cervical dys-

tonia had spread beyond the neck area in 26% of the patients after a mean of 6.7 years, but only 6% eventually developed dystonic involvement of four or more nearby body areas. Laryngeal dystonia spread to other body areas infrequently, most often to the lower face or neck. Brachial dystonia progressed to involve other body areas in 41% of patients, usually spreading into the neck, lower face, trunk, or opposite arm (Table 30-1). Ethnic background, in particular Ashkenazi Jewish ancestry, was found to be associated with likelihood of spread, especially in patients with cervical dystonia.

The estimated occurrence of spontaneous remission has been assessed in several retrospective studies of cervical dystonia. These reports indicate a large variability in spontaneous remission rate, ranging from 4 to 40% of patients. Most investigators believe that some 20% of cervical dystonia will have a partial or complete remission. However, most remissions are transient, with a duration of 2 months to 18 years. The rate of permanent remission is unknown but is estimated to be less than 1%. Most remissions occur within the first 1 to 5 years after dystonia onset. Although it is much less common, patients with remission beginning 5 years after disease onset tend to have longer, more permanent resolution of symptoms. Remissions may be more frequent in patients presenting with tonic rather than clonic cervical dystonia, although this observation has not been consistent.

Symptoms may be worsened by stress, intercurrent illnesses and, in many patients, positional factors or certain activities. Patients with blepharospasm may report that the most severe symptoms are provoked by driving a car, exposure to bright lights or wind, or attempting tasks in which keeping eyes open is important. Patients with cervical dystonia or truncal dystonia may find that sitting up, walking, or trying to use their arms and hands exacerbates symptoms, whereas lying down or reclining improves symptoms.

Factors Affecting Prognosis

Factors associated with a good prognosis include adult onset in a single body area and the lack of any other neurologic abnormality suggesting a diagnosis other than idiopathic dystonia; in particular, no evidence of progressive cognitive decline, spasticity, weakness, neuropathy, or parkinsonism. The exception is dopa-responsive dystonia, an inherited disorder combining parkinsonism and dystonia. Dopa-responsive dystonia is exquisitely responsive to low doses of levodopa for prolonged periods of time and has an excellent prognosis.

The presence of a *geste antagonist* had been associated in some cases with a reduced likelihood of a spontaneous remission. However, a comparative study between cervical dystonia patients with a *geste antagonist* and those without has shown a reduction in overall disability and an increased employability associated with a *geste antagonist*.

Disability and psychosocial functioning has been studied by Jahanshahi and colleagues. Of 100 cervical dystonia patients assessed, 22 were classified as permanently sick with regard to employment. Patients with cervical dystonia, however, did not differ from those with cervical spondylosis in terms of personality or other important psychosocial dimensions, indicating that the disabilities found in cervical dystonia arose from the presence of a chronic disorder rather than from any specific, associated, psychologic dysfunction. Factors contributing to disability arising from cervical dystonia included position, pain (68%), and reduced head mobility. Pain was present in 60 to 70% of patients with cervical dystonia and, in many, was the most disabling aspect. Moderate to severe depression was present in one of four of the patients, and 48% were moderately to severely disabled by the disorder. Effective treatment of cervical dystonia symptoms by botulinum toxin injections resulted in a corresponding improvement in psychological function, indicating that movement of the head and associated pain played the pivotal role in the disability and depression.

Therapies Affecting Prognosis

No cure for dystonia exists. That early diagnosis and initiation of treatment alter the course of dystonia and increase the chance for a remission has been speculated but not shown.

Therapies for dystonia are divided into three categories: oral medications, intramuscular injections, and surgical procedures. Although these therapies do not offer a definitive cure, improvement of symptoms of dystonia improves quality of life and alleviates disability in many patients. Standard oral pharmacologic therapy includes anticholinergic agents, baclofen, clonazepam, and levodopa. Tetrabenazine, a catecholamine-depleting agent, also has been shown to improve symptoms but is not available easily in the United States and may be difficult to use in patients, as often it causes dysphoria and depression as a side effect. A variety of other medications have been tried anecdotally and found to be of some benefit in an occasional patient. These agents include gabapentin, other benzodiazepines, carbamazepine, and dantrolene. Overall, approximately 40% of patients will improve on oral therapy, but side effects limit many oral agents. With the exception of levodopa, all these agents must be initiated at low doses, with a gradual increase in dose as tolerated until benefit occurs or side effects intervene.

Intramuscular injection of botulinum toxin is the most effective way to treat focal dystonia. Botulinum toxin is a potent neurotoxin that acts to prevent the release of acetylcholine at the neuromuscular junction. It accomplishes this effect by specific action on the proteins responsible for fusion of acetylcholine-containing vesicles with the presynaptic membrane. The effect of botulinum toxin is to weaken injected muscle. Little effect is seen on the central nervous system, so the centrally mediated limitations of the oral agents do not play a role. The effect of botulinum toxin is not permanent. The onset of action of botulinum toxin occurs within 3 days of injection, and peaks at 2 to 4 weeks after injection. The duration of benefit is 3 to 6 months. Patients then require treatment with botulinum toxin, or symptoms will reappear. No evidence suggests that botulinum toxin alters the natural history of dystonia, but repeated injections may provide long-term symptomatic relief. The limitations of botulinum toxin include the inability to treat large numbers of muscles because of dose considerations; involvement of muscles that are inaccessible or unsafe to inject, such as prevertebral muscles involved in anterocollis; and unwanted adverse effects, including excess weakness of injected muscle and diffusion of toxin into nearby, uninvolved muscles. This finding is particularly important in the treatment of writer's dystonia, as writing requires fine-motor skills that may be disrupted by even a small amount of undesired weakness.

Surgical procedures, including thalamotomy, rhizotomy, and selective peripheral denervation, usually are reserved for patients in whom no other treatment has been effective. Thalamotomy has an advantage in that it can ameliorate generalized dystonia. However, bilateral thalamotomies are necessary and frequently result in significant surgical morbidity, such as hemiparesis or dysarthria. Selective peripheral denervation with partial rhizotomy is applicable only to cervical dystonia. This procedure may be beneficial in appropriately selected patients but may require long postoperative recovery periods and may cause excessive neck weakness. Procedures such as pallidotomy currently are being explored. A good outcome from surgical procedure rests heavily on the training and experience of the surgeon and the careful selection of patients.

Short-Term Prognosis

In children with autosomal dominant dystonia and onset in the leg, spread of dystonia to other body areas is almost inevitable. Symptom onset in late childhood and adolescence, affecting the limb or neck, is associated with a slightly better prognosis.

In adults with onset of focal dystonia of the neck, eyes, face, or limbs, the prognosis generally is better. Although dystonia may spread to other areas in the same region, the likelihood of developing generalized dystonia is small. During the first 5 years after onset, the symptoms may fluctuate dramatically. Symptoms may be most pronounced at onset and then improve, or onset may be mild, with a gradual worsening. Remissions, although most likely to occur during the early years, tend to be transient.

Long-Term Prognosis

The prognosis for childhood-onset dystonia remains guarded. No therapy can halt the spread of symptoms or cure dystonia, and the majority of affected children progress to generalized dystonia. However, pharmacologic interventions can provide some relief in many children. Children are able to tolerate high doses of both anticholinergics and baclofen without serious side effects. Trihexyphenidyl in doses to 120 mg and baclofen doses up to 320 mg have been used successfully in controlling symptoms. Botulinum toxin injections can be administered in focal areas in which dystonic symptoms are most disabling.

The presence of generalized dystonia in a family with autosomal dominant dystonia is not necessarily a harbinger of ill for future children. The gene has a low penetrance, indicating that other factors must play a role in the development of symptoms. Genetic analysis of the DYT1 gene has shown that if one parent carries the DYT1 gene, 50% of his or her children will inherit the gene, but only 30% of the gene carriers actually will develop symptoms of the disorder. In inherited dystonia, the severity and extent may vary considerably, with some family members manifesting generalized symptoms and others having only mild focal areas of involvement.

Adult-onset dystonia likewise usually is a chronic disorder. Genetic analysis of the families of patients with cervical dystonia have shown that the DYT1 gene does not underlie this disorder. However, cervical dystonia appears to be a genetic disorder, possibly autosomal dominant in nature but with a penetrance so reduced that often it appears to be sporadic. The prognosis for focal dystonia patients depends on successful symptom treatment.

Additional Reading

Bressman SB, de Leon D, Brin MF, et al. Idiopathic dystonia among Ashkenazi Jews: evidence for autosomal dominant inheritance. Ann Neurol 1989;26:612–620.

Bressman SB, Warner TT, Almasy MA, et al. Exclusion of the DYT1 locus in familial torticollis. Ann Neurol 1996;40:681–684.

Chan J, Brin MF, Fahn S. Idiopathic cervical dystonia: clinical characteristics. Mov Disord 1991;6:119–126.

Fahn S, Marsden CD, Calne DB. Classification and Investigation of Dystonia. In CD Marsden, S Fahn (eds), Movement Disorders 2. London: Butterworth, 1987;332–358.

Greene P, Kang UJ, Fahn S. Spread of symptoms in idiopathic dystonia. Mov Disord 1995;10:143–152.

Jahanshahi M, Marion MH, Marsden CD. Natural history of adult-onset idiopathic torticollis. Arch Neurol 1990;47: 548–552.

Jahanshahi M. Psychosocial factors and depression in torticollis. J Psychosom Res 1991;35:493–507.

Lowenstein DH, Aminoff MJ. The clinical course of spasmodic torticollis. Neurology 1988;38:530–532.

Nutt JG, Muenter MD, Aronson A, et al. Epidemiology of focal and generalized dystonia in Rochester, Minnesota. Mov Disord 1988;3:188–194.

Van Zandlijcke M. Cervical dystonia (spasmodic torticollis): some aspects of the natural history. Acta Neurol Belg 1995;95:210–215.

Chapter 31

Gilles de la Tourette's Syndrome

Eric J. Pappert

Gilles de la Tourette's syndrome (GTS) is a neuropsychiatric disorder characterized by the onset of multiple motor—and one or more phonic—tics before adulthood. The tics may occur intermittently but, to qualify for the diagnosis of GTS, must be present for at least 1 year. Furthermore, no other neurologic disorder can explain the presence of the tics. In addition to tics, GTS commonly is associated with other signs and symptoms, including attentional difficulties, obsessive-compulsive and antisocial behaviors, depression, anxiety, cognitive difficulties, and explosive episodes of rage.

Natural History

As part of GTS, tics commonly present in childhood or early adolescence, with a typical onset near age 7. Three-fourths of GTS patients have symptoms by age 11; however, the inception of tics occurs from infancy to as late as early adulthood. At onset, two-thirds of GTS patients have simple motor tics affecting primarily the face and head, and less than one-fourth will first present with tics in the upper body, legs, or trunk. These simple motor tics may be brief jerks or more sustained contractions and affect such individual body areas as the eyelids, neck, face, or shoulders. Fewer than one-fifth of GTS patients have phonic tics, such as sniffing, grunting, squeaking, or throat clearing noises, as their initial sign. Individual word tics or coprolalia are rarely presenting signs. The tics may begin suddenly, though a gradual onset is more common.

During childhood, patients generally cannot predict or control the point at which their tics will occur. With early adolescence, GTS patients may report a premonitory sensation, such as a vague discomfort or urge to move that intensifies before the tic.

Over subsequent years, patients experience multiple simultaneous tics that come and go. At the time of adolescence and the subsequent 5 to 10 years, GTS symptoms generally become fully expressed. The motor tics become more complex, involving body turning, squatting, jumping, or touching. Some tics are sustained dystonic movements and can be self-injurious. Vocal tics may evolve beyond inarticulate noises to include formed words or coprolalia. Such a complex vocal tic typically occurs in only one-third of patients and usually appears 5 to 7 years after onset of symptoms. Vocal intrusions consisting of altered syllables (loudness or emphasis) of normal words, palilalia (the repetition of a phrase or word with increasing rapidity), or echolalia (the automatic repetition of what is said to him) also can occur. In later teenage years, the tics can be more unpredictable and seemingly can change from day to day, while at the same time becoming less severe. Older children may note brief relief of premonitory sensations immediately before the tic, yet describe its return shortly after the tic. Teenage and adult GTS patients may have a limited capacity to delay or suppress tics for a period of time, until the build-up of the urge overcomes them and they must produce the tic. Other symptoms can present during this time, including mental coprolalia (intrusive coprolalic thoughts) or copropraxia (involuntarily making obscene gestures).

Some evidence suggests a genetic link between various psychiatric disorders and GTS, specifically attention-deficit disorder (ADD) and obsessive-compulsive disorder (OCD). ADD, usually in association with hyperactivity (ADHD), typically occurs before age 5 in GTS patients, preceding clinically apparent tics. This disorder is more common in males, and some investigators report one-half to three-fourths of GTS patients meet the criteria for ADHD.

In most patient cohorts, obsessive-compulsive symptoms (sudden, intrusive, repetitive thoughts or urges for action) or OCD are reported in one-fourth to one-half of GTS patients. A waxing and waning course, complex movements or rituals, and repetitious behavior associated with urges and partial suppressibility can characterize both tics and OCD, making their distinction at times difficult. Though some GTS patients may have classic OCD symptoms, such as washing rituals and hygiene concerns, among the more typical obsessive-compulsive symptoms are touching, tapping, rubbing, counting, and symmetry worries. In contrast to ADD and ADHD, these behaviors are more likely to present at 3 to 6 years after onset of tics in GTS. Both ADD (or ADHD) and OCD may be far more disabling than tics and can be the reason for bringing GTS patients to the clinician.

Non-OCD anxiety and mood disorders also are described in GTS patients, though whether these conditions are related directly to GTS or merely represent secondary responses or maladaptive efforts to cope with the disorder remains unknown. Finally, self-abusive behaviors (bruxism, picking at scabs, punching objects, hitting or biting oneself) and explosive episodes of rage occur in a small percentage of GTS patients. Due to a lack of formal prospective studies, the natural history of the behavioral disorders associated with GTS is unknown. Temper tantrums, aggressiveness, and explosiveness may emerge in the preadolescent period, worsen in the teenage years, and then abate.

Factors Affecting Prognosis

No clinical features or laboratory findings are linked definitively to short- or long-term prognosis in GTS. Childhood symptom severity is suggested by some to predict tic intensity during adulthood, and one report indicated that two-thirds of children with moderate tics had mild symptoms as adults, whereas more than three-fourths with severe tics had moderate or severe symptoms in adulthood. Goetz et al., however, proposed that childhood tic severity cannot be used to predict later course but that adolescence functioning may be more predictive.

Evaluation for Prognosis

The evaluation for the prognosis of GTS involves little beyond proper clinical diagnosis and determination of associated behavioral abnormalities. Numerous neurologic and psychiatric disorders can produce tics and similar behavioral abnormalities as part of their clinical spectrum, and they should be considered. Overall prognosis in these cases will be linked to the underlying disorder. These conditions include inherited neurodegenerative disorders (Huntington's disease, neuroacanthocytosis, and juvenile neuroaxonal dystrophy), trauma, encephalitis (encephalitis lethargica, herpes simplex, human immunodeficiency virus), stroke, rheumatic fever, and toxic-metabolic encephalopathies. Tics may precede or accompany psychosis as part of the stereotypies or unusual mannerisms seen in schizophrenia. Similarly, autistic children may have mannerisms that could be interpreted as tics. Finally, various drugs are reported to induce or exacerbate tics, including stimulants (amphetamines, pemoline, cocaine, and methylphenidate), anticholinergics, antipsychotics, carbamazepine, and tricyclic antidepressants.

As many of the behavioral abnormalities associated with GTS contribute directly to long-term prognosis and can be the primary cause of disability, a thorough evaluation for their presence and severity should be undertaken. A number of psychometrically reliable and valid objective scales that measure OCD symptoms can be used. The Leyton Obsessional Inventory and the Yale-Brown Obsessive-Compulsive Scale (adult and children's versions) are used widely and are sensitive measures for documenting OCD. Neuropsychological tests that evaluate vigilance, impulsivity, and attentional (sustained, focused, selective, and divided) ability are similarly useful in the documentation of ADD and ADHD in patients with GTS.

Therapies Affecting Prognosis

Neuroleptics, including haloperidol and pimozide, are considered the most consistently helpful treatment in the suppression of tics, but no studies indicate that their use favorably affects long-term prognosis. The incidence of drug-induced side effects is high, frequently including weight gain, dysphoria, and sedation. Other movement disorders may occur as a result of neuroleptic use, including acute dystonia, bradykinesia, and akathisia. Both the chronic use and the discontinuation of these medications can lead to tardive dyskinesias at any age, though its incidence in younger patients is much less.

Stimulants (methylphenidate, dextroamphetamine, and pemoline) are the mainstays of treatment for ADD and ADHD, yet evidence for beneficial long-term outcome of these agents in GTS remains uncertain. The use of these agents has been associated with both precipitation of GTS and tic exacerbation; however, more recent studies have suggested that this association is unfounded or is a small risk. Data on other medications, including tricyclic antidepressants, clonazepam, and clonidine, is limited. Patients with GTS and OCD may benefit from treatment with clomipramine or other selective serotonin-reuptake inhibitors. Again, the long-term outcome of patients receiving these agents is not known.

In addition to medical management, social and educational resources may have an impact on the academic, behavioral, and psychosocial outcomes of patients with GTS. These resources include family support and assistance in understanding and parenting children with GTS. Selected studies have demonstrated that GTS children's self-concept correlated with their parents' reaction to their disorder. Patient, teacher, and peer education significantly may affect patients' ability to cope with the disorder and to be more successful academically and socially. The early identification of learning disabilities can have an impact on a child's education and ensure that proper teaching procedures are instituted. In conjunction, the GTS child's social developmental level should be assessed, and appropriate counseling should be provided. Overall, an effort should be made to keep all GTS patients in the classroom, rather than providing them with outside tutoring or placing them within a "special education" structure. Information on family, patient, and teacher-peer education resources is available from many chapters of the Tourette Syndrome Association.

Short-Term Prognosis

Over time, individual tics in GTS patients wax and wane in their intensity and frequency and even may alter in character. Though the presenting tics may disappear, they are replaced by new ones. New tics again may fluctuate, and past tics may or may not return. Many patients may have single or multiple tics that are persistent and remain unchanged in character. Tic symptom severity can fluctuate over hours, days, or weeks during prepubescence, adolescence, and adulthood. The degree of tic severity fluctuation, however, tends to diminish with age. Though increases in severity and improvement may occur for no apparent reason, multiple factors have been associated with increases in tic severity, including emotional stress, excitement, hormonal changes associated with menses, pain, allergies, temperature changes, and certain bacterial or viral infections.

Long-Term Prognosis

More than 100 years ago, Gilles de la Tourette stated that

> [T]he establishment of a tic is never followed by its ultimate disappearance; it may be modified in all sorts of ways, yet the expert observer will not fail to mark its presence. A complete cure is not to be expected, for however much paroxysms may be alleviated and their frequency reduced, the morbid condition has become a sort of function, a product of the patient's mental constitution.

According to Goetz, both Gilles de la Tourette and Charcot believed that tic disorders carried a poor overall prognosis, owing in part to their conviction that the tics were associated with serious psychiatric illnesses and in part to the observed tenacity of the disorder. Though these opinions and studies in the 1960s and early 1970s characterized GTS as a chronic, lifelong illness, this view was based on patients from the more severe end of the clinical spectrum. Because the major treatment of GTS involves potent neuroleptic drugs that can have irreversible side effects (e.g., tardive dyskinesia), a clear knowledge of the prognosis of this condition may influence both short- and long-term therapeutic decisions.

Although prospective longitudinal studies in GTS are limited in scope, retrospective studies indicated that many patients' tics improved in late adolescence or early adulthood, with an overall observation that approximately one-third had a "complete" remission and another one-third experienced a substantial improvement. These conclusions were based on primarily subjective reports, and objective data remain limited. In one questionnaire study, 73% of respondents believed that their tics had diminished considerably by late adolescence. The median age at which this improvement occurred was 16 years. The degree of improvement, however, was influenced neither by the maximal severity of the GTS nor by the patients' response to therapy. Lucas followed 20 subjects for 2 to 15 years into early adulthood and found that 14 had experienced improvement in their tic disorder, leading to the conclusion that "the tics almost invariably diminish in late adolescence...." Similarly, Zausmer reported that 75% of 41 patients rated themselves as improved, with 10 noting complete remission for more than a year. In a similar study, all patients older than 15 clinically improved as compared to their earlier function.

Lifelong "complete" remissions are rare, and occasional recurrence of mild tics during adult life is more common. Erenberg and coworkers found that 88% of adults continued to have impairment of activities of daily living as a result of tic symptoms alone, with 33% having severe interference. In this same study, 41% of all GTS patients older than 18 years continued to require pharmacologic therapy for their tics.

Data on long-term prognosis of concomitant behavioral symptoms in GTS are limited and at times conflicting. Commings and Commings noted that obsessive-compulsive symptoms became most problematic at mid-adolescence and reached a plateau thereafter, whereas other psychiatric conditions, such as depression, anxiety, and alcoholism, peaked in early adulthood. In contrast, Park and associates reported that nearly one-half of patients with ADHD, OCD, or disruptive behaviors improved on pharmacologic treatment over time. Erenberg also reported that nearly 60% of patients with previous learning disabilities or behavioral problems (mood swings, extreme anxiety, temper outbursts, and obsessive-compulsive behavior) no longer were having these difficulties or that they interfered only to a mild degree in their daily life.

In an effort to better understand the impact of GTS on patients' lives, Bruun and Budman combined their data and that of Stefl on 293 adult patients to evaluate the social and occupational status of the individuals. Nearly one-half never married or were divorced or separated, and only 57% were employed full- or part-time. Of Stefl's 114 patients, 14% graduated from or had some graduate-school experience, 34% completed or had some college experience, 32% had a high-school diploma, 18% had 9 to 11 years of education, and 4% had 8 or less years.

The development of better assessment measures for GTS since 1990 has focused on patient reports and objectively observed data. Objective data include direct observation of patients and evaluation of videotape-recorded tics. The latter methodology is advantageous as it allows for data assessment by multiple observers in the absence of direct involvement with patients and their care. It further may avoid the confounding effects of conscious or unconscious tic suppression seen during direct patient examinations. The use of such combined data in longitudinal assessments of GTS patients will provide additional important information regarding prognosis in the future.

Additional Reading

Bruun RD, Budman CL. The Natural History of Gilles de la Tourette Syndrome. In R Kurlan (ed), Handbook on Tourette's Syndrome and Related Tic Disorders. New York: Marcel Dekker, 1993.

Bruun RD. The Natural History of Tourette's Syndrome. In DJ Choen, RD Bruun, JF Leckman (eds), Tourette's Syndrome and Tic Disorders. New York: Wiley, 1988.

Commings DE, Commings BG. A controlled study of Tourette syndrome: I. Attention deficit disorder, learning disorders and school problems. Am J Hum Genet 1987;41:701–741.

Erenberg G, Cruse RP, Rothner AD. The natural history of Tourette syndrome: a follow-up study. Ann Neurol 1987;22:383–385.

Goetz CG, Tanner CM, Stebbins GT, et al. Adult tics in Gilles de la Tourette's syndrome: description and risk factors. Neurology 1992;42:784–788.

Goetz CG. Charcot, the Clinician: The Tuesday Lessons. New York: Raven, 1987.

Lucas AR. Follow-Up of Tic Syndrome. In FS Abuzzahab, FO Anderson (eds), Gilles de la Tourette's Syndrome. St. Paul, MN: Mason, 1976;47–67.

Park S, Como PG, Lu Cui MS, et al. The early course of Tourette's syndrome clinical spectrum. Neurology 1993;43:1712–1715.

Stefl ME. The Ohio Study: Initial Report of Data Prepared for the Tourette Syndrome Association. New York: Tourette Syndrome Association, 1983.

Zausmer DM. The treatment of tics in childhood: a review and a follow-up study. Arch Dis Child 1954;29:537–542.

Chapter 32
Hemifacial Spasm

Paul E. Greene

Hemifacial spasm (HFS) is a disorder in which involuntary contractions occur in muscles innervated by the facial nerve (cranial nerve VII). Three separate kinds of abnormal muscle activity are possible in HFS: individual muscle twitches, trains of muscle twitches, and episodes of tonic muscle contraction. Most patients with HFS have muscle contractions in the orbicularis oculi, although synchronous contractions often are seen in other ipsilateral facial nerve innervated muscles, such as the frontalis, zygomaticus major, risorius, depressor anguli oris, and mentalis. The etiology of HFS is thought to be compression of the facial nerve as it exits the brain stem, usually by an aberrant artery, such as the posterior inferior cerebellar artery, anterior inferior cerebellar artery, or by branches of these arteries. Irritation of the nerve at this site is believed to generate both spontaneous electrical activity and "cross-talk," or simultaneous activation of axons going to different parts of the face. Occasionally, HFS has been associated with compression of the facial nerve at the same location by arteriovenous malformations or tumors; it has been associated also with plaques of multiple sclerosis involving central myelin at the same location. On rare occasions, however, HFS seems to be associated with more peripheral lesions of the facial nerve (e.g., after Bell's palsy) or with pontine infarcts involving the facial nucleus. This finding has led to speculation that a peripheral lesion of the facial nerve may induce a change in the facial nucleus and that this change is necessary for HFS to occur.

HFS is rare: An estimated incidence of 0.78 per 100,000 was reported in Olmsted County, MN, between 1960 and 1984, a figure that was 3% of the incidence of Bell's palsy (25.2 per 100,000). However, HFS seems to be much more common in Asia, possibly related to a genetically based variation in vascular anatomy, placing the anterior inferior cerebellar artery closer to the facial nerve.

Natural History

The natural history of HFS was discussed in a series of 106 cases presented by Ehni and Woltman in 1945. They found that HFS was a disease that progressed very slowly, if at all, and had a benign outcome. HFS usually began around the eye and spread to the lower face, and twitching usually was the initial symptom, progressing to sustained spasms in a minority of patients. Twitching and spasms were the only symptoms of HFS in most patients, though a few patients also developed facial weakness or hearing loss. The duration of disease and length of follow-up was not given for the patients in that series.

Characteristics of patients in the Ehni and Woltman series are shown in Table 32-1. Symptoms around the eye were present at the onset in 90% of cases. In 70% of cases, periorbital muscles were involved before lower facial muscles and, in 25% of cases, the spasms initially involved only the lower eyelid (18%) or upper eyelid (7%). In 15%, no spread of symptoms occurred after onset of the disease. Twitching was the initial symptom in 95% of patients, and 20% of these eventually developed

Table 32-1. Comparison of the Clinical Characteristics in Two Series of Hemifacial Spasm Patients

Characteristic	Ehni and Woltman's Study	Columbia University Study
Number of patients	106	158
Age of onset	17–70 yrs (mean, 45 yrs)	9–79 yrs (mean, 51 yrs)
Ratio of women to men	1:5	1:5
Duration of disease	Not given	<1 yr–40 yrs (mean, 5.7 yrs)
Develop sustained eyelid closure	23.6%	38.2%
Develop facial weakness	15.1%	9.2%

sustained spasms, but the time required to develop these spasms was not recorded. However, in five patients, sustained spasm was present at onset, to which twitching was added later in one. In 15% of patients, the authors reported facial weakness but did not comment on the degree of weakness or the duration of disease at time of examination. In addition to facial weakness, these authors' patients reported several symptoms possibly related to their HFS. Hearing loss was present in 14% of patients on the side of the spasms. One or two patients reported increased tearing, facial numbness, loss of taste, vertigo, or tongue weakness on the side of the spasms. Six patients (6%) went on to develop asynchronous hemifacial spasm in the contralateral face after an interval ranging from less than 1 year to a maximum of 15 years. Nine patients (8.5%) went on to develop remissions lasting weeks to 3 years.

At the Movement Disorders Center at Columbia-Presbyterian Medical Center in New York, we have seen 204 patients with HFS, including 158 patients with available data regarding onset and progression of the disease. On the basis of examination at the first visit before botulinum toxin injections, some data can be provided about the natural history of HFS. As shown in Table 32-1, the characteristics of our patients were similar to those of Ehni and Woltman. Ninety-six patients had magnetic resonance imaging or computed tomography scans of the head, which was normal in 66%, showed an ectatic posterior fossa vessel in 12.5%, and revealed a posterior fossa arteriovenous malformation or tumor in 6%.

Symptoms began around the eye in 93% of our patients; 6% started in the lower face, and clicking in the ear was the first symptom in one patient. The exact site of onset was not specified in most patients, but 16 patients reported initial twitching in the lower eyelid, whereas only two patients reported initial twitching in the upper eyelid; all eventually developed twitching in upper and lower lids. In 14% of patients, twitching was intermittent at onset of disease, but most of these patients were constantly aware of twitching by the time they consulted us. Sustained eyelid closure developed in 38% of patients after a mean 5.6 years. The other 62% of patients had minimal or no sustained spasms after a mean 5.4 years of disease. Only 9% of our patients had marked facial weakness. The other 91% of patients had normal facial strength or had only an asymmetric face at rest. We had 26 patients with disease duration of 10 or more years. The outcome in these patients was similar to that of the group: Some 62% had no sustained eyelid closure after a mean 18.6 years, and 88% had no significant facial weakness after a mean 16.8 years.

As in the previous series, some of our patients developed other symptoms besides facial movements and weakness. Hearing loss or some form of tinnitus was present on the side of the HFS in 25%. Ipsilateral facial pain was present in 11%, ipsilateral facial numbness in 8%, and slurred speech with severe spasms in 3%. One or two patients also associated the following complaints with their HFS: drooling, decreased taste or smell, and vertigo. Eight patients (5%) reported remissions lasting 1 month to 1 year (mean duration, 6 months).

Therapies Affecting Prognosis

Since 1945, two effective treatments for HFS have been developed: removal of a blood vessel from the root exit zone of the facial nerve (microvascular decompression) and botulinum toxin injections. Several very large series of patients with HFS have been reported with these treatments, but few data about the clinical course of the disease have been presented. Both of these treatments significantly alter the course of HFS. From 70% to more than 95% of patients undergoing microvascular decompression have been reported completely free of spasms after the operation. Botulinum toxin injections have been reported to improve (but usually not to eliminate) spasms in 100% of injected patients. In addition, botulinum toxin injections can cause facial weakness, and even though the effects of the injections wear off after 3 to 6 months, most patients are reinjected before the effects completely wear off. This finding renders difficult the interpretation of residual spasms and facial weakness in patients undergoing chronic botulinum toxin injections.

Short- and Long-Term Prognosis

The course of HFS in our patients was similar to the course described by Ehni and Woltman. Somewhat more of our patients developed sustained eyelid closure, and fewer developed facial weakness, but these differences may be owing to different criteria for weakness and eyelid closure. In both groups, HFS was a static or slowly progressive illness. Despite the confounding effects of repeated botulinum toxin injections, my impression is that few patients develop progressive spasms or facial weakness over time. Although hearing loss, tinnitus, and facial numbness develop in some patients, a relationship between these symptoms and HFS remains to be confirmed.

Additional Reading

Auger RG, Whisnant JP. Hemifacial spasm in Rochester and Olmsted County, Minnesota, 1960 to 1984. Arch Neurol 1990;47:1233–1234.

Ehni G, Woltman HW. Hemifacial spasms: review of one hundred and six cases. Arch Neurol Psychiatry 1945; 53:205–211.

Illingworth RD, Porter DG, Jukabowski J. Hemifacial spasm: a prospective long term follow up of 83 cases treated by microvascular decompression at two neurosurgical centres in the United Kingdom. J Neurol Neurosurg Psychiatry 1996;60:72–77.

Jannetta PJ. Microsurgical exploration and decompression of the facial nerve in hemifacial spasm. Curr Top Surg Res 1970;2:217–220.

Savino PJ, Sergott RC, Bosley TM, Schatz NJ. Hemifacial spasm treated with botulinum A toxin injections. Arch Ophthalmol 1985;103:1305–1306.

Tolosa E, Marti MJ, Kulisevsky J. Botulinum toxin injection therapy for hemifacial spasm. Adv Neurol 1988;49: 479–491.

Zhang K-W, Shun Z-T. Microvascular decompression by the retrosigmoid approach for idiopathic hemifacial spasm: experience with 300 cases. Ann Otol Rhinol Laryngol 1995;104:610–612.

Part VI

Demyelinating Disorders

Chapter 33

Optic Neuritis

Valerie Biousse and Nancy J. Newman

Optic neuritis is an inflammation of the optic nerve typically occurring in young patients. It is characterized by subacute, painful loss of central vision. Multiple causes underlie inflammatory optic neuritis, including such infectious diseases as syphilis, cat-scratch fever, and Lyme disease, and such non-infectious inflammations as sarcoidosis and systemic lupus erythematosus. However, in most cases, optic neuritis remains idiopathic or is associated with multiple sclerosis (MS).

Idiopathic demyelinating optic neuritis is the most common acute optic neuropathy in people younger than 45. At least two-thirds of patients are women. In high-risk areas, such as northern Europe and the northern United States, the yearly incidence is 3 per 100,000 and, in lower-risk areas, the incidence is 1 per 100,000.

The Optic Neuritis Treatment Trial (ONTT), a large, multicenter trial, was designed to evaluate the effects of corticosteroid treatment on acute idiopathic optic neuritis. It continues to provide important information regarding the natural history, prognosis, and treatment of this disorder (see Beck and associates).

Natural History

Visual Outcome

Patients with idiopathic inflammatory optic neuritis typically improve spontaneously over several weeks, regardless of treatment. In the ONTT, improvement began within the first 2 weeks in most patients and within the first month in nearly all patients. At 6 months, 94% of all patients had vision of 20/40 or better, and in 75%, vision had improved to 20/20 or better. The majority of visual field defects also returned to normal. Therefore, lack of some visual improvement within the first month of optic neuritis should be considered atypical and warrants further investigation. Recurrence of optic neuritis ranges from 20 to 35%, depending on length of follow-up. The ONTT reported recurrences in either eye within 2 years in 16% of the patients treated with placebo.

Conversion to Multiple Sclerosis

The risk of subsequent development of MS after an isolated attack of idiopathic optic neuritis varies from 19 to 75%, depending on the series and the length of follow-up. One study by Francis et al. and another by Rizzo and Lessel of predominantly white female subjects from northern latitudes reported a risk of developing MS at approximately 20% at 2 years and 40% at 5 years. Life-table analysis suggested an approximate 74% risk of developing MS within 15 years of an optic neuritis attack, with the majority developing MS within 5 years. In the ONTT, 18% of optic neuritis patients treated with placebo had a second MS-defining neurologic event at 2 years, the number increasing to 27% at 4 years.

Table 33-1. Percentage of Patients with Multiple Sclerosis According to Baseline Brain MRI After 4-Year Follow-Up

Follow-Up	Normal MRI (%) (n = 202)	1–2 Signal abn (%) (n = 61)	>3 Signal abn (%) (n = 89)
6 mos	1.0	6.8	17.2
1 yr	2.6	14.0	25.6
2 yrs	4.9	19.7	31.7
3 yrs	9.3	27.7	43.1
4 yrs	13.3	35.4	49.8

MRI = magnetic resonance imaging; signal abn = periventricular signal abnormalities.
Source: Reprinted with permission from RW Beck, J Trobe, for the Optic Neuritis Study Group. What have we learned from the Optic Neuritis Treatment Trial? Ophthalmology 1995;102:1507.

Table 33-2. Percentage of Patients with Multiple Sclerosis within 2 Years by Treatment Group and Baseline Brain MRI in the ONTT

Baseline Brain MRI	Treatment Groups		
	IV Steroids (%) (n = 120)	Placebo (%) (n = 113)	Oral Steroids (%) (n = 119)
Normal	3	3	7
1–2 Signal abnormalities	15	23	23
>3 Signal abnormalities	16	39	38

MRI = magnetic resonance imaging; ONTT = Optic Neuritis Treatment Trial.
Source: Reprinted with permission from RW Beck, J Trobe, for the Optic Neuritis Study Group. What have we learned from the Optic Neuritis Treatment Trial? Ophthalmology 1995;102:1507.

Factors Affecting Prognosis

Visual Outcome

In the ONTT, poor baseline visual acuity was the only valuable predictor of poor visual outcome, but visual recovery still was good in most patients, even those with no light perception. Of 160 patients starting with a visual acuity of 20/200 or worse, all had at least some improvement, and only 8 (5%) had visual acuities that still were 20/200 or worse at 6 months. Of 30 patients whose initial visual acuity was light perception or no light perception, 20 (67%) recovered to 20/40 or better.

Recurrence of Optic Neuritis

The ONTT reported an incidence of optic neuritis recurrence at 2 years among patients treated with oral prednisone alone (30% in either eye) greater than that among those treated with intravenous steroids followed by oral prednisone (13% in either eye) or those treated with placebo (16% in either eye). Therefore, treatment of optic neuritis patients with oral prednisone alone should be avoided.

Conversion to Multiple Sclerosis

The ONTT confirmed that white-matter abnormalities on brain magnetic resonance imaging (MRI) were a powerful predictor of the subsequent risk of MS. Patients with three or more lesions on MRI had a 2-year risk of MS of 32%, whereas patients with a normal MRI had a risk of 5%. At 3-year follow-up, the risk of MS was 43% in patients with three or more lesions on the MRI and 9% for patients with normal MRI. At 4-year follow-up, the risk was 50% and 13%, respectively (Table 33-1). These findings are in accordance with Francis et al.'s study showing that 82% of patients with abnormal MRI scans developed definite MS versus 6% with normal MRI at the time of optic neuritis. In the ONTT, most of the beneficial effect of intravenous steroid treatment in reducing the 2-year rate of MS (see Therapies Affecting Prognosis) was seen in patients with an abnormal brain MRI at study entry (Table 33-2). Other, less powerful predicting factors for the development of MS among ONTT patients included nonspecific previous neurologic symptoms, history of optic neuropathy in the fellow eye (as previous optic neuropathy in the study eye was an exclusion criterion and therefore not evaluated), white race, and family history. Rizzo and Lessel suggested that the risk of developing MS after optic neuritis was greater for women than for men (74% and 34%, respectively) 15 years after their attack of optic neuritis. This prospective study also suggested that onset of optic neuritis between the ages of 21 and 40 modestly increased the risk of developing MS. However, in the ONTT, gender and age at onset of optic neuritis were not predictive of subsequent development of MS at 2-year follow-up. The ONTT confirmed that cerebrospinal fluid abnormalities had little predictive value for development of MS.

Evaluation for Prognosis

At a first attack of optic neuritis, evaluation for prognosis should include measurement of visual acuity and determination of previous nonspecific neurologic symptoms, previous optic neuritis in the fellow eye, and family history of MS. An MRI of the brain is useful, as it is a powerful predictor of the development of MS after an isolated attack of optic neuritis.

Therapies Affecting Prognosis

Until recently, patients with optic neuritis were treated empirically and received either oral or intravenous steroids—or no treatment—depending on the severity of the visual loss and the doctor's preference. The ONTT provided important information on the prognosis of optic neuritis depending on treatment. Patients in the ONTT were assigned randomly to three treatment arms: (1) oral prednisone, 1 mg per kg per day for 14 days; (2) intravenous methylprednisolone, 250 mg four times daily for 3 days, followed by oral prednisone, 1 mg per kg per day for 11 days; or (3) oral placebo for 14 days. Each regimen was followed by a short oral taper (see Beck and associates, 1992).

Visual Outcome

Compared with placebo and oral prednisone regimens, intravenous therapy provided more rapid recovery of vision but no long-term benefit. Most of the difference in rate of recovery among groups was seen in the first 2 weeks. Thereafter, differences in visual function among groups were small. After 1-year follow-up, no significant differences were seen among groups for visual acuity, contrast sensitivity, color vision, or visual field.

Table 33-3. Percentage of Patients with Multiple Sclerosis by Treatment Group After 4-Year Follow-Up in the ONTT

Follow-Up	Treatment Groups		
	IV Steroids (%) (n = 134)	Placebo (%) (n = 126)	Oral Steroids (%) (n = 129)
6 mos	3.1	7.4	7.2
1 yr	6.4	13.4	10.5
2 yrs	8.1	17.7	15.6
3 yrs	17.3	21.3	24.7
4 yrs	24.7	26.9	29.8

ONTT = Optic Neuritis Treatment Trial.
Source: Reprinted with permission from RW Beck, J Trobe, for the Optic Neuritis Study Group. What have we learned from the Optic Neuritis Treatment Trial? Ophthalmology 1995;102:1507.

Recurrence of Optic Neuritis

The regimen of oral prednisone alone not only provided no benefit to vision but was associated with an increased rate of new attacks of optic neuritis in both the initially affected and the fellow eyes. Within the first 2 years of follow-up, new attacks of optic neuritis in either eye occurred in 30% of the patients in the oral prednisone group, contrasted to 16% in the placebo group and 13% in the intravenous group.

Conversion to Multiple Sclerosis

The ONTT also found that the group receiving intravenous corticosteroid had a rate of development of MS within the first 2 years (7.5%) lower than that of the placebo or oral prednisone groups (16.5% and 14.7%, respectively). However, this protective effect no longer was appreciable after 3 years: Some 17.3% of patients treated with intravenous steroids and 20.7% of those treated with placebo had developed MS (Table 33-3).

Short-Term Prognosis

The short-term prognosis for optic neuritis patients is good, with a large majority of patients recovering nearly normal visual function within the first month. However, even patients with visual acuity of 20/20 or better often experience persistent subjective visual complaints such as dimming of colors, diminished sense of brightness, and lack of contrast. The ONTT showed that patients treated with intravenous steroids recovered vision sooner, but ultimately no differences were seen in visual function among the three treatment groups.

Long-Term Prognosis

The long-term prognosis for optic neuritis patients is dominated by the risk of development of MS. The risk varies from 13% at 4 years in patients with normal brain MRI at the time of optic neuritis to 50% at 4 years in patients with more than three periventricular signal abnormalities on MRI. Intravenous steroids have only a temporary protective effect on the development of MS. Ongoing studies are seeking to determine whether the administration of other agents useful in the treatment of MS will delay the onset or modify the course of MS after presentation with isolated optic neuritis.

Additional Reading

Beck RW, Arrington J, Murtagh R, et al. Brain magnetic resonance imaging in acute optic neuritis. Experience of the optic neuritis study group. Arch Neurol 1993;50:841–846.

Beck RW, Cleary PA, Anderson MM Jr, et al. A randomized, controlled trial of corticosteroids in the treatment of acute optic neuritis. N Engl J Med 1992;326:581–588.

Beck RW, Cleary PA, Backlund JC, et al. The course of visual recovery after optic neuritis: experience of the Optic Neuritis Treatment Trial. Arch Ophthalmol 1994; 101:1771–1778.

Beck RW, Cleary PA, Trobe JD, et al. The effects of corticosteroids for acute optic neuritis on the subsequent development of multiple sclerosis. N Engl J Med 1993;329:1764–1769.

Beck RW, Optic Neuritis Study Group. The Optic Neuritis Treatment Trial: three-year follow-up results. Arch Ophthalmol 1995;113:136–137.

Beck RW, Trobe J, for the Optic Neuritis Study Group. What have we learned from the Optic Neuritis Treatment Trial? Ophthalmology 1995;102:1504–1508.

Francis DA, Compston DAS, McDonald WI. A reassessment of the risk of multiple sclerosis after extended follow up. J Neurol Neurosurg Psychiatry 1987;50:758–765.

Morrissey SP, Miller DH, Kendall BE, et al. The significance of brain magnetic resonance imaging abnormalities at presentation with clinically isolated syndromes suggestive of multiple sclerosis: a 5-year follow-up study. Brain 1993;116:135–146.

Newman NJ. Optic neuropathy. Neurology 1996;46: 315–322.

Rizzo JF, Lessel S. Risk of developing multiple sclerosis after uncomplicated optic neuritis: a long term prospective study. Neurology 1988;38:185–190.

Chapter 34

Multiple Sclerosis

Patricia K. Coyle

Multiple sclerosis (MS) is an immune-mediated disorder affecting the central nervous system (CNS). It is characterized by inflammation and demyelination. Activated T cells enter the CNS across small veins and produce an immune cascade. This cascade results in localized areas of myelin loss and oligodendrocyte destruction. Microglia and macrophages are critical participants in the destructive immune process. The resultant pathologic lesions, called *plaques*, accumulate over time and produce an increasing total lesion burden. One or more infectious agents are implicated as environmental triggers for this immune-mediated process. In addition, host genetic factors play an important but as yet unidentified role.

MS is the major acquired neurologic disorder of young adults. An estimated 300,000 to 350,000 MS patients reside in the United States. Disease onset in 90% of patients occurs between the ages of 15 and 50, with a mean onset age of 30. Women make up at least 70% of cases.

Natural History

The natural history of MS is highly variable. Autopsy studies indicate that MS can be asymptomatic, with subclinical disease perhaps as common as clinical disease. Symptomatic MS involves a spectrum of severity, ranging from very mild to very severe. Disease course varies depending on the clinical type of MS.

The clinical classification of MS not only describes disease course but has prognostic significance. Most MS patients (85%) begin with relapsing disease, characterized by acute attacks and exacerbations of neurologic problems. Between attacks, relapsing MS patients appear clinically stable. A subgroup of relapsing patients (approximately 10 to 20%) is considered to have especially mild (benign) disease. A minority of MS patients (10 to 15%) have primary progressive disease. They never experience acute relapses but rather have slow worsening of deficits. Ultimately, some 50% of relapsing patients also develop slow progression with or without superimposed acute relapses. At this point, such patients are classified as having changed from relapsing to the secondary progressive form of MS. The final clinical type, progressive relapsing disease (≤5%), describes MS patients who are progressive from onset (similar to the primary progressive form) but later experience one or more relapses.

Overall, MS has little direct effect on survival. The life span of MS patients as a group is shortened by only 2 years as compared to age- and gender-matched controls. At 25 years into the disease, 76% of MS patients are alive, contrasted to 85% of matched controls. In several different MS populations, the mean survival after disease onset was 25 years, and the median survival was 27 to 38 years. However, survival is linked strongly to degree of disability. For MS patients with severe disability, the probability of death is increased more than fourfold. Survival is highest for MS patients with unrestricted activity, is decreased for wheelchair-bound patients, and is lowest for bed-confined patients. The overall observed-to-expected MS mortality ratio (standard-

Table 34-1. Prognostic Factors in Multiple Sclerosis

Factor	Favorable	Unfavorable
Gender	Female	Male
Age at onset	<40 yrs	≥40 yrs
Clinical type	Relapsing	Progressive
Relapse type	Monosymptomatic	Polysymptomatic
Relapse system	Optic nerve, sensory, brain stem	Motor, cerebellar, sphincter involvement
Relapse rate	Low	High (>5 in first 2 years)
Relapse recovery	Complete	Incomplete
Disability at 5 and 10 years	Minimal	Moderate to severe
Magnetic resonance imaging	Decreased T2 lesion load	Increased T2 lesion load
	Decreased active lesions	Increased active lesions
		Increased demyelination, axonal and tissue loss

ized for age, disability, and gender) is 2. With suicide excluded, the ratio falls to 1.29. For MS patients with mild disability, the observed-to-expected mortality ratio is 1.5 and falls to 1.36 with suicides excluded. For MS patients who are wheelchair- or bed-confined, the observed-to-expected mortality ratio is 4.4, with or without suicides excluded. Ten years into the disease, mortality is only 6% in patients with unrestricted activity, contrasted to 69% and 83%, respectively, in wheelchair- and bed-bound patients. Mortality in an MS population can be attributed to secondary complications of the disease (50 to 66%), to suicide (up to 29%), to primary complications of the disease, or to non-MS causes. The suicide rate among MS patients is up to seven and a half times that of the general population.

MS produces significant morbidity. Ultimately, 30% of MS patients become wheelchair-bound, 50% require a unilateral assistive device to ambulate after 15 years, and at least 70% experience neurologic disability that disrupts vocational careers.

The attack rate for relapsing MS varies over time. On the average, relapsing MS patients experience 1.2 clinical relapses annually. Relapse rate is highest early in the disease course and falls over time. After a first attack, more than 25% of patients have a relapse within 1 year, 50% within 3 years, 75% within 5 years, and 95% within 15 years.

Relapses typically develop over hours to days but occasionally occur over minutes or over several weeks. Recovery generally occurs within 3 months.

Usually, recovery is good following early attacks. Less than 3 to 4% of early relapses are severe enough to make the patient nonambulatory. In these very severe attacks, however, almost 40% of patients will have no improvement.

Magnetic resonance imaging (MRI) studies find that most MS lesion formation is clinically silent. New brain lesions outnumber clinical attacks 5 to 10 times. According to serial cranial MRI studies, relapsing and secondary progressive MS patients average 20 new lesions per year, benign relapsing patients 9 lesions per year, and primary progressive patients 3 lesions per year.

Factors Affecting Prognosis

Although not all studies uniformly agree, a number of prognostic demographic, clinical, and laboratory factors underlie MS (Table 34-1). The most important overall prognostic factor is the extent of disability 5 years into the disease. Clear-cut impairment at this point correlates with a more severe disease course. The relapsing disease subtype, in particular the benign or mild relapsing form, is more favorable than are the progressive forms of MS. Early onset age and female gender also favor a better prognosis than do onset after age 40 and male gender. Specific types of relapses (those involving optic nerve, brain stem, or sensation), monosymptomatic involvement, and complete recovery from relapses indicate a more favorable prognosis. The frequency of relapses early in the disease course also has prognostic significance. Patients with five or more relapses in the first 2 years reached a Kurtzke extended disability status scale (EDSS) of 6 (unilateral assistive device required to walk 100 meters) by 7 years, whereas those with two to four relapses required 13 years, and those with one attack required 18 years to reach this same level of disability. MRI features have been correlated with prognosis. Prognostic features are T2 lesion load, active lesions (defined as new, enlarging, or enhancing lesions), and extent of demyelination and tissue loss.

Most studies have found that pregnancy has no prognostic consequences. However, one Scandinavian study reported that the risk ratio for MS was

Table 34-2. Therapies for Relapsing Multiple Sclerosis That Affect Disease Course

Drug	Dosage	Actions
Interferon-β1b (Betaseron)	8 mU SC every other day	Clinical relapses decreased by 30% (all data) and 34% (2-yr data)
		Moderate-severe relapses decreased by 51%
		Decreased time to first relapse
		Decreased MRI T2 lesion burden
		MRI active lesions decreased by 75%
Interferon-β1a (Avonex)	6 mU IM weekly	Decreased sustained neurologic deterioration
		Clinical relapses decreased by 18% (all data) and by 32% (2-yr data)
		MRI active lesions decreased by 50%
Glatiramer acetate (Copaxone)	20 mg SC daily	Clinical relapses decreased by 32% (all data) and 29% (2-yr data)

MRI = magnetic resonance imaging; IM = intramuscularly; SC = subcutaneously.

higher in nulliparous women than in parous women. The risk ratio increased over time, ranging from 1.5 to close to 3. Moreover, pregnancy significantly lowered the risk of secondary progression. The researchers also found a trend for pregnancy to be associated with a more prolonged time to reach a disability status scale of 6.

Cerebrospinal fluid (CSF) findings have no documented effect on prognosis. However, a recent study reported that lack of oligoclonal bands correlated with a good prognosis.

Evaluation for Prognosis

The evaluation for prognosis involves appropriate disease classification, accurate demographic and clinical data, close monitoring of relapses, serial neurologic evaluations, and specific laboratory assessment. Cranial MRI to look at total lesion burden accumulation and at active lesion formation is helpful to suggest prognosis in all the clinical types except primary progressive disease. This form of MS seems particularly to affect the spinal cord and to involve axonal damage and tissue loss rather than extensive inflammatory lesion burden. MS patients with primary progressive disease are more likely to be older at onset, to be of the male gender, and to present with progressive myelopathy.

Therapies Affecting Prognosis

Three treatments now available for MS affect the disease course (Table 34-2). Both of the available recombinant interferon-βs have been shown to decrease clinical relapses and cranial MRI disease. The data are more robust for interferon-β1b (Betaseron), but this finding likely is attributable to a dosage higher than that for interferon-β1a (Avonex). Interferon-β shows a dose-related response, which was confirmed in a recent study using a third product, interferon-β1a (Rebif). Interferon-β1a slows worsening on the neurologic examination, as measured by the EDSS. At 2 years, 22% of the interferon-β–treated group had worsened, contrasted to 35% of the placebo-treated group in the interferon-β1a phase III multicenter study.

Both interferon-β1b and glatiramer acetate (Copaxone) also appear to have a positive effect on neurologic deterioration. In the case of interferon-β1b, this finding was a statistical trend (at 5 years, 35% worsened in the treated group, contrasted to 46% in the placebo group). In the case of glatiramer acetate, at 2 years, 21% of treated patients had worsened, contrasted to 29% of placebo-treated patients. In the glatiramer acetate study, MRI was not evaluated routinely and, therefore, whether this drug has a positive effect on MRI lesion burden and activity is not known. This question is being addressed in an ongoing European study.

For progressive forms of MS, such cytotoxic therapies as cladribine and methotrexate may slow worsening. In one placebo-controlled methotrexate study, a composite clinical rating scale was used to show a modest benefit of methotrexate therapy on upper-extremity function. For cladribine, an initial phase II study showed significant slowing of progression compared to placebo. Once the drug was stopped, patients rapidly deteriorated to the same disability level as that of the placebo group. This study led to a multicenter placebo-controlled trial. The preliminary report found no significant effect on disability, although treatment reduced volume of enhancing lesions on MRI. Primary and secondary progressive MS patients were entered into the trial and, therefore, may have been underpowered to show an effect on disability.

Corticosteroids can hasten the time frame of recovery from acute relapses. However, they have not been shown to affect overall prognosis.

Short-Term Prognosis

Short-term prognosis is favorable for most MS patients. At onset, only a small minority show an acute fulminant course (the malignant or Marburg variant of MS). Most relapsing MS patients show some recovery from acute attacks and, particularly early on, recovery often is complete. Recovery begins most typically within 4 to 6 weeks. Primary progressive MS patients, in contrast, show slow deterioration, with occasional periods of clinical stabilization or, rarely, mild improvement.

In one analysis, early progression and motor involvement were the predictors of short-term deterioration. In another analysis, baseline EDSS of 3 to 5 and disease duration of less than 20 years were associated with higher probability of short-term worsening. A number of factors are postulated to induce MS worsening, including viral infection, pregnancy, heat exposure, and stress. Infection and pregnancy are the best-defined relapse triggers. Approximately 27% of acute relapses clearly are associated with viral (especially respiratory) infection, and viral infections are associated temporally with up to 60% of attacks. Anecdotal data suggest that bacterial infections also may trigger relapses. These infection-related attacks must be differentiated from pseudoexacerbation, which refers to transient neurologic worsening coincident with fever. Pseudoexacerbations clear once the infection is treated and do not reflect new lesion activity. Most studies have found a 30 to 40% rate of relapse in the postpartum period. However, two more studies found no increased risk of relapse after birth. They found a protective effect during pregnancy, particularly in the latter part. Heat exposure can produce temporary worsening of MS-related abnormalities,

presumably owing to conduction failure at increased body temperature. Stress is related frequently as a precipitant of relapses by many patients, but this effect has not been documented in formal studies. Trauma has not been shown to be a factor in either onset or worsening of MS.

Long-Term Prognosis

The majority of MS patients ultimately develop disability from their disease. At least 50% of relapsing patients enter a secondary progressive stage. Progressive disease does not indicate inexorable worsening. Up to 30% of progressive patients stabilize for several years, and a smaller proportion even may show improvement. The rate of progression seems to be greater for secondary progressive patients than for primary progressive patients. Once patients enter a secondary progressive stage, 75% remain ambulatory after 5 years, and 40% remain ambulatory after 15 years. The strongest predictor for progression is baseline disability (EDSS 3 to 5). In the recent interferon-β1a study, treatment with interferon-β was the single prognostic variable that correlated with risk for progression. Weaker predictive correlations were seen with an upper-extremity functional test (box and blood test for the nondominant hand) and with the ambulation index for more severely affected MS patients.

A subgroup of relapsing patients have a benign MS course. They have minimal permanent neurologic impairment 10 years or more into the disease, infrequent relapses, and excellent recovery from relapses. Although the exact proportion of relapsing patients who fall into this benign subgroup is not known, several studies have suggested approximately 20%.

Clinical and MRI and CSF data influence the long-term prognosis for development of MS in patients with monosymptomatic events (isolated optic neuritis, brain stem or cerebellar lesion, transverse myelopathy). Patients who have these isolated syndromes and in whom a brain MRI demonstrates typical MS lesions have a 70 to 90% risk of developing MS within 5 years, contrasted to a 4% risk for patients with normal MRI. The risk for MS is increased with a greater number and load of MRI lesions and with infratentorial lesions. When the lesion volume is greater than 1.23 cc, the risk of MS within the next 5 years is 90%, contrasted to 55% when lesion volume is less than 1.23 cc and 6% when MRI is normal. Higher lesion load also is associated with earlier onset of MS. Patients who have monophasic syndromes and show abnormal CSF (positive oligoclonal bands or intrathecal IgG production) also have an increased risk of developing MS. The predictive value of such abnormal CSF is 92%. Clinical risk factors for MS after isolated optic neuritis include young onset age (26 to 40 years), venous sheathing, recurrent optic neuritis, and (possibly) female gender. For transverse myelopathy, the major clinical risk factor is an incomplete (as opposed to a complete) myelopathy.

Additional Reading

Kraft GH, Freal JE, Coryell JK, et al. Multiple sclerosis: early prognostic guidelines. Arch Phys Med Rehabil 1981;62:54–58.

Lublin FD, Reingold SC. Defining the clinical course of multiple sclerosis: results of an international survey. Neurology 1996;46:907–911.

Phadke JG. Clinical aspects of multiple sclerosis in northeast Scotland with particular reference to its course and prognosis. Brain 1990;113:1597–1628.

Poser S, Poser W, Schlaf G, et al. Prognostic indicators in multiple sclerosis. Acta Neurol Scand 1986;74:387–392.

Runmarker B, Andersen O. Pregnancy is associated with a lower risk of onset and a better prognosis in multiple sclerosis. Brain 1995;118:253–261.

Runmarker B, Andersen O. Prognostic factors in a multiple sclerosis incidence cohort with twenty-five years of follow-up. Brain 1993;116:117–134.

Sadovnick AD, Eisen K, Hashimoto SA, et al. Pregnancy and multiple sclerosis: a prospective study. Arch Neurol 1994;51:1120–1124.

Visscher BR, Liu KS, Clark VA, et al. Onset symptoms as predictors of mortality and disability in multiple sclerosis. Acta Neurol Scand 1984;70:321–328.

Weinshenker BG. The natural history of multiple sclerosis. Neurol Clin 1995;113:119–146.

Weinshenker BG, Issa M, Baskerville J. Long- and short-term outcome of multiple sclerosis: a three-year follow-up study. Arch Neurol 1996;53:353–358.

Part VII

Neoplastic Disease

Chapter 35
Glioma

Mark T. Brown

Gliomas are primary brain neoplasms that derive from glial cell precursors and include astrocytomas, oligodendrogliomas, and ependymomas. In this chapter, the three gliomas are considered separately because their biological behavior and prognosis vary. Each type is graded further on the basis of various histologic characteristics that, to a greater or lesser extent, determine the biological behavior of the tumor.

Astrocytic neoplasms are the most common primary brain neoplasms in adults and can be characterized by cellular morphology as fibrillary or nonfibrillary, with roughly 90% having a fibrillary morphology. Fibrillary astrocytic tumors can be graded further in a three-tiered system as astrocytomas, anaplastic astrocytomas (AA), and glioblastoma multiforme (GBM) on the basis of such histologic characteristics as increasing cellularity, mitoses, vascular proliferation, and presence of necrosis. *Nonfibrillary astrocytomas* include such morphologic variants as pilocytic and protoplasmic astrocytomas. In this chapter, *malignant astrocytomas* refer to AA and GBM. *Astrocytoma* means well-differentiated fibrillary astrocytoma unless otherwise specified.

Oligodendrogliomas account for 4 to 8% of cerebral gliomas and are graded as well-differentiated or anaplastic on the basis of increasing cellularity, nuclear pleomorphism, mitoses, vascular proliferation, and necrosis. Oligodendroglial neoplasms may dedifferentiate into GBM.

Ependymomas occur intracranially (5% of intracranial gliomas) primarily in the region of the fourth ventricle or as spinal cord neoplasms (15% of spinal cord tumors) usually in the lumbosacral region. Ependymomas are graded as well-differentiated or anaplastic on the basis of the same histologic features as those for oligodendrogliomas.

Natural History

The natural history of malignant astrocytomas is understood well, with the course being one of progressive neurologic dysfunction and death and a median survival of 3 to 6 months. The natural history of well-differentiated astrocytomas is not understood as well. Their biological behavior is variable, with some tumors remaining quiescent for years and others progressing to more malignant forms. The incidence of astrocytoma progression to AA or GBM varies between 13 and 87% in assorted series, with the average interval to progression being roughly 4 years. However, predicting in given patients the point at which this may occur is not possible. The natural history for oligodendroglial neoplasms also is understood poorly. Oligodendrogliomas vary biologically similar to astrocytomas, though their overall natural history is less aggressive than that of astrocytic neoplasms. Some authors have suggested two periods in the life history of benign oligodendrogliomas. In the first (onset) phase, patients are asymptomatic or have only seizures, and the tumor is consistent with long survival. In the second phase, intracranial hypertension or neurologic deficits are produced, and the tumor correlates with shorter survival. Progression from well-differentiated oligodendrogliomas to anaplastic oligodendrogliomas or GBM carries with it the poorer prognoses of the more malignant forms. Patients with intracranial infratentorial ependymomas have shorter disease-free intervals and shorter survivals after treatment than those with spinal ependymomas.

Factors Affecting Prognosis

Factors affecting prognosis have been defined best for malignant astrocytomas. The most important factors in this group include age at diagnosis, histologic grade (GBM versus AA), and postoperative Karnofsky performance status (KPS). Age is especially important, with patients older than 45 to 50 having a poorer prognosis than younger patients independent of tumor grade. GBM patients have a worse prognosis than AA patients. Patients with a KPS of 70% or greater have a more favorable prognosis than those with a KPS of less than 70%. (Some analyses show that a KPS of 90% or greater is better than a KPS of less than 90% for subsets of patients with GBM.)

The most significant prognostic factor for low-grade fibrillary astrocytomas is age, with a significant improvement in survival for patients younger than 40 as compared to older patients. Other variables correlating with increasing survival are gross total surgical resection, lack of major postoperative deficit, and surgery performed since the 1970s.

Pilocytic astrocytomas are nonfibrillary astrocytomas with a patient prognosis significantly better than that for patients with fibrillary astrocytomas. These neoplasms may be cured if total surgical excision is possible. This procedure occurs most often when the tumor is located in noneloquent cerebral cortex. When pilocytic astrocytomas are located in their characteristic locations near the hypothalamus and third ventricle and cannot be resected completely, they carry a less favorable patient prognosis because of their tendency to progress slowly, though malignant degeneration is less common than in fibrillary astrocytomas.

Favorable prognostic factors for patients with oligodendrogliomas include well-differentiated histology compared to anaplastic histology, age 40 years or younger, more extensive surgery, and presentation with seizures and normal neurologic examination.

For intracranial ependymoma patients, favorable prognostic factors are being of an age beyond 16 years (in contrast to other gliomas wherein younger age is favorable) and having a postoperative KPS of greater than 70. Histologic anaplasia definitely is not associated with a poorer prognosis, possibly because of the relatively unfavorable location in the posterior fossa. Spinal ependymomas have been described as arising from the filum terminale (40 to 50% of cases) or at other spinal regions. In filum terminale ependymomas, factors having a favorable influence on prognosis are clinical history of less than 1 year, confinement of the tumor to the filum terminale, and total tumor removal. For other intramedullary spinal ependymoma patients, favorable prognostic factors include well-differentiated histology, location below C5–C6 cervical region, mild preoperative symptoms, and total tumor removal. Tumor size and age at diagnosis are not useful prognostic factors.

Evaluation for Prognosis

Accurate histologic diagnosis is the most important factor in evaluation for prognosis. Though more specialized tests may be valuable in research settings to determine labeling indices, presence of epidermal growth factor receptors, or chromosomal-genetic abnormalities, they are not used routinely to determine prognosis. Preoperative neuroimaging, preferably with magnetic resonance imaging (MRI), is vital, as it allows an informed decision about resectability of the lesion. Recent work suggests that the presence of residual tumor enhancement on early postoperative MRI scanning in malignant glioma patients is significant for prognosis. Such residual tumor enhancement on MRI was associated with a risk of death in GBM patients 6.6 times higher than that in patients without residual tumor enhancement. In patients with intracranial ependymoma, evaluation with cerebrospinal fluid cytology and spinal MRI or myelography should be performed to rule out drop metastases (occurring in 5 to 30% of cases), which change the underlying prognosis and mandate more extensive radiotherapy. Prognostic factors of age and postoperative performance status should be documented.

Therapies Affecting Prognosis

More extensive surgery and radiotherapy with more than 5,400 cGy are associated with significantly improved survivals in most studies of malignant astrocytomas. The benefit of these modalities is demonstrated best in certain patient subgroups, such as those with GBM and better performance status. Demonstrating the benefit of adjuvant chemotherapy has been more difficult. Early trials of nitrosoureas suggested that certain subgroups would benefit from adjuvant chemotherapy but did not demonstrate statistically significant survival advantages. One meta-analysis of 16 clinical trials with more than 3,000 patients selected randomly to receive either radiotherapy or radiotherapy and adjuvant chemotherapy has shown survival improvements for both AA and GBM patients treated with chemotherapy. The estimated increase in survival for patients treated with combination radiotherapy and chemotherapy was 10.1% at 1 year and 8.6% at 2 years.

For low-grade astrocytomas, gross total resection clearly is associated with improved survival. Considerable controversy remains regarding the efficacy of external-beam radiotherapy for low-grade astrocytomas. Retrospective analyses have not shown convincing benefit for radiotherapy, though it may benefit a subset of older patients with incompletely resected fibrillary astrocytomas. A prospective randomized clinical trial of radiotherapy for astrocytomas is under way, but the results will not be known for a number of years. The lack of clear benefit must be weighed carefully against the known long-term risks of radiation.

Total resection of pilocytic astrocytomas can be curative. Postoperative radiotherapy does not appear to improve survival. Some evidence suggests that pilocytic astrocytomas may respond to chemotherapy, but not clear is whether this confers a survival advantage.

For oligodendrogliomas, subtotal or total resection (instead of minimal resection or biopsy) and surgery since 1970 significantly prolong survival. As with astrocytomas, the role of radiotherapy is controversial. No randomized prospective clinical trials have evaluated radiotherapy for oligodendroglial neoplasms. Several retrospective reviews have failed to demonstrate benefit for either histologic grade. A large retrospective analysis suggested that a subset of oligodendroglioma patients with neurologic deficits (as opposed to those with seizures and normal neurologic examination) benefited from radiotherapy. This analysis did not show radiotherapy benefit for anaplastic oligodendrogliomas. Such

oligodendrogliomas are chemotherapy-sensitive neoplasms, though unclear is whether chemotherapy significantly prolongs survival in comparison to other treatment modalities.

For intracranial ependymomas, a more complete surgical excision tends to improve survival, and presence of postoperative residual disease on computed tomography (CT) or MRI is a statistically significant risk factor for poorer survival. Postoperative radiotherapy to the posterior fossa significantly improves survival. Standard treatment is 54 Gy to the tumor bed with wide margins. For spinal ependymoma patients, total surgical excision is associated with a more favorable prognosis regardless of whether the tumor is located in the filum terminale or elsewhere. The role of radiotherapy is controversial. If complete resection of the tumor is possible, radiotherapy probably is not advantageous, but it may be beneficial with subtotal removal, anaplastic histology, and doses of 45 to 50 Gy.

Short-Term Prognosis

Currently, the short-term prognosis is determined by the preoperative condition of the patient and the patient's perioperative course. With the advent of CT and MRI and improvements in neurosurgical technique, surgical morbidity and mortality continue to decline as ability to achieve more complete resections improves. Many series demonstrate that surgery in the modern era of neuroimaging (since the 1970s) carries a more favorable prognosis than did surgery before this time. Aggressive nursing care, physical therapy, and rehabilitation services will maximize short-term functional ability. The short-term prognosis remains less favorable for those patients in whom only biopsy is possible because the tumor is unresectable.

Long-Term Prognosis

Median survival times (MSTs) for GBM are 12 to 15 months and for AA are 24 to 36 months, though these figures do not take other prognostic factors into account. A recent recursive partitioning analysis of prognostic factors in malignant gliomas (GBM and AA) treated with conventional radiotherapy with or without adjuvant chemotherapy

Nonparametric Recursive Partitioning

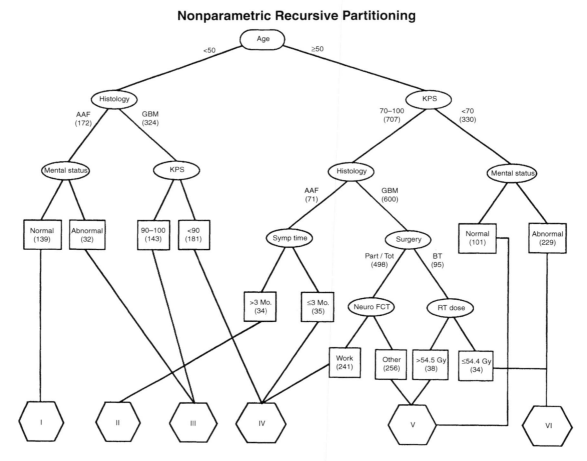

Figure 35-1. Results of a recursive partitioning analysis indicating prognostic factors leading to classification into six groups, with class I having the best prognosis and class VI the worst. (AAF = astrocytomas with anaplastic or atypical foci; GBM = glioblastoma multiforme; KPS = Karnofsky performance status; Symp time = symptom time [duration]; Part/Tot = partial/total; BT = biopsy; Neuro FCT = neurologic function; RT dose = radiotherapy dose.) (Reprinted with permission from WJ Curran Jr, CB Scott, J Horton, et al. Recursive partition analysis of prognostic factors in three Radiation Therapy Oncology Group malignant glioma trials. J Natl Cancer Inst 1993;85:707.)

found six patient classes with distinct differences in survival (Fig. 35-1). The prognostic factors that determined a patient's class included age (age <50 years carrying a better prognosis), histology (AA better than GBM), mental status (normal better than abnormal), KPS (higher KPS more favorable), duration of symptoms (>3 months better than <3 months), extent of resection (partial or complete resection better than biopsy), amount of radiotherapy (more than 54.4 Gy better than lesser amounts), and ability to work (those able to work had a better prognosis). Patients in class I had the best survivals, whereas those in class VI had the poorest survivals.

The MST for each class was as follows: class I MST, 58.6 months; class II, 37.4 months; class III, 17.9 months; class IV, 11.1 months; class V, 8.9 months; and class VI, 4.6 months.

In most series before 1990, patients with fibrillary astrocytomas had a 40 to 50% 5-year survival and a 20 to 30% 10-year survival. In more recent series, with patient disorders diagnosed since the advent of CT, the MST is 7.5 years, with 5- and 10-year survivals of 65% and 40%, respectively. The prognosis is better for those with pilocytic astrocytoma, for which 85% 5-year survival and 79% 10-year survival have been reported.

Survival figures for patients with oligodendrogliomas vary widely depending on the series. MSTs range from 35 to 85.2 months, with 5-year survivals ranging between 23 and 97% and 10-year survivals from 13.3 to 34%. In series that distinguish between histologies, 5-year survivals range between 45 and 70% for well-differentiated tumors and between 19 and 32% for anaplastic ones.

For intracranial ependymomas, 5-year survival after surgery and radiotherapy is 49 to 83% for adult patients. Some series report better 5-year survival for adults than for children (83% for those older than 18 years versus 29% for those younger than 18). For fourth ventricular ependymomas, 3-year, 5-year, 10-year, and 15-year survival rates of 60%, 41%, 27%, and 12%, respectively, have been reported. The 5-year survival rate for patients with spinal ependymoma is roughly 75 to 80% regardless of postoperative function, but those with minor deficits have a 20-year survival of 50% versus 33% for those with major postoperative deficits.

Additional Reading

Burger PC, Scheitauer BW, Vogel FS. Surgical Pathology of the Nervous System and Its Coverings. New York: Churchill Livingstone, 1991;193–437.

Celli P, Cervoni L, Cantore G. Ependymoma of the filum terminale: treatment and prognostic factors in a series of 28 cases. Acta Neurochir (Wien) 1993;124:99–103.

Celli P, Nofrone I, Palma L, et al. Cerebral oligodendroglioma: prognostic factors and life history. Neurosurgery 1994;35:1018–1035.

Curran WJ Jr, Scott CB, Horton J, et al. Recursive partition analysis of prognostic factors in three Radiation Therapy Oncology Group malignant glioma trials. J Natl Cancer Inst 1993;85:704–710.

Ferrante L, Mastronardi L, Celli P, et al. Intramedullary spinal cord ependymomas—a study of 45 cases with long-term followup. Acta Neurochir (Wien) 1992;119:74–79.

Fine HA, Dear KBG, Loeffler JS, et al. Meta-analysis of radiation therapy with and without adjuvant chemotherapy for malignant gliomas in adults. Cancer 1993;71:2585–2597.

Harsh GR IV, Wilson CB. Neuroepithelial Tumors of the Adult Brain. In JR Youmans (ed), Neurological Surgery. Philadelphia: Saunders, 1990;3097–3101.

Laws ER Jr, Taylor WF, Clifton MB, Okazaki H. Neurosurgical management of low-grade astrocytoma of the cerebral hemispheres. J Neurosurg 1984;61:665–673.

Medbery LA III, Straus KL, Steinberg SM, et al. Low-grade astrocytomas: treatment results and prognostic variables. Int J Radiat Oncol Biol Phys 1988;15:837–841.

Shaw EG, Daumas-Duport C, Scheithauer BW, et al. Radiation therapy in the management of low-grade supratentorial astrocytomas. J Neurosurg 1989;70:853–861.

Chapter 36
Meningiomas

Gerhard M. Friehs and Beverly C. Walters

In 1879, William McEwen (1848 to 1924) performed what was probably the first neurosurgical operation on a human being in modern times. Although histologic substantiation does not exist, the *fungus cerebri* he removed and described was most likely a meningioma. Likewise, Horsley was the first to remove an intraspinal meningioma in 1888. These tumors usually are benign and slow-growing and arise from the arachnoid cap cells. They account for 13 to 20% of brain tumors. The incidence increases with age, ranging from 0.3 per 100,000 per year in childhood to 8.4 per 100,000 per year at old age. On average, the incidence is 2.3 per 100,000 per year for benign meningiomas and 0.17 per 100,000 per year for malignant types. Meningiomas can arise wherever meninges are found, with the majority being found in or around the brain and 5 to 12% located in the spinal canal. The male-to-female ratio is 1:2 for cranial meningiomas and 1:5 for spinal meningiomas, and the age of highest incidence is 43 years for female and 52 years for male patients. Most commonly, depending on location, meningiomas of the cerebral meninges present clinically with a wide range of symptoms, including cranial nerve deficits, altered affect, seizures, hemiparesis, or speech difficulties. For spinal meningiomas, the typical sign leading to detection of spinal meningiomas is gradual myelopathy, with an occasional presentation of root symptoms.

Meningiomas can appear as classic benign, atypical, anaplastic, and sarcomatous types. The exact histopathologic criteria determining the malignancy of meningiomas remain to be developed. Whether meningeal hemangiopericytomas and fibrous histiocytomas should be included in the group of meningiomas or whether they present a distinctly different category of tumors remains unclear.

The occurrence of meningiomas has been linked both to previous cranial trauma with injury to the meninges and to previous radiation. A genetic cause appears to be at work in neurofibromatosis type II, with partial deletion on chromosome 22. Another possibility is a positive correlation between breast cancer and meningiomas and a suspected relationship with estrogen and progesterone.

Natural History

Despite more than 100 years of accumulated knowledge on meningiomas, the natural history of the disease basically still is unknown. No prospective study has ever been conducted. The closest to a natural history of meningiomas is summarized in two retrospective studies of asymptomatic meningiomas. Olivero and colleagues described the fate of patients who had incidentally detected meningiomas and did not undergo any form of therapy. The authors report that the tumors in 35 of 45 patients did not show any growth at 3 to 72 months after detection. In 10 of 45 patients, the tumors grew an average of 0.24 cm per year. In a German study, 17 patients with incidentally detected meningiomas were analyzed retrospectively. After a follow-up period of 2 to 89 months, a median annual growth rate of 3.6% was found, with a range between 0.5 and 21%.

Table 36-1. Simpson Grading System for Removal of Meningiomas

Grade	Degree of Removal
I	Macroscopically complete removal with excision of dural attachment and abnormal bone (including sinus resection when involved)
II	Macroscopically complete with endothermy coagulation (Bovie, or laser) of dural attachment
III	Macroscopically complete without resection or coagulation of dural attachment or of its extradural extensions (e.g., hyperostotic bone)
IV	Partial removal leaving tumor in situ
V	Simple decompression (or biopsy)

Jääskeläinen and coworkers reported data from the Finnish cancer registry on a subgroup of meningioma patients who were followed without therapy. No information can ascertain whether these tumors were incidental findings or symptomatic meningiomas. Additionally not clear was whether patients were untreated owing to personal choice, surgical inaccessibility (as in large skull-base tumors), or their underlying health or overall poor functional status. However, the authors reported a 1-year mortality rate of 61.1% for patients with untreated meningiomas.

Because of the wide range in outcomes for untreated intracranial tumors, a wide variability appears possible in the growth rate of the tumors. Some may be watched carefully and perhaps never undergo operation, with excellent outcomes.

The natural history of spinal meningiomas is completely unknown, but as those patients who do present for treatment usually do so with progressive neurologic deficit, one may assume that their disease has a relentless, albeit histologically benign, course. For progressive myelopathy, surgical treatment may be assumed to be preferable to progressive paralysis. In addition, a report from the Norwegian cancer registry indicates that intraspinal meningioma is the most common intraspinal neoplasm and that the outcome in intraspinal meningioma treatment is superior to that for intracranial meningioma, with survival rates being 15% higher. Improvement in neurologic outcome with surgery has been seen with the introduction and use of microsurgical technique, and gross total removal is associated with a recurrence rate of 6%. Subtotal removal has a recurrence rate of 17%.

The natural history of malignant meningiomas has not been documented, but as such disorders are incurable even with aggressive treatment, a reasonable assumption is that no treatment would afford an even worse prognosis for the patient, in life expectancy and progressive neurologic deficit.

Factors Affecting Prognosis

Of all meningiomas, regardless of location, the histologic type may affect prognosis greatly. Malignant meningiomas carry a much worse prognosis and cannot be cured. Patients with malignant meningiomas have 4.6-fold risk of death compared to patients with benign tumors. Other intracranial meningioma factors that determine a good patient prognosis include a good preoperative Karnofsky performance score, young age, complete surgical resection (Simpson grade I, II; Table 36-1) with removal or coagulation of the dural attachment, and the addition of adjunctive therapy in the event of incomplete surgical resection. Tumor location has not been reliable for prognosis despite consideration of skull-base meningiomas as therapeutically more challenging. Absence of seizures has been found to be a poor prognostic sign, but this limitation probably is an epiphenomenon, as tumors of the convexity, even when they are small, commonly present with seizures and usually are removed easily, whereas the most involved skull-base meningiomas may never become epileptogenic, and their removal may be difficult—or impossible.

In intraspinal meningioma patients, early diagnosis, complete removal, and use of microscopical technique appear to be the most relevant factors in producing a good outcome, as measured by longevity, recurrence, and neurologic function. Clearly, the fewer the symptoms, the better is the ultimate outcome with respect to neurologic deficit. A scale for the classification of deficits has been suggested by Solero (Table 36-2).

Evaluation for Prognosis

The first step in evaluating prognosis is to record a history and to perform a physical examination. An elderly patient experiencing tremendous neurologic deficit or other health problems will not enjoy the same prognosis as that for someone who is young and presents with a single seizure. A careful evaluation of the patient is followed by an examination of all necessary imaging studies, which may include computed tomography, magnetic resonance imaging, and angiography. This process determines the treatment algorithm, beginning with size and location of the lesion, surgical accessibility, surgical exigencies (e.g., proximity or involvement of vascular structures), preoperative treatment (e.g., endovascular therapy), and consideration of alternative therapeutic programs. A multidisciplinary approach is best, with the involvement of neurosurgeons, neurologists, radiation oncologists, and radiosurgeons. The information gathered can be combined to estimate an overall prognosis for the individual patient.

Therapies Affecting Prognosis

Prognosis with treatment requires consideration of treatment risks. The mainstay of treatment for meningioma is neurosurgical removal. Surgical mortality is quoted between 0 and 14%, and no reliable data indicate a significant increase in mortality with old age. A 5.4% mortality rate was reported in one study in patients age 70 or older, whereas other authors found a much increased mortality of 23% in patients older than 70. Not a single well-designed study has focused on morbidity after surgery of meningiomas, with the possible exception of a publication on the incidence of postoperative seizures in patients with supratentorial meningiomas. In this excellent study, the authors developed a formula by which the likelihood of postoperative seizures could be calculated. The following variables were found to be predictive of postoperative seizure occurrence: preoperative seizure history, preoperative language disturbance, extent of tumor removal, parietal location of tumor, postoperative anticonvulsant medication status, and postoperative hydrocephalus.

The mainstay of therapy and treatment of choice is surgical exploration and attempted complete surgical removal of the meningioma. Adjuvant therapy may be indicated after incomplete resection (Simpson's grades III through V). One study indicated that patients with subtotally resected meningiomas can have a good 5-year overall and a progression-free survival rate of 85% and 89%, respectively, with adjuvant radiotherapy; figures that compare favorably to

Table 36-2. Classification of Neurologic Disability According to Symptoms and Signs

Classification	Symptoms and Signs
Group I	Pain only (local, radicular)
	Pain and pyramidal signs
	Pain and slight radicular or funicular motor-sensory deficits
Group II	Slight motor deficit: walking with aid
	Slight motor deficit or radicular and funicular sensory deficits
	Slight motor deficit or sphincter disturbances
Group III	Severe motor deficit: flexion-extension against gravity
	Sensory deficits
	Severe motor deficit, sensory deficits, or sphincter disturbances
Group IV	Very severe motor deficit: flexion-extension without gravity, paraplegia
	Sensory deficits
	Sphincter deficits

the 45% recurrence-free survival after subtotal resection without adjuvant radiotherapy.

Though the addition of postoperative radiotherapy clearly has its place and value, the morbidity associated with this treatment modality cannot be ignored. Probably the most complete analysis of postoperative radiation reported a 3.6% morbidity, including sudden blindness due to retinitis and radionecrosis. Morbidity associated with radiosurgery has been reported to be near 6% with gamma-knife radiosurgery and almost 40% with linear accelerator-based radiosurgery.

The treatment of choice for malignant meningiomas is surgical resection followed by radiotherapy. The addition of chemotherapy with cyclophosphamide, doxorubicin, and vincristine has been proposed but no controlled study shows additional benefit over adjuvant radiation alone. However, a median survival rate of 5 years can be expected. Complete surgical removal is the only reasonable treatment for spinal meningiomas.

Short-Term Prognosis

Only one available prospective study charted the overall short-term prognosis of meningioma patients with all treatment-related risk factors taken into account. The survival rates are 91% at 3 months and 89% at 1 year of cumulative observed survival.

Long-Term Prognosis

In the Finnish registry, the overall survival rate for intracranial meningioma patients is quoted to be 82.5% at 5 years, 71.7% at 10 years, and 62.6% at 15 years. When complete surgical removal can be achieved, the actuarial recurrence-free survival rates were 93% at 5 years, 80% at 10 years, and 68% at 15 years. In another study, the 5-year survival rate for patients with benign meningiomas after incomplete surgical resection and adjuvant therapy was 85% and the 10-year rate was 77%. With incomplete surgical resection alone without adjuvant radiotherapy, the 5-, 10-, and 15-year recurrence-free survival rates were 63%, 45%, and 68%, respectively. Some 58% of patients with malignant meningiomas treated with surgery and radiotherapy still were alive at the 5-year mark. This finding is confirmed by a prospective study wherein a treatment combination of surgery, radiotherapy, and adjuvant chemotherapy resulted in a median survival of 5.3 years for patients with malignant meningiomas.

Recurrence of benign intracranial meningiomas occurs in 19% of patients within a 20-year period. Risk factors for recurrence include invasion of bone, dural insertion, and soft consistency of the tumor. If none of the risk factors are present, the recurrence rate is estimated to be 11%, with a 15 to 24% recurrence rate and a 34 to 56% recurrence rate with one and two of these risk factors, respectively. For malignant (anaplastic) meningiomas, the recurrence rate is 78% at 5 years. For spinal menin-

giomas, the recurrence rate is 6% with total surgical removal and 17% in patients with subtotal resection 4 to 17 years after resection.

Additional Reading

Chamberlain MC. Adjuvant combined modality therapy for malignant meningiomas. J Neurosurg 1996;84:733–736.

Chozick BS, Reinert SE, Greenblatt SH. Incidence of seizures after surgery for supratentorial meningiomas: a modern analysis. J Neurosurg 1996;84:382–386.

Firsching RP, Fischer A, Peters R, et al. Growth rate of incidental meningiomas. J Neurosurg 1990;73:544–547.

Goldsmith BJ, Wara WM, Wilson CB, et al. Postoperative irradiation for subtotally resected meningiomas. A retrospective analysis of 140 patients treated from 1967 to 1990. J Neurosurg 1994;80:195–201.

Jääskeläinen J. Seemingly complete removal of histologically benign intracranial meningioma: late recurrence rate and factors predicting recurrence in 657 patients. A multivariate analysis. Surg Neurol 1986;26:461–469.

Kallio M, Sankila R, Hakulinen T, Jääskeläinen J. Factors affecting operative and excess long-term mortality in 935 patients with intracranial meningioma. Neurosurgery 1992;31:2–12.

Olivero WC, Lister JR, Elwood PW. The natural history and growth rate of asymptomatic meningiomas: a review of 60 patients. J Neurosurg 1995;83:222–224.

Sankila R, Kallio M, Jääskeläinen J, Hakulinen T. Long-term survival of 1986 patients with intracranial meningioma diagnosed from 1953 to 1984 in Finland. Comparison of the observed and expected survival rates in a population-based series. Cancer 1992;70:1568–1576.

Simpson D. The recurrence of intracranial meningiomas after surgical treatment. J Neurol Neurosurg Psychiatry 1957;20:22–39.

Solero CL, Fornari M, Giombini S, et al. Spinal meningiomas: review of 174 operated cases. Neurosurgery 1989;25:153–160.

Chapter 37

Childhood Brain Tumors

William D. Brown

Eighty-five years ago, Howard Henry Tooth noted the variation in prognosis for patients with brain tumors and a relationship between the morphology of a tumor and the clinical course of the patient. Subsequent attempts to refine these observations identified clinical, surgical, and pathologic variables that seem to have prognostic importance in specific situations, but a complete understanding of Tooth's original observation remains elusive.

Introduction

Intracranial tumors are the second most common neoplasias in childhood, the leukemias being the most common. With an overall incidence of 2.4 per 100,000 children (age <15 years), more than 1,500 new cases of intracranial tumor are identified in the United States each year. Clinical experiences and modest successes in the treatment of childhood brain tumors (CBTs) are documented extensively, but morbidity and mortality associated with tumor biology and therapeutic manipulation of it remains substantial. Interpretation of reported experiences must be modified by the understanding that clinical trials, studies of tumor biology and genetics, and epidemiologic surveys in children with brain tumors are limited by a persistent inability to explain outcome differences for histologically identical tumors on the basis of age, gender, race, location, known tumor biology, or intervention.

This limitation arises from the dependence of current brain tumor classification schemes on tumor morphology and their failure to account for the effects of tumor location, histologic features, clinical presentation, operative findings, or patient age on prognosis. Astrocytic tumors with identical histologic appearances, for example, have very different prognoses, depending on location (e.g., cerebellum versus hypothalamus), whereas certain clinical signs, such as lethargy or focal neurologic deficit, may influence outcome negatively. The presence of specific histologic features, such as indistinct tumor margins, large size, extension, necrosis, or cysts, influences the surgeon's impression of surgical success and is often used as discriminating criterion to direct treatment. Finally, though CBTs are understood widely to behave differently from identical tumors in adults, current classification schemes make no allowance for patient age. Because so many clinical and management decisions depend on histologic diagnosis, critical evaluation of the process of assigning a diagnosis is important to understanding why such schemes provide an incomplete prognostic picture.

Tumor Heterogeneity

The histologic appearance of CBT often is heterogeneous, with several distinct tumor morphologies appearing within the same specimen. In one study, histologic criteria for as many as four disparate tumors were present in a single specimen. When this situation occurs, common practice directs treatment on the basis of the most malignant component. Yet, the location of the surgeon's biopsy needle within the tumor can have a significant effect on the choice of diagnosis offered, and the size of the initial surgical resection or biopsy is related inversely to the chances of a missed diagnosis. Incorrect identification of the tumor may lead to inappropriate treatment and can have important negative consequences on prognosis.

Geographic Variability

Living on a farm is a significant CBT risk factor, and rural living in general increases in all populations the risk for gliomas. Yet such associations are rare, for the recognition of CBT varies according to geographic location, a poorly understood phenomenon. The incidence of brain tumors in Japan, for example, is less than one-third that of the United States. Glioblastomas have an incidence of 0.8% of CBT in Denmark but account for 26.4% of CBT in Connecticut. Germinomas constitute 15 to 18% of CBT in Japan but only 3 to 5% in North America. Medulloblastomas vary in incidence from one-fifth to one-third of all CBT depending on locale, and specific world populations, such as the Maoris of New Zealand, have an unexplained increased incidence of this tumor. Ependymomas have an incidence of either 5 or 20%, depending on the registry. Astrocytic tumors vary from one-fourth to more than one-half of all CBTs, and one childhood population-based brain tumor registry gives different incidences for glioblastoma in two different descriptions of a common database. Whether the incidence of specific tumors truly is different or the tumors are identified differently is unknown, but reproducible tumor recognition is necessary for determining prognosis, and the effect of geographic differences on CBT prognosis must be explored further.

Reliability of Diagnosis and Malignancy Grading

The World Health Organization manual is the descriptive brain tumor atlas most commonly used to assign diagnosis. It does not list defining histologic features for each tumor but enumerates those that are allowable. The manual offers no operationally defined definitions of histologic boundaries between or among diagnostic classes, nor does it offer guidance on how to distinguish the extent to which certain morphologic features must be present to qualify for designation as *mixed* or *malignant*. When the histologic pattern is not obvious, neuropathologists must make subjective interpretations of what they see in the microscope before offering a diagnosis.

Formal evaluation of the process by which a diagnosis is assigned suggests that histologic features are not identified reliably by experienced neuropathologists, even when teams of readers are used. Histologic criteria may be applied inconsistently or interpreted differently by different observers using the same or separate data. Many diagnoses are subject to considerable disagreement or misidentification, and some common tumors, such as anaplastic astrocytoma, anaplastic ependymoma, astrocytoma *nos*, fibrillary astrocytoma, glioblastoma, and oligodendroglioma, are identified reliably by teams of observers less than 50% of the time.

Different CBTs are associated with different grading schemes. Some tumors have multiple grading schemes in common use; more than 14 separate schemes are available for use to assign a malignancy grade for astrocytic tumors, 3 of which are used routinely. The current World Health Organization manual does not offer a system of grading for these tumors but nevertheless does arrange them into a scale of ascending malignancy (astrocytoma, anaplastic astrocytoma, glioblastoma). Histologic descriptions (mitosis, necrosis, endothelial proliferation, and nuclear atypia) used for the determination of diagnosis are the same features used to assign a grade. This situation can lead to confusion when a tumor marked as low-grade in one scheme is ranked as high-grade in another or a glioblastoma on biopsy behaves clinically as a lower-grade tumor.

If CBTs are heterogeneous and identified unreliably, and if tumor grade is an inconsistent predictor of biological behavior, then uniform patient populations cannot be selected for treatment protocols. Rational interpretation of existing clinical data for patients with medulloblastoma or anaplastic astrocytoma, for example, may not be as useful as previously believed, limiting the prognostication process.

Reporting Study Cohorts

Survival data are reported variously in the literature, and the method of patient exclusion has an important influence on the way in which survival data are analyzed. Some authors eliminate from analysis all patients who die within a month of initial surgery, so as to exclude surgical deaths from cohort analysis. Others exclude patients dying as late as 3 months after surgery for the same reason. Progression-free survival and disease-free survival are outcomes different from simple survival, and resulting conclusions are drawn differently. Large study populations often are accumulated over many decades and may pool data from many geographically distant institutions. New methods of imaging, such as computed tomography (CT), magnetic resonance imaging (MRI), and positron emission tomography have become useful in the diagnosis and management of CBT during the accumulation of many of these databases, allowing earlier diagnosis and more aggressive intervention to occur in patients enrolled later. Advances in radiotherapy (RT) and novel chemotherapeutic regimens may become available to patients during long periods of observation, influencing both prognosis and outcome. Changing technology and differing methods of patient reporting mandate cautious interpretation of available literature and a measured application of published conclusions to any individual patient.

Factors Affecting Prognosis

Two separate meanings of the word *prognosis* often are interchanged in modern medicine. The more common concept is the likelihood of recovery from disease, whereas a less-appreciated meaning is the ability to foresee the course and probable outcome of a disease. Specific clinical variables are outlined further in the light of this second meaning of prognosis. These variables include age at presentation, complications, histologic appearance, location, neuroimaging appearance, race and ethnicity, special techniques, symptom duration, therapy, and underlying conditions (Table 37-1).

Age

The prognosis for children with brain tumors is better than that of adults. Infants and children younger than 2, however, have a worse prognosis independent of the type or location of brain tumor. Children in whom medulloblastoma or ependymoma has been diagnosed have a poor prognosis when they are younger than 3 years and are designated as high-risk. Children who are younger than 10 years and in whom glioma has been diagnosed have more undifferentiated, aggressive tumors, whereas children older than 10 have a better prognosis; in this group, though, the increased survival occurs in younger children. The value of Collins Law—the concept that survival is related to the age of the patient plus 9 months—has been assessed in a variety of CBTs and has been found to be applicable for anaplastic astrocytoma, glioblastoma, pineoblastoma, medulloblastoma, primitive neuroectodermal tumor (PNET), teratoma, germinoma, ependymoma, choroid plexus papilloma, and tumors that cannot be classified. However, it does not apply to craniopharyngioma, oligodendroglioma, and plain, fibrillary, pilocytic, or protoplasmic astrocytoma when the age is younger than 8 years at diagnosis.

Underlying Conditions

The prognostic importance of an underlying predisposition to tumor formation now is being recognized. Mounting evidence of a genetic influence on tumorigenesis suggests that a sequential loss of genetic material is critical. In the transformation of a plain astrocytoma to glioblastoma, for example, no fewer than six molecular genetic steps are required to convert the normal glial cell to a glioblastoma. This sequence includes the loss of loci from chromosomes 17p, 13q, and 22 in normal glial cells, resulting in a low-grade astrocytic tumor. An additional loss of material at chromosome 9p and the p53 gene provide one transition to anaplastic astrocytoma. Deletions from chromosome 10q (the glioma suppressor gene) and amplifications of the epidermal growth factor receptor gene are almost universal in glioblastomas. The number of genetic alterations seems to be more important than is their chronology. Genetic alterations may be found also in other tumors. Loss of heterozygosity at 17q inactivates the p53 tumor suppressor gene and has been reported in oligodendrogliomas, mixed tumors, and medulloblastomas. Its presence is a consistently poor prognostic sign only for medulloblastomas and astrocytic tumors. CBT may be associated with inherited conditions and specific chromosomal defects (Table 37-2); the occurrence of brain tumors in these syndromes sug-

Table 37-1. Prognostic Variables for Specific Pediatric Brain Tumors

Diagnosis	Age	Complications: Presence of Endocrinopathies	Histologic Appearance	Location	Neuroimaging Appearance	Special Diagnostic and Prognostic Techniques	Symptom Duration Before Diagnosis	Response to Chemotherapy	Therapy Response to Radiotherapy	Therapy Degree of Surgical Resection	Presence of Ventricular Shunt
Astrocytoma	DH	—	VI	I	I	I	I	U	LI	VI	—
Anaplastic astrocytoma	I	—	VI	I	I	I	—	LI	I	VI	—
Brain stem gliomas	—	—	LI	VI	I	—	LI	DH	LI	LI	—
Cerebellar astrocytoma	—	—	VI	—	—	—	—	—	LI	VI	I
Choroid plexus tumors	—	—	—	—	—	—	I	—	—	—	—
Craniopharyngioma	DH	VI	DH	LI	VI	I	—	—	I	VI	—
Ependymoma	I	—	VI	I	I	I	I	LI	LI	VI	LI
Glioblastoma	LI	—	VI	I	I	—	—	LI	LI	L	—
Hypothalamic tumors	—	VI	—	—	—	—	—	—	—	—	—
Malignant neoplasm nos	VI	—	LI	I	—	—	—	LI	I	LI	I
Medulloblastoma	VI	—	LI	I	VI	LI	—	LI	I	VI	I
Oligodendroglioma	DH	—	—	—	LI	DH	—	U	U	VI	—
Optic gliomas	—	—	—	—	I	—	LI	—	—	—	—
Pilocytic astrocytoma	—	—	LI	I	I	I	—	LI	U	LI	—
Pineal region tumors	I	—	I	I	I	I	—	I	VI	—	I
Pituitary tumors	—	—	LI	VI	VI	I	—	—	—	—	—
PNET	VI	—	LI	VI	VI	—	—	I	I	VI	I
Thalamic tumors	—	—	—	—	—	—	—	—	I	—	—

VI = very important; DH = does not help; I = important; U = unknown effect; LI = less important; PNET = primitive neuroectodermal tumor; nos = not otherwise specified.

Note: This table represents necessarily subjective interpretations of available clinical data. The importance of a particular variable to *prognosis* should not be confused with its importance to *diagnosis*. The value of histologic appearance, for example, may be very important in diagnosis but have less value in predicting outcome. Other variables, such as age, may not help in making a diagnosis but are useful in predicting outcome.

Table 37-2. Central Nervous System Tumor Associations with a Negative Impact
on Childhood Brain Tumor Prognosis

With Associated Disorders

Syndrome	Tumor Type
Gardener syndrome	Multiple types
Gastrointestinal and genitourinary anomalies	PNET
Mental retardation	Astrocytoma
Multiple dural arteriovenous malformations	Astrocytoma
Pulmonary arteriovenous fistulas	Glioblastoma
Sturge-Weber syndrome	Choroid plexus papilloma

With Chromosomal Abnormalities

Syndrome	Chromosome	Tumor Type
Bilateral acoustic neuromas	22q	Acoustic neuroma
Carcinoma	9q31	Medulloblastoma
Gorlin syndrome	1q22	Medulloblastoma
Neurofibromatosis 1	17q11.2	Astrocytoma, ependymoma, meningioma, neurofibroma, neurilemmoma, optic glioma
Neurofibromatosis 2	22q	Astrocytoma, ependymoma, meningioma, Schwannoma
Tuberous sclerosis	9q32–34	Astrocytoma, ependymoma, ganglioneuroma, glioblastoma
Trisomy 21	21	Astrocytoma
Turcot's syndrome	5q21–q22	Glioma
von Hippel–Lindau syndrome	3p25–26	Hemangioblastoma

PNET = primitive neuroectodermal tumor.

gests a relatively poorer outcome. The current prognostic importance of activators (proto-oncogenes), inhibitors of cellular division (tumor suppressor genes), and the four classes of oncogenes (growth factors, transmembrane receptors, intracellular transducers, and nuclear transcription factors) is unknown.

Race and Ethnicity

Ethnicity influences CBT incidence: Asians are less often affected than are blacks, who are less often afflicted than are whites; Israeli Jews are less often affected than are non-Israeli Jews. However, unlike such other childhood cancers as acute lymphocytic leukemia, in which race may influence prognosis, no such observation has been made in CBT.

Symptom Duration

For some CBTs, recent symptom onset is a poor prognostic sign. Rapid progression similarly is

ominous. Both are associated with decreased survival, and both correlate with histologic features of malignancy and aggressive tumor behavior. This effect may be a result of the tumor itself and of edema associated with it and is especially true for brain stem gliomas, ependymomas, and other tumors of the posterior fossa. Poor performance on the initial neurologic assessment is associated with decreased survival.

Neuroimaging Appearance

The value of modern neuroimaging methods to the early detection, diagnosis, and management of CBT cannot be overstated. MRI has greatly enhanced the ability to detect disseminated and metastatic disease in such tumors as medulloblastoma or ependymoma prone to spread within the subarachnoid space; this spread always is associated with a poor prognosis. MRI and CT are valuable also in the evaluation of surgical success, as they are better able than the surgeon's intraoperative estimate to detect residual dis-

Table 37-3. Histologic Cerebellar Astrocytoma Features Important for Prognosis

Glioma A	Glioma B
Microcysts	Pseudorosettes
Rosenthal fibers	Necrosis
Leptomeningeal deposits	High cell density
Oligodendroglial foci	Mitosis
10-Year survival: 94%	10-Year survival: 29%

ease within the first 24 postoperative hours. In one study of ependymomas, postoperative neuroimaging findings showed that the surgeon overestimated the degree of resection in one-third of cases.

Tumor appearance on neuroimaging may be useful in predicting clinical course. Evidence of herniation, heterogeneity, ring enhancement (CT), and size greater than 4 cm are poor prognostic findings in astrocytomas. The presence of cystic structures or necrosis within brain stem gliomas always is associated with significantly shorter survival times (median time to death, 6 months). This observation reflects not the effect of RT but part of the natural history of the tumor, independent of treatment. Though neuroimaging may be useful in making a diagnosis when appearance is typical, its value in determining prognosis must be considered in light of its limitations; CT, for example, is known to underestimate the degree of tumor invasion, as tumor may be found outside the area of contrast enhancement at autopsy.

Location

Histologically identical tumors may have very different prognoses on the basis of location alone, a particularly important consideration in CBT, wherein a 70% incidence of infratentorial tumors is contrasted to the 30% incidence in adults. An astrocytoma has a much better prognosis if it occurs in the cerebellum than if it occurs in the hypothalamus or thalamus. Brain stem gliomas may be histologically benign but are in a malignant location, and their prognosis is worse than that of a glioma in the hypothalamus. Optic gliomas have a much better prognosis, because the tumor tends to remain locally and grow slowly. This finding is true also for other so-called local tumors such as meningiomas, schwannomas, neu-

rofibromas, and oligodendrogliomas. Astrocytomas that are multifocal, involve the corpus callosum, or occur in the infratentorial space have a comparatively poorer prognosis than if they are solitary, lobar, and supratentorial, whereas supratentorial PNETs have a prognosis worse than that of those occurring in the posterior fossa.

Histologic Appearance

Most information about the effect of histologic appearance on prognosis comes from analysis of astrocytic tumors. The presence of necrosis usually (but not always) is associated with a higher grade of malignancy and a poorer prognosis. The degree of local invasion (astrocytic tumors, oligodendroglioma), the amount of encapsulation (craniopharyngioma, pilocytic astrocytoma), and the mode of distant spread within the subarachnoid space (PNET, ependymoma) may be visualized directly under the microscope, and all directly affect prognosis. Yet, histologically similar tumors in identical locations, such as cerebellar astrocytomas, do not always have the same prognosis, even though cerebellar astrocytomas generally are regarded as benign tumors with a good prognosis. Gilles and coworkers identified a distinct subset of cerebellar astrocytomas with poor prognosis on the basis of histologic features alone. The histologic features of glioma A conferred a good prognosis (10-year survival, 94%), whereas the features of glioma B— necrosis, high cell density, and mitosis—identified a population with a poor prognosis (10-year survival, 29%; Table 37-3). Various grading schemes use combinations of histologic features to assign a degree of malignancy and to predict outcome, but the applicability of these adult studies to CBT remains controversial and may not be as helpful as previously assumed.

Special Techniques

A resurgence of interest in markers of cellular division and their possible relevance to brain tumors has led to many published clinical studies. Monoclonal antibodies, histochemical stains, flow cytometry, labeling indices, and serial measures of such biological markers as alpha-fetoprotein, beta–human chorionic gonadotropin, and placental alkaline phosphatase are unproved as prognostic tools, as are such markers of cell differentiation as glial fibrillary acidic protein, vimentin, antineuronal filament antibodies, and proliferating-cell nuclear antigens, despite reports to the contrary. DNA flow cytometry has been disappointing as a prognostic tool, but such other forms of cell indexing as bromodeoxyuridine labeling are useful in predicting recurrence risk for astrocytic tumors and ependymomas. Although the Ki-67 labeling index may be useful for prognosis of anaplastic astrocytomas and pituitary tumors that lack other histologic or ultrastructural markers of biological behavior in adults, it plays an uncertain role in CBT. Epidermal growth factor receptor gene amplification in glioblastoma is associated with increased malignancy but is not correlated with outcome. The degree of N-*myc* and c-*myc* gene amplification in medulloblastoma has been similarly disappointing.

Complications

Complications associated with surgery, chemotherapy, RT, and tumor biology may have a significant impact on prognosis. Secondary seizures, neurologic deficits, respiratory compromise, and feeding difficulties adversely affect prognosis. The presence of endocrinopathies associated with hypothalamic tumors, such as astrocytomas and craniopharyngiomas, has a poor prognosis that worsens with the addition of chemotherapy. RT to the brain and spinal cord increases the risk of permanent growth hormone deficiency and a predictable loss in ultimate attained height. Gonadal dysfunction may occur and increases long-term morbidity associated with CBT. Permanent cognitive changes associated with a tumor are exacerbated by surgical removal of brain tissue and often are worsened by administration of chemotherapy or RT.

Therapies Affecting Prognosis

Chemotherapy

The concept of the log-kill hypothesis is important to modern chemotherapeutic interventions. It suggests that the average tumor comes to medical attention with a cell burden of 10^9 cells. If the surgeon achieves a 90% removal, it represents a logarithmic reduction of only one, to 10^8 cells. RT can contribute another 2 logs, reducing the cell burden to 10^6, which significantly adds to survival and chances for remission. The most that chemotherapy can add is another 1 to 2 log-kills for a remaining cell burden of 10^4, after which the body must eliminate the rest. Significant improvements in survival have been made in the chemotherapy of ependymomas and astrocytomas in children, an improvement even more dramatic for the treatment of PNET and pineal region tumors. To be weighed against these important benefits are the long-term risks of successful treatment. Methotrexate significantly increases the risk for cognitive impairment and dementia, seizures, focal motor signs, and leukoencephalopathy. The risk of second malignancies increases with the use of chemotherapeutic drugs, especially alkylating agents.

Radiotherapy

In only a very few instances does the response to RT have prognostic significance, and the literature is confusing. RT for astrocytomas, for example, has been reported as both effective and ineffective. Some CBTs may increase in size despite RT. Germinomas are a notable exception as the most radiosensitive of all malignant CBTs, and a significant majority may be cured with RT. In some centers, a tumor typical in appearance and location is presumed to be a germinoma and proved without biopsy by a test dose of RT. In this practice, an inherent danger is the possibility that the germinoma is not pure but instead is a nongerminomatous tumor that has a similar appearance but a dismal prognosis. RT frequently follows surgical resection, but a response to RT does not predict response to chemotherapy and may have no relevance to outcome. Any benefit of RT must be measured against the hazards of treatment. Prognosis depends on the volume of radiation, dose fraction, and whether spinal irradiation accompanies cranial irradiation.

Experience with RT in patients with acute lymphocytic leukemia provides some information about long-term effects of cranial radiation. These patients exhibit a measurable *nonprogressive* disturbance in cognition associated with an IQ lower than that of control patients. Patients with CBT, however, experience a progressive deficit in cognition that worsens over a period of at least 10 years. This deficit is associated with learning problems, school dysfunction, and a postradiation dementia. The volume of radiation seems important, since whole-brain radiation has an effect more severe than that of local radiation. Radiation of the posterior fossa produces less of this effect than does radiation of the supratentorial space.

The long-term effects of RT are increasingly recognized as management of CBT improves. Its effects are not benign, significantly affect quality of life, and worsen the course of the disease. This finding is especially true for very young patients (age <3 years) in whom RT should be delayed as long as possible. Finally, RT may play a role in the induction of second central nervous system tumors that may themselves be malignant.

Surgery

For most CBTs, the more tumor the surgeon can remove, the better is the outcome for the patient. Mortality associated with modern neurosurgery is less than 5%. Novel surgical approaches, advances in microtechnique, and increasing use of intraoperative neurophysiologic monitoring have contributed significantly to the management of tumors considered previously to be inoperable. The ability of the surgeon to estimate a gross total resection has had a measurable positive effect on survival in infants younger than 3 months, in children with medulloblastoma, and in patients with low-grade astrocytomas. Tumors with capsules or sharp margins, such as pilocytic astrocytomas, often can be removed completely, and the patient can be declared cured, but others with more insidious and deceptive margins, such as craniopharyngiomas and anaplastic astrocytomas, may require multiple resections or cannot be removed completely.

Ventricular Shunting

The presence of a ventricular shunt adversely influences prognosis. Patients who require shunting have more neurologic sequelae, larger tumors, and are sicker when they first come to medical attention. Complications of ventricular shunting, such as acute hydrocephalus, ventriculitis, and hemorrhage, worsen prognosis. The creation of a new anatomic pathway increases the risk for distant metastases outside the nervous system in tumors that are so predisposed, such as choroid plexus carcinoma, PNET, and ependymoma. The risk of shunt and central nervous system infection is increased significantly during immunosuppressive therapy.

Short- and Long-Term Prognosis

The process of prognostication in CBT has severe limitations, and opinions offered to individual patients regarding the disease prognosis often prove inaccurate. The body of CBT is too diverse to be able to offer any but the most general advice to patients and parents regarding prognosis, and only short-term prognostication seems appropriate. Children with brain tumors have a more favorable outcome than do adults with similar tumors, and significant age-dependent differences in tumor biology directly (usually positively) influence tumor behavior. Improved surgical, medical, and RT management have lengthened short-term survival, but identification of those children with long-term survival and minimal morbidity remains difficult, because current methods of tumor identification include no clinical information and are based solely on morphologic features; clearly, tissue diagnosis alone is a poor predictor of outcome.

If the purpose of tumor identification is to communicate something about biological behavior and prognosis, obviously both biological and prognostic variables must be included in any future diagnostic and prognostic schemes, because current schemes do not allow for accurate long-term prognostication. This limitation already has been recognized in treating such tumors as PNET and ependymoma, for which the inclusion of biological variables in tumor categorization identifies patients who are at high and low risk for recurrence (Table 37-4). Future studies of prognosis in CBT should recognize the effect of biological variables on outcome so that rational, reasoned advice based on quantifiable, patient-specific factors may be offered to the child with a brain tumor.

Table 37-4. High- and Low-Risk Variables for Recurrence of PNET and Ependymoma

Lesion	High Risk	Low Risk
PNET	Age <2 yrs; partial resection; brain stem involvement	Age >3 yrs; complete resection; no metastasis or spread
Ependymoma	Age <3 yrs; partial resection; high grade; symptom duration <1 month	Age >15 yrs; complete resection; low grade; slow progression

PNET = primitive neuroectodermal tumor.

Additional Reading

Gilles FH, Sobel EL, Leviton A, et al. Childhood Brain Tumor Consortium. Histologic feature reliability in childhood neural tumors. J Neuropathol Exp Neurol 1994;53:559.

Gilles FH, Sobel EL, Leviton A, et al. Quantitative histologic factors for grouping childhood supratentorial neuroglial tumors. Pediatr Pathol Lab Med 1997;17:809–834.

Gjerris F, Klee JG, Klinken L. Malignancy grade and long-term survival in brain tumors of infancy and childhood. Acta Neurol Scand 1976;53:61.

Schoenberg BS, Schoenberg DG, Christine BW, Gomez MR. The epidemiology of primary intracranial neoplasms of childhood. Mayo Clin Proc 1976;51:51.

Chapter 38
Meningeal Carcinomatosis

Julie E. Hammack

Meningeal carcinomatosis (carcinomatous meningitis) is the metastatic spread of epithelium-derived malignancies to the leptomeninges. This term does not include either those patients with meningeal spread of hematopoietic tumors (meningeal leukemia or lymphoma) or those patients with meningeal spread of glial tumors (meningeal gliomatosis).

Natural History

The leptomeninges are one of the rarer sites of central nervous system (CNS) metastases, being far outnumbered by metastases to the brain parenchyma and the epidural space of the spinal cord. Data suggest that CNS metastases, including meningeal carcinoma, may be increasing in incidence, either as a result of improved diagnostic techniques or because patients with systemic cancer are surviving longer and have more opportunity to develop metastases to this relative "sanctuary" from systemic chemotherapy. Although exceptions are found, meningeal carcinomatosis rarely is the first sign of a cancer and rarely is the first sign of a disease relapse. Much more frequently, it occurs as another manifestation of widespread metastases and often late in the clinical course of the malignancy.

Breast and lung cancer are the tumors that spread most commonly to the meninges. Melanoma is a close third, followed by genitourinary, gastrointestinal, and head and neck cancers. Virtually all tumor types have been reported to metastasize to the meninges. In 2 to 4% of patients, the site of the primary tumor (usually adenocarcinoma) never is identified. The incidence of meningeal carcinomatosis in patients with cancer reported in the literature is 1 to 10%, depending on the underlying malignancy and the type of series consulted. Melanoma and small-cell lung cancer, although comparatively rare tumors, have the highest propensity to spread to the meninges.

The precise mechanism whereby cancer cells reach the pia-arachnoid is unknown. Entry along the perivascular spaces of radicular arteries and veins or the perineural spaces of spinal roots or cranial nerves appears most likely. When intraparenchymal metastases abut the pial or ependymal surface, they may shed malignant cells into the cerebrospinal fluid (CSF), or cancer cells may migrate outward along the perivascular spaces of cerebral arterioles. Direct spread from the lumen of a leptomeningeal vessel or the choroid plexus appears less likely and has not been demonstrated in autopsy studies.

The signs and symptoms of meningeal carcinomatosis typically affect multiple levels of the neuraxis (supratentorial, posterior fossa, and spinal), although single-level disease is common at presentation. The most common initial symptom is headache (in 30 to 51% of patients, depending on the clinical series) resulting from meningeal irritation or communicating hydrocephalus. The most common initial neurologic sign is altered mental status, including abnormalities in the level of consciousness (ranging from mild somnolence to delirium) and the content of consciousness (ranging from mild personality and behavioral changes to severe dementia). Tables 38-1

Table 38-1. Symptoms at Presentation

Symptom	Percentage of Patients
Headache	51
Spine or radicular limb pain	37
Nausea and vomiting	34
Weakness	34
Sensory disturbance	33
Altered mental status	26
Diplopia	20
Incoordination	20
Seizures	18
Sphincter disturbance	18
Reduced visual acuity	9
Dysarthria	7
Dysphagia	5

Source: Adapted from M Balm, J Hammack. Leptomeningeal carcinomatosis. Presenting features and prognostic factors. Arch Neurol 1996;53:629.

Table 38-2. Signs at Presentation

Signs	Percentage of Patients
Altered mental status	27
Meningismus	13
Cranial nerve abnormality	
II*	19
III	11
IV	5
V	6
VI	13
VII	10
VIII	7
IX	2
X	6
XI	3
XII	5
Cerebellar signs	15
Upper motor neuron deficits	9
Cerebral deficits	3
Myelopathy	6
Lower motor neuron deficits	37
Cauda equina syndrome	20
Multilevel polyradiculopathy	15
Anal sphincter dysfunction	5

*Includes both diminished visual acuity and papilledema.

and 38-2 detail the spectrum of signs and symptoms and their frequency.

Examination of the CSF with cytologic confirmation is essential to making the diagnosis of meningeal carcinomatosis. Neuroimaging, however, may identify the presence of meningeal tumor and exclude other causes of CNS dysfunction. Magnetic resonance imaging (MRI) with gadolinium is superior to computed tomography scanning with contrast in the identification of meningeal enhancement (a common but not universal finding in patients with meningeal carcinomatosis). Yet, only 30 to 50% of head and spine MRIs will show this abnormality. Both computed tomography and MRI are effective in identifying hydrocephalus or an intraparenchymal or epidural mass lesion. Myelography rarely is required.

The CSF profile is rarely, if ever, normal in these patients. The most common abnormality is elevated protein, followed in incidence by an increase in nucleated cells (reactive lymphocytes, polymorphs, or atypical cells), a low CSF glucose, and a raised CSF opening pressure. Some adenocarcinomas are associated with the tumor marker carcinoembryonic antigen, which may be detected in the CSF. With the first lumbar puncture, the cytology is positive in only 50 to 75% of patients. The cumulative positive cytology rate is 94% by the third lumbar puncture. Occasionally, cisternal CSF will yield a positive cytology when the lumbar CSF does not. Some patients may require a meningeal biopsy to confirm the diagnosis. Although a positive CSF cytology absolutely confirms the diagnosis of meningeal carcinomatosis, it may not be required before instituting treatment. In some cases, a lumbar puncture may be contraindicated, as with coagulopathy or an associated intracranial mass lesion. If the MRI findings are diagnostic in these cases, it may be appropriate to treat the patient empirically, without cytologic confirmation.

Treatment of meningeal carcinomatosis never is curative and must be considered strictly palliative. The treatment includes radiotherapy to the symptomatic level of the nervous system. As radiation is not curative, entire neuraxis radiation rarely (if ever) is indicated and carries prohibitive toxicity. Most systemically administered chemotherapy agents do not cross the blood-brain barrier in sufficient amounts to be useful. Chemotherapy administered directly into the ventricles via an Ommaya reservoir or intrathecally into the lumbar CSF may be helpful to some patients. However, only a limited number of chemotherapy agents can be introduced directly into the CSF with acceptable neurotoxicity. Such agents include methotrexate, cytarabine, and thiotepa.

Factors Affecting Prognosis

One-half of all patients with meningeal carcinomatosis die from causes attributed to progression of their systemic (extra-CNS) cancer. The remainder die from causes related to CNS disease (progressive coma, aspiration pneumonia, etc.). Spontaneous regression or stabilization of disease virtually never occurs, although some patients may survive for many months or even a few years without treatment of their CNS cancer. This result is extremely rare, however.

Some clinical factors appear to influence survival. Patients who have extensive, progressive systemic cancer (especially with metastases involving the liver or lung) tend to fare less well than do those with minimal or no apparent systemic tumor burden. Some 60 to 84% of patients have a significant systemic tumor burden at the time their meningeal carcinomatosis is diagnosed. Some reports suggest that meningeal carcinomatosis from breast cancer often follows a more indolent course than do other malignancies. Perhaps 15 to 20% of patients with leptomeningeal spread of breast cancer will survive for 1 year. An occasional patient with lung cancer or melanoma may survive for more than 1 year, if the patient has limited systemic disease. Patient age did not appear to affect the prognosis in some studies, although in one study, age of 55 or older was associated with shorter survival times (Boogerd and coworkers). In a retrospective study at the Mayo Clinic, we found that female gender was a small but significant ($p <0.02$) independent predictor of longer survival, even in patients with malignancies other than breast cancer. The numbers were small, however, and other investigators have not noted a gender difference in survival. A poor performance status, neurologic or otherwise, was associated (not surprisingly) with a worse prognosis. Similarly, the presence of cerebral or cranial nerve symptoms (as opposed to pure spinal symptoms) was a negative predictor of survival in patients in both the Mayo study ($p = 0.05$) and the study of Clamon and Doebbeling ($p = 0.026$). Patients with a longer history of neurologic symptoms before diagnosis, suggesting more indolent disease, have

been reported to survive significantly longer than do those with a short history of symptoms.

An elevated CSF protein level at the time of diagnosis was associated with shorter survival times in several studies, and at least one study noted a low CSF glucose was a negative predictor of survival (Boogerd and coworkers). The CSF cell count and number of malignant cells present on the cytologic specimen had no prognostic value, and no other CSF parameter was useful in prediction of survival. Radiographic findings, such as location and extent of meningeal enhancement and presence or absence of hydrocephalus, are not known to be helpful in predicting the outcome.

Evaluation for Prognosis

A thorough history and general physical and neurologic examination of the patient are the most important tools for predicting patient outcome in meningeal carcinomatosis. Patients with a long duration of neurologic symptoms (>6 months) before diagnosis tend to have more indolent disease. Patients who are disabled significantly (e.g., unable to perform self-care) on the basis of either their systemic or their neurologic disease will have the shortest survival. The neurologic examination will identify those patients with single or multilevel meningeal spread.

At least one-half of patients with meningeal carcinomatosis will die from complications of their systemic tumors. All patients, therefore, should receive restaging of their cancers. MRI with gadolinium of the head or spine usually is essential for diagnosis but is not very helpful for making a prognosis. A CSF examination should be performed and may yield useful information in determining the prognosis (see Factors Affecting Prognosis).

Therapies Affecting Prognosis

A prospective, randomized, controlled trial of radiation and systemic or intra-CSF chemotherapy in the treatment of meningeal carcinomatosis never has been published. Ample retrospective, anecdotal data suggest that radiotherapy and chemotherapy are helpful in providing palliation and may prolong survival. No patient with meningeal carcinomatosis is cured by these treatment modalities. Virtually all patients should receive radiotherapy to the symptomatic area, unless their life expectancy is deemed to be so short they may not survive a 2-week course of treatment. Radiation is regarded as the therapy most useful in improving or at least stabilizing neurologic symptoms. The Mayo Clinic series suggested that radiotherapy had a modest effect on prognosis, prolonging median survival from 3 weeks without radiation to 3 months with radiation alone. However, Boogerd and coworkers found no prolongation of survival with radiation. The efficacy of intra-CSF chemotherapy in prolonging survival is even less certain. Several studies noted median survivals of 4 to 6 months in patients who had received intra-CSF chemotherapy in addition to radiation. A study by Grossman and associates compared intra-CSF thiotepa with methotrexate in a prospective, randomized study and found no significant advantage of one over the other. Median survival in both groups was less than 4 months, and the authors concluded that intra-CSF chemotherapy did not prolong survival. Many more long-term (>12 months) survivors are found among those who have received radiation or chemotherapy. Notably, the aforementioned studies revealed an inherent bias toward selecting higher-functioning patients with more favorable pretreatment prognostic factors. Patients who were debilitated or moribund were unlikely to be subjected to such aggressive therapies and, hence, the data erroneously may suggest that a treatment is beneficial.

Short- and Long-Term Prognosis

Meningeal carcinomatosis has been termed the disease of "40 days and 40 nights" and, without treatment, the median survival is only 4 to 8 weeks from diagnosis. Even with treatment, very few patients will survive for 6 months. Most patients have widely metastatic cancer at the time they develop neurologic symptoms, and one-half will die from complications of their systemic tumors. The other half will die from complications of their neurologic disease, including progressive coma with respiratory arrest and aspiration. Treatment is at best palliative. Little or no rationale is found in treating patients who are moribund, as they likely will die during the course of therapy. Radiation and possibly intra-CSF chemotherapy are indicated in young, relatively high-functioning individuals with limited systemic tumor.

Additional Reading

Balm M, Hammack J. Leptomeningeal carcinomatosis. Presenting features and prognostic factors. Arch Neurol 1996;53:626–632.

Boogerd W, Hart AAM, van der Sande JJ, et al. Meningeal carcinomatosis in breast cancer. Prognostic factors and influence of treatment. Cancer 1991;67:1685–1695.

Clamon G, Doebbeling B. Meningeal carcinomatosis from breast cancer: spinal cord vs. brain involvement. Br Cancer Res Treat 1987;9:213–217.

Grant R, Naylor B, Greenberg HS, et al. Clinical outcome in aggressively treated meningeal carcinomatosis. Arch Neurol 1994;51:457–461.

Grossman SA, Finkelstein DM, Ruckdeschel JC, et al. Randomized prospective comparison of intraventricular methotrexate and thiotepa in patients with previously untreated neoplastic meningitis. J Clin Oncol 1993;11:561–569.

Jayson GC, Howell A, Harris M, et al. Carcinomatous meningitis in patients with breast cancer. Cancer 1994;74:3135–3141.

Kokkoris CP. Leptomeningeal carcinomatosis. How does cancer reach the pia-arachnoid? Cancer 1983;51:154–160.

Sorensen SC, Eagan RT, Scott M. Meningeal carcinomatosis in patients with primary breast or lung cancer. Mayo Clin Proc 1984;59:91–94.

Wasserstrom WR, Glass JP, Posner JB. Diagnosis and treatment of leptomeningeal metastases from solid tumors: experience with 90 patients. Cancer 1982;49:759–772.

Chapter 39

Central Nervous System Lymphoma

Lloyd M. Alderson

Primary central nervous system lymphoma (PCNSL) is a high-grade, diffuse non-Hodgkin's lymphoma that can involve the brain, eyes, leptomeninges, and spinal cord. There are two distinct forms of this disease that differ in both etiology and prognosis. PCNSL in immunocompetent patients most often presents in the sixth decade of life either as a single or a multiple periventricular brain lesion that often responds to cytotoxic therapy. Histologically, it is a monoclonal, B-cell neoplasm similar to other extranodal lymphomas. PCNSL in immunosuppressed patients (typically, organ transplant recipients or patients with acquired immunodeficiency syndrome [AIDS]) presents at any age, often is disseminated more widely in the central nervous system (CNS), and is much less likely to respond to cytotoxic therapy. This disease is a polyclonal lymphoproliferative disorder driven by the unchecked dissemination of the Epstein-Barr virus.

Natural History

PCNSL was first described by Bailey in 1929 as a form of sarcoma. Brain histiocytes were thought to be the cells of origin, giving rise to the name *primary reticulum cell sarcoma of the brain*. The first demonstration that this tumor was composed of lymphocytes appeared in 1963. Until recently, PCNSL has been a rare disease, comprising only 1% of all brain tumors, with an incidence of less than one case per 1 million person-years. However, since the 1970s there has been a dramatic and unex-

plained rise in the incidence of PCNSL among immunocompetent patients, particularly in the elderly. In 1974, the incidence in the United States overall was less than 0.5 cases per 1 million person-years. Now, it is approximately 3 and, in persons older than 60, it approaches 10. In addition, PCNSL is 100 to 350 times more likely in patients with acquired or deliberate immunosuppression. The AIDS epidemic and the growing number of organ transplantation recipients has added to the number of PCNSL patients in the United States.

In immunocompetent patients, PCNSL typically presents with a focal neurologic deficit and a homogeneously enhancing parenchymal brain lesion on gadolinium-enhanced magnetic resonance imaging. In 40% of these patients, more than one brain lesion is seen. Ocular involvement occurs in 20% of patients. Patients who initially present with visual loss and ocular lymphoma have an 80% chance of developing parenchymal brain lesions at some point. Clinical evidence of cerebrospinal fluid dissemination occurs in 12% of patients, but autopsy studies suggest that leptomeningeal spread is much more common. Spinal cord involvement is rare. The need to exclude the possibility that organs other than the CNS and eyes are involved is controversial. The experience at Massachusetts General Hospital was that computed tomography scan of the chest and abdomen is unlikely to be positive for tumor in patients who present with CNS or ocular disease.

Unlike patients with other brain tumors, patients with PCNSL can have a history of sentinel lesions. Sentinel lesions are focal neurologic deficits and enhancing brain lesions that develop and spontaneously resolve, months or years before the diagnosis of PCNSL at another site. A few of these sentinel lesions have undergone biopsy, revealing demyelination and T-lymphocyte infiltrates. This finding suggests that the immune system plays an important role in preventing the development of PCNSL. It also suggests that the cell of origin may not reside in the CNS but simply may have an affinity for small blood vessels of the brain. In some patients, brain lesions can resolve with corticosteroid treatment alone, and these drugs should be avoided before biopsy if PCNSL is suspected.

PCNSL occurs in 6% of patients with AIDS. It is the AIDS-defining disease in 2% of patients and usually does not develop until CD4+ lymphocyte counts are less than 100 cells per square millimeter. Most patients have multifocal disease at presentation, and often the lesions have a necrotic center that does not enhance. It is often difficult to distinguish brain lesions associated with PCNSL from intracerebral toxoplasmosis. A trial of empiric anti-toxoplasmosis therapy is recommended before biopsy in most AIDS patients. The clinical presentation of PCNSL is more likely to include systemic and nonlocalizing symptoms (e.g., fever, weight loss, headache, lethargy, and mental status changes) in AIDS patients than in immunocompetent patients.

Histologically, PCNSL in immunocompetent and immunosuppressed patients does not differ, and the vast majority are designated high-grade tumors. More than 80% are classified as diffuse large-cell tumors (most commonly large-cell immunoblastic) by the Working Formulation of Non-Hodgkin's Lymphoma. High-grade, small, noncleaved-cell and intermediate-grade, small, cleaved-cell histologies make up much of the remainder. Although recent studies suggest that intermediate-grade CNS lymphomas are becoming rare, this histology suggests a better prognosis.

Treatment and Prognosis

Immunocompetent Patients

In no other brain tumor have treatment and prognosis changed so dramatically since the 1980s than in PCNSL in the immunocompetent patient. Unlike other extranodal lymphomas confined to a single organ, PCNSL is an aggressive disease often refractory to local treatment. If the disease is left untreated, the median survival of patients with PCNSL is 2 to 4 months. Surgical resection does not add significantly to survival and is not indicated unless palliative decompression is needed. External-beam whole-brain radiotherapy (RT) significantly increases patient survival. Patients treated with 60 Gy have a median survival of 17 months, but the 5-year disease-free survival remains low (3%). Favorable prognostic indicators are Karnofsky performance status and age. Median survival of patients who are older than 60 years or have a Karnofsky performance status score of less than 70 will have median survivals of less than 8 months. Older patients also are at higher risk of developing significant radiation-induced leukoencephalopathy.

Survival of immunocompetent patients with PCNSL is increased further with treatment regimens combining radiotherapy and chemotherapy. A median survival of 41 months has been reported in 16 immunocompetent PCNSL patients treated with procarbazine, lomustine (CCNU), and vincristine after RT. Similar results were reported for patients treated with intravenous and intrathecal chemotherapy in combination with whole-brain RT (Table 39-1). Patients who received less chemotherapy did less well. However, subsequent evaluation of these and other patients treated with an aggressive multimodality approach has revealed that a large proportion developed debilitating leukoencephalopathy. The combination of methotrexate and RT is clearly toxic to central white matter. The degree of leukoencephalopathy in these patients appears out of proportion to similarly treated patients with other diseases and raises the question of whether the radiation-induced death of lymphocytes infiltrating the brain is particularly toxic to oligodendrocytes.

Because of this toxicity, new treatment approaches that defer RT have been investigated. In a large series of patients treated at Massachusetts General Hospital, Glass and coworkers demonstrated that high-dose intravenous methotrexate alone is as effective as is multimodality therapy and is less toxic (see Table 39-1). More than 80% of patients achieve a complete response after the induction phase, and median survival for these patients has not been reached (Fig. 39-1). Again, unfavorable prognostic indicators are Karnofsky performance status and age. Methotrexate-induced renal toxicity

Table 39-1. Results of Various Treatment Trials for Central Nervous System Lymphoma

	Preradiation Chemotherapy	Radiotherapy	Postradiation Therapy	Median Survival (mos)
Natural history	None	None	None	2–4
Study				
Berry and Simpson 1981	None	45 Gy	None	17
Chamberlain and Levin 1992	None	54 Gy	Procarbazine-lomustine-vincristine	41
DeAngelis et al. 1992	IV Methotrexate IT Methotrexate	54 Gy	Cytosine arabinoside	42.5
Glass et al. 1994	IV Methotrexate	Deferred	—	>40

IT = intrathecal.

is a major concern in patients on this protocol, particularly in those older than 70 years.

When PCNSL involves the eyes, it necessitates local therapy. In one-half of such patients, ocular lymphoma is the initial manifestation of disease. Usually, both eyes are involved and should be treated. Despite treatment, ocular lymphoma often recurs. However, eye involvement in patients with PCNSL does not indicate a more aggressive disease or reduced median survival. Involvement of both eyes suggests an 80% chance of parenchymal brain lesions developing at some point. However, no role is known for prophylactic whole-brain RT or chemotherapy in these patients.

Even with optimal therapy, parenchymal brain lesions often recur in patients with PCNSL. Often they are not contiguous with the primary site of disease, again suggesting that the cell of origin does not reside in the CNS. Tumor recurrence is a poor prognostic factor, and median survival from the time of recurrence is less than 3 months.

Immunosuppressed Patients

In AIDS patients with PCNSL, treatment options are much more limited, and the prognosis remains poor. The prognosis reflects not only the virulence of the disease but that it occurs when the immune system is impaired severely. The diagnosis requires pathologic confirmation because of the high rate of concomitant infections, such as toxoplasmosis and cytomegalovirus. Corticosteroids can induce the involution of brain lesions and, again, should be avoided before biopsy. If the disease is left untreated or is treated with corticosteroids alone, the median

survival for AIDS patients with PCNSL is less than 2 months. The use of external-beam RT has been investigated in retrospective studies. The median survival in treated patients increased to 4 to 6 months. Similar studies concluded that AIDS patients who have PCNSL and are treated with RT often die of other opportunistic infections, whereas patients who are not treated die from progression of PCNSL. Chemotherapy protocols that used methotrexate or cytosine arabinoside have unacceptably high toxicity for most AIDS patients. Long-term survivors who have tolerated chemotherapy and have had durable responses have been reported. New antiviral strategies directed at human immunodeficiency virus and Epstein-Barr virus are more likely to benefit these patients.

The approach to PCNSL in transplant recipients and other patients who are immunosuppressed deliberately is very different, reflecting the very different prognosis. The biology of the disease is similar to that of PCNSL in AIDS patients. Tumors are polyclonal and Epstein-Barr virus–positive and will regress with reversal of the immunosuppression. Prognosis then becomes more dependent on the systemic consequences of normal immune function in a transplant recipient.

Long-Term Prognosis

The prognosis of PCNSL in the immunocompetent patient has improved dramatically since 1987. Durable, complete responses to intravenous chemotherapy alone are common, and median survival exceeds 3 years with most protocols. Clinical research efforts now focus on avoiding toxicity of the treatment. In contrast, the prognosis for PCNSL patients

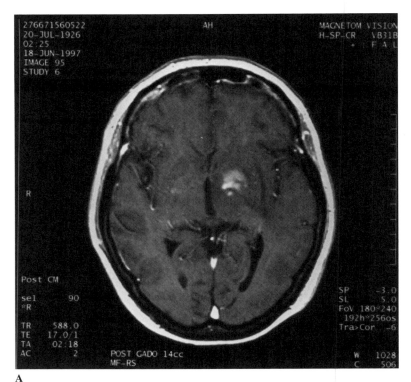

A

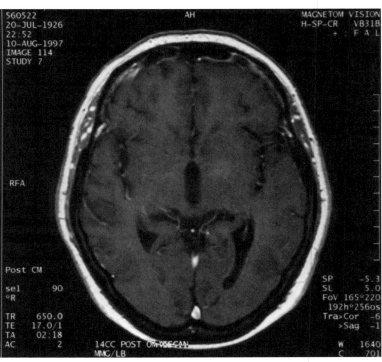

B

Figure 39-1. Gadolinium-enhanced, T1-weighted magnetic resonance imaging (MRI) scan from a 70-year-old immunocompetent woman with a history of ocular lymphoma. The patient presented with right-arm clumsiness, unsteady gait, and loss of memory. A. MRI of the brain shows periventricular lesions before chemotherapy. Patient was treated with three cycles of high-dose methotrexate, and her neurologic function returned to normal. B. MRI of the brain after the patient's third cycle shows resolution of the enhancing lesions.

with AIDS remains poor, and progress likely will reflect improvements in the treatment of the underlying immunodeficiency.

Additional Reading

Ahmed T, Wormser G, Stahl R, et al. Malignant lymphomas in a population at risk for acquired immune deficiency syndrome. Cancer 1987;60:719–723.

Berry M, Simpson W. Radiation therapy in the management of primary malignant lymphoma of the brain. Int J Radiat Oncol Biol Phys 1981;7:55–59.

Chamberlain M, Levin V. Primary CNS lymphoma: a role for adjuvant chemotherapy. J Neurooncol 1992;14:271–275.

DeAngelis L, Yahalom J, Thaler H, Kher U. Combined modality therapy for primary CNS lymphoma. J Clin Oncol 1992;10:635–643.

Fine H, Mayer R. Primary central nervous system lymphoma. Ann Intern Med 1993;119:1093–1104.

Glass J, Gruber M, Cher L, Hochberg F. Pre-irradiation methotrexate chemotherapy of primary central nervous system lymphoma: long-term outcome. J Neurosurg 1994;81:188–195.

Hochberg F, Miller D. Primary central nervous system lymphoma. J Neurosurg 1988;68:835–853.

Patchell R. Primary central nervous system lymphoma in the transplant patient. Neurol Clin 1988;6:297–365.

Peterson K, Gordon K, Heinemann M, DeAngelis L. The clinical spectrum of ocular lymphoma. Cancer 1993;72:843–849.

Remick S, Diamond C, Migliozzi J, et al. Primary CNS lymphoma in patients with and without acquired immune deficiency syndrome. Medicine 1990;69:345–360.

Chapter 40

Metastatic Central Nervous System Disease

Roy A. Patchell

Metastases to the central nervous system are the most common metastatic neurologic complications of systemic cancer. The most common sites of neurologic involvement are the brain parenchyma, the spine, and the spinal cord.

Parenchymal Brain Metastasis

Parenchymal brain metastases are tumors that originate in tissues outside the brain and spread secondarily to involve the brain. Metastasis to the brain is the most common metastatic complication of systemic cancer. Autopsy studies show that as many as 25% of patients who die from cancer have intracranial metastases at the time of death.

Natural History

Brain metastases are associated with a poor prognosis, regardless of treatment. Untreated patients have a median survival of only 4 weeks, and nearly all untreated patients die as a direct result of the brain tumor, with death due to the effects of increased intracranial pressure. The survival figure quoted here must be interpreted with caution because the information comes from retrospective studies done before the age of computed tomography and magnetic resonance imaging (MRI). Also, in the past as now, patients who receive no treatment for their brain metastases usually are patients with poor performance status, extensive systemic

disease, and (generally) very poor prognoses. In all likelihood, the average patient in whom the disease was diagnosed today would live longer than 1 month even if untreated.

Factors Affecting Prognosis

Data from large prospective clinical trials indicate the factors that correlate with better prognosis are (1) Karnofsky performance status scores in the range of 70% or greater, (2) absent or controlled primary tumor, (3) patient age younger than 60 years, and (4) metastatic spread limited to the brain. Although evidence also shows that single metastases have an intrinsically better prognosis than do multiple metastases, increases in survival in the single-metastases group likely result from more effective treatment being available to patients with single metastases than to patients with multiple metastases. Among comparably treated patients (radiotherapy alone), survival did not differ regardless of whether a single or multiple brain metastases were present. The type of underlying primary tumor also does not make a significant difference in survival.

Evaluation for Prognosis

The best diagnostic test for brain metastasis is the contrast-enhanced MRI scan. This procedure will identify the presence of multiple metastases. A general search for the presence of other systemic metastases (beyond the primary tumor in organ systems other than the central nervous system) usually is done, although the yield is low.

Therapies Affecting Prognosis

For patients with intracranial metastases, several methods of treatment are available. Corticosteroids, radiotherapy, surgery, and radiosurgery have a place in the management of metastases. Chemotherapy rarely is useful.

Corticosteroids are the first treatment usually given to patients with brain metastases, and more than 70% of patients improve symptomatically. Symptoms reflecting generalized neurologic dysfunction or brain edema respond more consistently to treatment than do such focal symptoms as hemiparesis. Treatment with steroids alone also has a slight effect on survival; the median survival time of patients is approximately 2 months. Most of these patients die from increased intracranial pressure.

Whole-brain radiotherapy (WBRT) is the treatment of choice for most patients with brain metastases. WBRT increases median survival to 3 to 6 months. Data from large retrospective studies have shown that more than one-half of patients treated with WBRT ultimately die from progressive systemic cancer and not as a direct result of brain metastases.

Surgical therapy usually is not an option for most patients with brain metastases, because of the presence of unresectable multiple lesions or extensive systemic cancer. In the subgroup of patients whose only metastasis is in the brain, however, death is more likely to be caused by the brain metastasis than by progressive systemic disease. Therefore, in patients who have controlled systemic cancer and develop brain metastases, the treatment of the brain disease is the factor that will most influence the length of survival. In this group, the question of more aggressive therapy, particularly surgery, for the brain metastases usually is raised. The results from two randomized trials clearly show that surgical resection is beneficial in selected patients. Patients treated with surgery plus WBRT have a median survival of 8 to 10 months. The best results with surgery are achieved in those patients with a single surgically accessible lesion and either no remaining systemic disease (true solitary metastasis) or with controlled systemic cancer limited to the primary site only.

The development of stereotaxic radiosurgery, a new method of delivering intense focal irradiation by using a linear accelerator (LINAC) or multiple cobalt-60 sources (gamma knife), has added a new method of treatment for brain metastases. Radiosurgery is not a substitute for WBRT but may be a replacement for surgical therapy in selected patients. Current prospective clinical trials may help to determine the role of radiosurgery both in the primary treatment of patients with single and multiple metastases and in the management of recurrent brain metastases. Reports from several uncontrolled series suggest that the local control rate for radiosurgery in the treatment of single metastases is perhaps 80 to 90%, similar to that achieved by conventional surgery. However, 5 to 15% of patients develop focal radiation necrosis and often require surgical removal of the necrotic debris.

Short-Term Prognosis

Paradoxically, the short-term prognosis for patients who develop brain metastases is excellent, owing to advances in treatment. Most patients experience symptomatic improvement and, in most patients, the brain tumors are able to be eliminated or at least stabilized and survival extended, with an acceptable quality of life.

Long-Term Prognosis

Despite advances in therapy and the relatively good short-term prognosis achieved after treatment, the long-term prognosis for patients with brain metastases is extremely poor. The median survival remains less than 6 months. However, the poor long-term prognosis is not due to failure of therapy of the brain disease; with modern treatment, most patients do not die as a result of their brain metastases. The poor prognosis is due to the underlying cancer and its tendency to spread and metastasize widely.

Spinal Metastasis

Metastasis affecting the spinal cord (and its nerve roots) is the second most common neurologic complication of systemic cancer and occurs in 5 to

10% of patients with cancer. Although spinal metastases usually occur in patients with advanced disease, it may complicate any stage of the illness and, in as many as 8% of patients who have spinal involvement, it is the first manifestation of the underlying malignancy.

Spinal cord damage may result from either compression by the tumor in the epidural space or by direct invasion of the spinal cord parenchyma. Of the two, metastatic epidural spinal cord compression is much more common. Metastatic tumor reaches the epidural space and compresses the spinal cord in one of two ways. In most cases, an initial metastasis to the vertebral body later spreads to the epidural space. Less commonly (but characteristic of lymphomas and neuroblastomas), a paravertebral tumor grows into the spinal canal through an intervertebral foramen. Metastatic epidural cord compression damages the cord by direct compression (with demyelination and axonal damage) and by secondary vascular compromise (causing ischemia, edema, and infarction).

Natural History

If untreated, metastatic epidural spinal cord compression results in the rapid development of permanent paraplegia (or quadriplegia). This condition usually results in complete loss of spinal cord function below the level of the lesion.

Factors Affecting Prognosis

The prognosis depends on the neurologic status of the patient at the start of treatment. Patients who are ambulatory when they begin treatment will remain ambulatory, and patients who are not ambulatory before treatment almost never regain useful function after treatment. The period during which patients are paraparetic before coming to treatment also is significant. Little improvement occurs after 24 hours.

Evaluation for Prognosis

An MRI of the spine is the best test to detect the number of areas involved and the extent of compression and potential cord damage. A standard neurologic examination also is useful for determining strength, reflexes, and sensory loss.

Therapies Affecting Prognosis

The standard treatment of spinal cord compression includes steroids and radiotherapy. The role of surgery is controversial. However, surgery has a clear place in several instances, including cord compression from an unknown primary tumor (for diagnosis), relapse after maximum radiotherapy, and progression while receiving radiotherapy. Simple laminectomy probably is not effective in most instances, but vertebral body resection has shown promise. In all cases, therapy is more successful at preventing further loss of function than in restoring lost function.

Short-Term Prognosis

The short-term prognosis generally is good if the patient is ambulatory and definitive treatment is started early. Most patients can expect stabilization of the spinal disease with treatment.

Long-Term Prognosis

The long-term prognosis for patients with spinal cord compressions is poor, owing to the presence of widespread systemic disease that afflicts most patients. The median survival of patients in whom metastatic epidural spinal cord compression is diagnosed is 3 to 4 months.

Additional Reading

Auchter, RM, Lamond JP, Alexander E, et al. A multiinstitutional outcome and prognostic factor analysis of radiosurgery for resectable single brain metastasis. Int J Radiat Oncl Biol Phys 1996;35:27–35.

Borgelt B, Gelber R, Kramer S, et al. The palliation of brain metastases: final results of the first two studies by the Radiation Therapy Oncology Group. Int J Radiat Oncol Biol Phys 1980;6:1–9.

Gilbert RW, Kim JH, Posner JB. Epidural spinal cord compression from metastatic tumor: diagnosis and treatment. Ann Neurol 1978;3:40–51.

Grant R, Papadopoulos SM, Greenberg HS. Metastatic epidural spinal cord compression. Neurol Clin 1991;9: 825–841.

Patchell RA. The treatment of brain metastases. Cancer Invest 1996;14:169–177.

Patchell RA, Tibbs PA, Walsh JW, et al. A randomized trial of surgery in the treatment of single metastases to the brain. N Engl J Med 1990;322:494–500.

Sorensen PS, Borgesen SE, Rohde K, et al. Metastatic epidural spinal cord compression. Cancer 1990;65: 1502–1508.

Vecht CJ, Haaxma-Reiche H, Noordijk EM, et al. Treatment of single brain metastasis: radiotherapy alone or combined with neurosurgery? Ann Neurol 1993;33:583–590.

Zimm S, Wampler GL, Stablein D, et al. Intracerebral metastases in solid-tumor patients: natural history and results of treatment. Cancer 1981;48:384–394.

Part VIII
Infections

Chapter 41

Human Immunodeficiency Virus and Related Opportunistic Infections

David B. Clifford

Human immunodeficiency virus (HIV) results in neurologic disease at each level of the nervous system both as a result of the primary infection and owing to opportunistic infections that occur because of deficient immunologic surveillance. The primary HIV-associated neurologic conditions include HIV-associated dementia (also known as *acquired immunodeficiency syndrome [AIDS] dementia complex*); vacuolar myelopathy; peripheral neuropathies that include most prominently a distal sensory neuropathy; and inflammatory myopathy. Opportunistic infections may be of almost any type, but the predominant forms include cryptococcal meningitis, toxoplasmic encephalitis, progressive multifocal leukoencephalopathy (PML), cytomegalovirus (CMV) encephalitis and radiculomyelitis, Epstein-Barr virus–associated primary central nervous system (CNS) lymphoma, and more aggressive neurosyphilis. In addition, varicella zoster virus reactivation, in the form of shingles, varicella zoster virus encephalitis, or myelitis, is more common in the setting of HIV.

Natural History

The natural history of HIV infection appears to be yielding to progress in therapy and, as only a short period of experience with newer therapies is available, investigators do not yet know the full impact. Infection with HIV results in a short viral syndrome often including fever, headache, myalgias, and sometimes a rash, which subsides spontaneously and is followed by a long period of clinical latency.

Good evidence suggests that the virus enters the cerebrospinal fluid (CSF) and brain during acute infection and may be recovered from these compartments throughout the infection. Thus, HIV is a neurologic infection from the onset.

During the latent period, which without treatment varies from a few years to in excess of 10 years, subjects may be asymptomatic but experience gradual erosion of their immune defenses, a condition that may be tracked by declining numbers of CD4 lymphocytes. During this period, subjects have increased risk of aseptic meningitis and probably have greater incidence of demyelinating motor neuropathy similar to Guillain-Barré syndrome.

When CD4 lymphocyte counts reach an approximate level of 200 cells per cubic millimeter, clinical symptoms typically begin to appear, including weight loss, fever, diarrhea, and increasing frequency of opportunistic infections. At this stage of infection, overt neurologic complications begin to arise as well, with HIV-associated dementia, myelopathy, and neuropathy being the most common. The neurologic opportunistic infections may occur also at this stage, particularly cryptococcal meningitis, PML, and toxoplasmic encephalitis. However, the remainder of complications, especially CMV-associated neurologic disease and lymphoma, commonly are not seen until CD4 counts fall below 100 (Table 41-1). Generally, once symptomatic disease occurs, survival is 2 years or less. However, advent of much more effective antiretroviral therapy rapidly appears to be changing this grim prognosis for many patients.

Table 41-1. CD4 Lymphocyte Count and Risk of Neurologic Complications in Human Immunodeficiency Virus (HIV)

Neurologic Complication	CD4 Lymphocyte Count			
	>200	100–200	50–100	<50
Aseptic meningitis	X	X	X	X
HIV-associated dementia	—	X	X	X
Peripheral neuropathy	—	X	X	X
Cryptococcal meningitis	—	X	X	X
Toxoplasmic encephalitis	—	X	X	X
Progressive multifocal leukoencephalopathy	—	X	X	X
Primary CNS lymphoma	—	—	X	X
CMV encephalitis	—	—	—	X

X = likely to occur; CNS = central nervous system; CMV = cytomegalovirus.

Factors Affecting Prognosis

The overall prognosis for HIV infection is affected by characteristics of both the host and the virus. In some cases, the host mounts a highly effective immune response that maintains viral levels in blood and tissues at very low levels. In this case, long-term survival may occur without therapy. In others, either because of virulence of the virus or because of inadequacy of host response, persistent high levels of virus RNA may be recovered from the blood. In these cases, the prognosis is poor, and rapidly declining CD4 counts with development of symptomatic disease results in brief survival of only a few years. During the course of infection, the virus itself may change, with development of "syncytium-forming" strains that appear to be associated with a more progressive course of infection. Recent investigations of viral dynamics reveal that complete turnover of the plasma RNA occurs in 1 to 2 days. Thus, to maintain steady state, a remarkably large number of new virions are being released continuously, accounting for the potential for rapid development of directed mutations that cause resistance to therapy.

Prognostic factors for development of neurologic disease are rather limited. Some investigators have suggested that possibly certain specific strains of the virus may be more likely to cause neurologic disease, but replicating these findings has been difficult. The Multicenter AIDS Cohort Study showed that such markers of advanced disease as anemia, more constitutional symptoms, lower body mass index, and more advanced age were associated with greater likelihood of developing dementia. Anemia before the onset of AIDS was particularly prognostic of subsequent development of dementia. Also, women may be more susceptible to dementia than are men. Clearly, the chance of dementia is increased greatly with CD4 counts less than 200. Though the course of HIV-associated dementia generally is considered to be progressive with perhaps a 6-month survival, individual subjects progress at variable rates, resulting in survivals varying from a few months to several years. To date, the difference in course has not been explained, although some longer survivals appear to be associated with drug-naïve patients in whom an effective antiretroviral regimen is initiated successfully.

Myelopathy often develops in the presence of dementia, although it may occur independently also. Prognosis for the myelopathy is unknown. My experience is that myelopathy is associated most often with uncontrolled systemic infection and, if modification of therapy achieves substantial control of HIV viral load, myelopathy may be arrested (though rarely reversed).

Neuropathy appears to be associated with advancing immunodeficiency but is more common in people with underlying independent causes for neuropathy, such as diabetes, alcoholism, vitamin B_{12} deficiency, or nutritional deficits. HIV-associated peripheral neuropathy has not been responsive to antiviral therapy. Often the prognosis is worse where combinations of neuropathologic processes converge, such as the use of neurotoxic therapies (e.g., didanosine [DDI], zalcitabine [DDC], or stavudine [D4T]), diabetes, or alcohol abuse. Identification and reversal of ancillary neuropathologic processes probably are most important in minimizing progression of this problem.

The risk for development of opportunistic complications is a function of the state of the underlying disease (see Table 41-1), the multiplicity of complications encountered, prior exposure to pathogens, and the outlook for therapy of the individual opportunistic pathogen. In HIV-infected patients, unlike much of medicine, multiple problems typically are encountered together, causing difficulty in attaining a secure diagnosis, potentially augmenting the disease virulence, and complicating the ability to tolerate needed therapy.

Cryptococcal meningitis is a serious complication, and its presentation may be confusing. It has a more serious prognosis if the infection is advanced at the time of diagnosis, reflected by very high fungal titers in the CSF, plasma cryptococcemia, and elevation of intracranial pressure. Though prognostic factors of significance have varied somewhat between different studies, impaired mental status at the time of diagnosis is a poor prognostic indicator. A low CSF white blood cell response also predicts a poorer outcome.

Generally, toxoplasmic encephalitis is a reactivation of prior exposures. In countries where ingestion of raw meats is common, a majority of the population is toxoplasma exposed, leading to higher risk for toxoplasmic encephalitis. Risk of this complication is decreased with negative antibodies, indicating absence of prior exposure, and is decreased also when sulfa drugs are used for *Pneumocystis carinii* pneumonia prophylaxis. Toxoplasmic encephalitis may present subacutely, and prompt diagnosis and therapeutic intervention are essential to reversing the disease. Often, the ability of patients to tolerate the antibiotic therapy is an important factor in the ability to treat toxoplasmic encephalitis. Up to 40% of AIDS patients are intolerant to sulfa drugs that generally are considered to be the cornerstone for therapy of toxoplasmic encephalitis. Currently, as sulfa drugs are used widely for prophylaxis against *P. carinii* pneumonia and also for reducing the incidence of toxoplasmic encephalitis, most cases are encountered in sulfa-allergic individuals for whom second-line therapy must be employed. Enough alternatives are available so that more than 80% still will enjoy an excellent clinical response. However, prognosis for survival for more than 1 year generally is considered poor, owing to the advanced stage of HIV at which this complication occurs.

Prognosis for the JC virus infection resulting in PML is exceedingly poor in AIDS patients. Exposure to JC is almost ubiquitous, yet only some 5% of HIV patients develop this fatal complication. In a recently completed controlled treatment trial wherein the best antiretroviral therapy was compared with use of cytosine arabinoside either intravenously or intrathecally, the mean survival was 2.5 to 3 months. The intervention did not appear to have any beneficial survival effect. However, widely known is that 10% of PML cases have a significantly better outcome, with long-term survival and occasional remission. This finding has been reported most commonly in cases in which the cause for immunodeficiency has been reversed (e.g., in kidney transplantation wherein the immunosuppression could be sacrificed). Some investigators hope that successful therapy for HIV will allow reversal of this otherwise fatal complication. Case reports from initiation of zidovudine therapy suggest that this might be the case and, more recently, multiple cases of remission have been associated with initiation of highly active antiretroviral therapy. The presence of enhanced inflammatory response on biopsy or of relatively preserved CD4 status are indicators of a somewhat better prognosis. However, to date, these factors have not been sufficient to result in improved survival in most patients.

CMV encephalitis and radiculomyelitis also have a grim prognosis. Risk for developing this complication is increased by prior exposure to CMV, which is widespread in the gay male population affected by HIV. Often, neurologic involvement follows viremia and other organ involvement, including the retina, adrenals, lungs, and gastrointestinal tract. In the case of encephalitis, a compilation of reported cases suggests that mean survival is 2 to 4 months from diagnosis, with most of the cases gleaned from autopsy series. This prognosis may be biased, because substantiating the diagnosis antemortem is difficult; thus, cases reported likely were the most aggressive end of the spectrum. With more rapid diagnosis during life, using a combination of clinical, radiologic, and CSF polymerase chain reaction testing for CMV DNA, my experience suggests that early and aggressive therapy may permit a longer survival with this infection, but no controlled data are available. Radiculomyelopathy is associated with a subacute progression of paraplegia, loss of bladder and bowel control, and variable degrees of radicular pain. Its diagnosis is easier than that of encephalitis, because it has an unusual polymorphonuclear pleocytosis on CSF examination. In the setting of CMV disease elsewhere in the body, recognizing this complication is easy, and rapid treatment has achieved stabilization of the myelopathy and led to some improvement over the subsequent several months. However, the extremely advanced patients who develop CMV complications generally have less than 1 year to live.

Similarly, primary CNS lymphoma is a dismal complication leading to death in 3 to 6 months. Though the tumor responds to radiotherapy (a treatment modality often offered to subjects), this option generally has not resulted in a survival benefit. Recent efforts to provide induction chemotherapy failed to improve the outlook. Though earlier reports suggested that most deaths were due to additional opportunistic complications, recurrent and progressive lymphoma also appear to play a role in the bleak outcome almost uniformly shared by these patients.

Evaluation for Prognosis

The history of the patient is one of the best indicators of prognostic outlook in HIV. Patient evaluation should include staging of HIV by attaining an understanding of the probable time of seroconversion, CD4 count history, HIV RNA viral load history, complications of the infection encountered, and the therapeutic history. Patients without multiple active problems and in whom the immune system is relatively intact generally have a better prognosis. Furthermore, treating drug-naïve patients will be easier, and they are likely to have a much better response to current HIV therapy. If combination HIV therapy is initiated from the onset, viral replication is likely to be suppressed and emergence of resistance may be much delayed.

Therapies Affecting Prognosis

Proving an impact of therapy on the prognosis of the primary HIV-related complications has been dif-ficult. HIV-associated dementia has been shown clearly to respond to initiation of zidovudine therapy with improved neurologic performance but, in the largest natural history studies, zidovudine has neither reduced the incidence of dementia nor prolonged survival substantially. This finding may be due to development of resistant virus in advanced subjects on monotherapy, because of inadequate dosing for the CNS based on systemic therapy, or because the neurologic disease represents a separate pathophysiologic mechanism. However, the incidence of HIV-associated dementia may have been positively affected by the development of HIV therapy, as early studies suggested that 60 to 70% of subjects developed AIDS dementia complex, whereas more recent studies have reported an incidence of perhaps 7% per year of survival after the diagnosis of AIDS, which translates into approximately a 20% lifetime risk.

Myelopathy and neuropathy have increased since introduction of antiretroviral therapy, probably owing to more prolonged survival and better treatment of other potentially fatal opportunistic complications. At present, no restorative therapy is available for either of these complications. In the case of peripheral neuropathy, recombinant human nerve growth factor is being evaluated as a means of treating the distal sensory peripheral neuropathy.

Therapy for opportunistic infections can influence prognosis vastly. Without therapy, the opportunistic complications are fatal in weeks to a few months. Cryptococcal meningitis and toxoplasmic encephalitis are both highly treatable diseases. Prompt initiation of amphotericin B followed by permanent suppressive therapy with fluconazole has resulted in a good quality survival for a majority of subjects after cryptococcal meningitis. Similarly, more than 80% of patients with toxoplasmic encephalitis respond well to therapy and, with permanent suppression, live to die of other complications of advanced immunodeficiency.

In contrast, PML to date has not responded consistently to any therapy. Cytosine arabinoside appeared to be associated with the largest number of remissions, but a controlled trial of this therapy failed to show benefit in AIDS. An early report of interferon-β was not encouraging, but recent reconsideration of this therapy suggested that it still may warrant a larger controlled study. No other therapy holds wide support for efficacy, although exploration of topoisomerase inhibitors and cidofovir are under consideration at the present time. Therapy for lymphoma at present consists of radiotherapy, which may provide transient improvement in function and a window of preserved function but fails to result in substantial delay of mortality.

Short-Term Prognosis

HIV-related neurologic complications have a somewhat encouraging short-term prognosis. In the case of dementia, effective antiviral therapy often will result in measurable improvement in function. Myelopathy at least may be stabilized by antiviral therapy, whereas neuropathy generally is slowly progressive, causing discomfort but not fatal complications. The short-term prognosis is rather good for the treatable opportunistic infections, including toxoplasmosis and cryptococcal meningitis. Prognosis remains grim, with less than 6-month survival and generally progressive disability, for PML and lymphoma.

Long-Term Prognosis

Current published experience indicates that death will occur within 2 years of most of the neurologic complications of HIV. This progression occurs because virtually all the complications occur at the point of advanced disease, and a fatal complication typically occurs within a few years of reaching this disease stage. However, perhaps more than in any other area of medicine, this prognosis may be rewritten in the near future. Development of multiple new antiretroviral drugs in three different classes (to date) have allowed physicians to develop

much more effective suppression of this infection and may allow physiologic immune reconstitution. Prolonged survival or recovery from some of the neurologic complications may become possible if the promise of these therapies can be achieved.

Additional Reading

Arribas JR, Storch GA, Clifford DB, Tselis AC. Cytomegalovirus encephalitis. Ann Intern Med 1996;125: 577–587.
Bacellar H, Munoz A, Miller EN, et al. Temporal trends in the incidence of HIV-1 related neurological diseases. Multicenter AIDS cohort study 1985–92. Neurology 1994;44:1892–1900.
Baumgartner JE, Rachlin JR, Beckstead JH, et al. Primary central nervous system lymphomas: natural history and response to radiation therapy in 55 patients with acquired immunodeficiency syndrome. J Neurosurg 1990;73: 206–211.
Berger JR, Kaszovitz B, Post MJ, Dickinson G. Progressive multifocal leukoencephalopathy associated with human immunodeficiency virus infection. A review of the literature with a report of sixteen cases. Ann Intern Med 1987; 107:78–87.
Chuck SL, Sande MA. Infections with *Cryptococcus neoformans* in acquired immunodeficiency syndrome. N Engl J Med 1989;321:794–799.
Harrison MJG, McArthur JC. AIDS and Neurology. Edinburgh: Churchill Livingstone, 1995.
Holland NR, Power C, Mathews VP, et al. Cytomegalovirus encephalitis in acquired immunodeficiency syndrome (AIDS). Neurology 1995;44:507–514.
Porter SB, Sande MA. Toxoplasmosis of the central nervous system in acquired immunodeficiency syndrome. N Engl J Med 1992;327:643–648.
Price RW. Neurological complications of HIV infection. Lancet 1996;348:445–452.
Sidtis JJ, Gatsonis C, Price RW, et al. Zidovudine treatment of the AIDS dementia complex: results of a placebo-controlled trial. Ann Neurol 1993;33:343–349.

Chapter 42

Acute Viral Encephalitis

Kenneth L. Tyler

Viral encephalitis results from viral infection of and injury to cells within the brain parenchyma. The clinical presentation and the scope of associated abnormalities on laboratory and diagnostic studies can vary considerably and are influenced dramatically by such factors as the nature of the infecting virus and the age of the patient. Viruses commonly implicated in causing encephalitis belong to the family *Herpesviridae* and the *Alphavirus*, *Flavivirus*, and *Bunyavirus* genuses. Examples of common encephalitis-causing viruses found in North America and belonging to these groups include herpes simplex virus (HSV), Epstein-Barr virus (EBV), varicella-zoster virus (VZV), St. Louis encephalitis virus, Western encephalitis virus, Venezuelan encephalitis virus, Eastern encephalitis virus, and California encephalitis virus. The typical clinical picture of severe encephalitis is one of an acute febrile illness associated with headache, alteration in consciousness, focal neurologic deficits, seizures, and signs of increased intracranial pressure. Associated meningeal irritation can produce nuchal rigidity. In some patients, cerebellar, brain stem, spinal cord, or radicular signs and symptoms are joined to the basic picture of encephalitis and even can become the predominant feature. Almost invariably, viral encephalitis is associated with a cerebrospinal fluid (CSF) pleocytosis. Laboratory and diagnostic studies reflect the parenchymal central nervous system (CNS) dysfunction and frequently include abnormalities on electroencephalography (EEG) and in neuroimaging studies, including computed tomography (CT) and magnetic resonance imaging (MRI).

Natural History

Effective antiviral treatment for specific types of viral encephalitis did not become available until the documentation of the efficacy of vidarabine (adenine arabinoside) for the treatment of HSV encephalitis in 1977, followed by acyclovir in 1986. Additional antiviral drugs now are available, with efficacy against HSV, cytomegalovirus, EBV, VZV, and the human immunodeficiency virus. The natural history of HSV encephalitis thus is appreciated best in studies performed before the introduction (and now widespread use) of antiviral therapy.

Many types of acute encephalitis due to viruses other than HSV are not amenable to specific antiviral therapy and, as such, illustrate the natural history of disease altered primarily by supportive rather than specific therapy. The mortality of viral encephalitis varies exceedingly and depends in large part on the nature of the infecting agent. At one extreme are cases due to rabies, in which mortality is essentially 100%. Other types of viral encephalitis with exceedingly high mortality rates include untreated HSV encephalitis (60 to 80%) and encephalitis caused by the eastern encephalitis virus (35 to 70%). At the other extreme are cases of encephalitis caused by such viruses as mumps, EBV, California encephalitis virus, and VZV, in which death in immunocompetent individuals is unusual (<1%). In large series of unselected cases of encephalitis, mortality generally runs between 5 and 15%. The incidence of sequelae in survivors of specific types of encephalitis generally parallels the mortality figures. In large unselected series, the overall incidence of neurologic sequelae generally is reported as 25 to 50%, with severe sequelae occurring in 5 to 10%. Typical sequelae include cognitive and behavioral deficits (e.g., memory loss), alteration in mood (e.g., depression), dysphasia, headaches, seizures, and motor deficits. These figures vary tremendously in different studies because of variations in the infecting agents, the demographics of the patient population studied, the duration of follow-up after acute encephalitis, and the sensitivity of the methods employed to determine sequelae, especially in the cognitive sphere.

Factors Affecting Prognosis

In addition to etiology, several consistently identified factors influence prognosis in viral encephalitis. In the case of HSV encephalitis, the amount of virus present in brain tissue correlates with clinical outcome. Patients with large amounts of virus ($>10^4$ median tissue culture infective doses of virus per gram of brain tissue) had a poor prognosis. A similar observation has been made for Japanese encephalitis, in which culture of the virus from CSF, which presumably reflects higher levels of virus within the CNS, is associated with enhanced mortality. Prognosis is influenced by demographic, clinical, and laboratory findings that include patient age, level of consciousness, presence or absence of focal neurologic signs or seizures, and results of diagnostic studies, including CSF analysis, EEG, and CT or MRI.

Age

Poor short-term outcome (e.g., as indicated by neurologic status at time of hospital discharge) in children with encephalitis is inversely proportional to age, with younger children being at highest risk. Similar results apply to medium-term prognosis. In a prospective study of 25 patients with encephalitis, Kennedy and colleagues found that only 25% of patients aged 3 or younger who survived encephalitis had a developmental quotient of more than 80 and had no major neurologic signs or behavioral problems 7 to 8 months after hospital discharge. By contrast, the corresponding figure was 79% for those older than 3.

In a study of prognostic factors in 462 cases of childhood acute encephalitis, Rautonen and coworkers found a fivefold higher risk of death or "severe damage" in children younger than 1 year of age as compared to older children. These children were at particularly high risk for the development of psychological and language and speech difficulties in comparison with their older counterparts. Increased mortality has been described also in younger patients infected with Japanese and Eastern encephalitis viruses.

By contrast, in some viral infections, prognosis is better in younger individuals and worse in the elderly. In studies of antiviral therapy in HSV encephalitis performed by the National Institute of Allergy and Infectious Diseases Collaborative Antiviral Study Group (NIAID-CASG; reviewed by Whitley), age also was an important prognostic factor that influenced acute mortality and the degree of morbidity present at evaluation at 6 months postinfection. In these studies, patients younger than 30 fared significantly better than did older patients. Some 62% of acyclovir-treated patients younger than 30 were neurologically normal or had only mild impairment (e.g., decreased attention span) at follow-up, as compared to only 36% of those older than 30. Discriminate analyses of long-term survival in acyclovir-treated patients by age range indicate that the mortality is 11% in those younger than 20 years, 22% in those 20 to 59, and 62% in those older than 60. Increased mortality has been described also in elderly patients infected with St. Louis and Eastern encephalitis viruses.

Level of Consciousness

Level of consciousness at the time of hospital admission (or on initiation of therapy in the case of HSV encephalitis) is an important predictor of subsequent prognosis. In most studies, consciousness has been characterized either into broad general categories (e.g., normal, disoriented, or unconscious) or quantified using the Glasgow coma scale (GCS). In the GCS, patients receive points on the basis of their best level of verbal responsiveness (1 to 5 points), motor responses (1 to 6 points), and eye movements (1 to 4 points), with higher scores representing better neurologic function. As an approximation, patients with a GCS score of less than 6 are comatose, those with scores in the range of 7 to 10 are semicomatose, and those with scores of more than 10 are lethargic.

In Rautonen's series of acute childhood encephalitis, 1.6% of patients with normal consciousness died or survived with severe damage. The corresponding figures were 6.6% in those who were disoriented and 31.8% in those who were unconscious at the time of admission. In the prospective series of encephalitis in children and young adults (Kennedy and associates), 75% of those with a GCS score of 10 to 15 were essentially normal at time of hospital discharge, contrasted to 60% of those with a score of 5 to 9, and only 33% of those with a score of 5 or less. Other studies generally have confirmed the relationship between low GCS (e.g., ≤6) and poor outcome.

In some studies, the relationship between GCS score and outcome only applied to the subgroup of patients with extremely low GCS scores. In the NIAID-CASG trials of HSV encephalitis, all acyclovir-treated patients with a GCS of more than 10 survived; 50% of those with a GCS score of more than 6 at the time of initiation of acyclovir therapy survived with normal or only mildly impaired neurologic function. Conversely, the prognosis for patients with a GCS score of 6 or less was abysmal: Some 25% of this group died, and all the remaining survivors had severe neurologic impairment requiring continuous supportive care. Clearly, in HSV encephalitis, patient outcomes improve when antiviral therapy is initiated before deterioration in consciousness.

In addition to the degree of consciousness and its duration, the duration of time it takes for patients to recover full consciousness also may be a prognostic variable. In one study, 85% of children who had a depressed mental state for less than 1 week were normal at the time of hospital discharge, contrasted to only 30% of those with depressed consciousness of longer duration.

Focal Neurologic Deficits

The presence of focal neurologic deficits also has been suggested to influence prognosis. In a retrospective study of 106 children with encephalitis, Klein and colleagues found that 78% of patients with a nonfocal examination at hospital admission were neurologically normal at discharge, compared to only 30% of those with an initially focal examination.

Seizures are particularly common in viral encephalitis, occurring in approximately 50% of unselected cases of encephalitis and in up to 70% of cases of HSV encephalitis. The presence or absence of either focal or generalized seizures or both occurring in the acute phase has been identified as a prognostic indicator in some series but not others.

In Rautonen's series, generalized seizures were associated with the poorest prognosis, and 18% of patients with generalized seizures died or were damaged severely. Poor outcomes were seen in only 7% of patients with "minor" seizures and in 3.5% of patients without convulsions. In the series reported by Klein and colleagues, although the number of seizures, their duration, or clinical type were not found to be statistically significant clinical predictors of short-term neurologic outcome, patients with more than five seizures had poorer outcomes than did those with fewer or no seizures.

Diagnostic Studies

A variety of laboratory and diagnostic tests have been shown to be predictors of outcome. Among the CSF findings suggested to predict outcome are the degree of pleocytosis, the CSF–serum albumin ratio, the presence of autochthonous immunoglobulin production, the levels of creatine phosphokinase-BB isoenzyme, the CSF ratio of activated to nonactivated derivatives of clotting factor VII, the levels of CSF lactate, neuron-specific enolase, and interferon (IFN). However, the paucity of studies and the lack of a consistent association between any of these tests and survival or outcome measures in different series create difficulty in evaluating the value of any of these tests in predicting prognosis.

Surprisingly, a large study of the use of polymerase chain reaction in the diagnosis of HSV encephalitis revealed no correlation between the persistence of HSV DNA in the CSF with neurologic outcome. In some studies, patients with signs of infection within the CNS (e.g., positive CSF viral cultures, high CSF–serum IgG ratios, elevated CSF IFN levels) had a poorer prognosis than did patients with evidence of primarily systemic infection (e.g., positive viral cultures from sources other than CSF, seroconversion without intrathecal antibody synthesis, elevated serum IFN levels). This finding may have reflected a prognosis for postviral immune-mediated encephalitis more benign than that for primary viral encephalitis. A related observation has suggested that patients with a biphasic illness beginning with a nonneurologic prodrome (e.g., myalgia, respiratory symptoms, gastrointestinal symptoms, rash) followed by a neurologic illness may have a better prognosis than do patients with a monophasic, predominantly neurologic illness. The former group presumably is enriched for cases of postinfectious encephalomyelitis, whereas the latter group represents predominantly cases of primary viral encephalitis.

Typically, direct measurement of intracranial pressure (ICP) is obtained only in patients severely ill with acute encephalitis. In this subgroup, which is enriched for patients with HSV encephalitis, both elevation of initial ICP and elevated mean daily ICP are associated with a poor prognosis. In a study by Barnett and colleagues, all five survivors—but only one of five patients who ultimately died—of acute encephalitis had an initial ICP of less than 12 mm Hg. All four patients with a mean daily ICP of less than 20 mm Hg survived, whereas five of six patients with higher mean ICPs died.

Variability has been seen in attempts to correlate EEG findings with prognosis. In one large series, neither the presence of generalized slowing nor the existence of focal paroxysmal features predicted short-term neurologic outcome. In the case of HSV encephalitis, some have suggested that the presence on EEG of slow periodic or repetitive complexes over both hemispheres is associated with a particularly poor prognosis.

Almost invariably, neuroimaging studies, including CT and (more recently) MRI, are obtained in patients with suspected viral encephalitis. As might be expected, abnormalities on these studies generally are associated with a poorer prognosis. Common abnormalities on CT scan include signs of generalized brain edema, focal hypodensities, and areas of cortical contrast enhancement or hemorrhage. In the series reported by Klein and colleagues, 69% of patients with abnormal neuroimaging studies had abnormal short-term neurologic outcomes, compared to only 28% of patients with normal studies. In a retrospective study, Buttner and Dorndorf reported that 63% of patients with a "pathologic" CT scan died or had

severe disability, contrasted to 21% of patients with a normal CT scan.

The prognosis of neonatal HSV encephalitis also is influenced by the CT findings. Patients with severe changes on CT scan, such as areas of low attenuation or abnormal enhancement involving three or more lobes of the brain, typically have an extremely poor prognosis and either survive with severe sequelae or die. Many patients with only mild abnormalities on early CT scans (obtained <2 weeks after disease onset) still may develop severe sequelae, so a normal or mildly abnormal study is not a guarantee of a good prognosis.

Fewer studies correlate MRI findings with clinical sequelae than do those using CT scans. In cases of viral encephalitis, MRI consistently appears to be a more sensitive indicator of the magnitude and extent of CNS disease than does CT. In the case of HSV encephalitis, an MRI study of patients selected because they were left with pronounced memory impairment as their major residual sequelae suggested that this neuropsychological profile was associated with a high incidence of damage to the hippocampus and adjacent structures, the insula, the anterior and inferior portions of the temporal lobe, the fornix, mammillary bodies, and basal forebrain. In studies of patients with intractable seizures complicating encephalitis, it appears that patients who had encephalitis at a young age (<4 years) are more likely to develop MRI and neuropathologic evidence of medial temporal sclerosis than are their older counterparts. Patients who had encephalitis at older ages only rarely develop medial temporal sclerosis and more frequently have evidence of multiple neocortical foci. Although the number of cases studied has been extremely limited, abnormal brain perfusion identified by single photon emission computed tomography (SPECT) may be indicative of a poor prognosis for patients with acute encephalitis.

Evaluation for Prognosis

Based on the factors described, the evaluation for prognosis in cases of viral encephalitis should include a careful neurologic examination with particular attention to evaluating and recording the level of consciousness and searching for focal abnormalities. Use of the GCS may be helpful in recording the level of consciousness. After the acute phase of illness, neurocognitive disturbances can be evaluated with formal neuropsychological testing. Frequently used neuropsychological examinations include the subtests of the Wechsler Adult Intelligence Scale and of the Wechsler Memory Scale. Diagnostic studies in patients with encephalitis routinely include CSF examination, EEG, and neuroimaging studies. As noted, particular CSF findings may be of only limited value in predicting outcome. Perhaps the primary importance of the CSF is as a source for identifying the etiologic agent. The advent and widespread use of polymerase chain reaction techniques to amplify viral nucleic acid in CSF dramatically has improved early diagnosis and identification of specific viral agents causing encephalitis. Attempts to identify the etiologic agent using sources in addition to CSF and through serologic studies should be made. As noted in Natural History, the nature of the etiologic agent is an important determinant of both mortality and morbidity.

ICP monitoring may provide useful information concerning prognosis in patients with severe encephalitis. EEG and neuroimaging studies also should be performed, as they may add prognostic information. The presence of abnormalities on CT scan or MRI also suggest a poorer prognosis. As discussed in Diagnostic Studies, patients with severe memory disturbances after HSV encephalitis, and patients who develop intractable seizures following encephalitis may show particular anatomic patterns of MRI abnormality. Data on SPECT currently are too limited to recommend its routine use as an indicator of prognosis in encephalitis.

Therapies Affecting Prognosis

The most important therapy known to alter prognosis is the institution of specific antiviral treatment in patients with HSV encephalitis. The mortality of untreated HSV encephalitis exceeds 70 to 80%. The NIAID-CASG trials clearly indicate that early initiation of antiviral therapy improves prognosis. Treatment with vidarabine reduces mortality to approximately 54%, and treatment with acyclovir reduces mortality to 28%. Acyclovir also reduces overall morbidity in comparison to vidarabine. In the NIAID-CASG trial, 38% of patients with HSV encephalitis receiving acyclovir—but only 14% receiving vidarabine—returned to normal function-

ing. In the study by Marton and coworkers, younger patients (<17 years) treated with acyclovir or vidarabine had lower mortality and a higher rate of recovery but also an unexpectedly higher rate of neurologic sequelae as compared to older patients (18 to 74 years). In the NIAID-CASG trials, acyclovir-treated patients who had fever and focal neurologic findings for less than 4 days at the time therapy was begun all survived. When symptoms were present for more than 4 days before initiation of therapy, mortality increased to 35%.

In the study by Marton and colleagues, the incidence of neurologic sequelae was 25% in patients who had antiviral therapy initiated within 5 days of illness onset as contrasted to 64% in those in whom therapy was started at more than 5 days after onset. Full recovery occurred in 50% of the group receiving early treatment but in only 7% of those whose treatment began later. Surprisingly, mortality was not significantly different (25% versus 29%) in the two groups.

Postexposure use of rabies immune globulin and rabies vaccine clearly reduces the risk of developing rabies in exposed individuals. Information obtained from case reports and small series suggest that antiviral treatment also is valuable in encephalitis due to EBV, VZV, and cytomegalovirus. Either effective antiviral therapy is not available or existing data are too limited to draw conclusions for encephalitis due to arboviruses, enteroviruses, measles, and mumps. Although corticosteroids and other immunomodulatory therapies (e.g., plasma exchange, intravenous immunoglobulin) are used widely in the treatment of patients with postinfectious immune-mediated encephalomyelitis, data concerning their efficacy are largely anecdotal.

In patients with severe encephalitis, elevations in ICP are associated with a poor prognosis. One may reasonably assume that in this group of patients, therapy aimed at reducing ICP would be beneficial in reducing mortality and morbidity, although data directly establishing this point currently are not available.

Short-Term Prognosis

Acute mortality in untreated cases of HSV encephalitis generally is 70 to 80%. Among the arboviruses causing epidemic encephalitis in the

United States, Eastern encephalitis virus has the highest mortality (30 to 70%). Mortality in other forms of acute encephalitis typically is between 5 and 15%. Appropriate and early treatment of HSV encephalitis (<4 to 5 days after onset of symptoms) reduces mortality to approximately 25%, with full recovery in 50% of survivors.

Long-Term Prognosis

Many studies have suggested that neurologic sequelae present on initial or short-term evaluations subsequently improve with time. In two studies (Hokkanen and colleagues; Laurent and colleagues) involving a total of 11 patients with memory disturbances resulting from HSV encephalitis, 50% were found to have either normal memory or substantial improvement on follow-up at 1 year.

However, these results must be interpreted cautiously. Another long-term follow-up study (1.5 to 4.0 years) by Gordon and coworkers of four acyclovir-treated patients with HSV encephalitis suggested that long-lasting neuropsychological residua were common. These abnormalities, which included dysnomia and impaired new learning of both verbal and visual material, were obvious on formal neuropsychological testing but were not apparent with less sophisticated clinical screening. On a more practical level, none of the four patients was able to function at the prior level of achievement.

In a study of 42 children with nonbacterial meningoencephalitis, Donat and colleagues found that 5 of 40 survivors (12.5%) had residual focal neurologic deficits at the time of hospital discharge. On follow-up at 1 year, only one of these five patients had a persisting deficit. Ten survivors developed a "postencephalitic syndrome" characterized by headaches and behavioral alterations. This condition resolved within 6 months in nine patients and within 1 year in the remaining patient.

Long-term follow-up (2.4 to 12.9 years) by Rantala and colleagues of 73 children with viral encephalitis suggested that these children had lower performance and full-scale IQs, reduced visual acuity, more frequent focal EEG slowing, and more frequent electronystagmographic abnormalities than did age- and gender-matched controls but that these differences were not clinically significant.

Additional Reading

Barnett GH, Ropper AH, Romeo J. Intracranial pressure and outcome in adult encephalitis. J Neurosurg 1988;68:585–588.

Buttner T, Dorndorf W. Prognostic value of computed tomography and cerebrospinal fluid analysis in viral encephalitis. J Neuroimmunol 1988;20:163–164.

Donat JF, Rhodes KH, Groover RV, Smith TF. Etiology and outcome in 42 children with acute nonbacterial meningoencephalitis. Mayo Clin Proc 1980;55:156–160.

Gordon B, Selnes OA, Hart J, et al. Long-term cognitive sequelae of acyclovir-treated herpes simplex encephalitis. Arch Neurol 1990;47:646–647.

Hokkanen L, Salonen O, Launes J. Amnesia in acute herpetic and nonherpetic encephalitis. Arch Neurol 1996;53:972–978.

Kennedy CR, Duffy SW, Smith R, Robinson RO. Clinical predictors of outcome in encephalitis. Arch Dis Child 1987;62:1156–1162.

Klein SK, Hom DL, Anderson MR, et al. Predictive factors of short-term neurologic outcome in children with encephalitis. Pediatr Neurol 1994;11:308–312.

Laurent B, Allegri RF, Thomas-Anterion C, et al. Long-term neuropsychological follow-up in patients with herpes simplex encephalitis and predominantly left-sided lesions. Behav Neurol 1991;4:211–224.

Marton R, Gotlieb-Steimatsky T, Klein C, Arlazoroff A. Acute herpes simplex encephalitis: clinical assessment and prognostic data. Acta Neurol Scand 1996;93:149–155.

Rantala H, Uhari M, Saukkonen A, Sorri M. Outcome after childhood encephalitis. Dev Med Child Neurol 1991;33:858–867.

Rautonen J, Koskiniemi M, Vaheri A. Prognostic factors in childhood acute encephalitis. Pediatr Infect Dis J 1991;10:441–446.

Whitley RJ. Herpes Simplex Virus. In WM Scheld, RJ Whitley, DT Durack (eds), Infections of the Central Nervous System (2nd ed). Philadelphia: Lippincott–Raven, 1997;73–89.

Chapter 43

Chronic and Recurrent Meningitis

Patricia K. Coyle

Chronic Meningitis

Chronic meningitis is defined arbitrarily as a meningitis syndrome lasting 4 or more weeks. The syndrome involves varying combinations of meningoencephalitis features: fever, headache, stiff neck, mental status changes, and focal neurologic deficits. Occasional atypical presentations are characterized by acute psychosis, movement disorder, or a parkinsonian syndrome. These clinical features occur in the setting of a cerebrospinal fluid (CSF) pleocytosis. The characteristic CSF pattern of chronic meningitis is a mild-to-moderate mononuclear pleocytosis, increased protein level, and mildly depressed glucose level.

Many different causes are responsible for the chronic meningitis syndrome. The major infectious causes are *Mycobacterium tuberculosis* (tuberculosis, or TB) and fungal pathogens (especially *Cryptococcus neoformans*). The major noninfectious causes are neoplasm, sarcoidosis, and vasculitis (discussed in other chapters).

Natural History

The natural history of chronic meningitis most typically involves indolent symptoms that variously slowly worsen, fluctuate, or remain static but do not clear during an extended observation period. One major exception is TB meningitis, which can take a more acute, almost fulminant, course. Although by definition the duration of meningitis symptoms must last at least a month, the syndrome often persists for months to years. In several series, mean duration of symptoms ranged from 17 to 43 months, with isolated cases documented up to 12 years. Ultimately, over a several-year observation period, a high proportion of idiopathic chronic meningitis cases (at least 49%) spontaneously resolve. Some rare examples of TB meningitis even resolve spontaneously after several weeks. Most such cases are serous TB meningitis, a self-limited illness seen in children with active pulmonary TB. With this exception, the mortality rate of untreated TB meningitis is 100%. For the most common fungal causes of chronic meningitis (cryptococcal, coccidioidal, and histoplasma meningitis), untreated cases are uniformly fatal with very rare exceptions. Individual untreated patients have had disease courses lasting 18 to 25 years, although approximately 86% are dead within 1 year. In contrast, cases of spontaneous resolution of candidal meningitis have been reported. Overall, the mortality rate in unselected chronic meningitis cases ranges from 22 to 35%. For specific etiologies, mortality can approach 50%. The natural history of idiopathic chronic meningitis is better than that for the group as a whole. When an etiology is not established despite an extensive work-up, the reported mortality is as low as 5%.

Factors Affecting Prognosis

The major factors affecting prognosis in chronic meningitis are the underlying etiology and the timing of diagnosis and institution of appropriate treatment. Neoplastic meningitis, for example, has a very poor ultimate prognosis. Other factors that affect prognosis include age of the host, the presence of underlying health conditions, and the presence and management of complications. Although some studies suggest poor prognosis correlates with focal neurologic signs, cranial nerve palsies, and specific CSF findings (very low CSF glucose, very high CSF protein, very high CSF cell count), other studies have not found these clinical features or laboratory data to predict outcome.

Prognostic factors for chronic meningitis of specific etiology have been identified. For TB meningitis, prognostic factors include clinical stage of disease (see Short-Term Prognosis) at admission, clinical stage at time of treatment, delay in initiation of antituberculous treatment, age (the prognosis being worse in children younger than 5 and adults older than 50), presence of associated chronic medical or alcohol conditions, duration of illness before hospitalization, presence of cranial nerve palsy, and CSF protein level greater than 300 mg per deciliter. Prognostic factors on neuroimaging include the presence of hydrocephalus, ischemic infarcts (associated with a threefold increase in mortality), and basilar exudate. In the case of cryptococcal meningitis, poor prognosis is associated with certain CSF findings (positive India ink stain, high opening pressure, fewer than 20 white blood cells per cubic millimeter), an initial CSF or serum cryptococcal antigen titer of 1:32 or greater, nondetectable anticryptococcal antibody titer, cryptococci isolated from extraneural sites, low serum sodium, corticosteroid therapy, and underlying lymphoreticular malignancy. Good prognosis is associated with presence of headache as part of the meningitis syndrome (leading to more rapid diagnosis), normal mental status, and CSF cell count of greater than 20 white blood cells per cubic millimeter. For coccidioidal meningitis, poor prognosis is associated with hydrocephalus, underlying disease, pregnancy, and nonwhite race, whereas a good prognosis is associated with a low or absent CSF anticoccidioidal antibody titer at the end of treatment. For candidal meningitis, poor prognosis has been associated with a delay of more than 2 weeks in establishing the diagnosis, a CSF glucose of less than 35 mg per deciliter, intracranial hypertension, and focal neurologic deficits. Mortality is higher in neonates than in adults.

Evaluation for Prognosis

A systematic evaluation should be conducted to establish the underlying etiology and to institute appropriate treatment. The history attempts to determine pre-existent immunologic abnormalities, prior systemic diseases or specific infections that can involve the meninges, and concurrent extraneural involvement. Patients are screened for suggestive exposures or geographic risk factors.

The examination attempts to identify extraneural involvement, define the pattern of neurologic involvement, and survey for potential biopsy sites. Physical examination includes specific dermatologic and ophthalmologic evaluations for skin and eye lesions. Neurologic examination looks for evidence of spinal cord involvement, cranial nerve disease, focal lesions, hydrocephalus, peripheral nervous system involvement, or multilevel neuraxis involvement.

Generally, the laboratory investigation for chronic meningitis is extensive. The purpose is to confirm the diagnosis and to identify an etiology. CSF evaluation is a major focus. Usually, several (at least three) lumbar punctures are used, as negative culture, cytology, and stain tests should be repeated on large-sample volumes to increase the yield of these CSF assays. If lumbar CSF is unrevealing, particularly in basilar meningitis, ventricular or cisternal CSF should be examined. At least three cultures each should be sent from CSF, blood, urine, sputum, and (occasionally) such other sites as stool, nasopharynx, and bone marrow. Contrast MRI is performed to document meningeal enhancement, to determine a basilar meningeal process, and to look for hydrocephalus or focal lesions. Serologies are evaluated for specific bacteria (*Borrelia burgdorferi*, *Brucella* spp., *Leptospira* spp., *Treponema pallidum*), fungi (*Aspergillus* spp., *Coccidioides* spp., *Histoplasma* spp., *Sporothrix* spp., *Zygomycetes* spp.), parasites (*Cysticercus* and *Toxoplasma* spp.), and viruses (human immunodeficiency virus type 1 [HIV-1], human T-lymphotropic virus type 1).

Therapies Affecting Prognosis

For infectious causes of chronic meningitis, institution of appropriate antimicrobials as early as possible is associated with better prognosis. With treatment, the overall mortality rate for TB meningitis is 20 to 30%. Adjuvant therapy with corticosteroids is believed to improve the prognosis of more fulminant cases and of patients who have marked increased intracranial pressure. The mortality of cryptococcal meningitis is reduced to 17% with treatment, with recent trials showing an acute mortality rate as low as 6%. The mortality of candidal meningitis is reduced to 10 to 20% in adults and 0 to 29% in neonates, and the mortality of coccidioidal mycosis is reduced to 10 to 30%. Coccidioidal infection requires high-dose amphotericin and intrathecal installation of drug. The mortality of histoplasma meningitis is reduced to 21% with treatment.

Short-Term Prognosis

TB meningitis has been graded into stage I (normal level of consciousness, no deficits), stage II (lethargy or altered behavior, meningismus, such minor deficits as cranial nerve palsies), and stage III (seizures, abnormal movements, stupor or coma, such severe deficits as hemiparesis). Overall, TB meningitis mortality ranges from 20 to 30%. Stage II mortality is 4 to 55%, contrasted to a stage III mortality of 37 to 87%. Poor prognosis in TB meningitis is associated with higher stage, extremes of age, and coexistent miliary disease. Fungal meningitis, over the short term, is more likely to take a chronic, indolent, or sometimes relapsing course as compared to TB meningitis.

Long-Term Prognosis

The long-term prognosis of undiagnosed chronic meningitis is excellent, with 85% of patients ultimately recovering. Of children with TB meningitis, 25 to 50% show some permanent morbidity. Neurologic sequelae are seen in perhaps 25%. Age younger than 20 months, ischemic infarct, and ventriculomegaly are associated with a higher morbidity rate. For adults who survive TB meningitis, permanent morbidity is noted in 0 to 50% and neurologic deficits in up to 25%. Survivors of candidal meningitis may do well, with only 13% showing neurologic morbidity. Morbidity rates are higher for neonates, with more than 50% of survivors showing permanent damage. Several mycotic meningeal infections have high relapse rates. For coccidioidal infection (50% relapse rate), long-term suppressive therapy is indicated. Cryptococcal meningitis has relapse rates as high as 15 to 25% in non–HIV-1-infected individuals and relapse rates of 50% in AIDS patients. This finding necessitates long-term suppressive therapy in this patient population. *Histoplasma* infection also shows a high relapse rate (37 to 50%). Patients must be followed for at least 5 years, with repeat CSF studies 6 and 12 months after treatment is completed.

Recurrent Meningitis

Recurrent meningitis is defined as the occurrence of at least two discrete episodes of acute meningitis in the same individual. Clearance of symptoms and normalization of CSF must occur between the attacks. This infection syndrome is unusual, and no large-scale and long-term studies of recurrent meningitis patients exist.

The recurrent meningitis syndrome differs from chronic meningitis. It has a unique list of etiologies (Table 43-1). Drug-induced recurrent meningitis, for example, can be produced by a variety of agents, such as antibody preparations (intravenous immunoglobulins and monoclonal antibody), nonsteroidal anti-inflammatory agents (ibuprofen, naproxen, sulindac, tolmetin), antibiotics (ciprofloxacin, isoniazid, metronidazole, penicillin, phenazopyridine, sulfonamides, trimethoprim), carbamazepine, azathioprine, and cytosine arabinoside. Viruses are by far the most common type of organism among the infectious agents that cause recurrent meningitis. Two unconnected attacks of aseptic meningitis can occur, owing to different viruses or attacks due to the same agent. Herpes simplex virus (type 2 much more often than type 1) is the most frequent cause of recurrent viral meningitis and is recognized as the agent involved in many cases of idiopathic Mollaret's meningitis.

Natural History

By definition, recurrent meningitis is self-limited. The disease episodes last from days to a few weeks. Recovery is spontaneous, with the exception of the unusual cases of recurrent bacterial

Table 43-1. Causes of the Recurrent Meningitis Syndrome

Anatomic defects
    Congenital
    Postoperative
    Traumatic
Behçet's disease
Chemical meningitis
    Endogenous (cyst, tumor)
    Exogenous (dye, drug)
Collagen vascular disease
Drug-induced hypersensitivity
Familial Mediterranean fever
Idiopathic (Mollaret's)
    Herpes simplex virus
    Other causes
Immune defects
    Antibody deficiency
    Complement deficiency
    Splenectomy
Migraine with pleocytosis
Parameningeal infection with seeding
Recurrent bacterial-viral infections
Sarcoidosis
Vogt-Koyanagi-Harada disease
Whipple's disease

meningitis due to anatomic defects, seeding from parameningeal foci, or immunologic defects. These meningitis cases generally require appropriate antibiotic treatment. The number of recurrent meningitis attacks can range from as few as 2 to as many as 35 episodes. Multiple episodes are especially characteristic of idiopathic Mollaret's meningitis. The meningitis episodes recur over weeks to years, with 28 years the longest recorded duration. Symptom-free intervals last from days to years. Often, the recurrent meningitis syndrome will remit spontaneously. With the possible exception of untreated recurrent bacterial meningitis, virtually no mortality or permanent morbidity is associated with recurrent meningitis.

Factors Affecting Prognosis

No specific clinical, CSF, or other laboratory factors have been identified as affecting prognosis. Ultimate prognosis is determined by the underlying etiology. Recurrent meningitis due to systemic disease (such as Behçet's disease, collagen vascular

disorders, sarcoidosis, Vogt-Koyanagi-Harada disease) has a more guarded prognosis than does recurrent meningitis due to drug exposure, idiopathic Mollaret's meningitis, or migraine.

Evaluation for Prognosis

Similar to that for chronic meningitis, the evaluation of the recurrent syndrome begins with a careful history and a physical and neurologic examination. Dermatologic and ophthalmologic evaluations should look for dermal sinuses, suggestive rashes, ulcers, pigment changes, uveitis, and other abnormalities. The laboratory assessment relies heavily on CSF examination and complete neuraxis neuroimaging. Because herpes simplex has been implicated in many recurrent meningitis cases, polymerase chain reaction testing for herpes simplex virus DNA should be carried out on CSF and via paired anti–herpes simplex antibody studies.

Therapies Affecting Prognosis

Therapy affects prognosis when recurrent meningitis is due to a treatable pathogen, neuraxis anatomic defect, an endogenous chemical source, an underlying immune defect, or an underlying systemic disorder. Anecdotally, prolonged suppressive antiviral therapy has aborted recurrent attacks of herpes simplex meningitis. Correction of the predisposing condition can abort future attacks. In the case of anatomic defects, surgical repair is delayed until the meningitis has been fully treated medically. In the case of hypersensitivity-reaction recurrent meningitis, identification and withholding of the producing drug will prevent further attacks.

Short-Term Prognosis

The short-term prognosis of recurrent meningitis is excellent. Most cases recover within 3 weeks.

Long-Term Prognosis

In general, the long-term prognosis of recurrent meningitis, including that due to herpes simplex virus, is excellent, though relapses frequently occur. In rare exceptions, a poorer long-term prognosis reflects the underlying etiology.

Additional Reading

Anderson NE, Willoughby EW. Chronic meningitis without predisposing illness—a review of 83 cases. Q J Med 1987;63:283–295.

Berger JR. Tuberculous meningitis. Curr Opin Neurol 1994;7:191–200.

Cohen BA, Rowley AH, Long CM. Herpes simplex type 2 in a patient with Mollaret's meningitis: demonstration by polymerase chain reaction. Ann Neurol 1994;35:112–116.

Gripshover BM, Ellner JJ. Chronic Meningitis Syndrome and Meningitis of Noninfective or Uncertain Etiology. In WM Scheld, RJ Whitley, DT Durack (eds), Infections of the Central Nervous System (2nd ed). Philadelphia: Lippincott–Raven, 1997;881–896.

Hopkins AP, Harvey PKP. Chronic benign lymphocytic meningitis. J Neurol Sci 1973;18:443–453.

Katzman M, Ellner JJ. Chronic Meningitis. In GL Mandell, RG Douglas Jr, JE Bennett (eds), Principles and Practice of Infectious Disease (3rd ed). New York: Churchill Livingstone, 1990;755–762.

Perfect JR, Durack DT. Fungal Meningitis. In WM Scheld, RJ Whitley, DT Durack (eds), Infections of the Central Nervous System (2nd ed). Philadelphia: Lippincott–Raven, 1997;721–739.

Smith JE, Aksamit AJ Jr. Outcome of chronic idiopathic meningitis. Mayo Clin Proc 1994;69:548–556.

Tedder DG, Ashley R, Tyler KL, et al. Herpes simplex virus infection as a cause of benign recurrent lymphocytic meningitis. Ann Intern Med 1994;121:334–338.

Chapter 44
Bacterial Meningitis

Burk Jubelt and Stacie L. Ropka

Bacterial meningitis is an acute purulent infection of the cranial and spinal leptomeninges that can cause injury to the brain by a variety of mechanisms. The etiologic agents of bacterial meningitis are a variety of gram-positive and gram-negative bacteria acquired either in the community or nosocomially. Community-acquired bacterial meningitides generally are the result of infection with *Haemophilus influenza* type b, *Streptococcus pneumoniae*, *Neisseria meningitidis*, *Listeria monocytogenes*, and *Streptococci* group B (*Streptococcus agalactiae*). Major causes of nosocomial infection are *Staphylococcus aureus, Staphylococcus epidermidis*, and gram-negative bacteria.

Natural History

Left undiagnosed, bacterial meningitis has a poor prognosis, with mortality rates approaching 100%. Even with chemotherapy, bacterial meningitis remains a significant cause of mortality and morbidity, especially in the young and the elderly. In developed countries, the overall mortality rate has remained steady at 5 to 10% annually. Survivors have a 30 to 40% chance of long-term sequelae. In underdeveloped countries, the mortality rate remains high at 40%, with some reports of up to 67% annually. Sequelae may occur in as many as 60% of survivors.

In the 1970s, investigators realized that *H. influenza* type b was becoming resistant to antibiotic treatment. In certain parts of the United States, up to 50% of *H. influenzae* isolates reportedly exhibit drug resistance. Recent studies in underdeveloped countries have reported drug-resistant strains of pneumococci that have a 50% increase in mortality rates as compared to nonresistant pneumococcal isolates. The emergence of drug-resistant strains suggests that prognosis once again will worsen, with mortality rates increasing. Because of drug resistance, the use of third-generation cephalosporins has become routine in treating bacterial meningitis. Also, in light of new evidence suggesting that the inflammatory response may cause sequelae, steroids, such as dexamethasone, have been added to some treatment regimens.

Epidemiologic studies suggest that age, gender, and underlying immunodeficiencies are predisposing factors for infection. Specific predisposing host factors include age (with young and old at greater risk); gender (with male subjects at greater risk); socioeconomic status (with poor at greater risk); and immunodeficiencies, either genetic (in patients with deficiencies in the last factors of complement) or acquired (in patients that have had splenectomy, acquired immunodeficiency syndrome [AIDS], cancer treatment, organ transplantation). In addition, any situation in which sick people are in close proximity to each other (daycare centers, workplace, shopping malls) carries an increased risk for exposure to bacteria capable of causing meningitis.

In addition to mortality, permanent neuropsychological sequelae may result from infection.

Table 44-1. Prognosis of Specific Bacterial Causes of Meningitis

Organism	Fatality with Treatment (%)	Fatality without Treatment (%)	Sequelae in Survivors[a] (%)
S. pneumoniae	Elderly, 77; children and young adults, 20–60	All age groups, 100	Mostly children, 7
H. influenzae type b	3	95	40 (permanent, 8)
N. meningitidis	13	50–90	Mostly children, 3
Group B streptococcus (*S. agalactiae*)	Neonates, 55; infants, 23; overall, 12	—[b]	—
L. monocytogenes	19–22	Unknown	30
Gram-negative bacilli	17	Unknown	60

[a]Sequelae include developmental delay, hearing loss, motor deficits, epilepsy and seizures, hydrocephalus, and other less frequent neurologic deficits.
[b]With inappropriate antibiotic treatment, fatality increases to more than 50%.

These sequelae include hearing loss, mental retardation, epilepsy, hydrocephalus, seizures, visual impairment, impaired motor skills, cranial nerve palsies, and focal neurologic deficits. These sequelae may be permanent or may improve gradually over months to years after disease resolution (Table 44-1).

Factors Affecting Prognosis

The mortality, severity of infection, and type of sequelae depend on many factors that include early diagnosis and initiation of treatment; age (with a higher mortality rate in neonates and the elderly as compared to children and adults); clinical condition of the patient at initial presentation (with a higher mortality for patients presenting in coma or having focal seizures and an increased risk for sequelae in survivors); and the bacterial strain(s) involved. Although studies have indicated positive correlations between bacterial strain and prognosis, during epidemics more uncommon bacterial strains may be responsible for bacterial meningitis. In addition, geographic differences and year-to-year variations occur in causative bacteria. These aspects must be kept in mind when making a diagnosis, so that appropriate therapy is started as early as possible. Prognosis for specific bacterial agents follows (see Table 44-1).

Streptococcus pneumoniae

In the United States, *S. pneumoniae* causes 1,500 to 2,000 disease cases per year. The majority of cases of bacterial meningitis in the elderly (older than 70 years) also are due to *S. pneumoniae*, with a mortality rate in this age group of up to 77%. *S. pneumoniae* has been associated with 30 to 50% of cases in patients older than 15. It is also the most common cause of bacterial meningitis in adults older than 30. *S. pneumoniae* is responsible for some 10% of bacterial meningitis in children. Overall, *S. pneumoniae* meningitis has the highest fatality rate, with reports of 20 to 60% (untreated, 100%) and the most severe residual neuropsychological deficits in survivors. People with underlying conditions, such as chronic respiratory disease, splenectomy, sickle cell anemia, and alcoholism, are more susceptible to *S. pneumoniae* meningitis.

Haemophilus influenzae

H. influenzae causes 6,000 to 7,000 disease cases of bacterial meningitis per year in the United States. It is the most common cause of bacterial meningitis in children younger than 5 (60% of cases). *H. influenza* type b is responsible for 70% of cases for the 1-month to 4-year-old group. In developed countries, *H. influenza* type b–related bacterial meningitis has a 3% fatality rate; in less developed countries, the fatality rate increases to 20%. However, without appropriate therapy, the mortality rate is 95%. Of survivors, 40% have sequelae, but only 8% experience any severe permanent sequelae. *H. influenza* type b is a biphasic disease with outbreaks in the fall and spring. The effect of the new *H. influenzae* b vaccine on the bacterial strain profile for meningitis has yet to be determined.

Neisseria meningitidis

N. meningitidis is a common cause of bacterial meningitis primarily in children and young adults. Crowding, as in nursery schools, college campuses, and military installations, predisposes to outbreaks of the disease. In the United States, it causes 2,500 to 3,000 cases per year, with a 13% mortality rate. However, during outbreaks, the incidence rate can increase more than fivefold. Without treatment, the mortality rate of *N. meningitidis* meningitis is between 50 to 90%. Patients with underlying complement deficiencies are more susceptible to *N. meningitidis* infections.

Listeria monocytogenes

L. monocytogenes is rare in the general population but is one of the most common causes of bacterial meningitis in neonates. *L. monocytogenes* has become more prevalent in patients infected with the human immunodeficiency virus, occurring 60% more frequently in this population than in the general population. Listeria infections are seen also in other immunosuppressed conditions (e.g., patients treated with immunosuppressive agents, renal disease, cancer, and alcoholism and cirrhosis).

Streptococci Group B (S. agalactiae)

Streptococci group B (*S. agalactiae*) previously was only an important cause of bacterial meningitis in neonates; now it is prevalent in other populations. Though still responsible for 5 to 10% of bacterial meningitis in neonates, adults older than 60 are also at risk. In addition, underlying clinical conditions are important risk factors for meningitis caused by streptococcus group B bacteria, especially immunosuppressive conditions such as diabetes mellitus, AIDS, and immunosuppressive chemotherapy.

Gram-Negative Bacilli

Gram-negative bacilli are the most common cause of bacterial meningitis in the neonate (50 to 60% of cases). In addition, gram-negative bacilli are second only to *S. pneumoniae* as the cause of bacterial meningitis in the elderly. Bacterial meningitis from gram-negative bacilli has a 15 to 20% mortality rate and severe sequelae occur in 60% of survivors.

During the acute phase of bacterial meningitis, a number of complications are to be expected. Appropriate treatment of these short-term complications will have a major impact on the overall prognosis. A common short-term complication is increased intracranial pressure (ICP). Treatment to reduce ICP will reduce the risk of herniation and irreversible brain stem injury. Focal seizures also are fairly common, occurring in as many as 50% of children. Treating these seizures may prevent the development of more general seizures and status epilepticus with its inherent complications and may possibly prevent epilepsy. Accompanying hydrocephalus may occur also and may require shunting to prevent cerebral damage. Bacterial meningitis affects more than just the meninges. Such cerebrovascular complications as vasospasm, vasculitis, thrombosis, brain infarction, spinal cord infarction, aneurysmal formation, and subarachnoid hemorrhage often occur. Studies have reported that almost 7% of bacterial meningitis patients experience one or more of these vascular complications believed to result from the inflammatory angiodestructive process. The syndrome of inappropriate secretion of antidiuretic hormone also must have immediate treatment. Subdural effusion and subdural empyema also may occur, especially in children.

Evaluation for Prognosis

A prompt or early diagnosis allows for the initiation of broad-spectrum antibiotic therapy that correlates with a more favorable prognosis. Once the specific bacterial strain is elucidated, the antibiotic therapy can be tailored specifically. However, the initial diagnosis can be difficult. Certain specific presentations are based on age of the patient, duration of the illness, and the causative bacterial strains. The clinical diagnosis of bacterial meningitis in neonates can be difficult, because the patient presents with nonspecific clinical symptoms, including somnolence, irritability, seizures, respiratory distress, apnea, and poor feeding. Fever usually is present. A bulging fontanelle usually occurs later in the disease. The diagnosis is somewhat easier in children and young adults. Their symptoms include fever, headache, photophobia, and nuchal rigidity, including Kernig and Brudzinski signs. Altered mental status, other than lethargy from exhaustion, usually does not occur in this age group until near the end of the first week of infection. In the elderly, the presentation is more nebulous and includes a combination of fever, altered mental status (confusion to coma), and meningeal signs. Up to 89% of patients older than 50 will present with an altered mental status, which is significantly higher than in younger age groups. In the elderly, the early diagnosis of bacterial meningitis can be masked easily by underlying diseases.

If any of these manifestations of meningitis occur, especially with a suggestive history, a lumbar puncture must be performed. In patients presenting with altered mental status, focal deficits, or papilledema, a computed tomographic scan should be performed before lumbar puncture. The cerebrospinal fluid (CSF) profile usually will be diagnostic. A CSF pleocytosis of more than 10 to less than 10,000 cells per cubic millimeter of polymorphonuclear cells usually is seen. The protein is elevated (>50 mg per deciliter), and the glucose is reduced markedly (<40 mg per deciliter but usually 0 to 20 mg per deciliter). A Gram stain is positive 60 to 90% of the time, depending on the number of bacteria present. The ability to culture organisms from the CSF depends on the collection and storage of the sample (certain of the causative organisms being very susceptible to environmental conditions) and whether antibiotic therapy already has been initiated. Cultures are positive 80% of the time in untreated meningitis when the sample is handled properly. The culture can be positive when all other tests on the CSF are negative.

Therapies Affecting Prognosis

In addition to the timeliness of the institution of both nonspecific broad-spectrum and specific antibiotic therapy, other therapeutic strategies have proved efficacious for long-term prognosis. Owing to the inflammatory nature of bacterial meningitis, the use of corticosteroids in addition to antibiotics can reduce significantly the possibility of severe, permanent deficits in infants and children. One study suggested that dexamethasone can reduce the risk of neurologic or audiologic sequelae from 16% (placebo group) to 5% (dexamethasone group). The treatment and rapid resolution of acute complications (increased ICP, seizures, hydrocephalus, syndrome of inappropriate secretion of antidiuretic hormone, subdural effusion, subdural empyema) are of great import for prognosis.

Short-Term Prognosis

In the short term (days to several weeks), the outcome depends on rapid diagnosis and early treatment. Without early treatment, such complications as seizures, increased ICP, hydrocephalus, and vascular accidents are more likely to occur, resulting in greater morbidity and mortality. Seizures can occur within the first few days and for up to 6 months. They should be treated with standard anticonvulsants. A positive correlation is seen between focal seizures during the acute infection and long-term neurologic deficits.

Other short-term sequelae include hearing loss, motor deficits, and other neurologic deficits. In the majority of patients, barring the aforementioned complications and with appropriate antibiotic treatment, these sequelae will resolve in 6 to 9 months after infection.

Long-Term Prognosis

Long-term prognosis depends on residual deficits from the acute infection and from late complications. Major residual deficits include IQ of less than 70, seizures, spasticity, blindness, and profound hearing loss. Less severe deficits include IQ of 70 to 80, inability to read, mild to moderate hearing loss, abnormalities in speech discrimination, and school behavior problems.

Cognitive deficits are a frequent residual of bacterial meningitis. In one study of school-age children 6 to 7 years after recovery from bacterial meningitis, 25% had one or more deficits in fine-motor skills, IQ, school behavior, neuropsychological function, or auditory response. In addition, children with acute neurologic complications were at a greater risk for long-term sequelae.

Late complications include both obstructive and communicating hydrocephalus, late seizures, and increasing spasticity. Patients should be followed closely for several years after infection so as to formulate diagnosis of these complications and to institute prompt, appropriate therapy.

Additional Reading

Durand ML, Calderwood SB, Weber DJ, et al. Acute bacterial meningitis in adults. N Engl J Med 1993;328:21–28.

Grimwood K, Anderson VA, Bond L, et al. Adverse outcomes of bacterial meningitis in school-age survivors. Pediatrics 1995;95:646–656.

Jubelt B, Ropka SL. Infectious Diseases of the Nervous System. In RN Rosenberg (ed), Atlas of Clinical Neurology. Philadelphia: Current Medicine, 1998.

Loughlin AM, Marchant CD, Lett SM. The changing epidemiology of invasive bacterial infections in Massachusetts children, 1984 through 1991. Am J Public Health 1995;85:392–394.

Pomeroy SL, Holmes SJ, Dodge PR, Feigin RD. Seizures and other neurologic sequelae of bacterial meningitis in children. N Engl J Med 1990;323:1651–1657.

Roos KL. Meningitis as it presents in the elderly: diagnosis and care. Geriatrics 1990;45:63–75.

Schaad UB, Lips U, Gnehm HE, et al. Dexamethasone therapy for bacterial meningitis in children. Lancet 1993; 342:457–461.

Shattuck KE, Chonmaitree T. The changing spectrum of neonatal meningitis over a fifteen-year period. Clin Pediatr (Phila) 1992;31:130–136.

Unhanand M, Mustafa MM, McCracken GH, Nelson JD. Gram-negative enteric bacillary meningitis: a twenty-one-year experience. J Pediatr (Phila) 1993;122:15–21.

Wilfert CM. Epidemiology of *Haemophilus influenzae* type b infections. Pediatrics 1990;85:631–635.

Chapter 45

Lyme Disease of the Nervous System

John J. Halperin

For both biological and sociologic reasons, Lyme disease has been the subject of a great deal of controversy. The term was first coined in 1977 to describe a newly recognized syndrome that resembled juvenile rheumatoid arthritis occurring in Lyme, Connecticut. Now known is that this infectious disease is caused by the tick-borne spirochete, *Borrelia burgdorferi*. After inoculation with the organism, infection may remain localized, causing a pathognomonic, subacutely evolving rash known as *erythema migrans*, or may disseminate throughout the body, causing multisystem involvement. Despite frequent reference to the protean manifestations of this disease—suggesting that it can cause almost any phenomenon known to medicine—in fact, it generally follows one of several specific patterns, with involvement of joints, heart, and the nervous system being particularly common. Moreover, although it has been described popularly as a novel disease with which medicine has only limited experience, erythema migrans first was described early in this century, and the classic neurologic syndrome was first reported in the French literature 75 years ago. Although the responsible organism was identified only in 1982, the European literature throughout this century has described the clinical syndrome extensively as defined by a discrete set of neurologic phenomena occurring in patients with histories of bites by hard-shelled *Ixodes* ticks or as erythema migrans. In fact, in the 1922 description of the neurologic syndrome, Garin and Bujadoux proposed that the disease was caused by a spirochetal infection and, as early as the 1950s, European authorities recognized that symptoms improved with antimicrobial therapy.

The reasons for the controversies regarding this disease are complex. In large part, this situation can be attributed to difficulty in diagnosis. Particularly, the bias that diagnoses can be legitimate only if confirmed by laboratory tests has fostered a tendency to discount the clinical literature that predates the development of confirmatory laboratory techniques. Laboratory testing remains imperfect, constrained by several limitations peculiar to this infection and by others common to all serologic tests. The absence of laboratory tests with 100% sensitivity and specificity has permitted the dissemination of ideas that are at best irrational, giving rise to a sense that the prognosis of this disease can be extremely poor.

Its limitations notwithstanding, immunodiagnosis is the principle laboratory tool available for confirming the diagnosis. Particularly useful has been the detection of intrathecal production of anti–*B. burgdorferi* antibodies, a finding present in more than 90% of patients with acute central nervous system (CNS) infection. If false positives due to other spirochetal infections, such as neurosyphilis, can be eliminated, specificity of this technique is greater than 95%. Its only shortcoming is that apparent positivity may persist for years after adequate treatment, rendering it unreliable as a measure of treatment success or failure.

Natural History

As in all infectious diseases, severity of illness varies widely. Initial infection requires prolonged attach-

251

ment (longer than 24 to 48 hours) by an infected tick. Following such a bite, some individuals will not become infected, others will develop localized infection, and others will develop disseminated involvement. This variability is related to several factors. First, the *Borrelia* spirochete strains vary considerably. In Europe, two major subspecies of *B. burgdorferi* have been identified: *B. garinii,* which typically causes nervous system invasion, and *B. afzelii*, which is associated more consistently with dermatologic manifestations. In North America, only one subspecies occurs commonly: *B. burgdorferi sensu stricto*. However, multiple strains have been recognized, with varying pathogenic capabilities. Second, differences in host immunity presumably also contribute to disease severity. Patients with particular human leukocyte antigen phenotypes appear to be at increased risk of developing persistent rheumatologic difficulties; corresponding data regarding neurologic problems are inconsistent. Prior specific immune stimulation also may be a factor. One vaccine study in an animal model suggested that previously immunized hosts who then are re-exposed to particular strains of *B. burgdorferi* are at very high risk of developing arthritis. Finally, in some individuals, coinfection by other tick-borne pathogens (e.g., *Babesia* spp., *Ehrlichia* spp., tick-borne encephalitis virus) can lead to more severe disease.

After initial infection, disease may remain localized as an erythema migrans, or it may become disseminated. In this acute phase of the illness, dissemination tends to produce very specific syndromes. Patients may develop a multifocal erythema migrans, cardiac conduction abnormalities, lymphocytic meningitis, cranial neuropathies (particularly cranial nerve VII paralysis, which may be bilateral), or painful radiculoneuritis (first described in the European literature) consisting of radicular pain and weakness with a lymphocytic pleocytosis. All these syndromes tend to resolve spontaneously, although antimicrobial therapy tends to lead to more rapid recovery.

After resolution of the acute disseminated infection, in some patients organisms may be eliminated completely. In others, late forms of involvement may develop. Early, effective antimicrobial therapy clearly lessens the likelihood of development of these late manifestations. Other than this, the reasons that some individuals specifically are predisposed to develop particular late sequelae are not clear.

Chronic, persistent infection involves primarily the joints and the nervous system. A chronic, relapsing large-joint oligoarthritis was the late syndrome that first led to the recognition of Lyme arthritis. In the peripheral nervous system, a chronic, relatively mild mononeuropathy multiplex is the most common form of involvement. In the CNS, either focal brain or spinal cord inflammation (encephalomyelitis) or an encephalopathy are the typical manifestations. Although all these syndromes also usually improve with antimicrobial therapy, response may be less complete.

Factors Affecting Prognosis

A surprisingly limited amount of information is available concerning factors affecting prognosis, owing both to inaccurate diagnosis caused by the limitations in diagnostic technology and to the rather small number of good prospective, longitudinal epidemiologic studies. Much of the popular conception of the prognosis of Lyme disease actually relates to two (probably spurious) bodies of anecdotal data. The first consists of patients who have positive serologies and (typically) neuropsychiatric syndromes and who do not respond to what, in other circumstances, usually are curative antimicrobial regimens. The second includes patients who have negative serologic testing and nonspecific syndromes that have, on occasion, been linked to Lyme disease. Possibly in these patients, a diagnosis of Lyme disease has been made by process of elimination, other likely diagnoses having been eliminated and testing for Lyme being thought to be unreliable; these patients similarly fail to respond to appropriate treatment. The description of numerous such individuals, coupled with occasional true treatment failures, has led to the widespread notion that the prognosis of this infection can be very poor.

Epidemiologic studies have been limited. Some, looking at small, relatively closed populations at high risk of contracting Lyme disease, have provided valuable insights into disease incidence but have been too small to address issues of treatment response and development of infrequent, late-occurring disease manifestations. Other studies assessing treatment regimens have demonstrated successful treatment in some 90% of patients, with both early and chronic manifestations. However, most such treatment studies have had significant referral biases and limited long-term follow-up. Similarly, studies based on analysis of cerebrospinal fluid (CSF) samples are skewed toward patients who are likely to undergo lumbar puncture.

Probably the best studies have focused on pediatric populations. As many children see a pediatrician on a regular basis, longitudinal assessment of this population is possible without a referral bias. Such studies have demonstrated that early Lyme infection is diagnosed readily and treatment is virtually invariably successful. Again, to date, these studies have been too small to address issues related to more chronic and infrequently occurring forms of involvement.

Therapy Affecting Prognosis

A rational discussion of the outlook of this disease must start by examining only information concerning individuals in whom the diagnosis is clear-cut. Although undoubtedly the classic syndromes are not present in some patients, likely the therapeutic response should be no worse in individuals with a milder syndrome than in those with an infection sufficiently severe as to cause, for example, an encephalomyelitis.

Nonneurologic Manifestations

Several distinct syndromes have been identified as clearly caused by *B. burgdorferi* infection. Most respond well to antimicrobial therapy. Early in the infection, heart block may occur in up to 5% of patients and, although a temporary pacemaker may be required, almost invariably these patients respond well to antimicrobial therapy. Generally, Lyme arthritis also responds well to antibiotic treatment, except for a subgroup of individuals who develop persistent joint problems. The poor rheumatologic prognosis for these patients appears to be due to one of two factors. In some individuals, Lyme arthritis causes so much mechanical joint destruction that simply eradicating the infection cannot return joint function to normal. In others, apparently predisposed by HLA subtype, a persistent relapsing remitting arthritis continues, often

despite what typically would be curative antimicrobial therapy. These models well may prove instructive in assessing the prognosis in nervous system Lyme disease.

Neuroborreliosis

Neuroborreliosis can take one of several forms, and prognosis varies with the presenting syndrome. The disease can affect the peripheral nervous system, the CNS, or both. The most typical form is that first described 75 years ago: Early in the infection, the patient develops a *lymphocytic meningitis with or without a polyradicular syndrome* that typically is painful, with a significant but segmental motor deficit. Often evidence of a mild segmental myelopathy at the affected level is superimposed. In some patients, cranial nerves may be involved as well. Patients may have all or any component of this syndrome. In those with cranial neuropathies, approximately 90 to 95% will have complete resolution of their deficit. The lymphocytic meningitis almost always resolves with or without antimicrobial therapy. The radicular pain typically resolves over the course of several weeks although, with antimicrobial therapy, resolution may be more rapid. Some reports have suggested that corticosteroids used in conjunction with antibiotics may further speed recovery. The largest Danish prospective study of such patients reported that of 185 patients with neuroborreliosis evaluated on average 33 months after antibiotic treatment, 14 had persistent sensory symptoms, and 3 of the 14 still had significant pain. Only 10 of the 185 were unable to resume their previous activities, primarily because of residua of neuroborreliosis.

Other patients may develop a *peripheral neuropathy*, typically a mononeuropathy multiplex. Biopsies have demonstrated a vasculopathy with perivascular inflammatory infiltrates but without vessel-wall necrosis. Demyelination is relatively uncommon. If abnormal at all, CSF generally demonstrates a low-grade pleocytosis. Once the infection is treated, recovery generally is excellent. In one prospective study of 12 patients evaluated neurophysiologically before and after therapy, all improved clinically, and 11 of the 12 demonstrated significant neurophysiologic improvement.

Far more severe (but quite rare) is a focal encephalomyelitis. Patients with this disorder (probably occurring in approximately 1 in 1,000 infected, untreated patients) typically have focal CNS signs and significant abnormalities on brain or spinal cord magnetic resonance imaging (MRI) scans. A myelopathy tends to be particularly common. Clinically, such individuals can be confused with patients with a first episode of multiple sclerosis. As Lyme disease presumably does not protect patients from multiple sclerosis, in highly endemic areas a significant percentage of multiple sclerosis patients would be expected to have serologic evidence of exposure to *B. burgdorferi*, leading to potential misdiagnosis. However, if serum and CSF anti–*B. burgdorferi* antibodies are measured and compared appropriately and intrathecal production of anti–*B. burgdorferi* antibodies clearly is evident, a diagnosis of neuroborreliosis is fairly likely. In such patients, studies from the United States suggest that aggressive antimicrobial therapy usually will arrest progression of the disease, effecting a microbiological cure. However, as with patients with severe arthritis, those who have sustained significant CNS damage may have persistent symptoms referable to focal damage. European studies have been less positive, with significant numbers of patients continuing to deteriorate, although generally the antimicrobial regimens used have been less aggressive.

The most confusing group of patients in whom to assess prognosis consists of individuals with altered cognitive function. Such patients appear to fall into several subgroups. This disorder initially was identified in individuals with evidence of systemic Lyme disease—arthritis, carditis, peripheral neuropathy, constitutional symptoms—but no focal CNS abnormalities. In these individuals, brain MRI scans and CSF analysis usually were normal, although formal neuropsychologic testing typically confirmed the patients' subjective perception of difficulty with memory and cognitive limitations. In these individuals, the alteration of cognitive function likely represents a lymphokine-mediated "toxic metabolic" encephalopathy. Treatment of the non-CNS manifestations is successful in the vast majority of patients, and the altered cognitive function almost invariably resolves in parallel with the resolution of the non-CNS disease. A second group has similar cognitive difficulties but typically has (rela-tively minor) abnormalities on brain MRI and has mild CSF abnormalities, with a mild pleocytosis, minor increase in CSF protein, or intrathecal antibody production. In these individuals, the encephalopathy is likely due to a mild form of encephalomyelitis, and more aggressive antimicrobial therapy may be necessary.

In individuals with encephalopathy, recovery is to be expected. However, as in patients with more dramatic encephalomyelitis, some residua may persist. Generally, serial neuropsychologic studies of such patients have demonstrated excellent responses to antimicrobial therapy. One retrospective European study of 20 patients treated for Lyme meningoradiculitis revealed that all had some persistent cognitive difficulty several years after treatment. Antimicrobial regimens used in these patients generally were less aggressive than were those commonly used in the United States; whether these cognitive difficulties would be prevented by, or respond to, additional antimicrobial therapy has not yet been addressed. Finally, one U.S. study indicated that (1) a high proportion of patients treated for neuroborreliosis continue to describe persistent memory and cognitive difficulties, and (2) a significant percentage of treated patients have persistent deficits demonstrable on neuropsychologic testing. However, no statistically meaningful relationship was reported between the persistent symptoms and the persistent objective deficits, rendering the interpretation of chronic symptoms in such patients very difficult.

Short-Term Prognosis

Generally, the prognosis of Lyme disease is excellent, as the responsible spirochete is highly susceptible to commonly available antibiotics. Although the nervous system can be affected in a variety of ways and with a broad spectrum of severity, response to appropriate therapy usually is excellent. If treatment occurs early before significant tissue damage has occurred, cure is obtained in 90 to 95% of individuals.

Early in the infection, patients may have a variety of neurologic manifestations, including lymphocytic meningitis, cranial neuropathies, and painful radiculoneuropathies. All will resolve spontaneously in the vast majority of patients. With appropriate antimicrobial therapy, cranial neuropathies will resolve rapidly in 90 to 95% of patients and radiculoneuropathies in more than 90% (although some symptoms may persist, owing to persistent damage to affected nerves). The meningitis similarly resolves with or without treatment in the vast majority of patients. In general, full clinical response occurs over several months after effective therapy.

Long-Term Prognosis

The long-term prognosis for treated, infected individuals generally is excellent. If treatment delay leads to significant structural damage to nerves or the CNS, long-term sequelae may persist despite microbiological cure. A small percentage of patients may have persistent infection or persistent aberrant immune stimulation, leading to ongoing disease. The best approach to these few individuals, and their long-term prognosis, remain to be determined.

Additional Reading

Hansen K, Lebech A-M. The clinical and epidemiological profile of Lyme neuroborreliosis in Denmark 1985–1990. Brain 1992;115:399–423.

Lyme neuroborreliosis. Semin Neurol 1997;17.

Chapter 46

Neurocysticercosis

Oscar H. Del Brutto

Neurocysticercosis—defined as the infection of the central nervous system by the larval stage of *Taenia solium*, the pork tapeworm—is a rather common neurologic disorder in several areas of the world, including developing countries and industrialized nations with a high rate of immigrant population from disease-endemic areas. Clinical manifestations of neurocysticercosis are protean. This clinical pleomorphism is related to individual variations in the number and topography of lesions and to differences in the severity of the host's immune response against the parasites. Seizures, increased intracranial pressure, intellectual deterioration, and focal neurologic deficits, the most common clinical forms of presentation of neurocysticercosis, may be observed also in many other infectious and noninfectious diseases of the nervous system and do not permit the correct diagnosis without the aid of neuroimaging studies or specific immunologic diagnostic tests.

Natural History

From the moment a cysticercus invades the nervous system, it is exposed to a hostile environment. Should the host's immune system recognize the parasite as foreign, an appropriate reaction could be mounted to overcome the infection. However, in many patients this reaction develops slowly, and cysticerci live unchanged for many years. On the other hand, some cysticerci are rejected acutely after entering the nervous system. In those cases, the infection is eliminated, but the tissues of the host may be damaged as the result of this enhanced state of responsiveness. Between the extremes of immune tolerance and hypersensitivity exists a wide range of inflammatory changes and neuropathologic lesions induced by this complex host-parasite relationship. The severity of disease expression, and hence its prognosis, is related partly to the degree of inflammation around cysticerci.

Pathologic studies have shown four different stages of development and destruction of parenchymal brain cysticerci. Each stage correlates with distinctive histologic changes in the surrounding brain parenchyma, with characteristic findings on neuroimaging studies and, sometimes, with particular clinical manifestations. In addition, cysticerci located within the ventricular system or in the cerebrospinal fluid (CSF) cisterns at the base of the brain cause symptoms owing not only to the host's immune reaction but to the cysticerci's size, as they may grow enough to produce mass effect displacing neighboring structures or may block the CSF transit, causing hydrocephalus (Table 46-1).

Factors Affecting Prognosis

Host Age and Gender

Though neurocysticercosis affects men and women equally and from birth to senescence, the patient's gender and age have significant bearing on the outcome. In general terms, the disease in

Table 46-1. Pathologic Changes in the Nervous System, Neuroimaging Findings, and Clinical Manifestations, According to the Location and Stage of Development of Cerebral Cysticerci

Location and Stage	Parasite Appearance	Pathologic CNS Changes	Neuroimaging Findings	Usual Clinical Manifestations
Brain parenchyma				
Vesicular cysts	Translucent vesicular wall and fluid; viable scolex	Scarce inflammation in surrounding brain	Hypodense cystic lesions; no edema or enhancement	Seizures; possibly asymptomatic
Colloidal cysts	Thick vesicular wall; turbid fluid; degenerated scolex	Intense inflammatory reaction; thick collagen capsule around cyst	Hypodense, ring-enhancing lesions; marked edema	Seizures; headache; vomiting; focal signs
Granulomas, calcifications	Mineralized nodules; no scolex	Intense gliosis; giant cells	Hyperdense lesions; little or no enhancement	Recurrent seizures
Subarachnoid space				
Giant cysts in CSF cisterns	Racemose cysts; no scolex	Focal arachnoiditis; vasculitis; cerebral infarction	Multilobulated hypodense lesions; cerebral infarction	Seizures; intracranial hypertension; focal signs
Diffuse arachnoiditis	Hyalinized parasitic membranes	Hydrocephalus; fibrous arachnoiditis; cranial nerve damage	Hydrocephalus; abnormal enhancement of basal meninges	Focal signs; intracranial hypertension
Ventricular system				
Ventricular cysts	Translucent vesicular wall and fluid; viable scolex	Obstruction of Monro's foramina or cerebral aqueduct	Asymmetric hydrocephalus; cysts possibly visualized	Focal signs; intracranial hypertension
Ependymitis	Turbid fluid and thick vesicular wall	Inflammation of the ependymal lining	Enhancement of ventricular walls; hydrocephalus	Seizures; intracranial hypertension; focal signs

CNS = central nervous system; CSF = cerebrospinal fluid.

children usually runs a benign course and is characterized mostly by seizures that are easily controlled with standard antiepileptic medication. This benign course is related to the fact that children usually develop a single parenchymal brain cysticercosis and that hydrocephalus or ventricular cysts are rare. In contrast, neurocysticercosis in adults frequently is associated with multiple lesions, hydrocephalus, fibrous arachnoiditis, or ventricular cysts; as expected, mixed forms of the disease carry a worse prognosis than do pure, parenchymal forms. Paradoxically, the rare cysticercotic encephalitis—one of the most severe forms of neurocysticercosis—is more common in children than in adults. These cases are related to an enhanced state of responsiveness of the immune system against massive cysticerci infection of the brain parenchyma.

Some studies indicate that neurocysticercosis is more severe in women than in men, independent of the form of the disease. Indeed, cysticercotic encephalitis is seven times more frequent in young women than in men, and the prognosis of hydrocephalus due to cysticercotic arachnoiditis is worst in women. Such differences could be related to the fact that, in general terms, the immune system of women usually reacts to a greater degree than does that of men. Commonly, one can observe men who have multiple parenchymal brain cysts in the vesicular stage and present with mild symptoms that do not correlate with the burden of infection. In contrast, women with few cysts usually develop recurrent seizures, headache, and vomiting, owing to the edema that surrounds colloidal cysticerci. Multiple vesicular cysts on neuroimaging studies in women are uncommon.

Location and Number of Lesions

Together with the degree of the immune response, the location and number of lesions within the nervous system are main determinants in the prognosis of neurocysticercosis. With the possible exception of patients with cysticercotic encephalitis, the prognosis of parenchymal brain cysticercosis usually is good; most patients present with seizures that may be controlled easily with appropriate therapy. In contrast, patients with extra-parenchymal disease usually have protracted courses and a poor prognosis. Hydrocephalus secondary to cysticercotic arachnoiditis is associated with a 50% mortality rate at 2 years, and most survivors are left with irreversible sequelae. Giant subarachnoid cysticerci may induce inflammatory changes in the wall of blood vessels arising from the circle of Willis, with the subsequent development of a cerebral infarction. The same vasculitic changes are seen in patients with diffuse cysticercotic arachnoiditis; this form of the disease is associated also with entrapment and irreversible damage of cranial nerves at the base of the skull, producing diplopia, trigeminal neuralgia, and visual field defects. Ventricular cysticerci have been associated with recurrent episodes of loss of consciousness or even with sudden death due to acute hydrocephalus. Finally, cysticercosis of the spinal cord may cause severe root pain, motor weakness and sensory disturbances below the level of the lesion in a way similar to that observed in patients with other kinds of intramedullary or extramedullary tumors.

Parenchymal Brain Calcifications

The transformation of parenchymal brain cysts into calcifications is the most important risk factor associated with seizure recurrence after the withdrawal of antiepileptic drugs (AEDs) in patients with neurocysticercosis. Though the administration of standard doses of AEDs usually produces adequate control of seizures, recent studies have shown that up to 90% of patients have a relapse after AED withdrawal, even though they had remained free of seizures for 2 years as the result of therapy. This high risk of seizure recurrence is independent of other factors, such as the age of the patient, the type of seizures (generalized, simple partial, complex partial), or the

number of seizures before diagnosis. In some patients who have a relapse, neuroimaging studies performed immediately after the seizure have shown focal edema and abnormal uptake of contrast material around previously inert calcifications. These changes are related to a breakdown in the blood-brain barrier surrounding an epileptogenic focus (as has been demonstrated in patients with epilepsy due to other causes) and suggest that parenchymal brain calcifications actually represent permanent epileptogenic foci that may be reactivated when the inhibitory influence of an AED is withdrawn.

Evaluation for Prognosis

A proper classification of neurocysticercosis in terms of disease activity and location of lesions is essential for assessing the severity and the prognosis of the disease. Neuroimaging studies are highly valuable in this setting, as they provide accurate data on the number and topography of the lesions and on the degree of the inflammatory response around cysticerci. For patients with seizures, particular attention must be placed on the presence of parenchymal brain calcifications because, as was noted in the previous paragraph, they represent the most important risk factor associated with seizure recurrence after AED withdrawal. Magnetic resonance imaging is not as sensitive as computed tomography (CT) scan for the detection of small calcifications; therefore, every epileptic patient in whom the diagnosis of neurocysticercosis is suspected must undergo a CT. Immunologic tests have their role in the diagnosis of neurocysticercosis; however, every study attempting to correlate the positivity of such reactions with the severity of the disease or its prognosis has given disappointing results. Finally, cytochemical analysis of CSF can confirm the presence of cysticercotic arachnoiditis and can follow up the response to therapy.

Therapies Affecting Prognosis

Cysticidal Drugs

The introduction of two potent cysticidal drugs, praziquantel and albendazole, has changed the prognosis of neurocysticercosis. However, as the efficacy of these drugs was evaluated initially by counting the percentage of cyst destruction on CT scan, some have argued that these drugs improve only the CT scan without modifying the course of the disease. Recent studies have focused on the clinical outcome of the patients after therapy. In such studies, the control of seizures in patients with parenchymal brain cysts was better after a course of cysticidal drugs than when the cysts were left untreated (83% versus 26%; p <0.001). Moreover, the chance of remaining seizure-free after the withdrawal of AEDs seemed greater in those patients who previously were treated with cysticidal drugs. Other beneficial effects of cysticidal drugs include clinical improvement in focal neurologic deficits and normalization of the cellular immune function that most patients experience after therapy. Such studies have provided rational arguments favoring the use of cysticidal drugs in patients with viable parenchymal brain or subarachnoid cysticerci.

New Therapeutic Strategies for Hydrocephalus

The main problem negatively influencing prognosis for patients with hydrocephalus due to cysticercotic arachnoiditis is the high prevalence of shunt dysfunction. Indeed, these patients commonly can have two or more shunt changes or revisions during their lives, and their mortality has been related directly to the number of surgical interventions to change the shunt. A recent controlled study demonstrated that continued administration of prednisone for up to 2 years reduced the risk of subsequent shunt dysfunction from 60 to 13%. Prednisone was highly effective and was tolerated well in this setting, appearing as a promising drug for the management of this form of neurocysticercosis.

In addition, a new shunt device functioning at a constant flow without a valve mechanism has been developed to treat patients with hydrocephalus due to cysticercotic arachnoiditis. This shunt does not allow the entrance of spinal CSF into the ventricular system toward the shunt device. The inversion of CSF transit is one of the most common causes of shunt dysfunction, as it allows the entrance of subarachnoid inflammatory cells and parasitic debris within the ventricular cavities. In a preliminary report, 25 of 26 patients (96%) who had hydrocephalus due to cysticercotic arachnoiditis and in whom the new shunt was implanted had a functional shunt after a mean follow-up of 9 months.

Short- and Long-Term Prognosis

The short- and long-term prognosis of neurocysticercosis is not uniform and relies on the form of presentation and the occurrence of reinfections. Reinfection plays a major role, as some patients initially presenting with a relatively benign form of the disease may be evaluated several months or years later because of severe disease. Patients with cysticercotic encephalitis have a high mortality rate during the acute phase of the disease; in contrast, those who survive the acute episode recover almost completely. The same prognosis applies to patients with fourth-ventricle cysticerci, as they may die as the result of acute hydrocephalus but tend to recover completely after the cyst has been resected by surgery. In contrast, patients with hydrocephalus due to cysticercotic arachnoiditis usually have a poor long-term prognosis, owing to the frequent need of shunt revisions. In such cases, infection of the shunt device is another factor adding significant morbidity and mortality. The long-term prognosis for patients with epilepsy due to parenchymal brain calcifications or granulomas has not been settled, as possibly most such patients need prolonged therapy with AED.

Additional Reading

Del Brutto OH. Prognostic factors for seizure recurrence after withdrawal of antiepileptic drugs in patients with neurocysticercosis. Neurology 1994;44:1706–1709.

Del Brutto OH. Single parenchymal brain cysticerci in the acute encephalitic phase: definition of a distinct form of neurocysticercosis with a benign prognosis. J Neurol Neurosurg Psychiatry 1995;58:247–249.

Del Brutto OH, Santibañez R, Noboa CA, et al. Epilepsy due to neurocysticercosis: analysis of 203 patients. Neurology 1992;42:389–392.

Mitchell WG, Crawford TO. Intraparenchymal cerebral cysticercosis in children: diagnosis and treatment. Pediatrics 1988;82:76–82.

Rolfs A, Muhlschlegel F, Jansen-Rosseck R, et al. Clinical and immunologic follow-up study of patients with neurocysticercosis after treatment with praziquantel. Neurology 1995;45:532–538.

Roman RAS, Soto-Hernández JL, Sotelo J. Effects of prednisone on ventriculoperitoneal shunt function in hydrocephalus secondary to cysticercosis: a preliminary study. J Neurosurg 1996;84:629–633.

Sotelo J. Neurocysticercosis, Clinical, Prognostic and Therapeutic Aspects. In C Rose (ed), Recent Advances in Tropical Neurology. New York: Elsevier, 1995;87–97.

Sotelo J, Rubalcaba MA, Gomez-Llata S. A new shunt for hydrocephalus that relies on CSF production rather than on ventricular pressure: initial clinical experience. Surg Neurol 1995;43:324–332.

Vazquez V, Sotelo J. The course of seizures after treatment for cerebral cysticercosis. N Engl J Med 1992;327: 696–701.

Chapter 47

Creutzfeldt-Jakob Disease

Eugene C. Lai

Creutzfeldt-Jakob disease (CJD), also known as *human spongiform encephalopathy*, is a rare central nervous system disorder characterized by a relentlessly progressive course and an invariably fatal outcome. The disease occurs in adults throughout the world, with an annual incidence of 0.5 to 2.0 cases per 1 million population. Sporadic CJD constitutes most cases. Its exact etiology is unknown but has been hypothesized to involve a somatic mutation of the prion gene that causes a spontaneous conformational conversion of the normal host prion protein to an abnormal form. Some 5 to 15% of the cases, according to various reports, are familial and may arise from a germline mutation of the prion protein gene. The disease also is transmissible, as demonstrated in cases of iatrogenic CJD, but a traditional infectious agent never has been found. In addition, a new variant of CJD recently was identified in a small group of patients in Europe. Possibly a causal relationship exists with the bovine spongiform encephalopathy agent that affects cattle and is transmissible among animals. At this time, diagnosis of the disorder can be confirmed only by finding the typical spongiform vacuolar changes in brain tissue, particularly in the cerebral cortex.

Natural History

Sporadic CJD usually afflicts people in their late middle age, but the range can extend from 16 to 82 years (median, 60 years). Gender apparently produces no difference. Its initial clinical manifestations may be variable and confusing in the early stages of the disease. Memory decline, personality changes, and gait imbalance are the more common symptoms. Approximately one-third of patients present with mental deterioration that includes memory loss, behavioral abnormalities, and confusion; another one-third of patients have only physical complaints, most often cerebellar ataxia or visual disturbance; and the final one-third of patients have a mixture of both mental and physical symptoms. More than one-fourth of the patients report prodromal symptoms consisting of fatigue, disturbance of sleep patterns, appetite change, anxiety, or weight loss that may last for several weeks.

As a rule, the disease progresses rapidly, and symptoms advance within weeks. Memory decline usually progresses to profound and global intellectual deficits, often with prominent grasp, glabellar, palmomental, and snout reflexes. Such movement disorders as ataxia, tremor, dysarthria, bradykinesia, rigidity, or choreoathetoid movements may become pronounced. Myoclonus, often provoked by sensory stimuli or startle, usually appears in midcourse and is especially characteristic of the disease. Pyramidal tract involvement also is common, as manifested by hyperreflexia, extensor plantar reflexes, and clonus. Visual complaints include hallucinations, diplopia, dimming or blurring of vision, and visual distortions that may evolve into cortical blindness. The patient continues to deteriorate to mutism, complete helplessness, and a vegetative existence.

Factors Affecting Prognosis

Overall prognosis is poor, with severe mental deterioration occurring within 6 months of symptom onset. The patient becomes progressively incapacitated and incapable of self-care. Sporadic CJD typically ends in death from infections, dehydration, or starvation within 2 to 12 months. Only perhaps 4 to 5% of patients have clinical courses of more than 2 years. One study of 232 neuropathologically verified sporadic CJD cases reported that the mean duration of illness was 8 to 11 months (range, 1 to 130 months; median, 4.5 months). The recently identified variant CJD has a younger age of onset and death (median, 29 years) and a more prolonged disease duration (median, 12 months).

Although the literature contains many reports of clinical and pathologic manifestations of CJD, prognosis of the disease seldom is elaborated. The comments that follow are derived from available published information and my experience in caring for autopsy-proved cases of sporadic CJD over the last 10 years. This series consisted of patients whose ages ranged from 48 to 72 years and whose illness duration varied from 2.5 months to 5 years. Age, underlying systemic illnesses, mental status, and ability to swallow and control oral secretions are factors affecting prognosis.

The annual United States incidence of sporadic CJD in the 70- to 74-year age group is 1 per 167,000 population. The older patients apparently have a more rapid demise. Typically, they develop severe lethargy sooner; possibly, older and atrophic brains are more vulnerable to additional damage. These patients also are more likely to be triaged early and are apt not to receive aggressive treatment intervention.

Patients with systemic illnesses, such as hypertension, diabetes mellitus, and coronary artery disease, usually do not survive as long as do otherwise physically healthy patients. One reason for this finding may be that toward the more advanced stage of the disease, patients will not be able to take their medications orally and their systemic diseases will not be treated adequately.

Patients may become very agitated and aggressive, requiring heavy sedation. Often, they become progressively obtunded and incapacitated from either the disease itself or from sedative and antipsychotic medications. They then are more likely to develop aspiration pneumonia and other systemic infections, leading to a rapid demise.

Inability to swallow or control saliva quickly will cause such complications as aspiration, dehydration, or starvation. Often these conditions are not treated when the diagnosis of CJD is reasonably certain. Even with treatment, these disorders ultimately will cause death.

Therapies Affecting Prognosis

No known cure or effective treatment exists. One of my patients, a healthy 48-year-old woman, lived 5 years after the onset of symptoms because a percutaneous endoscopic gastrostomy was performed early. The family decided to feed her and keep her comfortable while withholding all other medical interventions. She was comatose for 4 years but, because of good home care, never developed an infection. Eventually, feeding was stopped, and she died 2 weeks later. Decisions to provide or withhold medications and feeding to the patient have a direct bearing on the duration of survival but not on quality of survival or function.

Short-Term Prognosis

The course of sporadic CJD is relentlessly progressive. Half of patients die within 5 months of symptom onset. Patients who have prodromal symptoms and are still cooperative by examination deteriorate more slowly and survive longer than do those who are agitated or obtunded. A steady progression to global dementia and physical incapacity within weeks to months is inevitable. Hospice care either at home or in an institution can provide comfort and support to the terminal patient and the family.

Long-Term Prognosis

Long-term survival is dismal. Younger and healthy patients who initially have a very gradual onset of symptoms, typically only personality changes, may survive longer. In one report, 9 of 232 patients (4%) with sporadic CJD had illness longer than 2 years (range, 2.5 to 4.5 years).

Additional Reading

Brown P. Transmissible Human Spongiform Encephalopathy (Infectious Cerebral Amyloidosis): Creutzfeldt-Jakob Disease, Gerstmann-Sträussler-Scheninker Syndrome, and Kuru. In DB Calne (ed), Neurodegenerative Diseases. Philadelphia: Saunders, 1994;839–876.

Brown P, Gibbs CJ, Rodgers-Johnson P, et al. Human spongiform encephalopathy: the National Institute of Health series of 300 cases of experimentally transmitted disease. Ann Neurol 1994;35:513–529.

Davanipour Z, Alter M, Sobel E. Creutzfeldt-Jakob disease. Neurol Clin 986;4:415–426.

Epstein LG, Brown P. Bovine spongiform encephalopathy and a new variant of Creutzfeldt-Jakob disease. Neurology 1997;48:569–571.

Ironside JW. Review: Creutzfeldt-Jakob disease. Brain Pathol 1996;6:379–388.

Kretzschmar HA, Ironside JW, DeArmond SJ, Tateishi J. Diagnostic criteria for sporadic Creutzfeldt-Jakob disease. Arch Neurol 1996;53:913–920.

Prusiner SB, Hsiao KK. Human prion diseases. Ann Neurol 1994;35:385–395.

Chapter 48

Herpes Zoster and Postherpetic Neuralgia

Rhonda G. Kost

Natural History

Herpes zoster is an infectious disease resulting from reactivation of varicella-zoster virus (VZV), the virus that causes chickenpox. Primary infection usually occurs in childhood, at which time the sensory ganglia are seeded with virus. VZV then persists latently for decades until it reactivates, descends the peripheral nerve axon, and causes its typical eruption. Herpes zoster is characterized by neuritis—pain, itching, paresthesias—and a vesicular rash classically demarcated by a unilateral dermatome. The rash typically crusts and heals in 1 to 4 weeks.

The most common and feared sequela of herpes zoster is postherpetic neuralgia (PHN). PHN is defined as neuropathic pain that persists beyond an agreed-on time, usually 1 or 3 months after rash onset. It is a common cause of chronic pain and may affect 50% of patients who are older than 60 years and develop zoster. PHN may overlap the pain of acute herpes zoster temporally but is considered a separate process, with distinct pathophysiology and natural history. The abnormal sensations in PHN are described most frequently as burning (49%), throbbing (40%), stabbing (40%), or shooting (38%) pain. Allodynia often is described. PHN can be severe and debilitating and may persist for months or years (<5%). Carefully selected treatment strategies can provide reasonable relief for up to two-thirds of patients with PHN.

Histopathologically, herpes zoster infection results in peripheral denervation, demyelination, and hemorrhagic necrosis of the sensory ganglion, with neuronal loss and scarring. These findings occur in the absence of PHN. Limited autopsy studies suggest that patients who develop PHN also have such evidence of central nervous system damage as atrophy of the dorsal horn of the spinal cord. The pathophysiology of PHN is unknown; however, animal models and other human pain syndromes suggest that in addition to peripheral damage, alteration occurs in the central processing of pain messages, perhaps through loss of descending noradrenergic and serotonergic inhibitory inputs onto second-order neurons. Central hyperexcitability is thought to be a key component in the development of PHN.

Factors Affecting Prognosis

More than 90% of adults are infected latently with VZV and, therefore, at risk for herpes zoster. The lifetime risk for herpes zoster is 20%, though the majority of cases occur in those older than 60 years. Immunocompromise, particularly declining cell-mediated immunity, increases the risk of herpes zoster; however, immunocompromise alone does not increase the age-adjusted risk for PHN. One exception may be the individual infected with the human immunodeficiency virus (HIV). However, the neuropathies caused by both HIV and many antiretroviral therapies have confounded estimates of PHN in these patients.

Several factors affect risk and prognosis in PHN. Age remains the most powerful and undisputed pre-

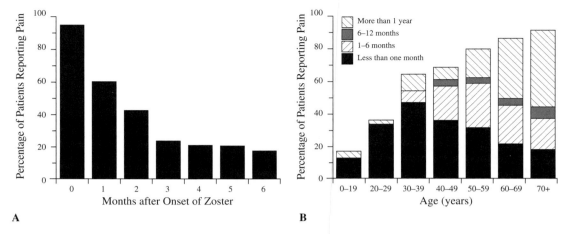

Figure 48-1. A. Pain in patients with zoster tends to resolve over time. Drawn from data obtained in the placebo arm of a zoster treatment study. (Adapted from MJ Wood, PH Ogan, MW McKendrick, et al. The efficacy of oral acyclovir treatment of acute herpes zoster. Am J Med 1988;85:79–83.) B. A retrospective analysis of 916 patients who were grouped arbitrarily by age and decade and by pain duration. Pain in patients with herpes zoster increases in frequency, severity, and duration with increasing age. (Adapted from JM DeMoragas, RR Kierland. The outcome of patients with herpes zoster. AMA Arch Dermatol 1957;75:193–196.)

dictor of PHN. The disease is unheard of in children, though it affects 27% of patients age 50 years and up to 73% of patients age 70 years and older. PHN also is more severe and of greater duration with increasing age (Fig. 48-1). Though most PHN resolves over time, 2 to 4% of individuals still will report pain at 1 year.

Several investigators have reported that pain severity measured prospectively at rash onset is correlated with risk for PHN, though not all researchers agree. In some studies, the frequency and severity of PHN is disproportionately high in ophthalmic zoster. One study reported that patients who experienced specific sensory deficits measurable at day 28 eventually met criteria for PHN, whereas patients without those deficits did not. It has been suggested also that the longer PHN has been present, the poorer is the prognosis.

Evaluation for Prognosis

Evaluation for prognosis entails a careful history and physical examination. Such factors as age, severity of initial pain, and the use of antiviral agents early in the course of disease should be determined. The loss of sensitivity to pinprick, touch, or cold and the presence of allodynia at or

adjacent to the zoster eruption, are correlated with PHN. These various factors carry more weight in evaluating a patient presenting within a month or two of rash onset and may be moot in the evaluation of a patient with established PHN of months' to years' duration. Additionally, a careful history of therapies tried to date is important. Though historically everything from snake venom to B vitamins has been tried, a limited number of reasonable therapies do exist. The prognosis is better for a patient who has not yet exhausted all remedies.

Therapies Affecting Prognosis

Many efforts have been made to intervene early during herpes zoster in hopes of limiting the subsequent development of PHN. Many conflicting claims have been made, and no panacea has emerged. This subject is reviewed extensively elsewhere (see Additional Reading). Universally, preventive interventions must be initiated within 72 to 96 hours of rash onset to be at all effective. When initiated promptly in patients age 50 years or older and continued for 3 weeks, corticosteroid treatment reduces acute pain and improves quality of life in the first month but does not affect the occurrence of PHN. The antiviral drug acyclovir also improves short-term pain and hastens healing but does not influence the development of PHN. The newer nucleoside analog antivirals—famciclovir and valacyclovir—definitely appear to shorten by days to weeks the duration of time until patients are pain-free and may reduce the duration of PHN in selected patients. In comparison with placebo, famciclovir significantly decreased the time until pain resolved (hazard ratio, 1.9; $p = 0.01$). In comparison with acyclovir, valacyclovir significantly reduced the proportion of patients reporting pain at 6 months by 26% ($p = 0.01$). Controversy persists as to when to begin measuring PHN, and the use of different pain definitions in various treatment trials greatly reduces the ability to compare them.

The limited retrospective data suggest that treatment with an antiviral agent early in acute zoster may facilitate a more robust response to tricyclic antidepressant (TCA) therapy administered later for PHN. These studies are provocative but require corroboration. Nerve blocks can provide short-term relief of pain during zoster, but reports that early nerve blocks can prevent the later development of PHN are uncontrolled.

Treatment of established PHN (i.e., PHN of many months' duration) rarely is curative. However, partial or complete relief of PHN can be achieved using a careful, systematic treatment plan (see Additional Reading). The mainstay of therapy for PHN is treatment with a TCA. In controlled trials, TCAs at relatively low doses provide partial or complete relief of the constant burning or aching component of PHN for 50 to 75% of patients. Amitriptyline is the best studied TCA, though nortriptyline, desipramine, and maprotiline have proved beneficial as well. Anticonvulsant agents (carbamazepine, phenytoin, and valproic acid) are more selective for the spontaneous lancinating component of PHN. Systematic sequential evaluation of several of the TCAs and their combination with an anticonvulsant agent may be necessary to achieve an optimal individualized treatment plan. Failure to benefit from one TCA does not preclude success with another agent.

Such topical agents as lidocaine or lignocaine-prilocaine gels, and neuroaugmentive therapies, such as transcutaneous electrical nerve stimulation, may provide relief for some patients, even if PHN is long-standing. Unpredictable responses to these nonpharmacologic interventions occasionally provide sustained relief, though the mechanism is unclear. Capsaicin, the substance P–depleting hot pepper derivative, causes intolerable burning in 30% of patients who use it. Capsaicin use does not alter prognosis.

Nerve blocks have not been studied prospectively in a controlled fashion for the treatment of established PHN, though anecdotes abound. Neuroablative procedures can be permanently disabling and have not been demonstrated to provide benefit.

Short- and Long-Term Prognosis

The short- and long-term prognosis for PHN of short duration is good. Overall, most pain related to zoster resolves over time (see Fig 48-1). An elderly patient who still has pain several months after rash onset has reason to hope that the pain will abate in the coming months. In the meantime, aggressive appropriate therapy with a TCA may make the pain bearable. Even after a year or more of PHN, the natural history is that of slow resolution. In the case of short-duration PHN that was relieved completely by therapy, periodically halting therapy is reasonable for determining whether the underlying process has resolved.

For the patient who has experienced PHN for years at the time of presentation, the prognosis is poorer. Before despairing, one must ensure that the patient has tried TCA and anticonvulsant medications in an adequate trial period with dose escalation every week until benefit or side effects limit the regimen. Failing that, an escalated trial of narcotics is appropriate. Narcotic therapy has been controversial in neuropathic pain; however, some data suggest that a subset of PHN patients do respond favorably to opiates, albeit to doses higher than those used for nonneuropathic pain.

Thus, for the chronic PHN patient with a history of inadequate therapeutic trials, proper treatment may offer more relief than was achieved previously. The patient who is a disappointed veteran of appropriate PHN remedies has a poor prognosis. Reasonable treatment expectations include reduction of symptoms in severity or frequency and attendant increase in the ability to resume normal activities and sleep. For the chronic patient, treatment that ameliorates PHN usually must be continued indefinitely. Though some speculate that early aggressive pain management may minimize the neurophysiologic conditions that lead to prolonged pain, no information ascertains whether successful late pain management alters the central pathophysiology of PHN.

Other Neurologic Complications of Herpes Zoster

A variety of other neurologic sequelae of herpes zoster have been described. Aseptic meningitis is common and usually asymptomatic. Motor paralysis is reported in fewer than 5% of zoster episodes, largely arising from cephalic, cervical, or sacral dermatomes. Most common is Ramsay Hunt syndrome, an ipsilateral facial palsy complicating zoster of the external ear or tympanic membrane. Tinnitus, vertigo, and deafness also occur and are variable in their resolution. Neurogenic bladder dysfunction may complicate sacral zoster, often resolving with the acute episode.

Ophthalmic complications of herpes zoster affecting the first branch of the trigeminal nerve (e.g., uveitis, iritis, and keratitis) largely result from the inflammatory response to virus. Prognosis is improved by early referral to an ophthalmologist and combination therapy with antiviral agents and corticosteroids.

Acute retinal necrosis (ARN) caused by VZV can occur with or without the cutaneous zoster rash. The risk of retinal detachment after VZV ARN is approximately 75%, and prophylaxis to the retina by photocoagulation of the edge of the necrotic retina is recommended. In untreated immunocompetent patients, the retinal lesions tend to enlarge over 1 to 2 weeks and then regress spontaneously over 4 to 8 weeks. Antiviral agents theoretically limit expansion and hasten regression, but their value never has been tested prospectively in normal patients. Often, corticosteroids are needed to blunt the inflammatory response as the lesions regress. The risk of progressive, sight-threatening disease from ARN is higher in immunocompromised patients, and the value of antiviral therapy is clearer. The risk of retinal detachment is perhaps the same as in normal patients. Seventeen percent of HIV-infected patients with zoster ophthalmicus develop ARN. Many respond to tapering antiviral therapy, some require chronic antiviral therapy and, in others, retinal lesions will progress relentlessly, even through foscarnet treatment.

In immunocompromised individuals, such as those with leukemia or lymphoma or those undergoing chemotherapy, instituting intensive antiviral therapy as early as possible is critical to minimize complications, including neurologic sequelae. Exuberant inflammatory response to viral antigens in tissue and immune complex deposition can precipitate myelitis, encephalitis, and angiitis with stroke; these events are rare and generally are limited to severely immunocompromised patients with cephalic zoster. The prognosis after CVA may depend more on collateral circulation and control of vasculitis than on VZV per se. Data are limited.

A variety of case reports have described subtle, unusual, or progressive neurologic complications of herpes zoster in patients infected with HIV. In one case, despite acyclovir treatment taken for another reason, the patient developed progressive VZV myelitis that was diagnosed postmortem in the absence of zoster rash. Several cases of progressive VZV encephalitis have been described. The profound deficits in cell-mediated immunity experienced in HIV infection may permit ongoing viral replication, even in the setting of antiviral therapy, as evidenced by the chronic atypical zoster eruptions often reported in acquired immunodeficiency syndrome (AIDS) patients. As these anecdotes emerge, the natural history and prognosis of these unusual neurologic complications in HIV patients may become clearer.

Resistance of VZV to antiviral drugs has been reported among immunocompromised patients, especially in AIDS patients undergoing prolonged therapy. Not known is whether antiviral resistance is playing a role in the unusual neurologic presentations described in the preceding paragraph. For the non-PHN neurologic complications of zoster, control of viral replication affects outcome and, therefore, the development of antiviral drug resistance is of increasing concern. Regarding PHN, antiviral resistance to acyclovir confers cross-resistance to famciclovir and valacyclovir, the two agents that hold the most promise for prevention of PHN. Overwhelmingly, aged persons who are at greatest risk for PHN are immunologically "normal" for their age and unlikely to develop resistant virus. Nonetheless, in the immunocompromised elderly patient, antiviral-resistant virus could alter the prognosis for

PHN. The alternative drug in the setting of acyclovir resistance—foscarnet—uses a different antiviral mechanism and thus is not cross-resistant; however, no information exists regarding foscarnet and the risk of PHN. Antiviral resistance has not been evaluated in PHN prevention and treatment studies.

Future Directions

The live attenuated varicella vaccine may change the face of zoster and PHN in the future. The vaccine boosts VZV-specific humoral and cellular responses not only in seronegative VZV-naïve children and adults but in seropositive adults (those who bear the risk of future herpes zoster). For the children now being vaccinated against VZV, it will not be known for another five or six decades whether their course of zoster has been altered (i.e., until they reach the age at which they would be at risk). It is anticipated that herpes zoster in the vaccinated generation may be rarer, or milder, or both. In the meantime, plans are afoot to vaccinate prospectively a large cohort of seropositive (naturally infected) adults age 60 years or older and to document the incidence and severity of zoster. Because the age-related increase in zoster incidence is thought to be due to declining cell-mediated immunity, the boost provided to cell-mediated immunity by vaccination might alter the risk and course of zoster and of such sequelae as PHN. This large multicenter trial awaits initiation, and the answer is not yet known; however, possibly in the future another evaluable factor in predicting prognosis will be whether a zoster patient has received a varicella vaccination.

Additional Reading

DeMoragas JM, Kierland RR. The outcome of patients with herpes zoster. AMA Arch Dermatol 1957;75:193–196.

Galer BS, Portenoy RK. Acute herpetic and postherpetic neuralgia: clinical features and management. Mt Sinai J Med 1991;58:257–266.

Harding SP, Lipton JR, Wells JCD. Natural history of herpes zoster ophthalmicus: predictors of postherpetic neuralgia and ocular involvement. Br J Ophthalmol 1987;71:353–358.

Hope-Simpson RE. The nature of herpes zoster: a long-term study and a new hypothesis. Proc R Soc Med 1965;58:9–20.

Jemsek J, Greenberg SB, Taber L, et al. Herpes zoster associated encephalitis: clinicopathologic report of 12 cases and review of the literature. Medicine 1983;62:81–97.

Kost RG, Straus SE. Postherpetic neuralgia: pathogenesis, treatment and prevention. N Engl J Med 1996;335:32–42.

Rentier B (ed). Updated proceedings of the Second International Conference on the Varicella-Zoster Virus. Neurology 1995;45(suppl 8):S54–S62.

Sacks SL, Straus SE, Whitley RJ, Griffiths PD. Clinical Management of Herpes Viruses. Washington, DC: IOS Press, 1995;175–261.

Watson CPN. Herpes Zoster and Postherpetic Neuralgia. Amsterdam: Elsevier, 1993;258.

Whitely RJ, Gnann JW. Editorial response: herpes zoster in patients with human immunodeficiency virus infection—an ever-expanding spectrum of disease. Clin Infect Dis 1995;21:989–990.

Part IX
Disorders of the Spinal Cord

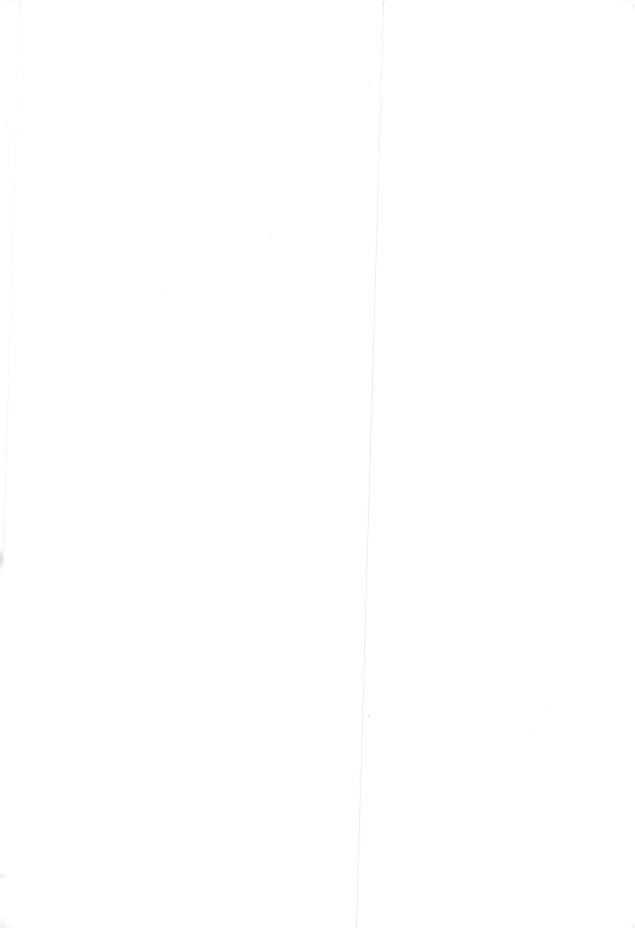

Chapter 49

Cervical Spondylosis

Michael Ronthal

The term *cervical spondylosis* is used to describe a disorder of the cervical spine with degenerative pathology involving discs, secondary osteophyte formation from the vertebral bodies, hypertrophy of the facet joints and ligaments and, sometimes, segmental instability or subluxation. It may be part of the aging process or can be triggered or aggravated by trauma. Some authors refer to anterior ridging osteophytes as *hard* disc pathology as opposed to *soft*, or recent, disc degeneration with herniation.

Hypertrophic cervical osteophytes are said to occur in as many as 30% of the adult population. The incidence rises with age but, for unknown reasons, the degree of anatomic abnormality is not correlated directly with clinical signs and symptoms. Of referred patients seen in a general neurology practice, perhaps one-half will have problems related to the neck or back.

Signs and symptoms of cervical spondylosis relate to compression and irritation of cervical nerve roots and the cervical spinal cord and to reactive neck-muscle spasm. Impingement on neighboring structures is less common but can produce a diverse and varied clinical picture. This chapter deals specifically with the natural history and prognosis of cervical spondylosis and its attendant clinical syndromes.

Natural History

Pain

Two main causes underlie pain in spondylosis: neck muscle spasm, which results in a painful stiff neck, and muscle contraction headache. The natural history of pain in cervical spondylosis never has been studied systematically but, in whiplash injury, a syndrome with pain based on a similar mechanism, 20 to 40% of patients have persistent pain for at least 2 years. Those with persistent symptoms have either more severe injuries or pre-existing spondylosis and headache. In general, the course of both signs and symptoms in cervical spondylosis may be summarized in one word: *fluctuation*, with each exacerbation of pain usually lasting 3 to 6 weeks. Most patients are treated at the judgment of the consulting physician; no prospective controlled trials of therapy have been reported.

Cervical Radiculopathy

Cervical radiculopathy may present with root pain, myotomal weakness, or dermatomal sensory loss. Symptoms may persist for months but tend to fluctuate. Even many asymptomatic patients continue to have clinical signs related to the nerve root involved: Slight wasting, weakness, a depressed or absent tendon reflex, and slight loss of sensation are commonly seen on careful examination. Electromyographic evaluation in this population shows chronic denervation in the affected muscles. Exacerbations and remissions may be spontaneous but frequently are related to trauma of one sort or another, often seemingly trivial. Often, patients report onset of an exacerbation or recurrent pain on awakening in the morning, likely relating to trauma sustained while tossing and turning during sleep and can be prevented with the use of good support at night, such as sleeping in a collar or on a hard pillow. The frequency of exacerbations and the effect of treatment never has been studied prospectively or retrospectively.

Spondylotic Myelopathy

The precise pathophysiology of myelopathy in cervical spondylosis is unknown. Clearly, cord compression must play a crucial role, but imaging studies often do not correlate well with clinical signs, and surgical decompression does not always alleviate the myelopathic signs; some patients progress despite decompression. Such other factors as ischemia or "rubbing" of the cord across bony ridges have, therefore, been invoked.

Because of general acceptance that cord decompression is the treatment of choice, reviews of the natural history of cervical myelopathy are sparse, and no recent studies have been reported. Ten of 14 patients treated with a collar by Campbell and Phillips improved. Lees and Turner reported spontaneous improvement in 6 of 15 patients with "severe" disability followed for more than 10 years. Their series included 28 patients treated with a collar; 17 improved, 7 were unchanged, and 4 were worse. Eighty-one patients with radicular symptoms never developed myelopathy. In a series reported by Nurick, 40% of 104 patients treated with a collar improved, 36% were unchanged, and 24% were worse. Symon and Lavender found that 67% of patients had a steady progressive deterioration, and of 102 patients followed by Phillips, the one-third who did not have an operation improved.

Factors Affecting Prognosis

Patients who develop myelopathy are likely to have a congenitally narrow neural canal, and the anterior-posterior diameter of the canal is the only sign that may predict whether any patient is likely to develop myelopathy. Adams and Logue reported a minimal "normal" canal width of 16 mm and in patients with myelopathy the width ranged from 9 to 15 mm. Though spinal canal diameter plays an important role in predicting myelopathy, an unstable spine also affects prognosis adversely, and subluxation may be an indication for spinal fusion in the presence of myelopathic signs.

Such extraneous features as pending litigation or psychiatric pathology often will be associated with continued complaints of pain and alleged disability in patients with headache or mild radiculopathy. These patients present an especially difficult diagnostic problem.

Evaluation for Prognosis

Because degenerative changes in the cervical spine in both the symptomatic and the asymptomatic population are common and because the natural history is one of fluctuation, evaluation for prognosis is often difficult. Although opinions vary, most patients with radicular syndromes improve with or without treatment, but myelopathy can become disabling.

The best tool for evaluation of the likelihood of myelopathy and analysis of its prognosis remains magnetic resonance imaging of the cervical spine to evaluate for cord compression and to measure canal diameter. The presence of segmental high T2 signal within the cord at the level of compression may be an indicator of poor prognosis either because it represents acute or subacute edema within the cord, implying more severe compression, or because it signifies the development of cord gliosis. Likewise, cord atrophy implies a poor outcome. Flexion and extension radiographs of the cervical spine provide a screen for spinal subluxation that adversely affects prognosis. Last, failure to respond to immobilization suggests a poor prognosis.

Therapies Affecting Prognosis

Mild pain is treated effectively with analgesics only. Neck muscle spasm and radicular pain usually respond to various combinations of immobilization, including local heat, massage, and mild cervical traction (5 to 6 pounds). Not infrequently, chronic pain-suppressive therapy is required: A combination of a muscle relaxant (e.g., diazepam, 2 mg three times per day) and a serotonergic antidepressant usually is effective. For acute and severe radicular pain, some treating physicians prefer a short course of oral steroid therapy or an injection of steroid into the cervical epidural space. Chiropractic manipulation is mentioned only to make the point that it is a potentially dangerous form of therapy. Approximately 12 million Americans undergo spinal manipulation therapy every year. One review described 138 cases with serious complications. The only published randomized controlled trial did not demonstrate that manipulation was significantly helpful.

The presence of myelopathy and cord compression on imaging studies is generally taken to be an indication for operative intervention. Although it is common (if anecdotal) knowledge that "patients improve after cervical decompression," proving that dictum from a review of the literature is difficult. The lack of available information prevents surgeons from predicting accurately when and for whom operative management is absolutely indicated. The common operative procedures are either cervical laminectomy, the "posterior" approach, or anterior discectomy and fusion, the "anterior approach." Laminectomy results in slightly greater morbidity figures, but the choice of surgery usually is based on the individual case: The spinal canal is approached from the direction of greatest compression. In a review of the literature, Rowland gave the following figures: Of 261 patients subjected to cervical laminectomy, 60% were improved, 34% were unchanged, and 6% were worse; of 385 patients subjected to anterior surgery, 52% were improved, 24% were unchanged, and 23% were worse; of 136 patients treated conservatively, 44% were improved, 33% were unchanged, and 23% were worse. One also should take into account perioperative morbidity. This factor varies from author to author but, in general, a 4 to 5% death or disability rate can be expected. Clifton and colleagues reviewed the probable reasons for poor surgical outcome in the treatment of cervical spondylosis. Fifty-six patients were studied with the following results: wrong diagnosis, 14.3%; spinal cord atrophy, 26.8%; diffuse spinal stenosis, 28.6%; and failure of decompression, 57.1%. Failed surgery, therefore, may be due to a technical fault in as many as 85% of patients who have a negative result.

Despite the uncertainty, and on the basis of the notion that in some way cord compression is integral to the pathogenesis of myelopathy in cervical spondylosis, experts generally accept that patients with myelopathy and demonstrable cord compression should be decompressed surgically. A controlled prospective trial is needed.

Short-Term Prognosis

Cervical spondylosis essentially is a chronic condition with an unpredictable and variable course. Even so, the patient can be reassured that the short-term course of any particular exacerbation of pain or radicular dysfunction is likely to be relatively brief. Myelopathy also often responds to neck immobilization, only to relapse when the collar is abandoned.

Long-Term Prognosis

Episodes of radicular dysfunction and pain can be expected to recur from time to time, but predicting the frequency of such exacerbations with any degree of accuracy is impossible. Myelopathy in cervical spondylosis generally is slowly progressive, but my practice has followed patients who, using a collar intermittently, have remained essentially static for 4 to 5 years. The best figures suggest a "50:50" prognosis, both in those submitted to surgery and in those treated conservatively (i.e., half will improve and half will not).

Additional Reading

Adams CBT, Logue V. Studies in cervical spondylotic myelopathy: II. Movement and contour of the spine in relation to the neural complications of cervical spondylosis. Brain 1971;94:569–586.

Bernhardt M, Hynes RA, Blume HW, White AA. Current concepts review: cervical spondylotic myelopathy. J Bone Joint Surg Am 1993;75:119–128.

Campbell AMG, Phillips DG. Cervical disc lesions with neurological disorder. Differential diagnosis, treatment, and prognosis. BMJ 1960;2:481–485.

Clifton AG, Stevens JM, Whitear P, Kendall BE. Identifiable causes for poor outcome in surgery for cervical spondylosis. Neuroradiology 1990;32:450–455.

Lees F, Aldren Turner JW. Natural history and prognosis of cervical spondylosis. BMJ 1963;2:1607–1610.

Nurick S. Natural history and results of surgical treatment of the spinal disorder associated with cervical spondylosis. Brain 1972;95:101–108.

Phillips DG. Surgical treatment of myelopathy with cervical spondylosis. J Neurol Neurosurg Psychiatry 1973;36:879–884.

Powell FC, Hanigan WC, Olivero WC. A risk/benefit analysis of spinal manipulation therapy for relief of lumbar or cervical pain. Neurosurgery 1993;33:73–78.

Rowland LP. Surgical treatment of cervical spondylotic myelopathy: time for a controlled trial. Neurology 1992;42:5–13.

Symon L, Lavender P. The surgical treatment of cervical spondylotic myelopathy. Neurology 1967;17:117–127.

Chapter 50

Syringomyelia

Grace A. Medeiros and James M. Gilchrist

Syringomyelia is composed of a complex group of conditions characterized by a cystic cavity with accumulations of fluid extending longitudinally over several segments of the spinal cord. If the syrinx extends into the medulla, the condition is known as *syringobulbia*. This abnormality has been classified broadly into communicating and noncommunicating types.

A communicating syrinx generally is associated with a craniovertebral junction abnormality, implying continuity at some time between the cerebrospinal fluid of the syrinx and the fourth ventricle, and accounts for 10% of cases at necropsy. The most common form of communicating syrinx is associated with the Chiari malformations. Other associated abnormalities include Dandy-Walker cyst, Klippel-Feil anomaly, basilar impression, and such acquired disorders as basal arachnoiditis, transverse myelitis, herniated intervertebral disc, posterior fossa neoplasm and cysts, cervical spondylosis, and idiopathic cases.

A noncommunicating syrinx (i.e., without continuity with the fourth ventricle) can be seen in association with spinal trauma, intramedullary and extramedullary neoplasms, tuberculous meningitis, spinal surgery, arachnoiditis, arachnoid cysts, multiple sclerosis, and Chiari malformations. Twenty-five to 60% of intramedullary tumors have an associated syrinx. Up to 38% of these syringes are idiopathic. Post-traumatic syringomyelia has an incidence of 3.4% or more after spinal cord injury but may not become clinically evident from several months to 36 years after injury.

Understanding of the evolution of the syrinx is clouded by multiple etiologies, varied clinical presentations, and unclear pathogenesis. It was not until 1965, when Gardener put forth the hydrodynamic theory to explain syrinx formation associated with hindbrain abnormalities, that management was directed toward a physiologic basis. Since then, this and other hydrodynamic theories have been accepted more widely as explanations of pathogenesis in the maintenance of the cavity.

Natural History

Up to 76% of syringomyelia presents in the second to fourth decades, although it may occur at any age. The disease affects both male and female populations equally. Presenting symptoms and signs include pain, headache made worse by stooping or coughing, a dissociated sensory loss, motor weakness, muscle wasting, hyperhidrosis, spasticity of the lower extremities, reflex abnormalities, neurogenic arthropathies, an ascending sensory level, sleep apnea, and drop attacks. Cranial nerve abnormalities include trigeminal sensory abnormalities, nystagmus, tongue atrophy, and Horner's syndrome. Scoliosis is present on radiographic scans in 57 to 64% of patients.

The highly variable nature of both treated and untreated syringomyelia renders prognostication difficult. The course runs a spectrum of complete stabilization to rapid evolution. Spontaneous resolution is reported rarely. A patient with a stable but distended syrinx may deteriorate acutely after a Valsalva maneuver from a cough or sneeze. This possibility is particularly a concern in traumatic paraplegic and quadriplegic patients who experience a Valsalva maneuver during transfers.

In general, the few studies of the natural history of untreated patients indicate a slowly progressive disease marked by years of relative stability. In Bowman's series of noncommunicating (spinal) syringes over a 10-year period, 40 to 50% of patients underwent spontaneous arrest of symptoms. Whether surgery has an effect on the natural history and long-term prognosis remains unclear.

Death due to syringomyelia is relatively rare. However, it can occur if the syrinx involves the brain stem, causing bradycardia and respiratory compromise.

Factors Affecting Prognosis

Duration of symptoms has a bearing on prognosis. Patients who have symptoms for longer than 2 years and then have posterior fossa decompression demonstrate an overall prognosis worse than those who receive the procedure within 2 years of becoming symptomatic. In one series, only 13% of such patients stabilized or improved clinically over a 10-year period. The presence of septations with loculation of the cavity along the syrinx before or after surgery also is a bad prognostic sign, as it precludes adequate drainage and may lead to further neurologic deterioration. Patients older than 40 years had a poor long-term outcome after surgery, regardless of symptom duration.

Etiology of the syrinx also has a bearing on prognosis. Although partial or completed collapse after surgery is demonstrated by 50 to 80% of patients with a syrinx associated with an intramedullary neoplasm, 20% may experience recrudescence associated with tumor recurrence. The presence on preoperative magnetic resonance imaging (MRI) of a syrinx associated with an intramedullary tumor favors resectability of the tumor and carries a better short-term prognosis, as it indicates a noninfiltrating tumor. An associated syrinx has no effect on the long-term prognosis. In contrast to intramedullary tumors, extramedullary lesions have a better prognosis. After surgical excision of the extramedullary tumor, which may include decompression, 85 to 100% of cases can expect complete clinical or radiologic improvement.

Although controversial, post-traumatic syringomyelia gives evidence of a higher incidence of syrinx formation after complete spinal cord injury than for incomplete lesions. Rarely, minor spinal cord injury may lead to a syrinx. However, severity of the injury has no correlation with syrinx size on the basis of MRI. The literature suggests that patients with the least neurologic deficit at presentation have the best prognosis and that patients with a normal examination after spinal trauma rarely develop syrinx. After spinal trauma, patients with earlier onset of syrinx occurrence tend to have more rapid clinical deterioration and require surgical intervention. No clear correlation ties the site of the syrinx to the magnitude of the neurologic deficits.

Reactive gliosis can result in failure of syrinx resolution and syrinx recurrence. Arachnoidal scarring before or after surgery portends a poor short- and long-term outcome.

Evaluation for Prognosis

MRI is the study of choice for prognosis. If an MRI is contraindicated clinically, a contrast computed tomography scan may be performed. The dimensions of the syrinx preoperatively have no bearing on prognosis, but a significant correlation exists between reduction or collapse of the cavity on postoperative MRI and good clinical outcome postoperatively. Clinical improvement may precede radiologic improvement by several weeks, and a cavity may be present before appearance of symptoms. Gadolinium-enhanced MRI is indicated when neoplasm is suspected. Also, a syrinx that appears radiographically to have collapsed but is associated with arachnoidal scarring or myelomalacia carries a poor prognosis. Persistence of a syrinx on postoperative MRI does not necessarily portend a poor clinical outcome.

Therapies Affecting Prognosis

Syringomyelia often requires surgical treatment. Management always has posed a clinical challenge, as no well-controlled prospective studies compare surgical techniques, and many of the studies involve small numbers of patients. Additionally, nonstandardization of surgical approach, multiplicity of etiologies, and variable criteria for good clinical outcome render posttreatment prognostication difficult. Some authors advocate close follow-up in clinically stable patients, with serial MRI and neurologic examination and delayed surgical intervention. Other authors advocate early intervention, as patients with the less severe deficit are more likely to have a good clinical outcome.

Generally, craniovertebral junction abnormalities with increased intracranial pressure are treated with posterior fossa decompression as a primary procedure, with or without such adjunctive procedures as closure of a patent canal, syringotomy, drainage of the fourth ventricle, and lysis of arachnoidal adhesions, among other procedures. Results vary but, in the most optimistic series, up to 86% of patients stabilized or improved postoperatively. Shunting is indicated if decompression fails. For primarily spinal, noncommunicating forms of syringomyelia, treatment options include laminectomy with syringotomy, simple drainage using either an open or percutaneous approach, subarachnoid space reconstruction and augmentation, and a variety of shunting procedures, including syringoperitoneal, subarachnoid, and syringopleural shunts. No consensus confirms the superiority of one shunting procedure over another. Shunting procedures are effective in more than 70% of patients in the short term if used as a primary mode of treatment, and they remain effective in 50% of patients after 10 years. Needle aspiration for syrinx decompression has been effective in 60 to 75% of cases in the short term, but only one-third of patients will maintain improvement over a median of 10 years. In patients with extramedullary neoplasm, tumor excision alone in one series resulted in complete resolution of the cavity in all cases, but long-term results are yet to be determined. For intramedullary neoplasms, syrinx drainage and appropriate adjunctive therapy are indicated.

Although no consensus is found for appropriate surgical technique, some evidence confirms that particular symptoms respond better to surgical intervention. Radicular and axial pain, occipital pain, and exertional headache respond well to surgery. In one series with syrinx associated with Chiari malformations, 75% of patients followed over 5 years experienced improvement in pain. Dysesthetic pain, however, is poorly responsive to treatment. Such sensory abnormalities as hypoesthesia respond variably but, in general, 75% of patients improve in the short term, a figure that falls to only 30% after 5 years. Improvement in weakness also is unimpressive. Fifty to 80% of patients may improve shortly after surgery, but only 25% remain improved after 5 years. Muscle atrophy also does not improve after treatment. In several series, spasticity improved in 72 to 80% after surgery, but long-term efficacy is uncertain. Bowel and bladder function are unlikely to be restored after surgery. Patients with a central cord syndrome associated with a Chiari malformation have a poor prognosis, as only one-third of patients will improve after surgery.

Arachnoidal scarring at the cervicomedullary junction increases surgical risk, and lysis of adhesions is indicated. Patients with an atrophic syrinx do not respond well to surgery. Another small series reported that although patients improved clinically after surgery, no radiologic improvement was seen. Operative mortality after posterior fossa decompression occurs in up to 15% of patients; many of these deaths include respiratory complications. Patients undergoing posterior fossa decompression also undergo transitory neurologic worsening in 6 to 8% of cases, and not all recover. Patients who have noncommunicating syringes and require a myelotomy may expect an increase in neurologic deficit that is transient in 80% or more of cases. However, despite adequate and aggressive surgical intervention, recurrence rates of syringomyelia are as high as 60% over a 5-year period.

Short-Term Prognosis

Syringomyelia is a chronic disease causing progressive neurologic dysfunction for which no medical therapy exists. Various surgical interventions are available, but comparing them is difficult, owing to lack of standardized techniques and standard criteria for outcome measurement. Most important, no good, well-controlled prospective studies compare surgery to nonsurgical management. Several studies have reported good results after surgery in up to 85% of patients, but many of these successes are temporary, with recurrence of symptoms and signs within a few years. Radicular and head pain are most amenable to surgery, but weakness, dysesthetic pain, and atrophy are less so. Only 20 to 30% of patients treated for syringomyelia improve rather than become clinically stable after surgery.

Long-Term Prognosis

Generally, patients with syringomyelia can expect long-term survival, with gradual increase in neurologic deficits regardless of whether they undergo surgery. Up to 50% of patients without surgery will have spontaneous stabilization of their deficits for 10 years or longer. Many of those patients who undergo surgical decompression of the syrinx will improve for a time after surgery, but at least one-half or more will experience recurrence of slow progression within 5 years. The mortality rate of 5 to 15% is similar in patients both with and without surgery. Overall long-term outcome is best in those patients with the least deficits at presentation and with the slowest progression.

Additional Reading

Anderson NE, Willoughby EW, Wrightson P. The natural history and the influence of surgical treatment in syringomyelia. Acta Neurol Scand 1985;71:472–479.

Barbaro NM, Wilson CB, Gatin PH, Edwards MS. Surgical treatment of syringomyelia. Favorable results with syringoperitoneal shunting. J Neurosurg 1984;61: 531–538.

Barnett HJM, Foster JB, Hudgson P. Syringomyelia. Philadelphia: Saunders, 1973.

Batzdorf U. Syringomyelia: Current Concepts in Diagnosis and Treatment. Baltimore: Williams & Wilkins, 1991.

Biyani A, El Masry WS. Post-traumatic syringomyelia: a review of the literature. Paraplegia 1994;32:723–731.

El Masry WS, Biyani A. In memory of Mr. Bernard Williams. J Neurol Neurosurg Psychiatry 1996;60:141–146.

Gamache FW, Ducker TB. Syringomyelia: a neurologic and surgical spectrum. J Spinal Disord 1990;3:293–298.

Garcia-Uria J, Guillermo L, et al. Syringomyelia: long term results after posterior fossa decompression. J Neurosurg 1981;54:380–383.

Mariani C, Cislaghi MG, et al. The natural history and results of surgery in 50 cases of syringomyelia. J Neurol 1991;238:433–438.

Samii M, Klekamp J. Surgical results of 100 intramedullary tumors in relation to accompanying syringomyelia. Neurosurgery 1994;35:865–873.

Sgouros S, Williams B. Management and outcome of post-traumatic syringomyelia. J Neurosurg 1996;85:197–205.

Chapter 51

Transverse Myelitis

Loren A. Rolak

Transverse myelitis (TM), an inflammation across the width of the spinal cord and usually spreading through several adjacent rostral-caudal segments, often affects both gray and white matter. Because it is associated frequently with immunologic alterations, such as systemic immune disorders (especially lupus), postinfectious conditions, and multiple sclerosis (MS), an immunologic cause is most likely. However, few immunologic studies ever have been performed, and details of the pathogenesis of TM are scant. Indeed, TM is rare, with an incidence of only one or two cases per million population per year.

Natural History

Transverse myelitis presents with acute spinal cord dysfunction, including motor weakness, usually with spasticity, hyperreflexia, and Babinski's signs; sensory loss, often with a discrete sensory level; and sphincter disturbances, especially bladder dysfunction. Symptoms develop rapidly, with approximately 20% of patients reaching their maximum deficit within 1 hour and 50% within 24 hours. It strikes the thoracic cord much more frequently than any other level, though the reasons for this selectivity are disputed. TM is equally common across all ages and races and both genders, and no difference between pediatric and adult TM is observed in the clinical picture or in the prognosis.

Although usually a monophasic syndrome, repeated or recurrent TM has been described. Up to

five recurrences in a period of 2 or 3 years may occur—often unaccompanied by any new changes on magnetic resonance imaging (MRI) scanning, spinal fluid examination, or evoked potentials—indicating isolated relapsing spinal cord disease. Such relapses may complicate those patients whose initial episode of TM was postinfectious and those patients with "idiopathic" TM. Evolving studies suggest that as many as 15% of TM cases ultimately may recur.

Factors Affecting Prognosis

Prognosis and counseling in TM centers around two concerns: prognosis for recovery of neurologic deficits after the attack of TM itself and prognosis for subsequently developing MS. Few studies specifically have addressed the prognosis for recovery of function after an episode of TM, and the limited data never have permitted any firm conclusions. Most studies agree that predicting outcome for individual patients is fraught with hazards, as no factors reliably correlate with recovery. The exception is the poor prognosis after spinal shock: Patients with an abrupt catastrophic onset with flaccid hyporeflexic paralysis seldom improve. One-half to two-thirds of such patients will remain paraplegic and nonambulatory. Conversely, those with a subacute onset over days or even weeks have a much better outcome, and two-thirds to three-fourths will recover substantially and will maintain ambulation. The lack of a complete cord syndrome, with preservation of reflexes and sensory function at initial presentation, characterizes these patients. Somewhat surprisingly, prognosis does not depend on age, gender, preceding febrile illness, the spinal cord level affected, the appearance of the cord on MRI scanning, or on any findings in the spinal fluid.

Because TM commonly complicates the course of MS, an initial presentation of isolated TM may raise suspicions that it actually represents the first attack of MS, in a fashion somewhat analogous to the relationship between optic neuritis and MS. The risk of developing MS after an idiopathic episode of TM is unknown. For the clinician who must counsel patients, studies addressing this relationship have produced contradictory results. Most of the studies before the widespread use of MRI scans in the mid-1980s, which include by far the largest series of TM cases on record, found the risk of progression to MS to be no greater than 10 to 15% and, at times, well below this range. For example, Berman and colleagues were able to identify every single case of TM occurring in Israel from 1955 to 1975, and only one of the 59 patients subsequently developed MS. During this same period, 747 patients in Israel were diagnosed with MS, and none of them presented with TM as their initial symptom. Thus, the probability that TM actually represented the first attack of MS in this population was negligibly small.

However, since the early 1990s, a number of prospective studies have followed small groups of patients with TM and have reported a very high rate of MS when initial MRI scans of the brain showed white-matter signal abnormalities typical of MS. A patient who presents with TM and whose MRI brain scan shows two or more white-matter lesions, especially periventricular or infratentorial in location, has a 65 to 90% chance of developing clinically definite MS within the next 3 to 5 years. Conversely, a similar TM patient whose MRI scan of the brain is normal has no more than a 5 to 10% chance of progressing ultimately to MS. The abnormal brain MRI thus confers a 10-fold increase in risk (Fig. 51-1).

Other laboratory tests are less useful for predicting the risk of MS. Oligoclonal bands in the spinal fluid most likely foreshadow an increased risk of MS, but most patients with oligoclonal bands also have abnormal MRI scans of the brain, and the overlap is so complete that a lumbar puncture provides little additional information than does the MRI scan alone. Evoked potentials, especially visual evoked potentials, are much less predictive. They show a high incidence of false-positives in patients who subsequently never develop MS and show a low sensitivity (near 30%) for those who do.

Evaluation for Prognosis

The most useful evaluations for prognosis are a detailed history and a physical examination. The abrupt onset of a complete bilateral cord syndrome with spinal shock portends little chance of recovery and implies permanent paraplegia and an inability to regain ambulation. A more subacute or gradual onset of a partial cord syndrome, with preservation of some spinal functions, suggests a good chance of ultimate recovery and preserved ambulation.

The MRI brain scan is a crucial determinant of the subsequent development of MS. However, patients who progress to MS still may have a mild course and ultimately may not develop any more disability than do patients with isolated severe TM. The arrival of MS does not always herald significant disability.

The spinal cord MRI scan itself offers little prognostic information. The presence of enhancement, cord swelling, or any other specific imaging abnormality never has correlated convincingly with a patient's ultimate clinical outcome (Fig. 51-2). Similarly, cerebrospinal fluid changes or evoked potential abnormalities do not provide useful prognostic information. Also, patients with postinfectious TM have the same ultimate outcome as those with idiopathic TM.

Therapies Affecting Prognosis

No therapy has altered the natural history of TM convincingly. The syndrome is sufficiently rare that no large controlled trials ever have been assembled, so conclusions must be extracted from small series and anecdotal information. Corticosteroids are used almost universally to treat the acute symptoms, but no study has been able to establish their effectiveness clearly. Also, no proof is available to substantiate that steroid therapy affects prognosis.

Figure 51-1. Magnetic resonance imaging brain scan of a patient presenting with transverse myelitis shows multiple white-matter lesions and periventricular signal changes indicating an increased risk for the subsequent development of clinically definite multiple sclerosis.

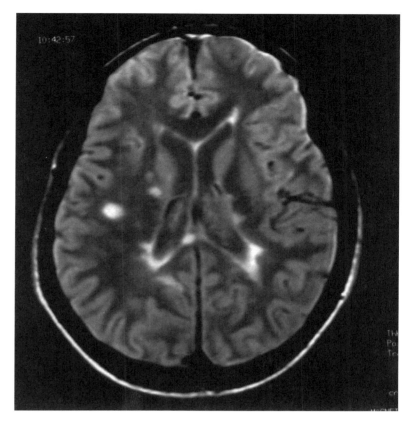

Before 1960, TM was almost uniformly fatal within months because of pulmonary emboli, respiratory problems, and infectious complications of sepsis, pneumonia, urinary tract infections, and decubitus. Proper nursing care and the use of antibiotics are the most effective therapies affecting prognosis.

Short-Term Prognosis

All studies, both old and modern, show a consistent uniformity of prognosis. Approximately one-third of patients with TM will recover well, generally defined as the ability to ambulate without any assistance and to control bowel and bladder function. One-third of patients recover modestly, with the ability to ambulate using some degree of assistance and with good (if not perfect) sphincter control. The remaining one-third of patients recover poorly and never regain the ability to walk or control bowel or bladder function.

The vast majority of recovery takes place within 2 or 3 months. However, some degree of recovery still may occur even 12 to 18 months later, and thus the usual pattern is a rapid initial recovery of considerable function in the first 2 or 3 months, followed by a more gradual persistent improvement in the remaining deficits over the next year or so. Patients who have shown little initial recovery in the first 2 or 3 months are, however, unlikely ever to improve substantially.

Long-Term Prognosis

The long-term prognosis for patients with TM now is reasonably good. Even for those patients who show little recovery within the first year, prognosis is for a nearly normal life span, as for most spinal cord injury patients. Patients who ultimately develop MS may do somewhat worse than the average MS patient, because of the disabling nature of spinal cord symptoms (see Chapter 34).

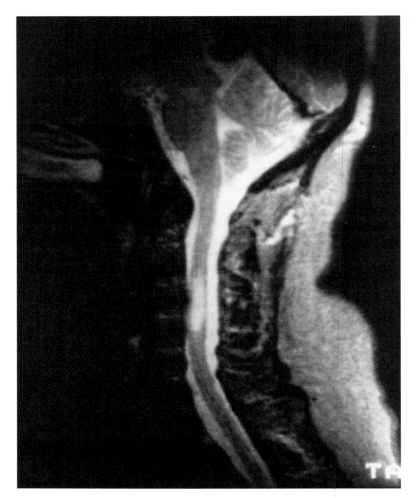

Figure 51-2. T2-weighted magnetic resonance imaging of the cervical spine shows increased signal extending over several segments of the cervical cord (very typical of transverse myelitis).

Approximately 15% of patients may develop relapsing or recurrent transverse myelitis without any other evidence of MS, but such relapses often improve completely, and many such patients still show little disability even after several recurrences.

Additional Reading

Altrocchi PH. Acute transverse myelopathy. Arch Neurol 1963;9:111–119.

Berman M, Feldman S, Alter M, et al. Acute transverse myelitis: incidence and etiological considerations. Neurology 1981;31:966–971.

Filippi M, Horsfield MA, Morrissey SP, et al. Quantitative brain MRI lesion load predicts the course of clinically isolated syndromes suggestive of multiple sclerosis. Neurology 1994;44:635–641.

Ford B, Tampieri D, Francis G. Long-term follow-up of acute partial transverse myelopathy. Neurology 1992; 42:250–252.

Jeffery DR, Mandler RN, Davis LE. Transverse myelitis: retrospective analysis of 33 cases, with differentiation of cases associated with multiple sclerosis and parainfectious events. Arch Neurol 1993;50:532–535.

Lipton HL, Teasdale RD. Acute transverse myelopathy in adults. Arch Neurol 1973;28:252–257.

Miller DH, Ormerod IEC, Rudge P, et al. The early risk of multiple sclerosis following isolated acute syndromes of the brainstem and spinal cord. Ann Neurol 1989;26:635–639.

Ropper AH, Poskanzer DC. The prognosis of acute and subacute transverse myelopathy based on early signs and symptoms. Ann Neurol 1978;4:51–59.

Simnad VI, Pisani DE, Rose JW. Multiple sclerosis presenting as transverse myelopathy. Neurology 1997;48:65–73.

Tippett DS, Fishman PS, Panitch HS. Relapsing transverse myelitis. Neurology 1991;41:703–705.

Chapter 52

Spinal Cord Injury

John F. Ditunno, Jr., and Christopher S. Formal

Traumatic spinal cord injury (SCI) can cause changes in motor, sensory, and autonomic function, resulting in disability and handicap. SCI is uncommon compared to many other neurologic conditions. The national annual incidence of SCI leading to hospital admission is between 30 and 40 per million population; the national prevalence is between 183,000 and 230,000. The associated economic burden is considerable. The lifetime direct costs for a person sustaining high tetraplegia can approach $2 million (in 1992 dollars). The average lifetime indirect costs (foregone earnings and fringe benefits) exceed $2.5 million. SCI affects young men more than any other group. The mean age at time of injury is 31 years, the median is 26 years, and 82% of patients are male. Motor vehicle crashes account for 45%; falls, 18%; acts of violence, 17%; and sports injuries, 13% of cases. The summer months have the highest rates of SCI, and Saturday and Sunday are the days of most frequent occurrence.

Seldom is the cord severed physically, even in cases in which the injury is physiologically complete and permanent. Processes that can worsen the initial injury occur within the cord in the hours or days that follow. The resulting "secondary injury" is an opportunity for intervention to decrease the permanent neurologic deficit.

Natural History

Initially, reflexes are lost with severe injury. The bulbocavernosus reflex often returns within hours in cases of upper motor neuron injury. The delayed plantar reflex, which consists of slow and protracted plantar flexion of the great toe and other toes after strong stimulation of the sole of the foot, also is observed early. Later, the extensor (Babinski's) reflex appears. It requires much less intense stimulation than does the delayed plantar reflex. Deep-tendon reflexes, such as the knee jerk, may return as late as 4 to 6 weeks. Spasticity develops over the months after trauma and is more severe with incomplete injuries.

The most rapid improvement after incomplete SCI occurs in the 4 to 6 months that follow and, though improvement can continue for a longer period of time, a plateau is reached at 1 year. (Cauda equina injuries may improve over a longer period of time.) The time course for lower-extremity motor improvement is similar for both incomplete paraplegia and incomplete tetraplegia. This finding is more consistent with improvement due to reversal of a focal spinal cord conduction block than with improvement due to axonal regeneration. If axonal regeneration were a prominent mechanism of improvement, lower-extremity motor function would improve more rapidly with incomplete paraplegia.

Neurologic decline in a person with a chronic, stable deficit is not expected. However, persistent spinal instability or post-traumatic cystic myelopathy can lead to further neurologic loss. Common morbidity after SCI includes urinary tract infection and pressure ulceration. In addition, musculoskeletal overuse syndromes commonly occur and can compromise function.

Table 52-1. American Spinal Injury Association Impairment Scale for Completeness

Grade	Description
A	Complete; no sensory or motor function in the sacral segments S4–S5
B	Incomplete; sensory but not motor function preserved below the neurologic level, including the sacral segments S4–S5
C	Incomplete; motor function preserved below the neurologic level; more than half of key muscles below the neurologic level with a muscle grade less than 3
D	Incomplete; motor function preserved below the neurologic level; at least half of key muscles below the neurologic level with a muscle grade of 3 or greater
E	Normal; sensory and motor function normal

Source: American Spinal Injury Association. International Standards for Neurological and Functional Classification of Spinal Cord Injury. Chicago: American Spinal Injury Association, 1996.

Though mortality after SCI has improved considerably, it remains higher than that of the general population. The most common causes of death for those surviving more than a day are pneumonia, nonischemic heart disease, and sepsis. If ischemic and nonischemic cardiac disease are grouped, cardiac disease is the most common cause. The frequencies of such causes as sepsis, pulmonary embolus, and pneumonia are increased most by SCI. SCI particularly increases by a factor of 210 the risk of death from pulmonary embolus during the first year.

Factors Affecting Prognosis

Neurologic Status

The degree of completeness of injury is described by the American Spinal Injury Association (ASIA) impairment scale (Table 52-1). A grade of A corresponds to a complete lesion; grades B through E are incomplete. The use of the scale is preferred over the use of verbal description, and the suffix -*paresis* is not used. The ASIA impairment scale grade is crucial for prognosis. Table 52-2 correlates admission and discharge grades. Apparently, improvement from grade A to a grade B or better is very unusual, and prognosis (in terms of improving grade) is poor. A decline in grade is equally unusual, as for example, prognosis is good for those admitted with a grade of D.

The prognosis for those admitted as grades B and C is less clear. Those admitted as grade B have a 28% chance of improving to grade D. However,

Table 52-2. Comparison of Hospital Admission Frankel Grade to Discharge Frankel Grade

		Discharge Frankel Grade			
		A	B	C	D
Admission Frankel Grade	A	89	5	3	3
	B	5	49	16	28
	C	2	1	41	53
	D	1	1	1	90

Note: Frankel grade closely corresponds to American Spinal Injury Association impairment grade. The rows and columns do not sum to 100 because data in some cases were incomplete, and cases involving a grade of E are not included.
Source: SL Stover, JA DeLisa, GG Whiteneck (eds). Spinal Cord Injury. Gaithersburg, MD: Aspen, 1995.

in one study, the subset of subjects with the ability to discriminate sharp and dull sensation performed better, with a majority gaining the ability to walk at least 200 feet with a reciprocal gait with or without the use of ankle-foot orthoses. (This ability may be explained by the proximity of the corresponding sensory tracts to the motor tracts.) Those admitted as grade C have a 53% chance of improving to D. One study considered subjects admitted as grade C and possessing initial quadriceps strength of 2/5 or less. All nine who developed quadriceps strength of more than 3/5 on one side by 2 months became functionally ambulatory. In another study of persons with incomplete paraplegia, all 29 subjects with a lower-extremity motor score (LEMS) of 10 or above at 30 days after injury later were able to ambulate in the community with a reciprocal gait. (The LEMS is determined by summing the muscle grades for each of the 10 key muscles for nerve roots L2 through S1.) Overall, 76% of those with incomplete paraplegia eventually were able to walk. In a similar study of persons with incomplete tetraplegia, all 15 subjects with a LEMS of at least 20 at 30 days after injury were able to walk in the community with a reciprocal gait at 1 year after injury; none of the 13 subjects with a LEMS of 0 at 1 month gained such ability. Overall, 46% of those with incomplete tetraplegia were able to walk.

Though persons with ASIA grade A injuries generally do not improve in terms of ASIA impairment grade, improvement can be seen in root function about the area of injury. Often, individuals gain one motor level. This motor improvement may occur through the mechanism of peripheral sprouting.

For a given neurologic impairment, functional prognosis is better for younger individuals than for older. After SCI with central cord syndrome, a majority of patients younger than 50 years will achieve ambulation, whereas this is not true of older subjects.

Functional Performance

Functional performance, including mobility and activities of daily living, can be predicted for persons with ASIA A (complete) injuries based on neurologic level. Those with spinal cord levels above C5 are dependent for transfers and for all activities of daily living. Such persons usually are able to operate a powered wheelchair, and they can locomote independently (in an appropriate environment). A reclining seat mechanism allows independence in the crucial activity of weight shifting to avoid pressure ulceration. A level of C5 or C6 allows the performance of some activities of daily living, such as upper-body dressing, but not others, such as bathing. Such a person can propel a manual wheelchair over limited distances. Operation of an adapted automobile or van also is possible. A person with a level of C7 can achieve independence in all activities of daily living and can transfer to a wheelchair and locomote in a suitable environment, which allows independent living. A person with paraplegia and a midthoracic level may be capable of ambulation, using bilateral knee-ankle-foot orthoses and a walker. However, this ambulation is not practical, and a

Table 52-3. Key Muscles

Nerve Root	Function
C5	Elbow flexors
C6	Wrist extensors
C7	Elbow extensors
C8	Flexor digitorum profundus to the middle finger
T1	Small-finger abductors
L2	Hip flexors
L3	Knee extensors
L4	Ankle dorsiflexors
L5	Extensor hallucis longus
S1	Ankle plantar flexors

Source: American Spinal Injury Association. International Standards for Neurological and Functional Classification of Spinal Cord Injury. Chicago: American Spinal Injury Association, 1996.

wheelchair provides superior performance in everyday activities. Through activity of the hip flexors, a spinal cord level of L2 allows a reciprocal gait pattern, and a level of L3, through the activity of the quadriceps, renders possible the stabilization of the knees without the need for knee-ankle-foot orthoses, though bilateral ankle-foot orthoses and bilateral canes or crutches may be needed for community ambulation.

Evaluation for Prognosis

The neurologic examination provides the most useful information for neurologic prognosis after SCI. The examination has been standardized by ASIA and includes measurement of motor and sensory function (Tables 52-3 and 52-4), allowing determination of the spinal cord level (the most caudal extension of continuous, normal function) and completeness as described by the ASIA impairment scale (see Table 52-1).

Information from magnetic resonance imaging also can contribute to prognosis. Findings associated with severe neurologic deficit and poorer prognosis are cord contusion involving more than one spinal segment and intramedullary hematoma. Less severe deficits and better prognosis are associated with normal spinal cord signal and small focal contusions associated with edema encompassing one spinal segment or less.

Table 52-4. Key Sensory Points

Nerve Root	Sensory Point
C2	Occipital protuberance
C3	Supraclavicular fossa
C4	Top of the acromioclavicular joint
C5	Lateral side of the antecubital fossa
C6	Thumb
C7	Middle finger
C8	Little finger
T1	Medial (ulnar) side of the antecubital fossa
T2	Apex of the axilla
T3	Third intercostal space
T4	Fourth intercostal space (nipple line)
T5	Fifth intercostal space (midway between T4 and T6)
T6	Sixth intercostal space (level of xiphisternum)
T7	Seventh intercostal space (midway between T6 and T8)
T8	Eighth intercostal space (midway between T10 and T12)
T9	Ninth intercostal space (midway between T8 and T10)
T10	Tenth intercostal space (umbilicus)
T11	Eleventh intercostal space (midway between T10 and T12)
T12	Inguinal ligament at midpoint
L1	Half the distance between T12 and L2
L2	Mid-anterior thigh
L3	Medial femoral condyle
L4	Medial malleolus
L5	Dorsum of the foot at the third metatarsal phalangeal joint
S1	Lateral heel
S2	Popliteal fossa in the midline
S3	Ischial tuberosity
S4–5	Perianal area

Source: American Spinal Injury Association. International Standards for Neurological and Functional Classification of Spinal Cord Injury. Chicago: American Spinal Injury Association, 1996.

Therapies Affecting Prognosis

Neurologic outcome of SCI is improved by the intravenous administration of methylprednisolone, 30 mg per kg, over a 15-minute period, followed by an interval of 45 minutes, then 5.4 mg per kg per hour for 23 hours. Treatment should begin within 8 hours of injury. Motor and sensory function are improved, regardless of whether measured 6 weeks or 6 months after injury and whether the injury initially causes partial or complete loss of motor and

sensory function. Treatment is not associated with significant increases in adverse events, such as wound infection or gastrointestinal bleeding. Treatment beginning more than 8 hours after injury is not effective.

Available soon should be results concerning other acute and subacute chemotherapeutic interventions, including such agents as GM_1 ganglioside and tirilazad. Also in progress is investigation concerning treatments for chronic, stable deficits, including transplantation of nerve and glial cells, and administration of such agents as 4-aminopyridine.

Spinal surgery can allow rapid mobilization after SCI and may decrease hospital length of stay. In such situations as an individual with declining neurologic status, surgery clearly may be indicated. No beneficial effect of surgery on neurologic outcome has been demonstrated for individuals with stable neurologic status.

Muscle paralyzed by upper motor neuron injury will respond to electrical stimulation of its nerve supply. Functional neuromuscular stimulation is patterned to cause muscle activity useful for exercise or function. Stimulation is produced by surface, percutaneous, or implanted electrodes. Such neuromuscular stimulation is better developed for lower-extremity function, and an available commercial system provides a reciprocal gait for those with paraplegia, using a walker and orthoses. Extensive training is necessary, and the system does not replace the use of a wheelchair for everyday activities.

Upper-extremity function after SCI can be improved by reconstructive surgery. In a typical procedure, a functioning but nonessential muscle is used to provide a lost motion. An example is the use of the posterior deltoid muscle to extend the elbow in a person with C5 or C6 tetraplegia.

Short-Term Prognosis

Acute SCI tends to affect the young male population. The neurologic status on presentation is very predictive of eventual neurologic function, with complete lesions doing poorest and mild, incomplete lesions doing much better (see Table 52-2). Treatment with intravenous methylprednisolone improves motor and sensory outcome. Common causes of early mortality are pneumonia and pulmonary embolus. More than 90% of those admitted for SCI survive to hospital discharge.

Long-Term Prognosis

More than 90% of individuals who are discharged from a hospital after SCI go to private residences in the community rather than to institutions. The rate of employment drops precipitously in the years after SCI but, by 10 years, has recovered to some 30%, which is half the rate of employment at the time of SCI. The educational level achieved rises in the years after SCI and comes to exceed that of the population in general. The educational level achieved by tetraplegic persons exceeds that of paraplegic persons. The rate of marriage in postinjury years for persons with SCI who are single at the time of SCI is lower than that of the general population. The rate of divorce for those who are married at the time of injury is increased, but a majority of those married at the time of injury still are married 5 years later. Women remain fertile after SCI, and available techniques can obtain semen from men with SCI for the purpose of insemination.

The suicide rate for those with SCI exceeds that of the general population. However, a majority of long-term survivors of SCI are glad to be alive, and severe impairment is compatible with a high degree of life satisfaction. In fact, life satisfaction may be less affected by the degree of neurologic impairment than by other factors, such as social integration.

Additional Reading

American Spinal Injury Association. International Standards for Neurological and Functional Classification of Spinal Cord Injury. Chicago: American Spinal Injury Association, 1996.

Bracken MB, Shepard MJ, Collins WF Jr, et al. A randomized, controlled trial of methylprednisolone or naloxone in the treatment after acute spinal cord injury: results of the second National Acute Spinal Cord Injury Study. N Engl J Med 1990;322:1405–1411.

Crozier KS, Cheng LL, Graziani V, et al. Spinal cord injury: prognosis for ambulation based on quadriceps recovery. Paraplegia 1992;30:762–767.

Crozier KS, Graziani V, Ditunno JF Jr, Herbison GJ. Spinal cord injury: prognosis for ambulation based on sensory examination in patients who are initially motor complete. Arch Phys Med Rehabil 1991;72:119–121.

Ditunno JF Jr, Formal CS. Chronic spinal cord injury. N Engl J Med 1994;330:550–556.

Donovan WH. Operative and nonoperative management of spinal cord injury. A review. Paraplegia 1994;32:375–388.

Stover SL, DeLisa JA, Whiteneck GG (eds). Spinal Cord Injury. Gaithersburg, MD: Aspen, 1995.

Waters RL, Adkins RH, Yakura JS, Sie I. Motor and sensory function following incomplete paraplegia. Arch Phys Med Rehabil 1994;75:67–72.

Waters RL, Adkins RH, Yakura JS, Sie I. Motor and sensory function following incomplete tetraplegia. Arch Phys Med Rehabil 1994;75:306–311.

Weinstein DE, Ko H, Graziani V, Ditunno JF Jr. Prognostic significance of the delayed plantar reflex following spinal cord injury. J Spinal Cord Med 1997;20:207–211.

Part X

Peripheral Nerve Disorders

Chapter 53

Guillain-Barré Syndrome and Related Demyelinating Neuropathies

Mark B. Bromberg

The demyelinating neuropathies represent a class of neuropathies in which the primary site of pathology is the myelin sheath, although axonal involvement also may be present in varying degrees. Within this class are subclasses that differ with respect to clinical presentation, degree of axonal pathology, and the presence of associated disorders. The prognosis and prognostic factors are unique for the different subclasses of demyelinating neuropathies. This chapter focuses on the more common demyelinating neuropathies and considers four questions:

1. What is the correct diagnosis?
2. What is the natural history of the neuropathy?
3. How does treatment affect long-term prognosis?
4. Do prognostic factors exist early in the course of the neuropathy?

The demyelinating neuropathies can be divided first by the clinical time course into acute and chronic forms. Guillain-Barré syndrome (GBS) is the most common demyelinating neuropathy and represents an acute, self-limited disorder. *GBS* is an eponym for acute flaccid paralysis due to damage of peripheral nerves. As originally described by Landry in 1859 and Guillain, Barré, and Strohl in 1916, this disorder is characterized by rapidly progressing weakness with areflexia and albuminocytologic dissociation. It had a favorable prognosis ("maladie bénigne et spontanément curable") if respiratory failure did not occur. Since the early recognition of the disorder, much new information that has become available focuses on the time course of progression, variants, and treatment. The syndromic

nature of GBS has been expanded and a new nomenclature proposed to describe subclasses (Fig. 53-1). Also, new information on pathophysiology relates to prognosis.

Chronic forms of demyelinating neuropathies are termed *chronic inflammatory demyelinating polyradiculoneuropathies* (CIDPs) or *chronic relapsing inflammatory polyneuropathies*. They follow a variety of clinical patterns and generally are believed to represent lifelong disorders. The long-term course and prognosis of CIDP are influenced strongly by treatment regimens. CIDP may be associated with several blood cell dyscrasias or other disorders, either at time of diagnosis or later in the course (Table 53-1). The nomenclature of CIDP should reflect the associated disorders, because the prognosis of the neuropathy is influenced strongly by the concomitant disorder.

Guillain-Barré Syndrome

Natural History

All forms of GBS follow a monophasic time course. Symptoms progress over a limited period, and more than 95% of patients reach their weakest state within 4 weeks of symptom onset. If symptoms progress over a longer time, the diagnosis of GBS should be questioned, and that of CIDP should be raised. The severity of symptoms at the nadir varies markedly, from mild limitations of function to paralysis and respiratory failure. The pathologic basis for the vari-

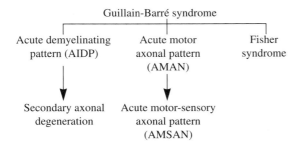

Figure 53-1. Relationships among forms of the Guillain-Barré syndrome. (Reprinted with permission from JW Griffin, CY Li, W Ho, et al. Pathology of the motor-sensory axonal Guillain-Barré syndrome. Ann Neurol 1996;39:26.)

ability in symptom severity depends on several factors, including the degree of demyelination, the degree of axonal damage, and the distribution of axonal damage along the course of the nerve fibers (proximal segments, including roots, or distal segments, including intramuscular branches).

Antecedent illnesses are reported in more than one-half of patients within 2 to 3 weeks of symptom onset. GBS is not thought to be a direct infection of the peripheral nervous system but is considered to represent an uncommon complication of a bacterial or viral illness. Recognized factors underlying the pathogenesis of demyelination and axonal damage have increased the understanding of the varying severity of dysfunction and ultimate outcome. These factors include the role of a specific antecedent illness, *Campylobacter jejuni* gastroenteritis, the formation of antibodies that recognize specific peripheral nervous system gangliosides that likely represent "molecular mimicry" between the bacterium and the neuronal gangliosides, and whether the antibody-mediated immune damage is directed primarily to myelin or to the axon.

The spectrum of acute flaccid paralysis includes a number of different types of GBS, each with unique pathologic features, prognosis, response to treatment, and prognostic factors.

Acute Inflammatory Demyelinating Polyradiculoneuropathy

Acute inflammatory demyelinating polyradiculoneuropathy (AIDP) is the form ascribed to

Table 53-1. Disorders Associated with Chronic Inflammatory Demyelinating Polyradiculoneuropathy

Monoclonal gammopathy of uncertain significance
Multiple myeloma
Plasma-cell cytoma
Waldenström's macroglobulinemia
Polyneuropathy, organomegaly, monoclonal gammopathy, endocrinopathies, skin changes (POMES syndrome)
Castleman's disease
Human immunodeficiency virus

Table 53-2. Disability Grading Scale

Grade	Disability
0	Healthy
1	Minor signs or symptoms
2	Able to walk 5 meters without a walker or equivalent support
3	Able to walk 5 meters with a walker or support
4	Bed- or chair-bound (unable to walk 5 meters with a walker or support)
5	Requires assisted ventilation (for at least part of the day)
6	Dead

Landry, Guillain, Barré, and Strohl. It is primarily a macrophage-mediated immune demyelinating disorder. Both distal and proximal (roots) nerve segments are affected preferentially. Axonal damage is thought to be a secondary pathologic process or an "innocent bystander." This form of GBS is the most common in North America.

The most detailed information about the course of AIDP and the effects of treatment come from formal therapeutic treatment trials in which the time required to change grades within a functional disability scale (Table 53-2) has been studied over a relatively limited (6-month) observation period. Fewer data focus on the ultimate level of functional disability achieved at the end of the recovery phase (18 to 24 months). Accordingly, a distinction is drawn between *rate* of recovery over an intermediate period (6 months) and final *extent* of recovery for AIDP patients.

Mortality from AIDP is less than 3% with recognition of impending respiratory failure and good intensive care. The long-term outcome after an average of 5 years of follow-up includes 60% with full functional recovery, 20% with residual leg weakness (ranging from mild to disabling), and 20% with residual sensory symptoms.

Acute Motor and Sensory Axonal Neuropathy

Acute motor and sensory axonal neuropathy (AMSAN) is the "axonal" form of GBS. A strong association is evident between an antecedent *C. jejuni* bacterial gastroenteritis and the production of antibodies to GM_1 gangliosides. The antibody-mediated attack is focused on the axon at the nodes of Ranvier, and the degree of axonal damage is severe. Sites of involvement include the entire length of the nerve. This disease represents a rare form of GBS in North America.

The prognosis of the AMSAN form is the least favorable because of its widespread axonal damage. Patients usually become respirator-dependent, and weaning them may require up to 6 months. Mortality may be higher than that in AIDP, usually owing to complications of prolonged intensive respiratory care. Improvement in disability rating is slow (12 to 18 months) and incomplete, with difficulty in ambulation a common sequel.

Acute Motor Axonal Neuropathy

Acute motor axonal neuropathy (AMAN) is the "paralytic China neuropathy." The clinical course is characterized by acute flaccid paralysis leading to quadriplegia with areflexia, frequent respiratory failure requiring ventilatory support, but no sensory symptoms. It is most common in rural areas, has a very high summer incidence, and preferentially affects children. This form has been seen most in northern China but also in Korea and Mexico. An antecedent *C. jejuni* infection is common, and the disease provides evidence of antibodies that recognize GM_1 gangliosides. The primary site of pathology is macrophage-mediated axonal injury at the nodes of Ranvier. Severe cases leading to death evince extensive proximal axonal damage. Antibody-mediated mechanisms may cause more distal denervation and regional conduction block to account for the relatively rapid and good recovery despite the axonal pathologic findings. The AMAN form is believed to be a less severe form of AMSAN.

The AMAN form of GBS is unique and includes a good prognosis. Early mortality (30%) was high but is less than 5% with good respiratory care. Recovery may begin within weeks. At 1 year, most patients can ambulate, although some have distal limb weakness. Older patients may have a slower rate of recovery.

Uncommon Variants

Uncommon variants of GBS exist. Although the clinical presentation may appear to differ from acute flaccid paralysis, all are thought to be variants of GBS because the course of progression is acute (reaching clinical nadir within 4 weeks), areflexia is found in the regions involved, and the cerebrospinal fluid protein is elevated. Segmental variants are characterized by weakness involving such regions of the body as pharyngeal-cervical-brachial nerves or lumbosacral nerves. Although autonomic dysfunction is common in AIDP, primary involvement of the autonomic nervous system occurs, albeit with some electrodiagnostic evidence for mild somatic nerve involvement. Pure pandysautonomia, without evidence of somatic nerve involvement, is exceedingly rare. Only the Fisher variant is considered in this chapter because the other variants are extremely rare, although the prognosis is considered to be good.

Fisher Variant. The Fisher variant is characterized by the triad of ophthalmoplegia, ataxia, and areflexia. Ophthalmoparesis is the presenting or early sign and may not become complete ophthalmoplegia. Motor weakness is not apparent on clinical testing. A strong association is seen between an antecedent *C. jejuni* infection and antibodies against the ganglioside GQ_{1b}. Electrophysiologic testing shows a greater degree of primary axonal changes in sensory nerves (reduced sensory nerve action potential amplitude) than in motor nerves (reduced compound muscle action potential [CMAP]) but a greater degree of axonal motor nerve involvement in cranial nerves. The overall prognosis of the Fisher variant is good, with the majority of patients showing no (or mild) residua assessed at 2 to 10 months. The contrast between axonal damage and rapid and full recovery has similarities to the clinical picture in the AMAN form of GBS, including evidence for an antecedent infection with *C. jejuni* and antibodies reactive to the ganglioside GQ_{1b}. The antibodies also react to cerebellar tissue, and both central and peripheral nervous systems may be involved in the Fisher variant.

Acute Inflammatory Demyelinating Polyradiculoneuropathy in Children.   Children of any age may develop AIDP (with cases seen in neonates), but it is more common after the age of 2. The clinical features are similar, but mortality is lower, and prognosis is good and may be better than that in adults. Long-term follow-up shows that more than 90% have good or full recovery of function. The poor prognostic finding in adults of low mean CMAP amplitude has not been tested fully in children.

Acute Inflammatory Demyelinating Polyradiculoneuropathy in Pregnancy.   A review of a limited number of cases indicates that AIDP has a minimal effect on the fetus and on the mother. No evidence substantiates transplacental transfer to infants of antibodies related to AIDP. The severity of weakness in the mother can include respiratory failure, but maternal mortality is no higher with good respiratory care. Termination of a pregnancy has little effect on the time course of weakness. Infant mortality, although very low (<4%), likely reflects factors other than maternal AIDP.

Factors Affecting Prognosis

Three inherent risk factors have been identified for a poor prognosis over the first 6 months in untreated patients: low mean CMAP amplitude, age older than 30 years, and respiratory failure requiring artificial ventilation. A fourth factor is the duration of symptoms before initiation of treatment (plasmapheresis).

Mean Compound Muscle Action Potential Amplitude

Statistically, low mean CMAP is the most powerful predictor of poor recovery rate. The mean CMAP amplitude is determined by summing the values obtained from the AIDP patient to routine distal motor nerve stimulation and expressing them as a percentage of the mean of the laboratories' lower limits of normal amplitude for the nerves studied. Mean amplitudes of 20% of normal are predictors of poor rate of improvement. Low CMAP reflects a reduced number of functioning motor units, either due to demyelination causing conduction block or due to axonal damage causing denervation. In AIDP, axonal damage with denervation is most likely. Thus, the prognostic value is a reflection of the degree of denervation.

In the AMAN form, the prognostic factor of a low mean CMAP amplitude does not predict outcome accurately as it does for AIDP and AMSAN. This limitation suggests that, although profuse denervation is present, it must be at a very distal site along the motor axon so that the time needed for regeneration is short. The poor risk factor of age in the AMAN form likely reflects a reduced capacity to regrow axons.

Age

Older age, not surprisingly, is a poor prognostic factor. In general, patients younger than 30 years fare better than do patients older than 60 years. The poorer outcome with age is not a reflection of greater electrodiagnostic abnormalities but more likely is a reflection of reduced capacity to regenerate new myelin or to grow new axons.

Respiratory Failure

As might be expected, ventilator dependency is a poor prognostic factor and most likely reflects a greater degree of axonal damage. The AMSAN, or axonal, form of GBS represents an extreme degree of axonal damage, and patients become quadriplegic and ventilator-dependent within days of symptom onset. The mean CMAP amplitude values are very low or zero in these patients, and their prognosis is the poorest of those for the different forms of GBS. Before the availability of intensive care units and positive-pressure ventilation, respiratory failure was the most common cause of death in GBS. Ventilator-dependent patients are at greater risk for life-threatening cardiac arrhythmias, pneumonia, pulmonary embolism, adult respiratory distress syndrome, and myocardial infarction. In reviews of GBS, the mortality rate for AIDP is near 3%.

Therapies Affecting Prognosis

Several randomized studies have demonstrated the efficacy of plasmapheresis and intravenous immune

Table 53-3. Time for Patients to Reach Grade 2 (Able to Walk Unassisted)

Group	Median Time After Treatment (days)		
	Plasmapheresis	Conventional	*p* Value*
All patients	53	85	<0.0001
Respirator patient subgroup	97	169	<0.01

*Determined from Kaplan-Meier curves.
Source: Adapted from The Guillain-Barré Syndrome Study Group. Plasmapheresis and acute Guillain-Barré syndrome. Neurology 1985;35:1096–1104.

globulin (IVIG) on the rate of improvement in AIDP over 6 months of follow-up. Efficacy endpoint measures were the time to change functional grades (see Table 53-2).

Compared to best supportive treatment, plasmapheresis has been shown to result in greater functional status (see Table 53-2) after 4 weeks, a shorter time to improve one grade, a shorter time to reach grade 2 (unassisted walking), and a better outcome at 6 months (Table 53-3). Patients who experienced respiratory support after starting plasmapheresis required support for a shorter period than did untreated patients with respiratory failure. Patients who required respiratory support before treatment did not experience a shortened time on the respirator. Differences were noted in outcome on the basis of when plasmapheresis was started. Patients who underwent treatment within 7 days of symptom onset showed the most rapid rate and greatest degree of improvement, as compared to patients who began treatment after the first week, but late plasmapheresis still was effective, as compared to untreated patients. Comparison studies have investigated the efficacy of plasmapheresis and IVIG. Both modes of therapy have been found to be approximately equally effective on the rate and degree of improvement over the first 6 months.

Treatment of AIDP in children is similar to treatment of adults, and plasmapheresis has been effective. Procedural difficulties attend plasmapheresis in children who weigh less than 30 kg because the priming volume of the pheresis machines competes with the child's small blood volumes. Priming with whole blood or exchange transfusions has been performed with good success under these circumstances but with the risks of transmitting infection inherent with whole-blood products. Difficulties also arise with venous access and acceptance of

central lines in children. IVIG has been used also with good therapeutic success to circumvent some of these problems.

Relapse in Acute Inflammatory Demyelinating Polyradiculoneuropathy

Several types of relapses have been described. A true relapse, or a recurrence of GBS, must be distinguished from CIDP. Although many aspects of AIDP and CIDP—such as immune-mediated demyelination—are similar, clear differences are seen in mechanisms, prognosis, and treatment. The primary difference is the immune mechanism; AIDP is a self-limited disease that follows a monophasic course because it is likely a response to an infection. CIDP has a protracted time course, with either an exacerbating and remitting course or a progressive course. Although the first symptoms of CIDP usually develop over several months, distinguishing between the two entities may not be possible if the first symptoms of CIDP are treated within the first 4 weeks.

True recurrent AIDP follows the same monophasic, self-limited time course as that of the initial event. Recurrence is rare—2 to 5% in large series. The interval between episodes ranges from months to more than 30 years. An occasional patient will experience recurrent episodes in the setting of infections.

Apparent relapses have been described after a good response to plasmapheresis. Some believe that when AIDP is recognized early and a series of plasmapheresis is started promptly, the monophasic immune mechanism still can be in effect in some patients when the series of phereses has been completed, a condition resulting in a rise of antibody

Table 53-4. Probability of Reaching Independent Ambulation

Patient Status	CMAP	1 Month		3 Months		6 Months	
		Pheresis (%)	None (%)	Pheresis (%)	None (%)	Pheresis (%)	None (%)
Not on respirator							
Prior illness >7 days							
Age 30	N	55	29	95	73	100	90
	A	25	11	67	38	86	56
Age 60	N	43	21	89	60	98	80
	A	18	8	54	28	59	44
Prior illness ≤7 days							
Age 30	N	39	19	85	56	96	76
	A	16	7	49	25	70	40
Age 60	N	29	14	74	43	90	63
	A	12	5	38	18	57	30
On respirator							
Prior illness >7 days							
Age 30	N	37	18	84	54	96	74
	A	15	7	48	24	68	39
Age 60	N	28	13	72	42	89	61
	A	11	5	37	18	55	29
Prior illness ≤7 days							
Age 30	N	25	12	67	38	86	57
	A	10	4	33	16	50	26
Age 60	N	18	8	54	28	75	44
	A	7	3	24	11	39	19

CMAP = compound motor action potential; N = normal (defined as >20% of normal lower limit); A = abnormal (<20% of normal lower limit).

Note: Pheresis is accomplished using a continuous-flow machine.

Source: Adapted from The Guillain-Barré Syndrome Study Group. Plasmapheresis and acute Guillain-Barré syndrome. Neurology 1985;35:1096–1104.

titers that mimic an apparent relapse. The plasmapheresis treatment protocol should be modified to include an extension of less frequent phereses out to 5 weeks from symptom onset. Several studies have reported relapse or failure after initial treatment with IVIG, and these patients have responded favorably to plasmapheresis.

Short- and Long-Term Prognosis

The short-term prognosis for AIDP—the probability of being ambulatory (disability grade 2) at 3 months—depends on the degree of axonal damage, severity of weakness, the patient's age, and promptness of treatment (Table 53-4). Overall, 70% of treated patients (plasmapheresis or IVIG) will be ambulatory at 3 months, but only 45% will be ambulatory if they required artificial ventilation.

Over the long term, the probability of being fully ambulatory (grade 0) at 3 to 5 years is 60%, and the probability of being ambulatory but with mild weakness (grade 1 or 2) is 20%.

Chronic Inflammatory Demyelinating Polyneuropathy

Natural History

Idiopathic Disease

CIDP with no associated disorders is called *idiopathic CIDP* and is the most common form. It is a chronic disorder that follows a number of time course patterns that are altered by treatment regimens. Formal diagnostic criteria apply to the disease. The immune-mediated damage in CIDP is believed to be directed primarily at myelin but, because of the chronic nature of the disease, the time for secondary axonal damage to occur is greater. As in AIDP and AMSAN, the most important prognostic factors are the degree of axonal damage and advanced age. Several blood cell dyscrasias may be associated with CIDP and may result in a greater degree of axonal damage (see Table 53-1).

The current prognosis of CIDP is linked strongly to treatment. The natural history of CIDP, before treatment with corticosteroids was introduced, includes several time courses: a relapsing and remitting course with variable degrees of disability during remissions; a slowly progressive course leading to total disability over months to years (and to death in some patients); and a stepwise progressive course. The wider recognition of chronic inflammatory neuropathies has led to earlier diagnosis and treatment, and distinguishing between remissions or relapses is difficult, owing to the natural history or to treatment.

The chronic nature of CIDP makes a cure unlikely, and the goals of treatment are to improve prognosis through individualized treatment regimens. Many treatment modalities and protocols are available. This review of prognosis focuses on reports of large series of patients with CIDP. The results of treatment of CIDP associated with more rare conditions frequently are reported as anecdotal examples and are not considered.

Disease with Monoclonal Gammopathy of Uncertain Significance

Approximately 30% of adult-age patients will have an associated monoclonal gammopathy of uncertain significance (MGUS). MGUS represents a monoclonal plasma-cell proliferation that formerly was considered benign because no abnormalities are noted on skeletal radiologic surveys and bone marrow biopsies at the time of diagnosis. However, MGUS may evolve into a recognized plasma-cell dyscrasia over time, and CIDP-MGUS patients must be followed indefinitely for a dyscrasia. An occasional patient will have CIDP-MGUS with an isolated plasma-cell cytoma detected on skeletal radiographic survey. The radiographic finding may be interpreted as equivocal, but these findings must be pursued, for these patients usually respond poorly to treatment until the cytoma

is treated specifically. Patients with CIDP-MGUS have a more indolent course as compared to that of patients with idiopathic CIDP.

Disease in Childhood

Although rare, CIDP occurs in childhood. Generally, treatment and prognosis are similar to those in adults. Approximately 25% of patients have a monophasic course with good functional recovery. Approximately 75% of patients have a relapsing course, with residual weakness in those with more frequent relapses.

Disease in Pregnancy

The onset of CIDP may occur during pregnancy or, in established CIDP, relapses may occur in association with pregnancies. The relapse rate with pregnancy appears to be greater than the relapse rate when not pregnant. Furthermore, relapses tend to occur during the third trimester.

Factors and Therapies Affecting Prognosis

The results of retrospective CIDP patient reviews indicate that most patients receive early treatment of their initial symptoms, with more than 80% responding to treatment within weeks, resulting in an improvement in functional grade. For approximately 40% of patients, treatment results in a monophasic course, whereas 40% have a relapsing course requiring adjustment of treatment. Approximately 15% of patients have a progressive course despite treatment. Overall, the mortality is approximately 10%. Poor prognostic factors are advanced age and marked degree of axonal loss.

Long-Term Prognosis

The long-term prognosis after 5 or more years for patients with CIDP is dependent on continued treatment, and no standards are available for immunosuppressive treatment regimens. Approximately 65% of patients with idiopathic CIDP will be without functional limitations or have only mild functional impairment (grade 0 or 1). Patients with CIDP-MGUS fare worse, and only 40% will function at grade 0 or 1.

Additional Reading

Ad Hoc Subcommittee of the AAN AIDS Task Force. Research criteria for diagnosis of chronic inflammatory demyelinating polyneuropathy (CIDP). Neurology 1991;41:617–618.

Bril V, Ilse WK, Pearce R, et al. Pilot trial of immunoglobulin versus plasma exchange in patients with Guillain-Barré syndrome. Neurology 1996;46:100–103.

Bromberg MB, Feldman EL, Jaradeh S, Albers JW. Prognosis in long-term immunosuppressive treatment of refractory chronic inflammatory demyelinating polyradiculoneuropathy. J Clin Epidemiol 1992;45:47–52.

Griffin JW, Li CY, Ho W, et al. Pathology of the motor-sensory axonal Guillain-Barré syndrome. Ann Neurol 1996;39:17–28.

The Guillain-Barré Syndrome Study Group. Plasmapheresis and acute Guillain-Barré syndrome. Neurology 1985;35:1096–1104.

McKhann GM, Griffin JW, Cornblath DR, et al. Plasmapheresis and Guillain-Barré syndrome: analysis of prognostic factors and the effects of plasmapheresis. Ann Neurol 1988;23:347–353.

Simmons Z, Albers JW, Bromberg MB, Feldman EL. Long-term follow-up of patients with chronic inflammatory demyelinating polyradiculopathy, without and with monoclonal gammopathy. Brain 1995;118:359–368.

Simmons Z, Albers JW, Bromberg MB, Feldman EL. Presentation and initial clinical course in patients with chronic inflammatory demyelinating polyradiculopathy: comparison of patients without and with monoclonal gammopathy. Neurology 1993;43:2202–2209.

van der Meché, Schmitz PIM, and the Dutch Guillain-Barré Study Group. A randomized trial comparing intravenous immune globulin and plasma exchange in Guillain-Barré syndrome. N Engl J Med 1992;326:1123–1129.

Chapter 54

Acquired Axonal Polyneuropathies

Daniel M. Feinberg and Eric L. Logigian

Axonal polyneuropathy is a syndrome of structural and functional deterioration of the peripheral nervous system (PNS) in response to a generalized exogenous or endogenous insult directed against PNS axons. Numerous causes are responsible for acquired axonal polyneuropathy. These neuropathies can be classified into three somewhat overlapping categories: (1) axonal polyneuropathies associated with systemic disease, (2) immune- or infection-mediated inflammatory axonal polyneuropathies, and (3) toxic axonal polyneuropathies. As difficulty attends making generalizations about prognosis of the many different acquired axonal polyneuropathies, this chapter addresses one representative example from each of these three categories.

Acquired Axonal Neuropathy Associated with Systemic Disease

The most common neuropathy in the category of acquired axonal neuropathy associated with systemic disease—and in the Western world—is diabetic neuropathy. Diabetes is associated with various cranial and limb mononeuropathies and with polyneuropathies. The two main diabetic polyneuropathies are a common, chronic, symmetric distal polyneuropathy and a less common, acute or subacute, asymmetric proximal neuropathy of the legs (i.e., diabetic amyotrophy).

Natural History

Approximately 50% of patients with long-standing diabetes mellitus, either insulin-dependent or non–insulin-dependent, develop a symmetric, distally predominant axonal polyneuropathy. The course of this neuropathy is variable but, in many patients, it evolves clinically from a sensory to a sensorimotor to a sensorimotor-autonomic neuropathy. The sensory disturbance often ascends over time from toes to knees, then to fingertips, then to the anterior trunk. Initially, annoying paresthesia predominates but, in some 10% of patients, incapacitating burning pain eventually develops.

An asymmetric proximal motor neuropathy, most commonly affecting hip, thigh, and ankle dorsiflexor muscles, occurs in elderly non–insulin-dependent diabetics. Sudden onset of deep, aching pain heralds the onset of weakness and wasting of proximal muscles. The patellar reflex usually is absent or diminished markedly. Except for severe pain, the majority of patients experience little sensory disturbance. Weight loss is common. Recovery occurs spontaneously over time. Within days to weeks, pain resolves regardless of whether it is treated. Muscle strength improves more slowly, usually within 6 to 12 months. Approximately 40% of patients have substantial residual disability due to muscle weakness and, less commonly, due to persistent pain. Not infrequently, the neuropathy recurs, this time on the unaffected side.

Factors Affecting Prognosis

In general, the severity and course of symmetric distal sensorimotor polyneuropathy parallels the course of diabetes mellitus. Clinically detectable neuropathy is correlated positively with duration of diabetes, serum glucose levels, age, height, and male gender. A genetic predisposition is suggested, but this hypothesis has not been proved.

By comparison, proximal diabetic neuropathy more commonly affects older patients. It is related less to disease duration and serum glucose levels.

Evaluation for Prognosis

Sensory nerve conduction abnormalities and denervation on electromyography (EMG) often are present even in subclinical symmetric diabetic neuropathy. In patients with more severe deficits, abnormalities in motor nerve conduction studies may be present as well. Several studies show correlations between clinical severity of neuropathy, increasing duration of diabetes mellitus, poor glucose control, and reduction in motor nerve conduction velocity.

The presence of active denervation in affected limb and associated paraspinal muscles is the electrophysiologic signature of proximal diabetic neuropathy. Often, such patients also have nerve conduction evidence of a mild, symmetric, distal polyneuropathy. In general, motor unit recruitment is reduced in proportion to muscle weakness. Prognosis likely depends in part on the number of residual motor units.

Therapies Affecting Prognosis

The morbidity of diabetic neuropathy is codependent on the presence of other end-organ damage, such as peripheral vascular, coronary, and renal disease. With tight control of serum glucose via multiple daily injections or an insulin pump or by pancreatic transplantation, the prognosis of diabetic neuropathy is improved. At a minimum, aggressive glucose control can delay the appearance of distal symmetric neuropathy by some 60% at 5 years and, therefore, its most severe complications: significant autonomic neuropathy (result-

ing in increased mortality) and small-fiber sensory neuropathy (resulting in foot ulcers and neurogenic arthropathy). Moreover, among diabetics who already have neuropathy, the restoration of euglycemia has been shown also to slow the progression of neuropathy. Trials of other therapies for diabetic neuropathy, including *myo*-inositol, aldose reductase inhibitors, and gangliosides, have been inconclusive in delineating efficacy. Ongoing clinical trials are investigating various neurotrophic growth factors that have proved efficacious in animal studies.

The control of serum glucose commonly is stated to be important for recovery of proximal diabetic neuropathy. However, many patients with this neuropathy have only slight elevation of serum glucose and improve regardless. Inflammatory nerve lesions have been reported in some proximal diabetic neuropathy patients. Treatment with intravenous immunoglobulin, corticosteroids, and cyclophosphamide apparently has resulted in improvement in pain and muscle strength. Though immunosuppressive therapy may be desirable for some patients, not yet clear is the impact that these therapies have on overall prognosis.

Immune- or Infection-Mediated Inflammatory Axonal Polyneuropathies

A representative example in the category of immune- or infection-mediated inflammatory axonal polyneuropathies is polyarteritis nodosa (PAN), the most common cause of vasculitic neuropathy. PAN is a systemic necrotizing vasculitis of small and medium-sized arteries and multisystem involvement (skin, liver, gastrointestinal tract, kidney, PNS, central nervous system, but generally sparing the lung), causing axonal polyneuropathy in approximately 50% of patients.

Natural History

Patients frequently present with constitutional symptoms in addition to neuropathy or other end-organ manifestations. Most frequently, PAN produces an evolving asymmetric polyneuropathy; less common presentations are a true mononeuropathy multiplex, a distal symmetric sensorimotor neuropathy, and a rapidly progressive ascending quadriparesis. Untreated, PAN usually is a fatal disease.

Factors Affecting Prognosis

Polyneuropathy is a major cause of morbidity in PAN. However, the major causes of mortality are the medical complications of systemic vasculitis. Therefore, not surprisingly, involvement of multiple organ systems, particularly renal disease and hypertension, is associated with a poorer prognosis.

Evaluation for Prognosis

The clinical diagnosis of vasculitic neuropathy due to PAN is suggested by an evolving asymmetric, painful polyneuropathy in a patient with constitutional or other, more specific systemic signs and symptoms. The severity of the neuropathy can be gauged by the reduction in amplitude of compound muscle and sensory nerve action potentials on nerve conduction studies and by the extent of denervation and reduction in motor unit recruitment on EMG. Although no studies correlate prognosis of PAN with severity of abnormalities on electrophysiologic testing or nerve biopsy, in general, patients with less evidence of axon loss are more likely to recover.

Therapies Affecting Prognosis

Corticosteroids were the first therapy shown to be effective for major manifestations of the disease and to prolong 5-year survival from 13% (untreated) to 48%. Subsequent retrospective studies have reported that the addition of cyclophosphamide or azathioprine to corticosteroid therapy further improves 5-year survival to perhaps 80%.

No modern treatment study of PAN provides long and careful follow-up of peripheral nerve function. Several relatively small retrospective studies have investigated treatment of systemic vasculitic neuropathy (including PAN patients) with corticosteroids and cytotoxic agents. Generally, these studies show that if the patient survives the medical complications of the vasculitis (and the immunosuppressive therapy), the neuropathy generally improves over several months to 5 years. The available data suggest that as many as 25% of the survivors make a full, or nearly full, recovery, and another 40 to 60% enjoy at least moderate improvement in their polyneuropathy.

Toxic Axonal Polyneuropathy

The most common toxic neuropathies seen by clinicians are those due to chemotherapeutic drugs. Of these, the vinca alkaloids have been used the longest. These drugs (vincristine, vinblastine, and vindesine) are derived from the *Vinca rosea* plant and are used widely in the treatment of many hematologic malignancies and of some solid tumors. They act as mitotic spindle poisons by binding to a microtubule subunit protein, impairing axonal transport and resulting in axonopathy. Besides triggering axonal polyneuropathy, the vinca alkaloids may cause gastrointestinal side effects, namely constipation and ileus, presumably due to autonomic dysfunction.

Natural History

Vincristine, the most widely used vinca alkaloid, predictably is neurotoxic. The clinical features of this neuropathy have been described in a prospective study. Onset of symptoms correlates with the initial dose of drug and frequency of administration. Often, paresthesias are the initial symptom, occurring in the hands before the feet. Objective distal sensory loss for all modalities usually develops but is not disabling. Muscle weakness is very common and typically involves the extensors of the fingers and wrists and, to a lesser extent, distal leg muscles. It is the most disabling feature of vincristine neuropathy. The earliest and most common sign is hyporeflexia; areflexia tends to occur in patients treated with higher initial doses.

Vincristine-induced axonal polyneuropathy improves with reduction in dose or with drug discontinuation. After discontinuation, paresthesias disappear; sensory loss and muscle weakness improve more slowly. Reflexes, except for ankle jerks, return. Although signs and symptoms of mild polyneuropathy often remain, vincristine polyneuropathy rarely results in long-term functional disability.

Factors Affecting Prognosis

The severity of vincristine-induced polyneuropathy increases with daily dose and with duration of therapy. Recovery from vincristine neuropathy depends on the severity of the polyneuropathy at the end of therapy (particularly the severity of muscle weakness), and on the elapsed time from termination of therapy.

Evaluation for Prognosis

Other than knowledge of treatment dose and duration, the most important indicator for recovery of vincristine polyneuropathy is the clinical severity of the polyneuropathy. Electrophysiologic studies are less useful in evaluation for prognosis. For example, amplitude of distal sensory nerve action potentials recovers less completely than do the signs and symptoms of the sensory disturbance.

Therapies Affecting Prognosis

Currently, no recommended therapy is available for vincristine neuropathy. A study examining the effect of a corticotropin analog showed improvement in sensory and autonomic symptoms and motor deficits but no improvement in sensory thresholds. Glutamate has been suggested as a neuroprotectant to prevent vincristine polyneuropathy, but this agent has not been tested in rigorous clinical trials.

Overall Summary of Prognosis

It is difficult to generalize about short- or long-term prognosis of acquired axonal polyneuropathies. However, prognosis will be better if axonal injury is less severe, if an offending exogenous agent can be removed (e.g., withdrawal of vincristine), or if available medical therapy is effective in controlling the underlying metabolic or structural insult (e.g., tight glucose control for diabetic neuropathy or immunosuppressive therapy for PAN). Finally, clinical recovery of axonal injury is slow, depending mainly on nerve regeneration. Months to years may be required to reach a plateau in clinical recovery.

Additional Reading

Casey EB, Jelliffe AM, Le Quesne PM, Millett YL. Vincristine neuropathy—clinical and electrophysiological observations. Brain 1973;96:69–86.

Chang RW, Bell CL, Hallett M. Clinical characteristics and prognosis of vasculitic mononeuropathy multiplex. Arch Neurol 1984;41:618–621.

Diabetes Control and Complications Trial Research Group. The effect of intensive treatment of diabetes on the development and progression of long-term complications in insulin-dependent diabetes mellitus. N Engl J Med 1993;329:977–986.

Dyck PJ, Thomas PK, Griffin JW, et al. (eds). Peripheral Neuropathy (3rd ed). Philadelphia: Saunders, 1993.

Fauci AS, Katz P, Haynes BF, Wolff SM. Cyclophosphamide therapy of severe systemic necrotizing vasculitis. N Engl J Med 1979;301:235–238.

Kennedy WR, Navarro X, Goetz FC, et al. Effects of pancreatic transplantation on diabetic neuropathy. N Engl J Med 1990;322:1031–1037.

Krendel DA, Costigan DA, Hopkins LC. Successful treatment of neuropathies in patients with diabetes mellitus. Arch Neurol 1993;52:1053–1061.

Mendell JR, Barohn RJ, Bosch EP, Kissel JT. Peripheral neuropathy (pt A). Continuum 1994;1:8–126.

Moore PM, Fauci AS. Neurologic manifestations of systemic vasculitis. A retrospective and prospective study of the clinicopathologic features and responses to therapy in 25 patients. Am J Med 1981;71:517–524.

Schaumburg HH, Berger AR, Thomas PK. Disorders of Peripheral Nerves (2nd ed). Philadelphia: FA Davis, 1992.

Chapter 55

Entrapment Neuropathies

William W. Campbell

Entrapment neuropathies can occur at any number of locations where a peripheral nerve must traverse a point of potential anatomic compromise. The most common entrapment by far is carpal tunnel syndrome (CTS), which can have an incidence as high as 308 in 100,000. Workers in situations of high ergonomic stress requiring forceful and repetitive wrist and hand motion may have an even higher incidence. Underlying medical conditions, such as diabetes mellitus or pregnancy, or ergonomic risk, may be important factors in as many as 25% of patients. Ulnar neuropathy at the elbow is seen in electrodiagnostic medicine laboratories at perhaps one-third the frequency of CTS. Peroneal neuropathy at the fibular head occurs much less frequently. These three entrapments account for the majority of cases.

Natural History

The natural history of most entrapment neuropathies is one of fluctuating progression. Patients with CTS tend to have flares and remissions related to such factors as the intensity of hand use. If the inciting cause is not identified and removed, the neuropathy tends to progress, and symptoms evolve, from mild intermittent paresthesias and pain to more constant paresthesias, more severe pain, sensory loss, weakness and, eventually, atrophy. The same evolution occurs with entrapments of the ulnar nerve at the elbow and the peroneal nerve at the knee, although the mix of pain, sensory complaints, and weakness tends to vary.

Concomitant with progression of signs and symptoms is increasing pathologic change. Early paranodal demyelination progresses to segmental demyelination and, eventually, to axon loss. In late stages, the added complication of intraneural fibrosis occurs and imposes a major limitation on recovery potential. Long-standing denervation of muscle may not permit recovery even if the nerve compression is relieved.

After surgical decompression, the prognosis is determined by time and distance considerations. Neurapraxia can be expected to resolve by 12 weeks. Any deficit after that time is due to axon loss. After decompression, the regenerating axons are in a race against time to reinnervate the target muscles before irreversible changes occur and cannot muster a rate of much over 1 inch per month. The implications of these limitations are significant. Leisurely decisions about a reasonable length of time for conservative management and about surgical exploration may not permit enough time for reinnervation, even if decompression is technically successful. The clinician in charge should calculate a worst-case scenario in which the compression is severe, major axon loss has occurred, and regenerating axons must travel the entire distance from the entrapment site to the target muscle. Surgical exploration must not be postponed beyond the time required for this process to occur.

Factors Affecting Prognosis

The primary factors affecting prognosis are the duration and the severity of entrapment. Long-standing, severe deficits have a much worse prognosis than do recent, mild conditions. Diseased peripheral nerves, such as those found in diabetics and alcoholics, cannot be expected to repair, regenerate, and recover with the alacrity of normal, young, healthy nerves.

Evaluation for Prognosis

The prognosis can be gauged by clinical and electrodiagnostic features. The clinical features suggesting a good prognosis include intermittent symptoms, lack of fixed sensory loss, and the absence of weakness or atrophy. Persistent sensory deficits and weakness imply a more severe process but still could be due to neurapraxia. Atrophy signals axon loss and indicates that the extent of recovery will depend on the efficiency of axonal sprouting and the time available for that process to occur. Failure of the Tinel's sign to progress down the nerve as expected after decompression of an axon-loss lesion implies rate-limiting intraneural fibrosis and a poor outcome.

Electrodiagnostically, the features suggesting a good prognosis include preservation of compound muscle action potential (CMAP) and sensory nerve action potential (SNAP) amplitude on distal stimulation, mild conduction slowing across the lesion, and minimal or no abnormalities on needle examination. Partial or complete conduction block or temporal dispersion on stimulation proximal to the entrapment does not imply a bad prognosis but is the expected finding in a primarily neurapraxic lesion, which has good potential for recovery if the compression is relieved. Significant slowing in the nerve segment distal to the lesion, decrease in CMAP and SNAP amplitude, and frank denervation on needle examination are the electrical markers of axon loss. They correlate with atrophy and fixed sensory loss and carry the same prognostic implications, but they are more precise and quantitative.

Individual Entrapment Syndromes

Carpal Tunnel Syndrome

Usually, the initial treatment of CTS is conservative. Available modalities include splinting, anti-inflammatories, steroid injections, and cessation of any inciting activities. Kaplan and coworkers treated 331 hands with splinting and anti-inflammatory agents and with follow-up for at least 6 months. Significant improvement was seen in 18%. Five factors predicted the response to treatment: age older than 50 years, duration greater than 10 months, constant paresthesias, stenosing flexor tenosynovitis, and a Phalen's test positive in less than 30 seconds. Two-thirds of the patients with none of these risk factors improved with conservative therapy. Only 40% of patients with one factor, 17% with two factors, 7% with three factors, and none with four or five factors responded.

Carpal tunnel release (CTR) is safe and effective surgery, with a high response rate in properly selected patients. The chances for substantial improvement are good after CTR, although residual numbness of the fingertips is common. Initial relief of pain is rapid, with subsequent improvement in numbness and weakness occurring more slowly. Symptomatic relief within the first 24 postoperative hours predicts a good or excellent result at 6 weeks' follow-up. Without subjective improvement at 24 hours, a good outcome still is possible, but a poor outcome becomes more likely.

Nancollas and colleagues reviewed 60 patients who underwent CTR at an average of 5.5 years postoperatively. A good or excellent overall outcome was reported by 87% of patients, with an average time of 9.8 months to maximum improvement. However, 30% of patients reported poor to fair strength and long-term scar discomfort, and 57% noted a return of some preoperative symptoms (most commonly pain) beginning an average of 2 years after surgery. The CTS was job-related in 42% of patients. The occupational cases improved more slowly, and patients remained off work longer, but the long-term subjective results were no different. Significant morbidity resulted from the surgical scar and decreased strength, and often considerable delay ensued until ultimate improvement, especially in patients with job-related CTS. Pain improves to a greater extent than do other symptoms after CTR. The prognosis is poor when pain has been present for more than 5 years before surgery.

In a study of 54 hands after CTR, Wintman and associates found that preoperative subjective hand weakness predicted less improvement of function and less satisfaction with overall symptom relief 3 months after surgery. Patients the most satisfied with their surgery were those with more preoperative night symptoms and intermittent paresthesias, and less preoperative hand-wrist pain, numbness, weakness, clumsiness, and difficulty with work-related tasks.

Severe and long-standing CTS is not necessarily a contraindication to surgery. The relative proportion of demyelination and axon loss and the duration of the disease will determine motor recovery, but lessening of pain and sensory dysfunction are not as predictable. Symptomatic improvement occurred after CTR in 14 of 15 hands with advanced CTS as defined by an absent median SNAP and absent or prolonged distal motor latency. Thenar atrophy resolved in 2 of the 10 patients in whom it was present. Even patients with advanced CTS may benefit from decompression.

Ulnar Neuropathy

The ulnar nerve may be compressed or entrapped at several locations, from the region of the medial intermuscular septum in the upper arm to the deep palmar branch in the hand. Most compressions occur at the elbow, either in the ulnar groove or beneath the aponeurosis of the humeroulnar arcade (the cubital tunnel) or as the nerve pierces the deep flexor-pronator aponeurosis as it exits from the flexor carpi ulnaris muscle (exit compression). The prognosis varies with each of these syndromes.

Patients with ulnar neuropathy at the elbow may improve with conservative treatment (Table 55-1). In Eisen and Danon's study of 30 patients who presented with ulnar distribution sensory complaints for at least 3 weeks but without motor abnormalities or objective sensory abnormalities on examination, only three (10%) showed progression of the disease and development of a motor deficit. Twenty patients (67%) were asymptomatic at follow-up, and 7 (23%) continued to have mild intermittent numbness. Electrodiagnostic studies accurately predicted those patients who would have a progressive and deteriorating course.

DeJesus and Steiner followed a group of patients managed nonsurgically for periods up to 4 years. The patients were divided by electrodiagnostic criteria into four groups: normal; abnormal conduction velocity limited to the ulnar groove (i.e., primarily

Table 55-1. Conservative Treatment of Ulnar Neuropathy at the Elbow

Minimization of elbow flexion
    Arms never crossed
    Forearm supinated and resting on thigh while sitting
    Telephone in asymptomatic hand only
    Book stand for reading
Avoidance of external pressure
    Elbow pads
    Night splints
    Elbow resting on pillow during desk work
    Nonsteroidal anti-inflammatory drugs for repetitive
      motion

neurapraxia); abnormal conduction velocity limited predominantly to the ulnar groove and with variable distal slowing (i.e., some element of axon loss); and involvement from above the elbow distally (i.e., severe axon loss). At follow-up, 46% of patients were normal after nonoperative management, and 15% were improved significantly. The likelihood of spontaneous recovery was greatest in those patients with the mildest electrophysiologic abnormalities.

Dellon and coworkers prospectively evaluated 128 patients with ulnar neuropathy at the elbow managed nonoperatively. Only 11% of patients with symptoms alone eventually had surgery as contrasted to 33% with mild to moderate abnormalities on examination and 62% with more severe abnormalities. The presence of persistent paresthesias, abnormal two-point discrimination, and any degree of muscle wasting moved patients into the category in which eventual surgery was likely. Electrodiagnostic abnormalities were not found to have predictive value. A history of elbow injury significantly worsened the outcome.

Patients who require ulnar nerve surgery may undergo any of several procedures, depending largely on the preference and habits of the surgeon. Complications are unlikely with simple decompression of the humeroulnar aponeurotic arcade (cubital tunnel). Anterior transposition usually is safe but can go terribly awry. Most ulnar nerve disasters occur in patients who have undergone transposition. However, simple decompression may not suffice for patients with moderate or severe neuropathies or for those with pathology in the ulnar groove. The overall good outcome rate for ulnar nerve surgery is about 70%.

Peroneal Neuropathy

In its arc across the fibular head, the peroneal nerve is superficial and vulnerable to external compression, and peroneal neuropathy at the knee most often develops in the setting of external pressure. The nerve may be susceptible also to stretch injury or entrapment at its point of passage through the fibrous arch at the origin of the peroneus longus muscle (the "fibular tunnel").

Habitual leg crossing is the classic cause of peroneal neuropathy at the knee, but external pressure damage may come from a variety of potential sources. Other causes include prolonged squatting and sudden, forceful plantar flexion or inversion of the ankle. Rarely, a mass lesion, such as a ganglion or peripheral nerve tumor, may compress the nerve, or it may experience entrapment at the fibular tunnel.

The most important element in the work-up is the medical detective work necessary to detect the mechanism of compression or stretch. In most patients, a meticulous history will uncover a likely explanation. Searching for a dimple, discoloration, or callus over the fibular head may help to confirm an external pressure mechanism. Failure to find a satisfactory explanatory mechanism of injury, failure of the neuropathy to resolve, or progression of the deficit under observation raises the possibility of mass lesion or fibular tunnel entrapment.

Electrodiagnostic studies are helpful in prognosis. The more nearly normal the motor conduction studies, the better the prognosis in general. Conduction block across the fibular head with normal or near normal distal conduction parameters implies a largely demyelinating lesion with high likelihood of recovery. Loss of CMAP amplitude recording from the extensor digitorum brevis is a mark of axon loss and an indicator that recovery will be more protracted. As the dorsiflexors of the foot and the long toe extensors are much more vital than are the short toe extensors, the CMAP recorded from the tibialis anterior correlates more reliably with functional capacity than does the CMAP recorded from the extensor digitorum brevis. The more profuse the fibrillations and the fewer the recruitable motor units during the early phases, the poorer the prognosis.

The prognosis in peroneal neuropathy at the knee is determined by the mechanism and severity of injury. Patients with simple external compression (e.g., habitual leg crossing) and an electromyogram (EMG) showing mostly demyelinating features and little axon loss have a good prognosis. The patient with a stretch injury due to an ankle fracture or dislocation, in which intraneural hematoma may be involved, and an EMG showing significant axon loss has a much more guarded prognosis.

Smith and Trojaborg found that only 6 of a group of 14 patients with peroneal palsy of compressive or spontaneous origin had a complete clinical recovery. The others had a variably incomplete recovery. Electrodiagnostic studies were valuable in predicting the outcome but found only partial correspondence between the clinical and the electrophysiologic findings in the group with incomplete recovery.

Short- and Long-Term Prognosis

In general, the best response to either conservative or surgical treatment of entrapment neuropathies occurs in patients with brief symptom duration and no clinical or electrical evidence of axon loss. Some two-thirds of CTS patients respond to conservative treatment, and perhaps one-third require surgical release. The presence or absence of certain risk factors can help to predict the likelihood of successful conservative management. Improvement of symptoms within the first 24 hours postoperatively portends a good outcome.

Long-term prognosis can refer to either the length of symptoms or to time after treatment. Patients with symptomatology of longer duration have a lesser chance of responding to any treatment modality. CTR produces a good to excellent overall long-term outcome, especially for pain relief, in 85 to 90% of cases, though often tempered by some loss of strength and scar discomfort. Many patients eventually note the return of some preoperative symptoms. Even patients with severe and longstanding CTS may have a degree of symptomatic improvement after surgery. Many patients with mild or moderate ulnar neuropathy may respond to conservative treatment or may improve spontaneously. Patients with severe neuropathies generally require surgery, and the overall good outcome rate is approximately 70%. Occasional patients, especially those undergoing transposition, have dreadful outcomes. Less than half the patients with peroneal palsy arising spontaneously or from compression have a complete clinical recovery. An EMG showing mostly focal demyelination and little axon loss is a favorable prognostic indicator.

Additional Reading

Clarke AM, Stanley D. Prediction of the outcome 24 hours after carpal tunnel decompression. J Hand Surg [Br] 1993;18:180–181.

DeJesus PV, Steiner JC. Spontaneous recovery of ulnar neuropathy at the elbow. Electromyogr Clin Neurophysiol 1976;16:239–248.

Dellon AL, Hament W, Gittelshon A. Nonoperative management of cubital tunnel syndrome: an 8-year prospective study. Neurology 1993;43:1673–1677.

Eisen A, Danon J. The mild cubital tunnel syndrome. Neurology 1974;24:608–613.

Haupt WF, Wintzer G, Schop A, et al. Long-term results of carpal tunnel decompression. Assessment of 60 cases. J Hand Surg [Br] 1993;18:471–474.

Kaplan SJ, Glickel SZ, Eaton RG. Predictive factors in the non-surgical treatment of carpal tunnel syndrome. J Hand Surg [Br] 1990;15:106–108.

Nancollas MP, Peimer CA, Wheeler DR, Sherwin FS. Long-term results of carpal tunnel release. J Hand Surg [Br] 1995;20:470–474.

Nolan WB III, Alkaitis D, Glickel SZ, Snow S. Results of treatment of severe carpal tunnel syndrome. J Hand Surg [Am] 1992;17:1020–1023.

Smith T, Trojaborg W. Clinical and electrophysiological recovery from peroneal palsy. Acta Neurol Scand 1986;74:328–335.

Wintman BI, Winters SC, Gelberman RH, Katz JN. Carpal tunnel release. Correlations with preoperative symptomatology. Clin Orthop 1996;326:135–145.

Chapter 56

Inherited Neuropathies

Jacqueline Crawford and Yuen So

The major hereditary neuropathies include hereditary motor and sensory neuropathies (HMSNs) and the more recently characterized hereditary neuropathy with liability to pressure palsies (HNPPs). The HMSNs are a heterogeneous group of conditions that historically were classified by their clinical and electrophysiologic characteristics. Since the early 1990s, molecular biology has produced a new method of classification that combines clinical phenotype with genotype. Studies evaluating prognosis on the basis of genetic defect now are possible.

Classification

To discuss this group of diseases, one must understand its nomenclature and genetics. HMSNs are known also as *Charcot-Marie-Tooth neuropathies*, in reference to the phenotypic description of childhood-onset distal weakness and atrophy associated with foot deformity as outlined by Charcot, Marie, and Tooth in 1886. As the underlying genetic defects are clarified, changes in nomenclature are evolving. For the purpose of this chapter, the HMSN nomenclature is used. Table 56-1 provides an index of the alternative nomenclature with reference to gene defect. The neuropathies are grouped broadly as demyelinating (HMSN Ia, Ib, X1, or X2) or axonal (HMSN II). HMSN Ia is the most common and is linked in most cases to duplication of a 1.5-kb segment of chromosome 17p containing the PMP22 gene. The PMP22 protein is expressed in myelin of peripheral nerves. HMSN Ib has been mapped to chromosome 1q,

where a point mutation occurs in the P_0 gene. The P_0 gene encodes another myelin protein expressed in peripheral nerve. HMSN II, the axonal form, is a genetically heterogeneous group of hereditary neuropathies. An autosomal dominant disorder, HMSN IIa, is linked to a deletion in chromosome 1 in some families. Presently, the genetic defect in other patients with HMSN II is unknown. Dejerine-Sottas syndrome or hypertrophic neuropathy of infancy initially was thought to be a genetically distinct demyelinating neuropathy characterized by early onset of severe weakness and was labeled HMSN III. Subsequent genetic investigations have revealed some cases to have the 17p duplication, as in HMSN Ia, and others may be due to mutations of either PMP22 or P_0 genes. HMSN X1 is linked to mutations in the connexon 32 gene and is characterized by X-linked dominant inheritance. Connexon is a protein involved in gap junctions that create intercellular channels. HMSN X2 and HMSN X3 are X-linked recessive but map to different locations on the X chromosome.

HNPP, or tomaculous neuropathy, manifests as recurrent nerve palsies, recurrent brachial plexopathies, or a sensorimotor polyneuropathy that may resemble HMSN I. The genetic abnormality is a deletion of the same 1.5-kb segment of chromosome 17 that is duplicated in HMSN Ia.

Clinical Features

The classic phenotype of distal weakness, atrophy, and areflexia most evident in the lower extremities

Table 56-1. Classification of the Hereditary Neuropathies

HMSN Nomen-clature	Alternate Nomen-clature	Patho-physiology	Inheritance Pattern	Abnormal Gene Product (Chromosome)	Type of Mutation	Approximate Frequency (%)
HMSN Ia	CMT 1A	Demyelination	Autosomal dominant	PMP22 (17p)	Duplication or missense	56–60
HMSN Ib	CMT 1B	Demyelination	Autosomal dominant	P_0 (1q)		1
HMSN II	CMT 2	Axon loss	Autosomal dominant or recessive	Many	Unknown	19
HMSN III	CMT 3 or Dejerine-Sottas	Demyelination	Unknown	Unknown	Unknown	Rare
HMSN X1	CMT X1	Demyelination	X-linked dominant	Connexon 32 (X)	Point mutation	}21
HMSN X2	CMT X2,3	Demyelination	X-linked recessive	Unknown (X)	Unknown	
HNPP	Tomaculous neuropathy	Segmental demyelination	Autosomal dominant	PMP22 (17p)	Deletion	Unknown

HMSN = hereditary motor sensory neuropathy; CMT = Charcot-Marie-Tooth disease; HNPP = hereditary neuropathy with liability to pressure palsies.

is seen in most of the HMSN subtypes. Delayed walking, new difficulty with walking or running, or foot deformity frequently are the first features that bring the patient to medical attention. Pes cavus, hammer toes, and inverted-champagne-bottle appearance of the calves are attributed to the distal atrophy. A wide spectrum of clinical severity is seen even in patients with the same gene defect. Some are completely asymptomatic, others have severe foot drop, and still others are confined to a wheel-chair. More severely affected patients have signifi-cant atrophy and weakness of distal upper extremities, sometimes to a degree that requires ten-don transfers to allow useful function of the hands.

Sensory loss is most prominent in the distal lower extremities. Unlike many acquired neu-ropathies, paresthesias or dysesthesias rarely are prominent, and many patients are unaware of any sensory loss until it is pointed out to them. The sen-sory loss affects all modalities and, in some cases, gives rise to sensory ataxia.

Some infrequent characteristics observed in occasional patients may be clinically important. Of the 595 patients ascertained in the Iowa Charcot-Marie-Tooth Study, one required intermittent mechanical ventilation. Thomas and coworkers described a variety of clinical features seen in their series of 61 patients with the 17p duplication (Table 56-2). Abnormal enlargement of peripheral nerves or spinal roots in HMSN Ia, secondary to recurrent

demyelination and remyelination, sometimes leads to entrapment neuropathy or radiculopathy. The Roussy-Levy syndrome—postural upper-extremity tremor in the setting of areflexia and foot defor-mity—once was considered a separate disease entity. However, many of these cases are now well established as simply a phenotypic variant of HMSN Ia. HMSN X2 is associated with mental retardation, whereas HMSN X3 is associated with spastic paraparesis. Some 5% of all patients with HMSN have sensorineural deafness. Although impaired distal sweating may be present, cardiovas-cular reflexes are intact in HMSN I and II.

HNPP patients with compression neuropathies often have areflexia, occasionally have pes cavus, but do not have the nerve enlargement seen in HMSN I. Some individuals who are proved to have the 17p deletion are clinically asymptomatic.

Natural History

Several studies address the question of clinical course. Killian and colleagues reported on eight HMSN Ia patients who were studied in 1967 and again 22 years later. Motor nerve conduction veloc-ity (NCV) declined by an average of only 2.2 m per second in the median nerve and 3.0 m per second in the peroneal nerve. Mild objective increase in leg weakness was noted in only one patient, even though half the patients complained of worsening leg weakness. One patient required the use of a leg brace in the last 3 years. Dyck and associates, on the other hand, documented more prominent progression of disease. They studied 31 patients with HMSN I and used the neurologic disability score to assess disease progression over 15 years. They estimated a decline of 0.6 neurologic disability score points per year in patients with ages between 5 and 14 years, 1.1 points per year in patients between 15 and 39 years, and 0.9 points per year in patients 40 years and older. Harding and Thomas found a mild increase in clinical severity proportional to the duration of symptoms. Hoogendijk and coworkers observed that NCV and clinical severity did not correlate with age in 44 patients with HMSN Ia. They concluded that the primary pathologic process is only slightly active past childhood. Overall, symptoms appear to worsen mildly with time.

The natural history of HNPP is not well delineated, as it received relatively little attention until 1993, when the genetic defect was identified. Some persons with the gene defect are clinically asymptomatic, whereas others sustain multiple, painless, acute focal neuropathies at common nerve compression sites. The acute neuropathies usually resolve within 6 months, but the recovery may be incomplete. HNPP is reported also to manifest as a distal amyotrophy of the lower extremities in some children.

Factors Affecting Prognosis

Demyelinating Versus Axonal Neuropathies

Harding and Thomas provided a comprehensive review of the clinical profiles in hereditary sensorimotor polyneuropathies in 1980. Their study predated the discovery of the gene defects; thus, they classified the neuropathies primarily on the basis of NCV. Median NCV of less than 38 m per second separated those with demyelinating neuropathy (HMSN I) from those with axonal neuropathy HMSN II (Table 56-3).

In patients with demyelinating neuropathy, the age of onset was primarily in the first and second decades, whereas those with axonal neuropathy had a broader distribution, with onset as late as the seventh decade of life. In general, patients with demyelinating neuropathy had a more severe dis-

Table 56-2. Uncommon Clinical Features in Hereditary Motor Sensory Neuropathy I

Focal neuropathies
    Entrapment neuropathies
    Radiculopathies
    Other focal neuropathies
Unusual pattern of weakness
    Bulbar palsy
    Diaphragmatic abnormalities
    Incontinence due to pelvic-floor weakness
Skeletal abnormalities
    Scoliosis
    Claw hand
    Pectus excavatum
    Acetabular dysplasia
    Patella dislocations
Hand tremor (Roussy-Levy Syndrome)
Deafness
Muscle cramps

ease with greater sensory loss and a greater frequency of upper-extremity weakness and total areflexia. Hoogendijk and colleagues and Thomas and coworkers found similar clinical characteristics in their studies of 44 and 61 individuals, respectively, with proved 17p duplication (HMSN Ia).

Nature of the Genetic Defect

The nature of the gene defect seems to be an imperfect predictor of disease severity. In Kaku and associates' study of 81 patients with the 17p duplication, 2 patients (aged 17 and 24 years) were unaffected clinically and had normal neurologic examinations. Another example is Garcia and colleagues' report on two sets of identical twins with the 17p duplication and divergent clinical severity. In one of the sets, one twin had hand weakness with atrophy and required leg braces, whereas the other's only manifestation was an inability to walk on his heels. The less affected twin in both pairs had the most prominent nerve enlargement. No other identifiable factors could account for the clinical variability. In HNPP, as many as 22 to 31% of individuals with the 17p deletion are clinically asymptomatic.

Although a genetic defect does not predict clinical outcome absolutely, it is helpful in certain clinical situations. Kaku and coworkers reported on a child who had onset of weakness in infancy and was

Table 56-3. Summary of Clinical Characteristics of Approximately 200 Patients with Hereditary Sensorimotor Neuropathies

Clinical Characteristic	Demyelinating (HMSN I) Median NCV: <38 m/sec (%)	Axonal (HMSN II) Median NCV: >38 m/sec (%)
Age of onset	60 in first decade, 25 in second	25 in first decade, 35 in second
Upper-limb weakness	67	51
Lower-limb weakness	87	94
Severe lower-limb weakness	34	33
Upper-limb tremor	39	16
Total areflexia	58	9
Vibration sensation loss	69	56
Pain sensation loss	53	31
Pes cavus	72	65
Scoliosis	10	2.7
Nerve thickening	29	0

HMSN = hereditary motor sensory neuropathy; NCV = nerve conduction velocity.
Source: Adapted from AE Harding, PK Thomas. The clinical features of hereditary motor and sensory neuropathy types I and II. Brain 1980;103:259–280.

homozygous for the duplication at 17p. She had atrophy of hand muscles, delayed walking, and very slow median NCV (10.4 m per second). Her severe manifestations probably are an example of gene-dosage effect.

Nerve Conduction Velocity and Clinical Severity

In HMSN I, wherein dysmyelination or demyelination is believed to be the primary pathologic mechanism, NCV correlates strongly with clinical severity. Dyck and associates observed that the degree of slowing correlated with eventual disability, as scored by the Neurologic Disability Score 15 years later. As NCV also correlated with the clinical severity at the time of the study, the clinical examination probably is also a helpful prognostic factor. As seen in many hereditary diseases, early age of onset of symptoms also correlates with severity of disease.

In HNPP, the median distal motor latency is prolonged, and motor NCVs are slowed moderately regardless of clinical state. Thus, electrophysiology is helpful for diagnosis but not for prognosis.

Evaluation for Prognosis

The clinical examination at time of presentation provides the most direct information regarding the even-tual outcome. For the most part, as the saying goes, "What you see is what you get." One can expect only mild increase in neuropathic weakness with time. NCVs may give additional prognostic information for the demyelinating hereditary neuropathies

Examination of family members, clinically as well as electrophysiologically, can help to determine the mode of inheritance. This finding is significant in the X-linked recessive forms, as they have associated mental retardation or spastic paraparesis. Identification of the exact genetic defect is helpful but, as mentioned in Nature of the Genetic Defect, a broad spectrum of clinical severity exists among persons with identical genetic defects.

Therapy Affecting Prognosis

No known therapy alters the course of hereditary neuropathies. Care for patients with these disorders includes appropriate bracing and occupational and physical therapy. Few patients with kyphoscoliosis require surgical intervention.

Some reports cite chronic inflammatory demyelinating polyradiculoneuropathy developing in persons presumed to have HMSN I. The patients had electrophysiologic evidence of segmental demyelination and severely elevated total protein in the cerebrospinal fluid and appeared to improve after steroid treatment or plasmapheresis. These reports highlight the importance of re-evaluation of HMSN patients who have an atypically rapid decline.

Short-Term Prognosis

Neurologic deterioration tends to be slow and imperceptible in the short term. An exception may be persons exposed to neuropathic toxins or those who develop concordant chronic inflammatory demyelinating polyradiculoneuropathy or other neuropathy. Pregnancy also may be associated with clinical deterioration in strength. Rudnik-Schoneborn and coworkers reported on 21 HMSN I patients who had one or more pregnancies. Among the women who had childhood-onset of neuropathic symptoms, 50% self-reported some increased weakness during pregnancy. Within that group, roughly 35% believed that the worsening reversed after pregnancy, whereas 65% thought it was persistent.

Long-Term Prognosis

A broad spectrum of severity occurs in the hereditary neuropathies, even among patients with identical genetic defects, with some being completely normal and a few being wheelchair-bound. In general, those who have noticeable weakness in infancy and childhood will have more disability as adults. Weakness progresses very slowly over a number of years. No definitive treatment avails for the hereditary neuropathies, but appropriate bracing allows most patients independent ambulation.

Additional Reading

Dyck PJ, Karnes MS, Lambert EH. Longitudinal study of neuropathic deficits and nerve conduction abnormalities in hereditary motor and sensory neuropathy type 1. Neurology 1989;39:1302–1308.

Dyck PJ, Swanson CJ, Low PA, et al. Prednisone-responsive hereditary motor and sensory neuropathy. Mayo Clin Proc 1982;57:239–246.

Garcia CA, Malamut RE, England JD, et al. Clinical variability in two pairs of identical twins with the Charcot-Marie-Tooth disease type 1A duplication. Neurology 1995;45:2090–2093.

Harding AE, Thomas PK. The clinical features of hereditary motor and sensory neuropathy types I and II. Brain 1980;103:259–280.

Hoogendijk JE, DeVisser M, Bolhuis PA, et al. Hereditary motor and sensory neuropathy type I: clinical and neurographical features of the 17p duplication subtype. Muscle Nerve 1994;17:85–90.

Ionasescu VV. Charcot-Marie-Tooth neuropathies: from clinical description to molecular genetics. Muscle Nerve 1995;18:267–275.

Kaku DA, Parry GJ, Malamut R, et al. Nerve conduction studies in Charcot-Marie-Tooth polyneuropathy associated with a segmental duplication of chromosome 17. Neurology 1993;43:1806–1808.

Killian JM, Tiwari PS, Jacobson S, et al. Longitudinal studies of the duplication form of Charcot-Marie-Tooth polyneuropathy. Muscle Nerve 1996;19:74–78.

Rudnik-Schoneborn S, Rohrig D, Nicholson G, Zerres K. Pregnancy and delivery in Charcot-Marie-Tooth disease type I. Neurology 1993;43:2011–2016.

Thomas PK, Marques W, Davis MB, et al. The phenotypic manifestations of chromosome 17p11.2 duplication. Brain 1997;120:465–478.

Chapter 57

Bell's Palsy and Other Facial Neuropathies

Joel C. Morgenlander

The facial nerve (cranial nerve VII) is one of the cranial nerves most frequently injured by disease. Dysfunction of motor innervation to the muscles of facial expression results in altered cosmetic appearance and inability to protect the cornea by blinking. Speech is slurred, owing to labial weakness; food may pouch into the cheek, owing to buccinator weakness; and involvement of the nerve to the stapedius muscle causes hyperacusis. Dysgeusia and decreased lacrimation and salivation may occur. Although some sensory fibers to the ear run with the facial nerve, numbness is an uncommon complaint. Pain due to facial nerve injury often is focused in a retroauricular location at which the facial nerve exits the stylomastoid foramen. Synkinesis, either motor or autonomic (e.g., crocodile tears), may arise from aberrant reinnervation.

The facial nerve may be injured alone or as part of multiple cranial neuropathies. Bilateral facial nerve involvement or multiple cranial nerve involvement usually indicates a need for more extensive diagnostic evaluation, often including magnetic resonance imaging of the brain and examination of cerebrospinal fluid (Table 57-1).

Natural History

Bell's palsy is the most common facial neuropathy, accounting for two-thirds of cases. Although Sir Charles Bell described cases that were idiopathic, he described cases also due to specific causes, such as trauma and syphilis. The term *Bell's palsy* is used for disease of uncertain etiology. Diagnosis depends on the typical presentation and course and on exclusion of other causes. The incidence of Bell's palsy is 20 per 100,000 population, with men and women equally affected. Peak age of occurrence is between ages 20 and 40. No facial-side predilection is evident. Bilateral onset occurs in 5%. Family history of Bell's palsy is present in 9%. The incidence is higher in women who are pregnant and in those with acquired immunodeficiency syndrome (although the mechanism may relate to the underlying human immunodeficiency virus infection). Several studies suggest that herpes simplex virus may be causal in most cases.

Maximal motor deficit in Bell's palsy usually occurs within days but may take 2 to 3 weeks. Recovery onset and degree depend on the severity of weakness. Patients with preservation of some facial movement usually begin to improve within 2 to 4 weeks, and recovery is complete. Completely paralyzed patients who begin to improve within 4 to 6 weeks have an excellent prognosis for full recovery, although some may have incomplete recovery or synkinesis. Those with no evidence of improvement at 6 weeks often have significant residual weakness and synkinesis. Overall, 85% of untreated patients will recover completely.

Herpes zoster oticus (Ramsay Hunt syndrome) is the cause of 5 to 10% of all facial neuropathies. Varicella-zoster infection is causal and may result in vesicles seen in the ear canal. Usually, multiple cranial nerves are involved, particularly the vestibulocochlear, resulting in concurrent hearing

Table 57-1. Causes of Bilateral Facial Neuropathies

Bell's palsy
Lyme disease
Sarcoidosis
Guillain-Barré syndrome
Syphilis
Tuberculous meningitis
Cryptococcal meningitis
Carcinomatous meningitis
Metastatic disease
Trauma

loss and vertigo. The prognosis for full recovery without treatment is less favorable than that for Bell's palsy, with as many as one-third of patients having residual dysfunction.

Lyme disease is a frequent cause of facial neuropathy, especially in endemic areas. Neurologic involvement occurs weeks to months after initial infection and may occur without prior rash or arthritis. Facial neuropathy is the most common neurologic sequelae, occurring in 50% of patients with neurologic involvement and in 11% of all patients with Lyme disease. Seventy-five percent of patients have a unilateral facial neuropathy, with the other 25% having bilateral involvement. Other neurologic involvement with Lyme disease, such as encephalitis or radiculitis, may be present. Without treatment, prognosis for the facial neuropathy due to Lyme disease is similar to that of Bell's palsy.

Tumors cause less than 5% of facial neuropathies. Tumor should be suspected when one of the following clinical features is present: progression of more than 3 weeks; absence of functional return at 6 months; partial weakness that is not lessening at 2 months; prolonged ear pain; or recurrent ipsilateral facial neuropathy. The most common tumors to involve the facial nerve are meningiomas, nerve-sheath tumors, parotid lesions, hemangiomas, and metastatic disease. Sudden loss of facial nerve function occurs in one-third of patients with tumor involvement, but tumors may involve the facial nerve without causing dysfunction. In contradistinction to non-neoplastic etiologies, facial twitching (e.g., myokymia or hemifacial spasm) often is seen. Enhanced magnetic resonance imaging or computed tomography scan of the brain aids in diagnosis. Prognosis

depends on the degree of nerve invasion by tumor. The nerve may be relatively unaffected but, if it is encased by malignant tumor, nerve resection may be necessary.

Trauma causes perhaps 5% of all facial neuropathies and is a more frequent cause in children. Perinatal trauma may occur in utero or by prolonged labor with or without forceps delivery. Signs of periauricular trauma or blood behind the tympanic membrane are clues. Excellent recovery occurs in most cases. When facial nerve injury is a result of cranial trauma, usually with concurrent skull fracture, complete paralysis may occur early. Prognosis for full recovery is guarded in the presence of a fracture along the facial canal due to presumed facial nerve transection.

Direct involvement with infection, such as suppurative otitis media or mastoiditis, can result in facial neuropathy, most frequently in children with partially treated or recurrent infections. Careful otologic examination is required in all patients with facial neuropathy. Facial weakness occurs over several days. Without medical treatment, prognosis for full recovery is poor.

Sarcoidosis is a systemic granulomatous disease that affects the nervous system in 5 to 10% of patients. Facial neuropathy is the most common neurologic manifestation and occurs in 50% of patients with neurologic involvement. Pulmonary involvement may be lacking in 10 to 20% of patients. Neurologic symptoms may be the presenting feature in 50% of those who will have neurologic sequelae. Usually, the course is monophasic, but it can be recurrent or progressive.

Melkersson-Rosenthal is a syndrome of episodic or progressive unilateral facial weakness, facial edema, and furrowed tongue. Usually, it begins in childhood or adolescence. A relapsing course is most common, and recovery from each episode usually occurs.

Unilateral and, more often, bilateral facial neuropathies occur as part of acute demyelinating polyneuropathy (Guillain-Barré syndrome). Guillain-Barré syndrome variants commonly involve the facial nerve and usually are associated with the presence of serum anti-GQ_{1b} antibodies. Diagnosis is suspected by the typical presentation of Guillain-Barré syndrome. Prognosis usually is good unless severe axonal degeneration occurs.

Factors Affecting Prognosis

Factors negatively affecting prognosis in Bell's palsy include complete paralysis, age older than 60 years, and presence of hypertension or diabetes mellitus. Hypertension and diabetes may induce microvascular changes that worsen ischemic injury from compression. Bell's palsy recurrence is more likely in the presence of a positive family history, possibly due to congenitally narrowed facial canal.

Multiple recurrences, regardless of etiology, worsen prognosis. Poor response to medical therapy, especially when contiguous infection or sarcoidosis is the cause, also portends a poor prognosis.

Evaluation for Prognosis

Evaluation for prognosis starts with a careful neurologic examination of the muscles of facial expression. The House-Brackmann grading system is used widely by otolaryngologists in following patients with facial neuropathy.

Electrophysiologic testing can aid in determining prognosis and in following recovery. It has been studied most thoroughly in treatment of Bell's palsy but can be applied to other causes of facial neuropathy. The major drawback is that studies often will be normal until 5 to 7 days after onset. The most useful technique is direct facial motor nerve conduction study. If the compound motor action potential amplitude of the affected side is less than 10% of the unaffected side, prognosis for good functional recovery is poor. Electromyography can be useful early in the course to detect voluntary motor unit potentials even when complete paralysis appears present. Electromyography is particularly useful to follow reinnervation later in the course or to assess success of facial nerve grafting. Nerve excitability tests are less reliable because of the qualitative nature of the testing. When the threshold of stimulation is increased significantly (>10 mA), prognosis for full recovery is poorer.

Therapies Affecting Prognosis

All facial neuropathies require careful eye care, such as the use of artificial tears and night patching, to protect the cornea from drying and trauma.

Steroids, particularly prednisone, have been used to treat Bell's palsy. No prospective, randomized, blinded study has been made, however. The most convincing evidence shows a decreased incidence of synkinesis, particularly autonomic synkinesis, in treated patients. Many studies suggest that patients treated with prednisone recover faster and to a greater extent than do those not treated. Treatment may be more beneficial if started early, particularly within 24 hours of onset of facial weakness. Despite the presence of diabetes mellitus in patients, prednisone therapy still improves outcome in patients with a typical presentation of Bell's palsy.

Often, prednisone is recommended to treat herpes zoster oticus both to hasten recovery and to prevent postherpetic neuralgia. Steroids should not be used for suspected Lyme infection. Steroids clearly are beneficial in the treatment of sarcoidosis affecting the nervous system. Steroids may be useful in hastening recovery in the Melkersson-Rosenthal syndrome, but conclusive data are lacking.

Acyclovir, given within 3 days of Bell's palsy onset, recently was suggested as beneficial in addition to prednisone. Numbers are small, and further prospective, randomized studies are needed. Early treatment with acyclovir clearly improves motor outcome and reverses hearing loss in herpes zoster oticus.

Antibiotics are useful in the treatment of Lyme disease. In an endemic area, a history of tick bite and facial neuropathy is sufficient to recommend therapy. Antibiotic therapy also is recommended for otitis media and mastoid infections.

Surgical treatment of Bell's palsy has not been shown to be effective. Surgery is indicated for tumor resection or facial nerve exploration after skull fracture with possible involvement of the facial canal. Often, myringotomy is used for otitis media associated with facial neuropathy. If facial nerve dysfunction persists despite antibiotic use, mastoidectomy may be performed. For acute demyelinating neuropathies, treatment with plasma exchange or intravenous immunoglobulin may hasten recovery from facial weakness.

Short-Term Prognosis

Most patients with facial neuropathies will manifest facial weakness for several weeks after onset.

Pain is relieved quickly with proper treatment. Patients with incomplete paralysis will have earlier recovery and infrequent occurrence of synkinesis. Patients having significant corneal injury can benefit from surgical treatment, such as weight implantation in the eyelid, that can be removed after recovery. When the typical course of Bell's palsy is not seen in short-term follow-up, other etiologies should be reconsidered, and further testing should be performed.

Long-Term Prognosis

Most patients with facial neuropathies will have full recovery. However, after 6 weeks, in the absence of recovery, significant residual weakness, synkinesis, and facial contracture become likely. For patients with significant functional and cosmetic impairment, microsurgical techniques can be used to improve facial movement and to regain symmetry, especially relative to the smile. Once again, in patients with presumed Bell's palsy, the diagnosis should be reconsidered in those not following the usual course of recovery.

Additional Reading

Adour KK, Ruboyianes JM, Von Doersten PG, et al. Bell's palsy treatment with acyclovir and prednisone compared with prednisone alone: a double-blind, randomized trial. Ann Otol Rhinol Laryngol 1996;105:371–378.

Coyle PK. Neurologic Lyme disease. Semin Neurol 1992;12:200–208.

Dumitru D, Walsh NE, Porter LD. Electrophysiologic evaluation of the facial nerve in Bell's palsy: a review. Am J Phys Med Rehabil 1988;67:137–144.

House JW, Brackmann DE. Facial nerve grading system. Otolaryngol Head Neck Surg 1985;93:146–147.

Morgenlander JC, Massey EW. Bell's palsy: ensuring the best possible outcome. Postgrad Med 1990;88:157–161,164.

Morgenlander JC. Neurosarcoidosis. In RT Johnson, JW Griffin (eds), Current Therapy in Neurologic Diseases. St. Louis: BC Decker, 1993;163–165.

Niparko JK. The Acute Facial Palsies. In RK Jackler, DE Brackmann (eds), Neurotology. St. Louis: Mosby, 1994;1291–1319.

O'Donoghue GM. Tumors of the Facial Nerve. In RK Jackler, DE Brackmann (eds), Neurotology. St. Louis: Mosby, 1994;1321–1331.

Saito O, Aoyagi M, Tojima H, Koike Y. Diagnosis and treatment for Bell's palsy associated with diabetes mellitus. Acta Otolaryngol 1994;(suppl 511):153–155.

Shafshak TS, Essa AY, Bakey FA. The possible contributing factors for the success of steroid therapy in Bell's palsy: a clinical and electrophysiological study. J Laryngol Otol 1994;108:940–943.

Chapter 58

Brachial Plexitis

David C. Preston

Brachial plexitis is a common, although underappreciated, disorder that frequently affects individual upper-extremity nerves or the brachial plexus proper. In the literature, this condition is known by a variety of names, including *Parsonage-Turner syndrome*, *brachial plexus neuropathy*, *shoulder girdle neuritis*, *brachial amyotrophy*, *brachial neuritis*, and *neuralgic amyotrophy*, among others. Although its etiology is unknown, some evidence suggests a self-limited inflammatory or immune-mediated disorder of peripheral nerve.

Natural History

The incidence of brachial plexitis has been estimated at 1.64 cases per 100,000 population. Affected ages range from 3 months to 75 years, with most cases occurring in an equal distribution from the third through the seventh decades. Generally, men are more affected than are women, ranging from 2:1 to 9:1, depending on the series reviewed. No difference is manifest regardless of whether the left or the right side is affected.

Evidence suggesting an immune-mediated process comes mainly from the observation that in many (though not all) cases, one can identify an antecedent event several days to a few weeks beforehand. Most often, the antecedent event is a viral infection (usually upper respiratory infection or flu) or immunization (especially tetanus toxoid). Other cases have followed surgery, minor trauma, strenuous exercise, or labor and delivery. In addition, the disorder has been associated also with connective-tissue diseases, including systemic lupus erythematosus and polyarteritis nodosa.

Brachial plexitis is heralded by the onset of shoulder pain, usually severe or excruciating, often awakening the patient from sleep. Patients describe the pain as sharp, stabbing, throbbing, or aching. The location of the pain is described as scapular (74%), radiating to neck (45%), shoulder (48%), arm (76%), and forearm (22%). The duration of the pain may be hours to several weeks. Commonly, the pain is maximal within the first day or two, bringing the patient to medical attention, often to the emergency room. Pain worsens with shoulder or arm motion but usually not with neck movement, coughing, or other Valsalva maneuvers. Often, orthopedic consultations are obtained initially and prove unrevealing. Early on, detecting muscle weakness may be difficult on examination because of the prominent pain. However, as the pain abates, typically within 1 or 2 weeks, significant underlying weakness becomes apparent. Muscle atrophy follows within a few weeks. Although any upper-extremity muscle can be affected, the muscles affected most often are the deltoid, supraspinatus, infraspinatus, serratus anterior, biceps, triceps, wrist, and finger extensors. In some cases, the diaphragm may be involved as well.

In brachial plexitis, the upper trunk and the nerves derived from the upper trunk of the plexus are affected most often. Less frequently, the entire plexus or the lower plexus can be affected. Brachial plexitis also can affect individual nerves in isolation. Certain nerves, especially the axillary, supra-scapular, anterior interosseous, and long thoracic, often are involved. A long thoracic palsy occurs most often in the setting of brachial plexitis, resulting in a characteristic syndrome of scapular winging from weakness of the serratus anterior muscle.

Weakness and atrophy are much more common than are paresthesias and sensory loss. This finding is explained partly by the tendency of brachial plexitis to affect predominantly or purely motor nerves (e.g., long thoracic, anterior interosseous). However, when sensory symptoms and loss are present, commonly only mild or minimal sensory abnormalities are found on examination. Sensory and motor deficits often are not found in the same nerve or same part of the brachial plexus, underscoring the multifocal nature of the disorder.

Brachial plexitis may affect one or both sides clinically but most often is primarily unilateral (two-thirds of cases). However, on close examination, especially with needle electromyography, abnormalities frequently are found on the contralateral side. Approximately 50% of patients with unilateral clinical findings will have abnormalities bilaterally on electromyography. When findings are bilateral, nearly always they are asymmetric.

Most cases are a one-time event. Recurrent episodes can occur but are distinctly uncommon. Recurrent episodes should suggest the possibility of the inherited form of brachial plexitis, a rare, dominantly inherited disorder that has both clinical presentation and prognosis similar to the idiopathic syndrome. In the familial form, men and women are affected equally. Other than a positive family history, minor dysmorphic features (e.g., hypotelorism) may be present on examination, suggesting the diagnosis.

Factors Affecting Prognosis

Prognosis varies with the degree and duration of initial symptoms. Patients with prolonged pain (i.e., >3 weeks) and those with severe atrophy have a worse prognosis. Similarly, patients with severe muscle weakness or paralysis have a longer recovery than do patients with mild or moderate weakness. Cases that are clinically unilateral fare better than do those with bilateral involvement. The distribution of muscle weakness and atrophy also affects prognosis. Patients with predominant

involvement of the upper trunk or nerves derived from the upper trunk fare better than do those with the lower trunk or entire plexus affected. This condition reflects axonal loss as the primary underlying pathophysiology and recovery occurring by axonal regrowth. As proximal muscles are located closer to the site of injury, they reinnervate first. Most patients with upper-trunk involvement recover in 1 year, but recovery in lower-trunk lesions often requires 1.5 to 3 years.

Prognosis is the same for both genders and regardless of the side affected. Similarly, the presence of an antecedent event does not affect prognosis, nor does the antecedent event (e.g., infection versus immunization).

Evaluation for Prognosis

With the exception of nerve conduction studies and electromyography, laboratory testing adds little to the evaluation of suspected brachial plexitis. Routine blood counts, chemistries, and sedimentation rate are normal. Orthopedic and x-ray evaluation of the shoulder and neck are unremarkable. Cerebrospinal fluid studies are negative, although rare patients will show a mildly elevated protein level. Nerve biopsy, although not indicated for diagnosis or prognosis in this disorder, typically shows evidence of severe axonal loss.

Nerve conduction studies and needle electromyography are useful in brachial plexitis, both in reaching a diagnosis and in assessing prognosis. It should be emphasized that after any acute axonal lesion, nerve conduction studies do not become abnormal until 4 to 7 days later (time required for wallerian degeneration), and denervation on electromyography does not develop until 3 to 4 weeks later. If testing is performed early on, the results must be interpreted with this knowledge. When performed after 3 to 4 weeks, nerve conduction studies and electromyography typically show a multifocal denervating process affecting the brachial plexus or individual peripheral nerves. Sensory nerve action potentials may be small if the recorded nerves are in the distribution of the symptoms. Needle electromyography typically shows an acute or subacute neuropathic pattern in weak muscles (fibrillations and positive waves, decreased recruitment of motor unit action potentials, but normal motor unit action potential morphology). Only after several weeks (and usually months) does reinnervation occur, resulting in changes in motor unit action potential morphology (i.e., increased polyphasia, longer duration, and higher amplitude).

One of the most helpful aids in assessing prognosis is whether axonal continuity to weak muscles is evident on electromyography. Muscles that are denervated completely, with no evidence of axonal continuity, have a longer recovery and more guarded prognosis. If no axonal continuity is present, reinnervation can occur only by axonal regeneration from the point of injury. However, in the presence of axonal continuity, reinnervation also takes place by collateral sprouting from adjacent intact motor fibers, which is not only highly effective but associated with a much shorter time to recovery.

Therapies Affecting Prognosis

Just as the underlying etiology in brachial plexitis is unknown, no proved therapy alters prognosis. For some patients, a short course of steroids is prescribed, though results are mixed; some patients report decreased pain. Otherwise, treatment is largely supportive. Analgesics, including narcotics, often are needed early on to treat pain. Physical therapy, especially range of motion and light exercise, is essential. Although most patients with brachial plexitis make a good recovery, the time to recovery commonly is months to years. During that time, prevention of contractures, especially around the shoulder, is important in ensuring a good functional outcome.

Short-Term Prognosis

The most pressing concern of the patient in the short term is pain. The prognosis regarding pain relief is very good, with the severe pain usually subsiding within 1 or 2 weeks. Occasionally, pain will last up to 3 weeks. After this, patients may be left with residual pain, which is partly musculoskeletal from muscle weakness and disturbed forces around joints. However, this residual pain usually is minor compared to the pain of the initial few days or weeks.

The short-term prognosis regarding muscle weakness and atrophy is not as good. Most patients will note improvement in muscular strength within the first month. However, lack of improvement within 6 to 12 weeks does not preclude a good long-term outcome.

Long-Term Prognosis

Overall, the long-term prognosis in brachial plexitis is excellent. By 1 year, 36% of patients have recovered fully; by 2 years, 75 to 80%; and by 3 years, 90%. Rare patients have reported continued improvement at up to 6 to 8 years after the event. Absence of signs of motor improvement after 3 to 4 months lessens the prognosis for full recovery. Such cases probably have complete denervation, and recovery is possible only from regrowth of the terminal axon. Risk of recurrence is low, typically in the range of 1 to 5%, though patients with the familial form of brachial plexitis are at increased risk for further events within their lifetime.

Additional Reading

Aymond JK, Goldner JL, Hardaker WT. Neuralgic amyotrophy. Orthop Rev 1989;18:1275–1279.

Beghi E, Kurland LT, Mulder DW, Nicolosi A. Brachial plexus neuropathy in the population of Rochester, Minnesota, 1970–1981. Ann Neurol 1985;18:320–323.

Bradley WG, Madrid R, Thrush DC, Campbell MJ. Recurrent brachial plexus neuropathy. Brain 1975;98:381–398.

Foo CL, Swann M. Isolated paralysis of the serratus anterior. A report of 20 cases. J Bone Joint Surg Br 1983;65:552–556.

Geiger LR, Mancall EL, Penn AS, Tucker SH. Familial neuralgic amyotrophy. Report of three families with review of the literature. Brain 1974;97:87–102.

Malamut RI, Marques W, England JD, Sumner AJ. Postsurgical idiopathic brachial neuritis. Muscle Nerve 1994;17:320–324.

Parsonage MJ, Turner JWA. Neuralgic amyotrophy: the shoulder girdle syndrome. Lancet 1948;1:973–978.

Smith BH, Ramakrishna T, Schlagenhauff RE. Familial brachial neuropathy. Two case reports with discussion. Neurology 1971;21:941–945.

Tsairis P, Dyck PJ, Mulder DW. Natural history of brachial plexus neuropathy. Report on 99 patients. Arch Neurol 1972;27:109–117.

Wiederholt WC. Hereditary brachial neuropathy. Report of two families. Arch Neurol 1974;30:252–254.

Chapter 59
Postpolio Syndrome

George M. Sachs

Postpolio syndrome (PPS), broadly defined, is the occurrence of new and otherwise unexplained weakness, fatigue, or muscular pain in patients who have recovered from acute paralytic polio. Most definitions require that 10 to 20 years of symptomatic stability intervene between acute polio and PPS. Similar symptoms are common in polio survivors experiencing rheumatologic, orthopedic, and psychiatric disorders and must be investigated vigorously in every case. From the neurologic standpoint, benefit is derived from distinguishing the diagnosis of postpolio muscular atrophy (PPMA) from other entities. PPMA requires objective demonstration of new muscular weakness with or without atrophy.

Natural History

Retrospective studies using patient questionnaires have noted late muscular pain, weakness, or fatigue in up to 60% of polio survivors. Studies employing more rigorous criteria for PPS (mostly through exclusion of other etiologies) have demonstrated rates of 20 to 30%. Of those with PPS, only a small fraction appear to have bona fide PPMA. The average time of onset is 30 to 40 years after acute polio. Although muscles with residual weakness usually become most symptomatic, PPS can affect previously strong (subclinically denervated) muscles. PPS rarely involves respiratory and bulbar weakness when such symptoms were not features of the original acute polio.

The pathophysiology of PPS is uncertain, but a number of mechanisms have been proposed. Loss of anterior horn cells likely plays a role. Naturally occurring, age-related loss has an exaggerated effect on the already diminished motor neuron populations in polio survivors. Whether the neuronal death rate is accelerated in PPS remains unclear. In a prospective study of polio survivors, electrophysiologic motor unit number estimation failed to document significant loss of motor units over the course of 5 years. However, this study's cohort showed stable strength during that period.

Loss of terminal branches from abnormally extended motor axon arborizations is another proposed mechanism for PPS. The finding of lone denervated muscle fibers in biopsies supports this hypothesis. Early studies with macro-electromyography (EMG) suggested shrinkage of motor unit territory in PPS. However, larger studies have demonstrated growth of motor unit territories in polio survivors with and without PPS (although the growth tends to be more marked in stable patients).

On the basis of histologic evidence of inflammation within the anterior horn and the presence of oligoclonal IgM bands in cerebrospinal fluid, viral reactivation has been considered as a cause of PPS. However, this hypothesis has not withstood scrutiny.

Factors Affecting Prognosis

Nearly all studies agree that the risk of developing PPS or PPMA increases with the severity of the original weakness. Patients contracting polio at a later age also are more likely to develop PPS. However this may not be an independent risk factor, as polio tends to affect older individuals more severely. Isolated studies have suggested other risk factors, including recent weight gain, involvement of lower extremities, time elapsed since acute polio, and female gender. These factors have not been confirmed consistently. The degree of recovery from polio frequently is cited as a risk factor. This theory would support proposed pathophysiology with markedly reinnervated motor units most susceptible to peripheral branch pruning or motor unit attrition. However, at least one study has pointed to an opposite effect (i.e., patients with less recovery at increased risk for PPS). The course of PPS has not been studied systematically, so factors determining rate of deterioration or eventual outcome are not known.

Evaluation for Prognosis

Laboratory investigations cannot predict the onset or the course of PPS. Standard EMG findings do not distinguish patients with PPMA from polio survivors with stable strength. Evidence of ongoing denervation and unstable motor unit potentials are common in both groups. Single-fiber EMG reveals the same degree of synaptic jitter and blocking in patients with PPMA and stable polio survivors. Macro-EMG, a specialized technique designed to evaluate the extent of motor unit territories in muscle, initially showed promise in demonstrating changes specific for PPS. Early studies revealed macro-EMG potential amplitudes in PPMA patients lower than those in stable polio survivors, presumably signifying shrinkage of motor unit territories. However, a larger study failed to confirm this finding.

Elevation of serum creatine kinase levels has not been investigated as extensively as a predictor of PPS. One study revealed modestly elevated creatine kinase levels in some 30% of newly symptomatic polio survivors with no elevation in stable survivors. Evaluating this finding is difficult, as no members of either group exhibited progressive neuromuscular failure, and late symptoms ultimately were attributed to other causes.

Therapy Affecting Prognosis

Exercise is the therapeutic intervention with the greatest potential for altering the course of weakness in PPS. Programs of low-level, nonfatiguing exercise have demonstrated improved strength in at least some muscles of PPS patients over courses ranging from 6 weeks to 2 years. However, a number of studies evaluating such programs did not use stringent criteria for determining PPS. Longer-term sequelae of exercise programs have yet to be determined. Isolated reports cite strenuous exercise as leading to acute deterioration in polio survivors. In a few instances, the resultant new weakness persisted indefinitely. Because of this, strength should be followed closely during exercise programs.

Weight loss and, occasionally, bracing or surgical correction of orthopedic deformities can slow the progression of muscular weakness in PPS. The benefit likely results from relief of muscular overuse. Patients will often note improvement in fatigue with aerobic conditioning programs. Tricyclic antidepressants can provide long-term benefit for muscular pain in PPS.

Short-Term Prognosis

PPS and PPMA generally follow slowly progressive courses. Cases of acute worsening are uncommon, and most have occurred after strenuous exercise or other muscle insult. When PPS affects respiratory or bulbar function, acute deterioration from pneumonia or other pulmonary disease poses considerable risk.

Long-Term Prognosis

Ten to 60 years after polio, 20 to 30% of survivors will experience the onset of PPS (including otherwise unexplained muscular pain). The incidence of PPMA is not known. A study following 50 randomly selected polio survivors revealed no neurologic deterioration over a 5-year interval, suggesting that PPMA is uncommon.

Longitudinal studies quantitating progressive limb weakness in PPMA have documented muscular strength decreasing at an average rate of 1 to 3% per year. Similarly, PPMA affecting respiratory muscles accounts for yearly decrements of approximately 2% in forced vital capacity. Ascertaining the long-term prognosis regarding pain and fatigue is more difficult, not only because they are less amenable to quantitation but because therapy can lead to lasting improvement.

Additional Reading

Jubelt B, Cashman NR. Neurological manifestations of post-polio syndrome. Crit Rev Neurobiol 1987;3:199–220.

Jubelt B, Drucker J. Post-polio syndrome: an update. Semin Neurol 1993;13:283–290.

Stalberg E, Grimby G. Dynamic electromyography and muscle biopsy changes in a 4-year followup: study of patients with a history of polio. Muscle Nerve 1995;18:699–707.

Windebank AJ, Litchy WJ, Daube JR. Lack of progression of neurologic deficit in survivors of paralytic polio: a 5-year prospective population-based study. Neurology 1996;46:80–84.

Chapter 60

Traumatic Nerve Injury

George M. Sachs

Traumatic nerve injury encompasses a wide range of severity. The mildest injuries involve no more than transient disturbance of impulse conduction. At the other extreme, complete division of major nerve trunks or avulsion of spinal roots leads to wallerian degeneration and permanent loss of both conductive and trophic nerve function. The extent of axonal degeneration and the potential for regeneration determine prognosis.

Natural History

Traditionally, nerve injury has been classified into three grades first defined by Seddon as *neurapraxia*, *axonotmesis*, and *neurotmesis*. The course of degeneration and recovery differs markedly for each grade, and they are best considered separately.

Neurapraxic injury involves conduction block with preservation of axonal and endoneurial continuity. Most often, pure neurapraxia is the result of mild compression, but it can be seen also with low-velocity penetrating injuries. Pathologically, the affected nerve demonstrates vacuolation and fissuring of myelin, with thinning or swelling of the underlying axon. Large, heavily myelinated axons are affected most and, therefore, motor and proprioceptive function are affected more than pain or temperature sensation. Recovery can occur within hours and almost always is complete by 2 months.

Axonotmesis entails axonal disruption with preservation of endoneurial sheaths. It occurs with moderate compression and stretch injuries. This condition leads to wallerian degeneration of axons distal to the site of injury, with variable retrograde degeneration. In axonotmetic injury, retrograde degeneration uncommonly progresses to the point of anterior horn cell death, but this effect has been noted, especially with proximal lesions. Recovery from complete axonotmetic injuries results entirely from regeneration of injured axons. Because endoneurial sheaths remain intact, regeneration typically is robust and well directed. The time course of recovery depends on the proximity of injury to target tissues. Axonal regeneration proceeds at a rate of 3 to 4 mm per day over proximal portions of limbs and slows to 1 mm per day more distally. Visible muscle contraction typically begins several weeks after axons reach their target. In general, recovery is maximal within 1 to 3 years. With partial axonotmetic injuries, peripheral sprouting of uninjured axons leads to quicker recovery, usually within months.

Neurotmesis refers to injuries that disrupt intraneural connective tissue and axons. This disruption includes severe lesions in continuity and complete transections. Stretch, crush, and high-velocity missile injuries and sharp trauma are common causes. Distal axons undergo wallerian degeneration, and retrograde degeneration can be marked with up to 80% loss of sensory and motor neurons in proximal injury. When spontaneous axonal regeneration is possible, often it is meager, delayed, and misdirected. Axons reconnecting with appropriate targets often demonstrate poor impulse conduction because constricted endoneurial sheaths inhibit effective myelination.

Factors Affecting Prognosis

The histologic grade of injury affects prognosis more than any other factor. Assessing the severity of axonal and endoneurial disruption is by far the most important focus in determining the outlook for spontaneous recovery. In addition, a number of other variables must be considered.

Proximal injuries show poorer recovery than do those occurring closer to peripheral target tissues. Several factors contribute to this trend. First, retrograde degeneration and neuronal death are more marked with proximal lesions. The length of axon remaining connected to the cell body presumably serves as a source of trophic factors important to neuronal survival. Second, proximal lesions require longer courses of regeneration. This necessity reduces the number of regenerating axons reaching target tissues. In addition, target tissues, especially muscle, undergo progressive degenerative changes with longer periods of denervation. Third, neurotmesis affecting proximal nerve trunks allows greater opportunity for diversion of regenerating axons toward inappropriate targets. Fourth, proximal injury may involve spinal root avulsion, whereupon spontaneous regeneration is impossible and surgical repair cannot be considered.

Sensory nerves tend to recover better than do motor or mixed nerves. The poorer recovery in motor nerves reflects the degeneration of target muscles and its effect on the complex process of re-establishing neuromuscular transmission. Nerve regeneration to small muscles is particularly problematic, because these muscles degenerate more rapidly and severely. Neurotmetic injuries in mixed nerves are complicated by aberrant regeneration of motor axons into sensory fascicles and vice versa.

The effect of age on prognosis has not been well investigated. Children show better recovery than do adults. This finding likely reflects the shorter distances required for regeneration and greater compensatory plasticity within the central nervous system. The impact of age on the rate and vigor of nerve regeneration remains unclear.

Underlying medical problems also affect prognosis. Polyneuropathy, either manifest or subclinical, worsens the initial injury and recovery. Pre-existing nerve compressions and scarring impede the recovery process. Complications from the presenting trauma, including infection, bone fractures, and compartment syndromes, can affect the prognosis adversely.

Evaluation for Prognosis

Most evaluation of nerve injuries focuses on the prognosis for spontaneous recovery, as this determines the choice between a conservative approach and surgical intervention. Certain findings on physical examination have a particularly important bearing on prognosis. Muscular atrophy and loss of autonomic function both indicate axonal disruption rather than neurapraxia. The detection of minimal voluntary contraction in severely weakened muscles is an important finding establishing at least some degree of axonal continuity. A Tinel's sign progressing distally over the nerve in the months after injury indicates a front of regenerating fibers. It is a favorable prognostic sign that demonstrates the rate of regeneration.

Electrodiagnostic studies serve both to localize the injury and to determine the degree of axonal loss. For the first few days after injury, electrodiagnosis cannot distinguish neurapraxia from axonal lesions. If significant axonal loss is present, motor conduction studies performed distal to the injury will demonstrate decreased compound muscle action potential amplitudes by 1 week. A decrease in sensory nerve action potential amplitude occurs a few days later if disruption of sensory axons occurs distal to the dorsal root ganglion. Conversely, preservation of sensory nerve action potential amplitudes within anesthetic areas indicates preganglionic injury, affording a poor prognosis.

With rare exceptions, electrodiagnostic evaluation is best delayed until 3 to 4 weeks after injury. This delay allows fuller assessment of abnormalities in conduction studies and electromyography (EMG). Needle EMG is indispensable for determining the degree of muscle denervation. It is sufficiently sensitive to demonstrate small numbers of intact motor axons. Any degree of preserved axonal continuity to a muscle on initial studies is an important prognostic feature that argues for conservative management. In cases of complete denervation, standard nerve conduction studies and EMG cannot differentiate axonotmesis from neurotmesis and, therefore, cannot predict the likelihood of successful regeneration. Surgical exploration can reveal partial or total nerve transection, but visual inspection may fail to identify intraneural fibrosis or other impediments to regeneration. Intraoperative nerve conduction studies often are the only way to assess early regeneration through an injured segment of nerve.

Radiographic studies also can aid in prognosis. The demonstration of traumatic meningoceles with myelography suggests root avulsion, although the correlation is not perfect. Similarly, hemidiaphragmatic paralysis on chest radiography or fluoroscopy indicates proximal brachial plexus or cervical root injury, generally a poor prognostic sign.

Therapies Affecting Prognosis

Surgical repair is the therapeutic intervention with the greatest impact on prognosis. In cases of complete denervation wherein intraoperative nerve conduction studies fail to show significant regeneration, resection with end-to-end suture or grafting can restore regenerative potential. When intraoperative studies demonstrate significant conduction across the lesion, surgical intervention usually does not go beyond external neurolysis. Internal neurolysis is reserved for cases undergoing split repair or those complicated by intractable neuropathic pain. Not clear is whether internal neurolysis improves regeneration. The prognosis after these various surgical procedures is discussed later (see Long-Term Prognosis).

Physical therapy affects outcome, particularly when muscles are denervated severely. The main impact of physical therapy is in preventing muscular contracture and fibrosis through passive stretching. Electrical stimulation of denervated muscle has not been proved to provide additional benefit.

Short-Term Prognosis

Two processes account for short-term recovery: resolution of neurapraxic conduction block and peripheral sprouting of uninjured axons. Recovery of neurapraxia can occur within hours and nearly always is complete by 2 months. Sprouting begins within days of injury and leads to progressive increase in strength over a few months. It can restore normal strength in muscles that have lost 50 to 75% of their innervating motor axons.

Long-Term Prognosis

Long-term prognosis is most at issue in cases of complete or nearly complete denervation. With axonotmetic injuries, the central question is whether regenerating axons will reach targets before they show irreversible degenerative and fibrotic changes. Once the location of injury has been determined, the length of time required for axonal regeneration to various targets can be estimated using regeneration rates of 3 to 4 mm per day in the upper arm or thigh, 2 mm per day in the forearm or calf, and 1 to 2 mm per day at the wrist and ankle. If regenerating axons can be expected to reach their target by 1 year, the outlook is favorable. By 2 years, most denervated muscles have undergone substantial fibrosis, and axons arriving beyond this time will have little effect.

Recovery from neurotmetic injuries depends on surgical intervention. The number of variables (surgical and nonsurgical) affecting recovery limits detailed prognostication for any individual case. However, case series from major centers for peripheral nerve surgery provide general outcome data. Under the best of circumstances, end-to-end suture or grafting leads to recovery of at least antigravity strength in 60 to 75% of upper-extremity nerve injuries without axonal continuity seen on intraoperative conduction studies. Return of antigravity strength occurs in 50 to 60% of similar cases in the lower extremities.

Even when muscular strength recovers well, aberrant regeneration may impede return of good motor function. In particular, hands often remain clumsy and exhibit pseudomyotonia after neurotmetic injury proximal to the wrist. Medical and physical therapy do little to ameliorate the sequelae of aberrant regeneration.

Additional Reading

Brown PW. Factors influencing the success of the surgical repair of peripheral nerves. Surg Clin North Am 1972;52:1137.

Friedman W. The electrophysiology of peripheral nerve injuries. Neurosurg Clin North Am 1991;2:43–56.

Kline DG, Hudson AR. Nerve Injuries. Philadelphia: Saunders, 1995.

Parry GJ. Electrodiagnostic studies in the evaluation of peripheral nerve and brachial plexus injuries. Neurol Clin 1992;10:921–933.

Sunderland S. Nerve Injuries and Their Repair. Edinburgh: Churchill Livingstone, 1991.

Part XI

Muscle Disorders

Chapter 61

Dystrophin-Related Muscular Dystrophies

George Karpati

Since the 1987 discovery of the dystrophin gene and its protein product and their relevance to Duchenne muscular dystrophy (DMD) and Becker's muscular dystrophy (BMD), impressive progress has been made in understanding the pathophysiology of these X-linked diseases. This understanding, in turn, has helped in planning and implementing new therapeutic strategies to counteract the deleterious consequences of dystrophin deficiency, in performing carrier detection and prenatal diagnosis, and in offering prognostication. This chapter focuses on the improved ability to provide a more refined short-, intermediate-, and long-term prognosis for the family and various health professionals so that they can deliver optimal care for the patient at various stages of the disease.

Duchenne Muscular Dystrophy

Natural History

Symptoms and signs of DMD are of insidious onset and slowly but relentlessly progressive. However, the rate of progression can be uneven and vary from case to case. The first convincing symptoms of muscular dysfunction usually become evident to the family after age 3 years, although walking often is delayed. Initial features include difficulty in getting up from a deep position, clumsy (waddling) gait and running, and enlargement of the calf and (sometimes) of other muscles. In some 30% of patients, slowing of cognitive development and learning difficulties may dominate the initial picture. The examination at this stage usually reveals a Gower's sign, exaggerated lumbar lordosis, and "slide-through" sign due to weakness of arm adductors. As the disease progresses, a tendency to toe walk supervenes, owing to tightness of the Achilles tendons.

By age 6 to 13 years (mean, near 9 years), the weakness of pelvic girdle and leg muscles reaches such a degree that independent or unassisted ambulation becomes impossible. As the disease progresses, contractures develop at the elbows, knees, hips, and ankles. Weakness of the axial trunk muscles may cause marked scoliosis and thoracic deformity. This condition, along with weakening respiratory musculature, leads to progressive respiratory deficiency and its complications (atelectasis, pneumonia, etc.), which results in a fatal outcome before age 20 years (mean, 17 years) unless some respiratory support is provided. Cardiac failure due to cardiomyopathy rarely is a problem unless survival into the third decade occurs.

Factors Affecting Prognosis

The diagnosis of DMD in phenotypically suggestive cases is made by showing a defect in the dystrophin gene at locus Xp21. In perhaps 65% of the patients, an out-of-frame deletion, detectable by multiplex polymerase chain reaction, is present. Two areas of deletion "hot spots" are defined. One is centered at the 3' end of the N-terminus, the other is within exons 44–45. A deletion may take out either one exon only or many exons. The out-of-frame deletion invariably creates a stop codon downstream and produces an unstable truncated dystrophin transcript and usually no detectable dystrophin protein. Some 5% of the DMD cases experience a reduplication of one or more exons leading to a subverted reading frame. The remaining DMD cases undergo presumed point mutations, causing stop-codon or splicing errors and the like.

As a rule of thumb, a deletion in the *N*-terminus or *C*-terminus region causes moderate to severe phenotypes, whereas deletions in the rod region tend to cause milder phenotypes. However, several exceptions to these rules have been reported but not explained fully.

In addition to gene mutation analysis, the demonstration of absence of dystrophin by microscopical immunocytochemistry or Western blot analysis must be obtained in all cases. Serum creatine kinase level is a rough guide for the activity of the necrotic process in the muscle, but its high degree of day-to-day variability precludes use of this parameter as a predictor of progression for the short term.

Ultimately, three major natural factors seem to determine the severity of phenotype: the amount of dystrophin, the evenness of its distribution among the muscle fibers, and possible compensating mechanisms for dystrophin deficiency (vide infra). The prevalence of revertant fibers (i.e., rare fibers containing sarcolemmal dystrophin presumably due to a second "corrective" or "reversing" mutation) is not a significant factor affecting prognosis.

DMD must be differentiated from α-sarcoglycan (SG) deficiency by appropriate immunocytochemical and gene mutation studies. The prognosis of SG deficiencies tends to be better than that of DMD, and genetic counseling is different, as SG deficiency is an autosomal recessive disorder (see Chapter 63).

A possible compensation for dystrophin deficiency may occur by upregulation of a dystrophin analog called *utrophin* and encoded on chromosome 6. This gene is intact in DMD. Normally, utrophin is expressed only at the neuromuscular and myotendinous junctions. However, in dystrophin deficiency, an apparent spontaneous upregulation of utrophin appears to occur, so that it is demonstrable not only in those restricted sites already noted but throughout the extrajunctional sarcolemma. Some

have hypothesized that this spontaneous upregulation of utrophin can be functionally important in DMD and that without such putative compensation, the severity of the disease would be even worse than it is. The notion that utrophin upregulation can be helpful in Duchenne dystrophy was confirmed by overexpression of utrophin in transgenic dystrophin-deficient (*mdx*) mice leading to abundant extrajunctional sarcolemmal utrophin, which impressively corrected the dystrophic phenotype. At the present, not clear is which factors are responsible for the spontaneous upregulation of utrophin in DMD. However, extensive efforts are attempting to find a pharmacologic agent that could enhance this natural process.

Presumably because of the cited factors (i.e., amount and distribution of dystrophin and utrophin upregulation) and, perhaps, other unrecognized factors, the severity of DMD can vary within a spectrum. Rare cases present with severe muscle weakness as a congenital muscular dystrophy. In most cases, the standard natural history takes its course as described in Natural History. In some cases, previously called *outliers*, the natural progression is slower in terms of wheelchair dependence and fatal outcome.

DMD can occur in female subjects as well (i.e., in manifest heterozygotes). Here, the severity of the disease depends on the amount and evenness of dystrophin present in the muscle. This condition, in turn, is determined by the pattern of X-chromosomal inactivation that, in most cases, is random and is not biased in favor of either paternally or maternally derived X chromosomes.

Therapies Affecting Prognosis

Physical Measures

Prolonged immobility from bedrest or casting can result in contractures, accelerated loss of muscle tissue, and faster decline of muscle force generation. In the ambulatory phase of the disease, regular stretching of the heel cords and the use of below-knee night splints are useful to improve and prolong ambulation. The adjustment of physical activities (i.e., avoidance of or reduction of lengthening contractions in leg muscles) tends to retard the rate of muscle fiber damage and dropout. Thus, DMD patients should be discouraged from climbing and descending steps or hills as much as possible. Long leg orthoses to stabilize the knee and ankle joints may prolong ambulation by 1 to 2 years. When the need for a wheelchair arises, proper seating is essential to minimize the risk of development of severe scoliosis that could shorten the life span of the patient. Appropriate respiratory exercises can minimize complications from respiratory insufficiency. In addition, nighttime assisted respiration or periodic daytime assisted ventilation can remove the element of respiratory muscle fatigue that compounds the respiratory muscle weakness–induced ventilatory insufficiency.

Anesthetic and Surgical Measures

Anesthesia, particularly with the use of depolarizing blocking agents and halothane, can cause two types of severe and potentially fatal complications: either cardiac arrest or an acute rhabdomyolytic crisis. Although the latter reaction has been compared to malignant hyperthermia, it evinces no associated rigidity or massive increase of the body temperature. DMD patients, therefore, should not be anesthetized with depolarizing muscle relaxants or fluorinated anesthetics; nitrous oxide and Ketamine appear to be safe.

Surgical measures may be necessary to improve comfort level, to prolong mobility, to correct severe scoliosis, and to minimize the risk of respiratory insufficiency. Tendon lengthening, particularly of the Achilles tendon, often is performed. Stabilization of the spine by rod-shaped metallic implants is a major operation and rarely is necessary currently, with proper wheelchair seating and careful monitoring of spinal alignment.

Drug Therapy

The only available drugs shown to have an objective, beneficial effect on muscle function in DMD are corticosteroids. On a daily dose of prednisone, 0.75 mg per kg orally, most DMD patients show a moderate but rapid improvement of muscle-force generation and on functional tests reflecting activities of daily living. Furthermore, the rate of decline of muscle force in key muscles is reduced substantially. These beneficial effects appear to be sustained for at least a couple of years. However, one cannot predict the long-term effectiveness of this type of therapy, as its pharmacologic basis remains obscure. The major drawback of prednisone therapy is its side-effects, including obesity, cataracts, and stunted growth. The most cumbersome of these is obesity, which substantially can compromise physical mobility and care. A lesser known analog of prednisone, Deflazacort, has fewer side effects than those of prednisone but has comparable therapeutic efficiency.

Miscellaneous

Dietary measures are useful in the care of DMD patients. An isocaloric balanced diet must be followed to avoid obesity, which has a negative effect on the course of the disease.

At various stages of the disease, DMD patients face a number of psychosocial problems that can affect the overall prognosis. One valuable support factor is to foster a proper relationship to peers in the school and social environment. DMD patients must not be isolated or castigated socially, and maintenance of self-respect is essential. Sexual frustration and lack of access to privacy must be addressed by parents, teachers, friends, and sometimes psychologists. Preoccupation with death in the later stages of the disease can produce significant depression that may necessitate pharmacologic and psychological therapy.

Future Perspectives

Although carrier detection in DMD has reduced prevalence, a very high spontaneous mutation rate of the dystrophin gene suggests that the incidence of DMD (1 per 3,500 live male births) will remain high. For these patients, the ultimate aim is to find a definitive therapy that, when applied early in the course of the disease, will have a decisive effect on prognosis. For the earliest possible implementation of any effective therapy, neonatal detection of DMD patients—by mass screening of all newborns for elevated serum creatine kinase activity—has been advocated strongly. At the present, two promising therapeutic approaches loom on the horizon for skeletal muscles: dystrophin gene replacement therapy and utrophin upregulation. Dystrophin gene replacement has been attempted by myoblast transfer; however, in its presently available form, it proved to be functionally inefficient in several human trials. Another means of dystrophin gene replacement is by direct gene transfer using a genetically modified adenovirus vector. In preclinical animal experiments, such a procedure produced promising short- and intermediate-term results. However, long-term beneficial effects required the concomitant use of immunosuppression, which is not ideal for human application. Improved adenoviral vectors and a safe and efficient route of administration of the therapeutic gene vector would raise hope that these obstacles will prove to be surmountable.

Reference to utrophin upregulation as a potential therapy for DMD has been made. Intensive search for a nontoxic molecule with the ability to sustain utrophin upregulation could be an elegant and cost-effective way of altering the prognosis radically. Definitive treatment of the cardiomyopathy may require cardial organ transplantation.

Short-Term Prognosis

DMD is a chronic, progressive disease of insidious onset. As such, little short-term deterioration is encountered unless immobility occurs (prolonged bedrest, casting, etc.). Disuse of muscle can result in enhanced contractures and accelerated muscle weakness.

Long-Term Prognosis

Progressive loss of muscle tissue leads to loss of ambulation (average age, 9 years) and death from respiratory insufficiency in the early twenties. Aggressive physiotherapy, bracing, and selected operations can improve the quality of life but have a limited effect on the ultimate prognosis. The effect of corticosteroid therapy on long-term prognosis is unclear. More definitive molecular therapies are required to avoid the dismal long-term prognosis.

Becker's Muscular Dystrophy

BMD is an allelic variant of DMD. In the majority of cases, an in-frame deletion is present in the dystrophin gene that gives rise to the generation of a reduced amount of a lower-molecular-weight dystrophin. Demonstration of such a reduced amount of a lower-molecular-weight dystrophin than normal on Western blot analysis is definite diagnostic evidence.

Natural History

The course of the disease is much more benign than that of DMD. It evinces a large variability in age of onset and in overall severity of symptoms and signs. In the majority of cases, leg weakness and a slow waddling gait first are noted between age 5 and 15 years (mean, 11 years). Curiously, exercise-induced muscle cramps are relatively common. Muscle hypertrophy and exaggerated lordosis is as common as that in DMD, but contractures and scoliosis are not. Mental subnormality is infrequent. Proximal upper-limb weakness often is delayed until the thirties. Independent ambulation usually is lost in the mid forties. Respiratory insufficiency is uncommon. In the later stages, cardiac failure can supervene, and it may be treated with appropriate medication or even by organ transplantation. No reliable data can indicate that BMD actually leads to premature death, unless intractable cardiac failure ensues.

Natural and Other Factors Affecting Prognosis

Cases having a small deletion of the dystrophin gene in the mid-rod portion of the molecule have the best prognosis, and some patients can remain only mildly symptomatic throughout life. Otherwise, very little information is available concerning other factors that have a major impact on prognosis. Late cardiac involvement must be recognized and treated.

Additional Reading

Emery AEH. Duchenne Muscular Dystrophy. Oxford, NY: Oxford University Press, 1987.

Griggs CR, Moxley RT, Mendell JR, et al. Prednisone in Duchenne dystrophy: a randomized controlled trial defining the time course and dose response. Arch Neurol 1991;48:383–388.

Hoffman EP. Clinical and histopathological features of abnormalities of the dystrophin-based cytoskeleton. Brain Pathol 1996;6:49–61.

Karpati G, Acsadi G. The principles of gene therapy in Duchenne dystrophy. Clin Invest Med 1994;17:499–509.

Karpati G, Brown RH. The dawning of a new era in the molecular biology of the muscular dystrophies. Brain Pathol 1996;6:17.

Moseley CF. Natural History and Management of Scoliosis in Duchenne Muscular Dystrophy. In G Serratrice (ed), Neuromuscular Diseases. New York: Raven, 1984; 545–549.

Rideau Y, Gatin G, Bach J, et al. Prolongation of life in Duchenne's muscular dystrophy. Acta Neurol 1983;5: 118–124.

Rideau Y, Glorion B, Duport G. Prolongation of ambulation in the muscular dystrophies. Acta Neurol 1983;5: 390–397.

Smith PEM, Calverly PMA, Edwards RHT, et al. Practical problems in the respiratory care of patients with muscular dystrophy. N Engl J Med 1987;316:1197–1205.

Chapter 62

Myotonic Dystrophy

James M. Gilchrist

Myotonic dystrophy, also known as *dystrophica myotonica*, *myotonica atrophica*, and *Steinert's disease*, is a multisystem disorder causing grip, percussion, and electrical myotonia; limb, facial, and pharyngeal skeletal muscle weakness; esophageal, gastrointestinal, and uterine smooth-muscle weakness; cardiac conduction abnormalities; endocrine dysfunction; frontal balding; cataracts; hearing loss; and mental retardation. Myotonic dystrophy is inherited as an autosomal dominant trait and, though 100% penetrant, shows marked variation in expression and age of onset, from intrauterine to middle age, most commonly becoming symptomatic in the second to fourth decades.

The gene for myotonic dystrophy resides on chromosome 19q and codes for a protein kinase that remains poorly characterized. The gene defect is an expanded trinucleotide repeat (CTG), which is unstable and commonly increases from generation to generation. Unaffected alleles have 40 or fewer repeats, whereas myotonic dystrophy alleles usually have more than 100. This expanded repeat on chromosome 19q is specific to myotonic dystrophy, though why it causes myotonic dystrophy remains a mystery.

Natural History

Myotonic dystrophy can present in many ways and to several different types of physicians. It is not uncommon for adult women to receive a diagnosis first shortly after giving birth to a neonate with congenital myotonic dystrophy. Patients also present for cataracts, infertility, lassitude, speech and swallowing difficulties, ptosis, and orthopedic problems, though the most common presenting complaint is distal limb weakness. This distribution, together with myotonia and the presence of systemic signs, makes for a relatively straightforward diagnosis, especially once one family member has had the disease diagnosed. Prominent proximal muscle weakness should raise suspicion of proximal myotonic myopathy (PROMM).

Symptoms can begin at almost any time but, for most adult patients, they begin in the second to third decade of life. Progression of weakness varies widely and can be rapid (into a wheelchair within 10 years) or very slow, with little change over decades. Most commonly, the disease steadily progresses, with patients needing ambulatory aids only after 15 to 20 years and requiring wheelchairs sometime later, if at all. Pain is an infrequent complaint, but stiffness (from myotonia) and fatigue, often debilitating, are frequent, especially in more mildly affected patients. The systemic nature of the disease also has an impact on the course, as cataracts occur in most patients, symptomatic cardiac conduction disturbance in some 10%, diarrhea or obstipation (occasionally leading to megacolon) in a few, and sleep apnea in many.

Frequently, life expectancy is shortened, and sudden death may occur from heart block. First-degree heart block is very common, as are bundle branch blocks. Second-degree block, atrial flutter, and complete heart block also occur. Most patients will experience slow progression of their electrocardiographic abnormalities, but perhaps 1 in 10 will become symptomatic. Heart failure is uncommon. Hypoventilation secondary to sleep apnea or diaphragmatic weakness is common. Dysphagia leading to poor nutrition and aspiration pneumonia can be another factor in early demise.

A distinct syndrome—congenital myotonic dystrophy—affects approximately 10% of affected children born to myotonic mothers (but not to myotonic fathers). Severe cases will present with neonatal hypotonia, hydramnios, respiratory distress, poor feeding, and arthrogryposis, resulting in an increased neonatal death rate. Myotonia uncommonly is present, and often the diagnosis is made by examining the previously undiagnosed mother. Surviving infants have severe disease, with facial and limb weakness, talipes, mental retardation, learning disabilities, and behavioral problems, from which they do not recover.

Factors Affecting Prognosis

Anticipation in genetic disease refers to subsequent generations having earlier onset and more severe disease. The discovery of enhanced trinucleotide repeat expansion in subsequent generations provided a genetic explanation for anticipation in myotonic dystrophy. Not uncommonly, multigenerational families with myotonic dystrophy will have a mildly affected oldest generation, a moderately affected next generation, and a severely affected youngest generation, and succeeding generations will have increasingly expanded trinucleotide repeat numbers. Studies correlating clinical severity with repeat number also have shown a strong correlation between number of trinucleotide repeats, age of onset, and severity (Fig. 62-1). Cardiac conduction defects correlate with increasing size of the triplet repeat as well, though whether this translates to increased risk of sudden death is uncertain. Mental retardation and gonadal dysfunction also correlate with increasing size of the expanded repeat. However, cataract formation, myotonia, and gastrointestinal dysfunction apparently do not.

Even before the ability to ascertain trinucleotide repeat number, earlier age of onset and greater severity at onset were indicators of poorer prognosis. Age of onset can help to predict the severity of specific features. For example, onset beyond age 50 years is associated uncommonly with weakness but is asso-

ciated almost always with cataracts. In childhood, onset is associated with mental retardation and weakness but not with cataracts. Earlier-onset adult cases (<age 30 years) are less likely to develop cataracts but more likely to have impaired mental abilities than are patients with later onset (>30 years).

Family history also is a factor, as the risk of congenital myotonic dystrophy increases from 10 to 40% for mothers with a previous congenitally affected child. As well, the incidence of symptomatic heart block seems to affect a minority of myotonic families (near 20%), with an increased risk in those families.

Asymptomatic women or those with only cataracts are unlikely to have children with congenital myotonic dystrophy. On the other hand, women with multisystem disease are most likely to have affected children. Age of the mother also may have an adverse effect on her children, as older women tend to have more severely affected children.

Evaluation for Prognosis

Combining a careful ascertainment of age of onset and a thorough examination will permit a general assessment of prognosis, with earlier age of onset and greater abnormality on examination being evidence for a faster and more symptomatic course. Assay for trinucleotide repeat number will establish the diagnosis and can confirm the clinical prognosis loosely. Triplet repeat number and severity overlap in population studies, such that repeat expansion may not be an accurate connotation in individuals. Examples of discordant clinical outcomes exist for similar degrees of triplet repeat expansion. This condition may result from somatic mosaicism, in which different triplet repeat expansions exist in different tissues. Triplet repeat testing commonly is performed on peripheral leukocytes, and the value there may be very different from muscle, brain, and the like. Electromyography, creatine phosphokinase, and muscle biopsy are of little help in prognosis.

Therapies Affecting Prognosis

No available treatments can change the course of myotonic dystrophy. Some drugs (e.g., phenytoin, carbamazepine, and mexiletine) may assuage symp-

Figure 62-1. An association is evident between DNA band size of the triplet repeat and age of onset-clinical severity of myotonic dystrophy. The band size increases as triplet repeat expansion increases. (Reprinted with permission from HG Harley, SA Rundle, W Reardon, et al. Unstable DNA sequence in myotonic dystrophy. Lancet 1992;339:1126.)

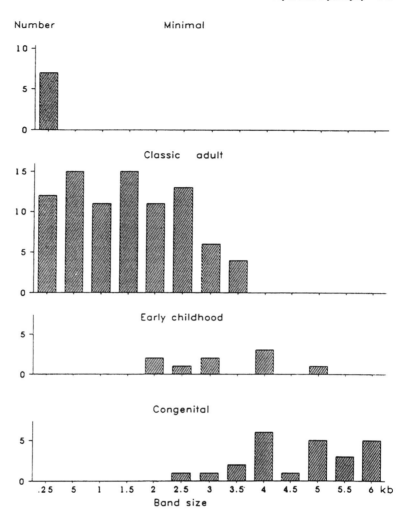

toms from myotonia, but effects on cardiac conduction must be considered first. Monitoring of electrocardiograms and periodic query after cardiac symptoms is necessary to warn of life-threatening cardiac conduction defects. Pacemaker insertion then may prevent sudden cardiac death. Evaluation and treatment of sleep apnea in the hypersomnolent patient also are beneficial for better well-being and to prevent pulmonary hypertension.

Short-Term Prognosis

Myotonic dystrophy will progress slowly, and little can be done to change that. Weakness, cataracts,

smooth-muscle involvement, and endocrine dysfunction advance on the order of years, not weeks or months. Preventive measures, such as periodic evaluations and electrocardiograms will lessen the chance of short-term downfalls. Otherwise, cardiac involvement can cause sudden and unanticipated arrhythmias resulting in syncope or death.

Long-Term Prognosis

The long-term prognosis is in part determined at conception, as the degree of CTG triplet repeat expansion plays a large role in determining the age of onset and the severity of the disease. Congenital myotonic dystrophy will have a stormy neonatal course that, if survived, will be the start of a shortened life characterized by mental retardation, delayed motor development, and physical disability. Adult-onset disease is more variable in its course, with a generally slower and more benign evolution. Severe cases will develop weakness (ultimately requiring ambulatory assistance) and cataract extraction, with additional possible complications of cardiac arrhythmias, dysphagia, disordered bowel function, infertility, diabetes, balding, ptosis, dysarthria, muscle wasting, sleep apnea, aspiration pneumonia, and hearing loss. Each of these complications also can affect later-onset cases but are less likely to do so. If they do have an effect, the effects are likely to be milder.

Additional Reading

Andrews PI, Wilson J. Relative disease severity in siblings with myotonic dystrophy. J Child Neurol 1992;7:161–167.

Gennarelli M, Novelli G, Andreasi Bassi F, et al. Prediction of myotonic dystrophy clinical severity based on the number of intragenic [CTG]n trinucleotide repeats. Am J Med Genet 1996;11:342–347.

Harley HG, Rundle SA, Reardon W, et al. Unstable DNA sequence in myotonic dystrophy. Lancet 1992;339:1125–1128.

Harper PS. Myotonic Dystrophy. Philadelphia: Saunders, 1989.

Harper PS, Rudel R. Myotonic Dystrophy. In AG Engel, C Franzini-Armstrong (eds), Myology (2nd ed). New York: McGraw-Hill, 1994;1192–1219.

Hawley RJ, Gottdeiner JS, Gay JA, Engel WK. Families with myotonic dystrophy with and without cardiac involvement. Arch Intern Med 1983;143:2134–2136.

Jespert A, Fahsold R, Grehl H, Claus D. Myotonic dystrophy: correlation of clinical symptoms with the size of the CTG trinucleotide repeat. J Neurol 1995;242:99–104.

Koch MC, Grimm T, Harley HG, Harper PS. Genetic risks for children of women with myotonic dystrophy. Am J Hum Genet 1991;48:1084–1091.

Melacini P, Villanova C, Menegazzo E, et al. Correlation between cardiac involvement and CTG trinucleotide repeat length in myotonic dystrophy. J Am Coll Cardiol 1995;25:239–245.

Redman JB, Fenwick RG, Fu Y-H, et al. Relationship between parental trinucleotide GCT repeat length and severity of myotonic dystrophy in offspring. JAMA 1993;269:1960–1965.

Chapter 63

Other Muscular Dystrophies

James M. Gilchrist

Muscular dystrophy is a term encompassing several different diseases, including three discussed in Chapters 61 and 62 (dystrophin-related muscular dystrophies [Duchenne muscular dystrophy and Becker's muscular dystrophy] and myotonic dystrophy). Three other dystrophies (Table 63-1) are discussed in this chapter: facioscapulohumeral dystrophy (FSHD), limb-girdle muscular dystrophy (LGMD), and oculopharyngeal muscular dystrophy (OPMD). FSHD and OPMD are inherited as autosomal dominant traits (LGMD is largely an autosomal recessive trait), and chromosomal locations are known. No effective therapies are available to delay, halt, or reverse the dystrophic process in any of the three.

Facioscapulohumeral Dystrophy

FSHD is inherited as an autosomal dominant trait, with high penetrance but with variable intrafamilial severity. Approximately 90 to 95% of families with FSHD are linked to chromosome 4q35, near the telomere.

Natural History

FSHD is a muscular dystrophy of characteristic and defining weakness involving the face and scapular muscles. The age of onset is variable, from childhood (when patients frequently are affected more severely) to the early third decade. The disease tends to progress from the face downward, affecting first facial muscles, then scapular muscles, proximal arm muscles, and pelvic girdle muscles, with the exception of the tibialis anterior, which is affected early when affected. Because the facial weakness often goes unnoticed and does not interfere with daily life, patients do not seek medical attention until the scapular muscles become noticeably weak, often several years into the disease.

At initial presentation, almost invariably the patient has facial weakness, with an expressionless face, horizontal or droopy smile, and few facial lines or wrinkles. The scapulae are winged and are rotated laterally and upward, giving the patient a webbed-neck appearance and causing the shoulders to be rounded and rotated forward. The clavicle is horizontal, and the axillary fold is reversed. The patient is unable to abduct the arm more than 15 to 20 degrees, though if the examiner can hold the scapula in place, abduction is improved. This inability to use the arms above the horizontal for activities of daily living (e.g., combing hair, brushing teeth, washing face) motivates most patients finally to see a physician.

The weakness is slowly progressive and, to a degree not seen in other dystrophies, may arrest for several years or more. However, the disease also may progress in sudden accelerations, and (in my experience) these rapid changes in strength and function are a common precipitant for seeking medical attention. Perhaps 20% of patients will become wheelchair-dependent and, except for the minority with severe disease, life expectancy is not affected.

Table 63-1. Muscle Involvement in Some Muscular Dystrophies

Site of Involvement	FSHD	LGMD	OPMD
Facial	++	–	±
Ptosis	++	–	++
Jaw muscles	+	–	±
Sternomastoids	+	±	–
Shoulder girdle	++	+	+
Pelvic girdle	+	++	+
Proximal limb	+	++	+
Distal limb	±	+	±
Myotonia	–	–	–
Dysphagia	–	–	++

FSHD = facioscapulohumeral dystrophy; LGMD = limb-girdle muscular dystrophy; OPMD = oculopharyngeal muscular dystrophy; + = common; ++ = universal; ± = can occur; – = does not occur.

Only approximately 10% of patients have severe ventilatory impairment, these being of younger onset. At least half of FSHD patients never will develop pelvic girdle weakness, and it is not uncommon to find relatives of any age with undiagnosed disease producing only facial weakness.

Factors Affecting Prognosis

As mentioned in the previous section, childhood onset usually is associated with more severe disease, including scoliosis, contractures, and wheelchair dependence, which occurs less often in later-onset patients. Sporadic cases also tend to have earlier onset and more severe disease.

In the region of 4q35 linked to FSHD is a series of tandem repeats. FSHD patients linked to this region have a deletion resulting in a fragment smaller than 35 kb, with normal controls usually being 50 to 300 kb. The area does not appear to make a protein and, hence, would not be the direct cause of FSHD, but a correlation has been found among fragment size, the age of onset (the smaller the fragment, the earlier the onset), and the age of loss of ambulation (the smaller the fragment, the earlier the loss of ambulation). The smallest fragments occurred in isolated cases.

A retinal vasculopathy and high-frequency hearing loss are associated with the muscle weakness in many FSHD patients, together and separately. It is mild in most, with severe involvement of the retina (Coats' disease) or of hearing in less than 2% of patients.

Evaluation for Prognosis

On muscle biopsy, a subset of FSHD patients have mononuclear cell infiltrates superimposed on the dystrophic process. This infiltrate is not characteristic of any stage of the disease but tends to be present within families, implying some genetic association. Presence or absence of the infiltrate is not helpful in prognosis. Creatine phosphokinase levels also do not correlate with prognosis but do tend to decrease to normal by the sixth decade. Electromyography (EMG) also is not helpful in establishing prognosis.

Therapies Affecting Prognosis

No therapy exists to alter the underlying genetic abnormality causing FSHD. Use of steroids to treat the occasional inflammatory infiltrate may result in temporary improvement but has no long-lasting effect on the course of the disease.

Certain interventions may help function and, hence, quality of life, including bracing, scoliosis surgery, and scapular stabilization surgery. However, pinning the scapula to the ribs should be performed only in a subset of patients who have a functioning deltoid muscle and whose occupation necessitates flexion and abduction of the shoulder higher than 90 degrees.

Short-Term Prognosis

FSHD is a slowly progressive, chronic disease. However, the disease does not necessarily progress at a uniform rate, and patients may experience periods both of more rapid worsening of weakness or of apparent stabilization. The overall course of the disease will not be altered by a course of steroids in those patients with inflammatory infiltrates on muscle biopsy.

Long-Term Prognosis

The weakness will accumulate over the course of many years, and functional abilities will be lost slowly. The affected muscles tend to progress from the face downward and do not affect function until the scapular muscles or the leg muscles become significantly weak. Fifty percent of patients will not have leg involvement. Except for the most severely affected patients who experience early, childhood onset, life expectancy is not affected, and many patients will not become wheelchair-dependent, though they may need aids to ambulation.

Oculopharyngeal Muscular Dystrophy

OPMD is another muscular dystrophy with a characteristic constellation of symptoms and signs. It is inherited as an autosomal dominant trait, and the defective gene has been localized to chromosome 14q11.2–q13. It was described first in 1915 in a French Canadian family, and subsequent studies have shown that all affected French Canadian families derive from a single individual who emigrated from France to Quebec in 1634. The disease is common also in Spanish Americans.

Natural History

The defining features of OPMD are progressive ptosis and dysphagia, beginning between the fourth and fifth decades. The ptosis usually starts first and is followed within a few years by dysphagia, but this order can be reversed. This unusual set of signs, coupled with the late onset and dominant inheritance, allows differentiation from myotonic dystrophy, myasthenia gravis, and mitochondrial myopathies. A study from Quebec (Brais and colleagues 1996) of 161 affected French Canadian patients revealed a mean onset age of ptosis at 48 years and of dysphagia at 46 years. The late onset age means most affected patients already have completed their families, making genetic counseling less useful. Localization of the genetic locus may allow presymptomatic carrier detection, but the relative mildness of the dystrophy renders genetic counseling less compelling than with other muscular dystrophies.

The ptosis always is bilateral, though occasionally asymmetric, and progresses over years, eventually to cover the pupil and to impede vision. Patients with severe ptosis often will compensate by extending the neck and contracting the frontalis muscles to allow vision beneath the drooped eyelids. Dysphagia involves the cricopharyngeal muscles, and patients usually can point to the exact spot in their neck at which food becomes stuck (i.e., the cricopharyngeal, or upper esophageal, sphincter). As the dystrophy progresses, the sphincter becomes increasingly resistant to opening and can impede swallowing to the point of starvation. Virtually all patients seeking medical attention will need swallowing evaluations, including esophageal manometry, esophagoduodenoscopy, and cine barium swallow.

Other features include dysarthria-dysphonia (58%); limitation of vertical and horizontal gaze (35% and 37%, respectively); and weakness of the arm (37%), the leg (74%), the tongue (47%), and the face (65%). Given the late onset age, life expectancy is the longest of the muscular dystrophies, and OPMD currently is less likely to be life threatening given improved management of dysphagia. I have yet to see a patient become wheelchair-dependent, though several patients have needed such aids to ambulation as canes and walkers. I have followed several large families, and mildly affected members who have not sought medical attention are common.

Factors Affecting Prognosis

Very little is known about which patients will do worse. Clearly, those patients with severe ptosis or dysphagia at a relatively early age (e.g., younger than 45) will have the most difficulty. Patients with limb weakness, particularly of the legs, will be more functionally impaired than those without weakness. Some reports have suggested an increased risk of cancer in patients with OPMD.

Evaluation for Prognosis

Laboratory examination adds nothing to prognostication. The muscle biopsy in OPMD often reveals rimmed vacuoles and unique intranuclear 8.5-nm diameter inclusions. Other intranuclear and cytoplasmic inclusions, 16 to 18 nm in diameter, also can be seen in OPMD but are seen also in inclusion body myositis. Beyond their diagnostic use, the inclusions do not convey a particular prognosis.

Therapies Affecting Prognosis

As with all other muscular dystrophies, no cure is available for OPMD, nor can any treatment affect the course of disease. Palliative management of the ptosis and dysphagia, however, may markedly improve the patient's quality of life and, in the case of severe dysphagia with impending starvation or recurrent aspiration, may prolong life. Blepharoplasty, either by resection of levator palpebrae muscle or by retraction of the levator palpebrae using silicon rods, will improve vision and appearance and is the surgery performed most often in OPMD patients. However, the ptosis usually recurs, sometimes within 2 or 3 years, and further surgery may not be possible without imperiling the cornea.

Various strategies may help the patient with symptomatic dysphagia. Avoidance of solid foods in favor of pureed food or liquids can be helpful, as can a speech and swallowing therapy consultation. Such techniques as bending and tucking the neck when swallowing often are beneficial. However, as the disease progresses, these noninvasive maneuvers become less satisfactory, and either esophageal dilation or cricopharyngeal myotomy may be necessary. Dilation works for less than 50% of patients (in my experience), usually because of transient benefit (less than a week). Even in those patients with more satisfactory results, dilation must be repeated every 3 to 5 months. Several reports in the literature cite very good responses to cricopharyngeal myotomy, but often patients are reluctant until their dysphagia becomes disabling or life-threatening. The ultimate treatment is parenteral feeding via gastrostomy.

Short-Term Prognosis

The symptoms of ptosis and dysphagia can be managed with a variety of both nonsurgical and surgical techniques. However, as the disease progresses, the invasiveness of the remedies necessary to provide relief increases.

Long-Term Prognosis

OPMD is a slowly progressive disease, and disability may arise from impaired vision due to severe ptosis, poor nutrition or pneumonia from dysphagia, or difficulty with ambulation and activities of daily living from limb weakness. The late onset of symptoms, the slow progression, and the restricted range of affected muscles allows for a life span nearer normal than that afforded by any other muscular dystrophy.

Limb-Girdle Muscular Dystrophy

Limb-girdle muscular dystrophy long was thought to be a term useful only as a repository for those myopathies not otherwise explained; in part, this concept was correct. Becker's muscular dystrophy, Emery-Dreifuss muscular dystrophy, spinal muscular atrophy, and lipid myopathy are among the diseases culled from LGMD in the last 50 years. Regardless, a core group of patients always experienced similar but nonspecific findings of a familial, proximal myopathy with dystrophic pathology. Since the early 1990s, much progress has been made not only in establishing LGMD as a legitimate entity but in establishing the genetic and pathophysiologic basis for the disease. This advance allows for a much more informed and reliable prognostication for patients with this diagnosis.

Several, but not all, of the LGMD diseases have been discovered to result from genetic defects in the dystrophin-associated glycoprotein complex, specifically involving the sarcoglycan complex (Table 63-2). This complex, along with dystrophin, is believed to be important in maintaining the structural integrity of the sarcolemmal membrane during contraction.

Natural History

In 1884, Erb described a muscular dystrophy with predominant shoulder girdle involvement, no facial involvement, a slow course, and onset in the second decade. At approximately the same time, Leyden and Moebius separately described a similarly slowly progressive dystrophy with the exception of pelvic girdle muscle involvement first and foremost. Since then, numerous attempts to classify LGMD syndromes have met with variable success. As with the spinocerebellar ataxias, a useful classification and a worthwhile sense of the natural history

Table 63-2. Nomenclature of Limb-Girdle Muscular Dystrophy

Inheritance	Designation	Also Known As	Chromosomal Location	Gene Product	Alternate Protein Names
Autosomal dominant	LGMD1	—			
	LGMD1A	—	5q31–q33	?	—
	LGMD1B	—	?	?	—
Autosomal recessive	LGMD2	—			
	LGMD2A	—	15q15.1–q21.1	Calpain-3	Muscle-specific calpain
	LGMD2B	—	2p13–16	?	—
	LGMD2C	SCARMD, DLMD	13q12	γ-Sarcoglycan	35DAG, A4
	LGMD2D	Primary adhalinopathy	17q21	α-Sarcoglycan	50DAG, A2, Adhalin
	LGMD2E	—	4q12	β-Sarcoglycan	43DAG, A3b
	LGMD2F	DLMD	5q33–q34	δ-Sarcoglycan	35DAG
	LGMD2G	—	17q11–12	?	—
	LGMD2H	—	?	?	—

LGMD = limb-girdle muscular dystrophy; SCARMD = severe childhood autosomal recessive muscular dystrophy; DLMD = Duchenne-like muscular dystrophy; ? = unknown.

awaited a genetic basis for the syndromes. In 1991, in a large inbred family on the island of Reunion, the first chromosomal location for autosomal recessive LGMD was discovered on chromosome 15q. Since then, other loci for autosomal recessive LGMD have been found on six other chromosomes and for autosomal dominant LGMD on chromosome 5q (see Table 63-2).

The disease's clinical course and characteristics can be divided roughly into two syndromes: a severe childhood-onset myopathy indistinguishable from Duchenne's dystrophy and a later-onset (second to third decade), slowly progressive proximal myopathy (Table 63-3). However, each of the genetic subtypes has some differences not discerned confidently before DNA localization.

The severe childhood autosomal recessive muscular dystrophy (SCARMD), also known as *Duchenne-like muscular dystrophy*, first was described in North Africa, where it is the most common type of muscular dystrophy, in large part owing to high rates of consanguinity. SCARMD has been seen in European, South American, and North American families. A series of Tunisian families with SCARMD were linked to chromosomal 13q and subsequently were discovered to have a defect in γ-sarcoglycan (LGMD2C). Subsequently, other families with SCARMD have been linked to other LGMD loci (LGMD2D, LGMD2E) coding for sarcoglycans, meaning that the clinical characteristics are not predictive of the

chromosomal defect, though severe cases are more likely to have a sarcoglycan defect than are milder cases. This syndrome has not been seen with autosomal dominant inheritance.

The first symptoms of the SCARMD phenotype usually begin before puberty and affect boys and girls equally with pelvic girdle weakness. Eventually and rapidly, shoulder girdle, distal limb, abdominal, and neck muscles become weak; and hip, knee, heel, and elbow contractures are common. Calf hypertrophy is common. The patellar, biceps, and triceps are lost, in that order, with the ankle reflexes being retained the longest. Independent ambulation is lost in all patients, with 20% losing that ability by age 15 years, another 55% by age 20, and the final 25% by age 30 (at least for the Tunisian families). Cardiac involvement is common, much as in Duchenne's dystrophy, but mental retardation is not. Facial weakness, macroglossia, and malocclusion can be seen in some advanced cases. Life expectancy is shortened dramatically.

The more commonly encountered syndrome of autosomal recessive LGMD has an onset somewhat later, between ages 5 and 25 years. The disease first affects the pelvic girdle muscles but eventually affects the shoulder girdle as well and, in more severe cases, the distal limb muscles. The rate of progression is variable but slower than that of SCARMD, with loss of independent ambulation occurring from the teens to the fifth decade (and sometimes not at all). Heel contractures are com-

Table 63-3. Clinical Characteristics of the Limb-Girdle Muscular Dystrophies

Designation	Onset Age	Progression	Weakness	CK	Other Signs
LGMD1A	18–40 yrs	Slow	Proximal	4–25×	Dysarthria Tight heel cords Absent ankle jerks
LGMD2A	5–20 yrs	Variable	Proximal	2–10×	Macroglossia Calf hypertrophy Scapular winging
LGMD2B	15–25 yrs	Slow	Proximal	2–55×	Absent ankle jerks Tight heel cords
LGMD2C	4–12 yrs	Fast	Proximal	25–50×	Calf hypertrophy
LGMD2D	2–25 yrs	Variable	Proximal	4–100×	Calf hypertrophy
LGMD2E	5–20 yrs	Variable	Proximal	2–200×	Calf hypertrophy
LGMD2F	2–7 yrs	Fast	Proximal	10–50×	?
LGMD2G	9–15 yrs	Slow	Distal and proximal	3–17×	Foot-drop; areflexia

LGMD = limb-girdle muscular dystrophy; CK = creatine kinase; ? = unknown.

mon, and other contractures ensue once ambulation is lost. Diaphragmatic and cardiac muscle are not involved clinically. Calf hypertrophy is common. Life expectancy is variable but is shortened particularly for those affected most severely.

The autosomal dominant form of LGMD differs somewhat from the autosomal recessive forms, although, without the family history, differentiation from recessive forms is not reliable. The age of onset is later, with a mean onset in the early twenties. Pelvic girdle muscles are involved first, with progression to shoulder girdle and distal limb muscles. Ambulation is lost in some but not all patients and rarely sooner than 15 to 20 years after onset. Heel contractures are universal, calf hypertrophy is less common, and dysarthria can be seen. Cardiac and diaphragmatic muscles are not involved. In my experience, only a minority experience significant impingement on life expectancy, those being the most severely affected (i.e., having lost ambulation).

Factors Affecting Prognosis

Much speculation and work has been directed at explaining such variability in clinical characteristics among families with the same defective gene. The answer may be found in the nature of the genetic defect (e.g., those patients with null mutations of a sarcoglycan protein, resulting in virtually no protein, will develop the SCARMD syndrome, whereas those patients with missense mutations will gener-

ate some level of protein and will have a milder syndrome). Additional support for this hypothesis comes from immunostaining of muscle for sarcoglycans. Absence of staining is indicative of no protein and is more likely in SCARMD, whereas partial staining is more likely in milder phenotypes. Neither technique—mutation analysis or sarcoglycan immunostaining—is widely available.

The most useful clues to prognosis are family history, age of onset, and rate of progression. A family history of SCARMD would portend a more severe case in any child affected before the age of 10 years. Absent any family history, early onset age by itself may not indicate the SCARMD phenotype but increases that likelihood. A rapid rate of progression, measurable over just 1 to 2 years, would be confirmatory of a severe LGMD syndrome, with a poor prognosis for independent ambulation and life expectancy.

Evaluation for Prognosis

Creatine phosphokinase, EMG, and muscle biopsy are useful in the diagnosis of LGMD, though the findings convey no particular prognostic information. Creatine phosphokinase is highest in the SCARMD syndrome, though it can be high early in the course of later onset forms. EMG and muscle biopsy convey a picture of a progressive dystrophic process, which does not differentiate the various subtypes. However, obtaining dystrophin quantitation on the muscle is essential to refute the possibility of Duchenne's or Becker's muscular dystrophy. If available, immunostaining for the sarcoglycan complex may provide useful prognostic information, as a complete lack of staining implies a total or near-total loss of protein and a more severe phenotype.

Therapies Affecting Prognosis

No cure is available for LGMD, nor is any method known to slow its progression. This limitation is no different from any other muscular dystrophy. However, as with the other dystrophies, certain palliative measures may allow for improved quality of life, including heel-cord lengthening, proper bracing, appropriate wheelchair fitting with a good spinal bracing system, and a regular stretching program to prevent contractures. Attendance at school and work is to be encouraged, and socialization of the patient may have the most beneficial effect on mood and quality of life of any intervention. The provision of a power wheelchair or scooter can provide a measure of independence such that patients can regain a sense of control over their own lives. Those patients with a positive sense of themselves will, for the most part, fare better.

Short-Term Prognosis

LGMD is a chronic disease and, in the short term, little will change. In those patients with early onset and rapid rate of progression, loss of function will occur such that significant changes in the patient's ability to perform independent tasks will take place on a yearly (or faster) basis. However, in the less severe phenotypes, such changes in function will take place slowly, over the course of years.

Long-Term Prognosis

For children with SCARMD, the ultimate prognosis is nearly as dismal as that for Duchenne's dystrophy. Patients will become wheelchair-bound by age 20 years and be dead before age 30. Once in the chair, contractures, scoliosis, cardiac disease, and pulmonary dysfunction will become issues to address.

The later-onset phenotypes of LGMD, both autosomal recessive and dominant, will have a more variable and usually more optimistic outcome. Loss of ambulation is less certain and often occurs only after many years of the disease. The ability to continue work depends on both the patient's desire and the employer's willingness to accommodate. Many patients can continue gainful employment for 10 to 20 years after onset. Life expectancy is shortened for those patients on the more severe end of the spectrum, such as those who lose independent ambulation, but as this may not occur in all cases, life expectancy is otherwise normal.

Additional Reading

Facioscapulohumeral Muscular Dystrophy

Kilmer DD, Abresch RT, McCrory MA, et al. Profiles of neuromuscular disease. Facioscapulohumeral muscular dystrophy. Am J Phys Med Rehabil 1995;74:S131–S139.

Munsat TL. Facioscapulohumeral Disease and the Scapuloperoneal Syndrome. In AG Engel, C Franzini-Armstrong (eds), Myology (2nd ed). New York: McGraw-Hill, 1994; 1220–1232.

Padberg GW. Facioscapulohumeral Disease (PhD thesis). Leiden, The Netherlands: University of Leiden, 1982.

Oculopharyngeal Muscular Dystrophy

Brais B, Tome FMS, Fardeau M, et al. The natural history of oculopharyngeal muscular dystrophy based on the study of a large cohort of French Canadian mutation-carriers. Neurology 1996;46(suppl):A309.

Tome FMS, Fardeau M. Oculopharyngeal Muscular Dystrophy. In AG Engel, C Franzini-Armstrong (eds), Myology (2nd ed). New York: McGraw-Hill, 1994;1233–1245.

Limb-Girdle Muscular Dystrophy

Ben Hamida M, Attia N, Fardeau M. Severe childhood muscular dystrophy affecting both sexes and frequent in Tunisia. Muscle Nerve 1983;6:469–480.

Duggan DJ, Gorospe JR, Fanin M, et al. Mutations in the sarcoglycan genes in patients with myopathy. N Engl J Med 1997;336:618–624.

Gilchrist JM, Pericak-Vance M, Silverman L, Roses AD. Clinical and genetic investigation in autosomal dominant limb-girdle muscular dystrophy. Neurology 1988;38:5–9.

Morandi L, Barresi R, DiBlasi C, et al. Clinical heterogeneity of Adhalin deficiency. Ann Neurol 1996;39: 196–202.

Shields RW. Limb Girdle Syndrome. In AG Engel, C Franzini-Armstrong (eds), Myology (2nd ed). New York: McGraw-Hill, 1994;1258–1274.

Chapter 64
Myasthenia Gravis

James M. Gilchrist

Myasthenia gravis is an autoimmune disorder in which polyclonal antibodies are directed against the postsynaptic acetylcholine receptor of the neuromuscular junction. The disease is characterized by fatigable weakness involving ocular, facial, pharyngeal, respiratory, and limb skeletal muscles. A bimodal incidence affects older male and younger female persons. The affected muscles may be focal (e.g., single extraocular muscles), regional (e.g., ocular and bulbar muscles), or generalized.

Natural History

The evolution of the natural history of myasthenia gravis can be divided into two eras: that before antiacetylcholinesterase and that after antiacetylcholinesterase. Before Walker's 1934 discovery of the benefits of anticholinesterases, mortality was as high as 40%. Since then, the mortality rate has declined steadily, in part owing to the use of anticholinesterases, thymectomy, and immune modulators but also, perhaps most important, related to the advent of antibiotics and positive pressure mechanical ventilation. Death attributable to myasthenia gravis now is uncommon, being less than 5%.

As in most other autoimmune disorders, the course in myasthenia gravis is characterized by spontaneous remissions and relapses, but the majority of patients experience a gradual increase in symptoms and affected areas over the first 3 years, with the disease usually reaching maximum severity by that time. According to the extensive experience of Grob and coworkers, generalized myasthenia gravis reached maximal severity in 55% of patients within the first year after onset, in 70% within 3 years, and in 85% within 5 years.

The remission rate depends on the definition of remission. The chance of at least a 1-year complete remission of symptoms after treatment withdrawal will reach 20% of patients by 10 years, whereas another 25% will be symptom-free on pharmacologic treatment. Recurrences can happen, less commonly after several years of remission. Many patients will stabilize after 3 to 5 years, though possibly at an impaired level of function. Only a small minority, perhaps 10%, will continue to worsen after several years. The majority (70 to 90%) of patients will improve over the course of time and with appropriate treatment.

More than one-half of all patients with myasthenia gravis initiate the disease with ocular symptoms, though nearly all patients have involvement of the extraocular muscles at some point in the course of the disease. In 25 to 33% of those patients whose initial involvement is ocular, the disease remains restricted to ocular muscles for the entire course and, in 15% of all patients, it remains solely ocular. Conversely, 85% of all patients manifest generalized disease at some point.

Exacerbation of the disease often is precipitated by intervening illnesses, such as infections, electrolyte imbalance, or thyroid disease; by changes in medication (either those used for treatment of myasthenia gravis or many drugs used for other conditions); or by pregnancy. However, even without such provocation, myasthenia gravis can worsen rapidly, occasionally to the point of respiratory failure. This myasthenic crisis is a relatively infrequent event in this era of aggressive immunosuppression and is encountered most commonly within the first year after diagnosis. Other autoimmune diseases are found in 25% of patients with myasthenia gravis.

Factors Affecting Prognosis

The thymus gland is abnormal in 85 to 90% of patients with myasthenia gravis, with the majority (70% of all myasthenics) having hyperplastic germinal centers. Thymoma is encountered in 15% of patients with myasthenia gravis; 30% of thymoma patients develop myasthenia gravis. This tumor most often is benign, though it may be locally recurrent and, in approximately 5 to 10% of thymomas, malignant. The course of patients with myasthenia gravis and thymoma is stormier (even when the tumor is benign) than when the thymus is hyperplastic or atrophic. Controlling the symptoms is more difficult, fewer patients have remission, and a lesser percentage improve after thymectomy (in the range of 30 to 50%). This prognosis worsens considerably with malignant thymoma, which can be disseminated and metastatic. In patients with invasive thymoma (stage 3 or 4), mortality is greater than 50% at 5 years and is not affected by the presence or absence of myasthenia gravis. In patients with thymoma of any stage, thymectomy is indicated more to prevent dissemination of the tumor than as a treatment of myasthenia gravis.

Beyond the obvious observation that more severe disease carries a more severe prognosis, the particular distribution of weakness (e.g., bulbar or respiratory muscle involvement) also conveys a more serious portent, and these patients should be monitored closely, particularly in the days and weeks after onset of these symptoms. Increased age at onset (>50 years) carries an increased risk of respiratory crisis and death and may convey less chance of remission.

As with any form of treatment, side effects may occur, and the immunomodulatory nature of many of the treatments of myasthenia gravis makes for potentially nefarious complications. Uniquely, corticosteroid treatment can adversely affect the course of myasthenia gravis in the immediate short term. The initiation of high-dose corticosteroids (e.g.,

prednisone, 60 mg per day) will precipitate in 50% of patients a worsening of myasthenic symptoms severe enough to require intubation or mechanical ventilation in 10%. This risk diminishes after 4 to 7 days but can occur up to 2 weeks after steroid induction, and these patients merit close inpatient observation. Initiation by gradual dosage increments largely seems to avoid this worsening but delays the eventual response.

Evaluation for Prognosis

The evaluation for prognosis of myasthenia gravis involves little beyond that necessary for diagnosis and management of the disease. An accurate delineation of the muscles involved and the time since onset are important. A search for thymoma via imaging studies of the anterior mediastinum is useful for therapeutic reasons as well. Single-fiber electromyography is a very sensitive measure of neuromuscular transmission (registering abnormal in 98% of myasthenia gravis), though not specific to this disease. It is useful in following the disease and may provide an objective measure of clinical response when this response otherwise is unclear. Single-fiber electromyography may show generalized abnormalities in strictly ocular myasthenia gravis, but this finding is not indicative of generalized disease nor of a propensity to develop generalized disease. Repetitive nerve stimulation and acetylcholine receptor antibody levels are not useful in determining prognosis.

Therapies Affecting Prognosis

Despite the lack of any prospective, well-controlled studies, thymectomy clearly has been a boon to the patient with myasthenia gravis, especially for those without thymoma and in whom disease duration is short. Substantial improvement will occur in 75% of patients, and symptom-free remissions will double roughly to 40 to 60% by 7 to 10 years. The age at thymectomy does not appear to affect response but may affect other parameters, such as surgical morbidity. Thymectomy usually is reserved for those between ages 18 and 55 years.

Immunomodulation is an important part of the treatment of myasthenia gravis but should be reserved for those patients unable to undergo thymectomy or for those with persistent symptoms after thymectomy. Corticosteroids provide a rapid response in up to 80% of patients, but these patients may fare better when concurrently given azathioprine, as the steroid taper is more likely to be successful. The benefit of azathioprine is delayed much longer (several months), but this agent is less likely to have side effects. The only controlled trial of immunosuppression used cyclosporin A, but its toxicity renders it a third- or fourth-line drug despite its proved clinical benefit. High-dose intravenous human immunoglobulin also has had considerable anecdotal success, but it is expensive.

Plasmapheresis is indicated in those patients needing immediate benefit, as it drops the acetylcholine receptor antibody titer by 75% within 24 hours. Antibody levels return to baseline within 2 weeks, so pheresis must be paired with other immunomodulation or be used in short-term situations, such as preparation for thymectomy or myasthenic crisis.

Last, supportive care, including the use of pyridostigmine (an anticholinesterase), must not be forgotten for symptom relief. Antibiotics and positive-pressure mechanical ventilators probably have had the most impact on prognosis of all therapeutic modalities. These devices must be allied with good nursing and pulmonary care, subcutaneous heparin in the nonambulatory patients, and close medical follow-up to minimize mortality and secondary morbidity.

Short-Term Prognosis

The course of myasthenia gravis will be the stormiest in the first 3 years for the majority of patients. Short-term remissions followed by exacerbations (which may be severe and include respiratory failure) are common. The first 6 months are crucial, as myasthenic crisis is most frequent then, and patients, doctors, and other caregivers may as yet be unfamiliar with the disease and may disregard important signs of failing neuromuscular transmission.

Long-Term Prognosis

Over the long term, the course of myasthenia gravis is not as woeful as its name implies. Up to 90% of patients can be expected to respond favorably to treatment, and 75 to 80% will have prolonged periods of improvement, with half of those free of symptoms. Only 10% of patients will continue to worsen over the 10 years after diagnosis, and fewer than 5% will die of the disease or of therapeutic complications.

Additional Reading

Beghi E, Antozzi C, Batocchi AP, et al. Prognosis of myasthenia gravis: a multicenter follow-up study of 844 patients. J Neurol Sci 1991;106:213–220.

Bever CT, Aquino AV, Penn AS, et al. Prognosis of ocular myasthenia. Ann Neurol 1983;14:516–519.

Grob D, Arsura EL, Brunner NG, Namba T. The course of myasthenia gravis and therapies affecting outcome. Ann N Y Acad Sci 1987;505:472–499.

Mantegazza R, Beghi E, Pareyson D, et al. A multicentre follow-up study of 1152 patients with myasthenia gravis in Italy. J Neurol 1990;237:339–344.

Oosterhuis HJGH. The natural course of myasthenia gravis: a long-term follow up study. J Neurol Neurosurg Psychiatry 1989;52:1121–1127.

Pascuzzi RM, Coslett HB, Johns TR. Long-term corticosteroid treatment of myasthenia gravis: report of 116 patients. Ann Neurol 1984;15:291–298.

Chapter 65

The Inflammatory Myopathies*

Paul E. Barkhaus

Inflammatory Myopathy

The inflammatory myopathies (IMs) are a heterogeneous group of diseases that have in common the element of inflammation present on the muscle biopsy. The inflammatory changes are considered to be the result of an autoimmune-disimmune process. Occasionally, IM may result from viral, bacterial, and parasitic causes (a subject outside the scope of this chapter). IM may affect individuals at a wide range of ages. Among the more common types of IM are polymyositis (PM) and dermatomyositis (DM). Other categories of IM have been described, such as those associated with neoplasm and connective tissue disease. Sporadic inclusion body myositis (S-IBM) also is a relatively common type of IM but is considered an entity separate from IM on the basis of biopsy findings and so is discussed separately in this chapter.

The nosology of IM has been periodically reviewed and proposed in the literature, but none of the theories or proposals has achieved uniform acceptance. For the purposes of this chapter, discussion of IM is confined to uncomplicated adult-onset cases of PM and DM (i.e., groups I and II as defined by Bohan and Peter). Regardless of cause or associated findings, weakness is the sine qua non for the diagnosis. Limb weakness typically is symmetric, proximal greater than distal. Among the cranial-

innervated muscles, the pharyngeal muscles occasionally are affected, the facial muscles uncommonly are affected, and the extraocular muscles almost never are involved.

Commonly used clinical criteria for uncomplicated PM and DM are those proposed by Bohan and Peter: chronic symmetric, proximal weakness; elevated serum creatine kinase (CK) levels; "myopathic" electromyogram (especially with the characteristic increase in insertional and spontaneous activity that may be seen earliest in the paraspinal muscles); and muscle biopsy showing inflammation. Choice of site for the latter is optimally made on the basis of electromyographic findings so as to reduce sampling error. Patients with suspected DM also should evince obligatory associated dermatologic changes. Patients meeting all criteria are considered as definite cases. Those lacking one criterion are considered as probable cases, and patients having only one criterion are considered as possible cases. In lieu of a more specific biological marker for IM, the foregoing criteria are used frequently for establishing the diagnoses of PM and DM.

Natural History

Since the 1950s, corticosteroid immunosuppression therapy has been believed to benefit such a large percentage of cases that no truly controlled treatment trials exist. However, retrospective data on IM remain from the precorticosteroid era. In one series (see Winkelmann and coworkers) that included pedi-

*The views expressed in this chapter are those of the author and do not necessarily represent those of the Department of Veterans Affairs or U.S. government.

atric patients, 122 untreated patients were assessed as 48 (39%) in remission, 13 (11%) improved, 12 (10%) unchanged, 14 (12%) worse, and 35 (28%) deceased. The minimal information available regarding those who died reveals that most had severe disease, some one-third were in the sixth decade of life, and half had their disease less than 7 months.

Another series (O'Leary and Waisman) of 38 cases of IM (predominantly DM) showed a mortality rate of 19 (50%), with the cause of death being ascertained in 10 of the 19. Most deaths appeared to be related to IM. Mortality was higher among patients older than 50 years. Of the surviving 19 patients, 4 with mild disease recovered spontaneously and completely. Some improvement occurred in seven patients who maintained a plateau of strength deficit. Of the remaining eight who showed no improvement, three had temporary improvement followed by relapse, and another three showed steady progression in weakness.

As diagnostic studies and methodologies have changed significantly since these reports, caution must be exercised against deriving too much interpretation. The results are impressive, however, for their rates of spontaneous remission, mortality, and variability in clinical course in the absence of immunosuppressive treatment. Given current standards of practice, it would be an exceptional physician who could delay treatment in a case of presumed IM.

In the corticosteroid immunosuppressive era, a number of clinical series have reported a range in mortality from 14 to 28%. Meta-analysis between studies is not possible, owing to variations in subgrouping of patients and inclusion of those with such associated disorders as malignancy and connective tissue disease. Most patients given immunosuppressive agents show some improvement.

Death in IM has been ascribed to numerous causes, including metastasis from carcinoma, profound muscular weakness, sepsis and infection (particularly pulmonary), cerebrovascular disease, and cardiovascular disease. How the latter two categories compare with mortality rates in older adults without IM remains uncertain.

Factors Affecting Prognosis

In IM, one may make the logical inference that increasingly severe clinical weakness is a propor-

tionately adverse factor in prognosis. Other factors adversely affecting prognosis include older onset age, presence of a malignancy, ischemic cardiac disease, connective tissue disease, interstitial lung disease, weakness of respiratory muscles, fever, and elevated sedimentation rate. Dysphagia and acute or recent onset of IM have been considered as minimal adverse factors in prognosis. Prognosis does not appear to be influenced by findings on muscle biopsy, presence of arthritis-arthralgia, CK levels, or findings on electromyography.

Evaluation for Prognosis

After a patient has been evaluated thoroughly for suspected IM and the diagnosis has been made, generally no additional testing—other than careful evaluation of clinical strength—is required for prognosis. Unless specific clinical symptoms and signs of underlying malignancy develop, monitoring for neoplasm does not appear warranted. Unless symptoms already are present at onset, patients should be watched for any signs of known associated problems in IM (e.g., dysphagia, pulmonary disease, connective tissue disorder).

Serial measurement of enzymes and repeat muscle biopsy are not indicated routinely. Serial routine needle electromyography likewise is not indicated in the absence of specific diagnostic problems (e.g., corticosteroid myopathy, focal compression neuropathy). Some data indicate that quantitative electromyography may be useful in monitoring disease progression, with a correlation between increased clinical weakness and decreasing motor unit action potential duration and area-amplitude ratio.

Therapies Affecting Prognosis

After a tenable diagnosis of IM has been established, treatment generally involves immunosuppression. In most cases, corticosteroid therapy in various dosages and routes of administration is the initial treatment. Exceptions might include patients showing signs of spontaneous improvement before initiation of therapy and patients who have very chronic, severe, but inactive disease and have not been treated. The latter situation is uncommon and, although the prognosis for improvement is dismal, a trial of immunosuppressive therapy is reasonable in the event that the patient may achieve a higher level of function. Patients beginning corticosteroid therapy should have appropriate anergy panel and tuberculosis skin testing before starting treatment. The treating physician is obliged also to observe the patient for potential systemic side effects of corticosteroids.

A common clinical dilemma that may affect prognosis is the differentiation between IM progression due to corticosteroid resistance and corticosteroid myopathy. The latter generally is not immediate in onset after initiation of corticosteroids and develops only after at least several weeks. Corticosteroid myopathy is not associated with progressively increasing CK levels, and muscle biopsy is not reliable in distinguishing it from IM. Needle electromyography also is not useful in differentiating the two entities on the basis of the alterations in the motor unit action potentials: Corticosteroid myopathy typically does not alter the shape or size of the potentials. In most cases of IM, the motor unit action potentials already have presumably undergone some degree of change (i.e., decrease in duration and increase in complexity) owing to remodeling of the muscle fibers within the motor unit. The persistence of increased insertional activity and fibrillation potentials would favor IM, as these elements are not features of corticosteroid myopathy. Absence of these findings does not exclude IM, however, as corticosteroid therapy may obscure them.

Failure to induce a clinical remission and delayed or inadequate therapy are obvious negative factors on prognosis. No consensus as to what defines steroid resistance in an individual case exists. In cases wherein the conventional therapeutic gambit of corticosteroids is judged ineffective or unable to sustain remission, such other agents as azathioprine, methotrexate and cyclophosphamide, chlorambucil, or cyclosporin A should be considered. These agents may be used as adjunct medications with steroids or as substitutes in various combinations. Other therapies reserved for cases refractory to the foregoing include plasmapheresis, leukapheresis, polyvalent human intravenous immunoglobulin, and total body irradiation. The precise role of immunosuppression in sepsis and its predisposition to hematologic malignancy in IM is unknown.

Beyond corticosteroid immunosuppressive therapy as the focal point of the patient's medical management, supportive care of the patient is critical for optimal prognosis to avoid controllable complications despite the underlying IM. This care must be individualized to each patient and includes assistive devices in ambulation, aids to daily living, contracture prevention, and the like. General medical management, particularly in older patients, also is important when such concurrent conditions as ischemic heart disease may affect prognosis. Prophylaxis for pulmonary emboli may be appropriate in selected cases.

Short-Term Prognosis

IM patients vary greatly as to type of onset (acute versus insidious). Patients having a relatively short, subacute progression with mild to moderate weakness at time of diagnosis, and no associated conditions or other organ system involvement, tend to respond best. The most important issue is prompt initiation of appropriate therapy and doses. Frequent clinical evaluation of the patient's strength in the first 6 to 12 months after initiation of therapy should corroborate efficacy of treatment and improved prognosis.

Long-Term Prognosis

IM remains a serious diagnosis owing in great part to the lack of understanding of the disease process. Until such time as definitive biological markers for IM are developed to refine diagnosis and controlled treatment trials are available, accurate prognostication for IM remains limited. Despite these limitations, clinical data from different series with adequate follow-up vary considerably but appear optimistic in uncomplicated IM.

Clinical remission lasting from 1 to 17 years after discontinuation of treatment occurred in 11 of 50 patients (22%) in one study. Clinical improvement required ongoing treatment in another 65% of PM patients and in 58% of DM patients (see Chwalinska-Sadowska and associates). Survival rates have improved, with the most optimistic figures from a series of 114 DM patients reported at 89% and 81% at 5 and 10 years, respectively (see Zhanuzakov and colleagues).

Invariably, good prognosis is linked to a favorable response to therapy. It also follows that as different or additional medications are needed to sustain a patient, the prognosis tends to worsen, regardless of response to treatment. In the same foregoing series of 17 PM patients and 33 DM patients (see Chwalinska-Sadowska and associates), 47% and 73%, respectively, required the addition of cyclophosphamide.

Although the literature is limited in its conclusions on prognosis in IM based on these additional treatment options, a few generalizations may be made. In various series, patients who are on corticosteroids and require secondary medications or therapies alone or in combination suggest that short-term response to treatment is fairly good. Given differences in study designs, dosages, and the like, good choices to achieve clinical improvement appear to be methotrexate (54 of 63 patients [86%] improved), cyclophosphamide (25 of 40 patients [63%] improved), azathioprine (84 of 103 patients [82%] improved), and cyclosporin A (27 of 31 patients [87%] improved). Plasmapheresis performed in a controlled, randomized trial (see Miller and colleagues) had no demonstrable effect, although sporadic positive reports occur. Improvement in both steroid-treated and non–steroid-treated patients indicate that polyvalent human intravenous gamma globulin exerts a favorable influence in some two-thirds of cases.

As prognosis invariably is linked to therapeutic efficacy, the preceding offers some hope of remission in IM, even in cases in which recrudescence of disease occurs. The caveat is that most of the foregoing cases are steroid-resistant, and clinical status on long-term follow-up is not available. Hence, the long-term prognosis in this multiple-therapy category of more severe or steroid-resistant IM remains uncertain.

Sporadic Inclusion Body Myositis

S-IBM is more common than previously was suspected and can be mistaken easily for one of the other types of IM (except DM), as dermatologic symptoms are not a part of S-IBM. S-IBM has been described in young adults and the elderly but is more common in the aged. S-IBM must be considered in the differential diagnosis of any older patient who has presumed IM and is a nonresponder to conventional therapy. This suspicion may necessitate thorough re-evaluation, including muscle biopsy on which the definitive diagnosis of S-IBM rests. Some patients show elements of active inflammatory changes on muscle biopsy, potentially obscuring the diagnosis further. Clinical weakness commonly is distal in S-IBM, especially in the wrist and finger flexors. Dysphagia may be present in up to 40% of cases, and CK levels are mild to moderately elevated. Though polyneuropathy may be present in fewer than 20% of patients, the overall process appears to be one of primary myopathy. Diabetes mellitus is described in some 20% of cases. Despite use of corticosteroids and other agents to treat IM, the clinical course generally is one of slow, inexorable progression and debilitation. Promising reports of immunosuppressive treatment, particularly intravenous gamma globulin, await confirmation. Mortality rate for IBM is uncertain, as most patients are older and die from other nonassociated conditions (e.g., ischemic heart disease).

Acknowledgment

I acknowledge the assistance of Ms. Joan K. Kappes.

Additional Reading

Inflammatory Myopathy

Barkhaus PE, Nandedkar SD, Sanders, DB. Quantitative EMG in inflammatory myopathy. Muscle Nerve 1990;13: 247–253.

Benbassat J, Gefel D, Larholt K, et al. Prognostic factors in polymyositis/dermatomyositis. Arthritis Rheum 1985;28: 249–255.

Bohan A, Peter JB. Polymyositis and dermatomyositis. N Engl J Med 1975;292:344–403.

Chwalinska-Sadowska H, Maldykowa H. Polymyositis-dermatomyositis: 25 years of follow-up of 50 patients' disease course, treatment, prognostic factors. Mater Med Pol 1990;22:213–218.

Lakhanpal S, Bunch TW, Ilstrup DM, Melton LJ. Polymyositis-dermatomyositis and malignant lesions: does an association exist? Mayo Clin Proc 1986;61:645–653.

Miller FW, Leitman SF, Cronin ME, et al. Controlled trial of plasma exchange and leukapheresis in polymyositis and dermatomyositis. N Engl J Med 1992;326:1380–1384.

O'Leary PA, Waisman M. Dermatomyositis. Arch Dermatol Syphil 1940;41:1001–1019.

Winkelmann RK, Mulder DW, Lambert EH, et al. Course of dermatomyositis-polymyositis: comparison of treated and untreated patients. Mayo Clin Proc 1968;43:545–556.

Zhanuzakov MA, Vinogradova OM, Soloveva AP. Effect of corticosteroid therapy on the survival of patients with idiopathic dermatomyositis. Ter Arkh 1986;58:102–105.

Inclusion Body Myositis

Amato AA, Gronseth GS, Jackson CE, et al. Inclusion body myositis: clinical and pathological boundaries. Ann Neurol 1996;40:581–586.

Barkhaus PE. Quantitative EMG studies in sporadic inclusion body myositis. Muscle Nerve 1997;20:1084.

Lotz BP, Engel AG, Nishino H, et al. Inclusion body myositis: observations in 40 patients. Brain 1989;112: 727–747.

Chapter 66

Lambert-Eaton Myasthenic Syndrome

Donald B. Sanders

The Lambert-Eaton myasthenic syndrome (LEMS) is a rare condition in which weakness results from a presynaptic abnormality of acetylcholine (ACh) release at the neuromuscular junction. It first was described in association with lung cancer and initially was considered to be a paraneoplastic syndrome. Recent developments demonstrate that LEMS results from an autoimmune attack directed against the voltage-gated calcium channels (VGCC) on the presynaptic motor nerve terminal.

Natural History

Usually, LEMS begins in later life, although it has been reported rarely in children. In early studies, diagnosis was much more common in men than in women. This predominance has been less pronounced in recent series, but the disease in men still outnumbers that in women almost 2:1 in most reports. In 50 to 70% of patients, a malignancy is found, is known to be present when the disease begins, or develops later. Usually, this malignancy is a small-cell lung cancer (SCLC). In patients with LEMS and SCLC (SCLC-LEMS), the cancer cells, which contain VGCC in high concentrations, probably induce the production of VGCC antibodies that cross-react with the nerve terminal VGCC. In LEMS patients without cancer (non–cancer disease [NCD]-LEMS), VGCC antibodies probably are produced as part of a more general autoimmune state.

Weakness is the major symptom of LEMS, and predominantly proximal muscles are affected, espe-cially in the lower limbs. The weak muscles may ache and occasionally are tender. Oropharyngeal and ocular muscles may be affected mildly. Although some patients have severe weakness, examination usually demonstrates less weakness than is expected from the severity of symptoms. In some patients, strength may improve after exercise and then weaken as activity is sustained. The cholinesterase inhibitors edrophonium chloride (Tensilon), neostigmine methylsulfate (Prostigmin), and pyridostigmine bromide (Mestinon) produce improvement in strength in some patients, though such improvement rarely is dramatic. Tendon reflexes are reduced or absent but frequently can be brought out or increased by activating the appropriate muscles or by tapping the tendon repeatedly. Most patients have dry mouth, which may precede other symptoms. Some patients have other manifestations of autonomic dysfunction, including impotence in men and hypotension.

LEMS may be discovered first when prolonged paralysis follows the use of neuromuscular blocking agents during surgery. Clinical worsening has been described after administration of aminoglycoside antibiotics, magnesium salts, calcium-channel blockers, and iodinated intravenous contrast agents.

The true incidence of LEMS is unknown, as frequently it is not recognized, especially in patients who are known to have cancer and in whom symptoms of LEMS may be attributed to cachexia or the effects of treatment. A prospective study found that 2 of 150 patients with SCLC had LEMS. This observation and results from other reports indicate that approximately 3% of SCLC patients develop LEMS. On the basis of this figure, the prevalence of SCLC-LEMS in the United States would be approximately 5 per 1 million. Even without considering the prevalence of NCD-LEMS, these numbers imply that in most LEMS patients, the disease is undiagnosed.

The diagnosis of LEMS is confirmed by demonstrating characteristic findings on electromyographic studies: The compound muscle action potentials (CMAPs) recorded with surface electrodes are small, and there is a decrementing response to repetitive nerve stimulation at low frequencies. During stimulation at frequencies from 20 to 50 Hz, the CMAP increases in size and characteristically becomes at least twice the size of the initial response. A similar increase in CMAP size is seen immediately after the patient voluntarily contracts the muscle maximally for 10 seconds.

Factors Affecting Prognosis

The prognosis in LEMS patients is determined largely by the presence and type of any underlying cancer, the presence and severity of any associated autoimmune disease, and the severity and distribution of weakness. Also, patients with rapidly progressive symptoms usually have more severe disease.

Evaluation for Prognosis

SCLC is the most frequent cancer in patients with LEMS, and the risk that a LEMS patient has SCLC is determined by that patient's smoking history and the duration of LEMS symptoms. A chronic smoker with recent-onset LEMS symptoms should be considered to have underlying SCLC until proved otherwise. In patients with SCLC-LEMS, weakness tends to begin more precipitously and to progress more rapidly than when cancer is not present, but many exceptions exist. Because LEMS frequently is the initial clinical manifestation of SCLC, an aggressive search for cancer, especially SCLC, should be part of the initial evaluation in all LEMS patients and should be repeated at appropriate intervals. This evaluation should include thoracic computed tomography scan or magnetic resonance imaging in all patients and bronchoscopy in those at high risk for SCLC. In most patients with SCLC-LEMS, the cancer is discovered within 2 years after the symptoms of LEMS begin; thus, the risk that any LEMS patient has cancer becomes less with time. However, this risk probably never is zero as lung cancer has been found as long as 12 years after onset of LEMS.

Autoimmune disorders that have been reported coincidentally with LEMS include systemic lupus erythematosus, rheumatoid arthritis, mixed connective tissue disease, polymyositis, Sjögren's syndrome, hyperthyroidism, pernicious anemia, celiac disease, juvenile-onset diabetes mellitus, and vitiligo. Autoimmune myasthenia gravis occurring with LEMS has been reported in rare cases. The initial evaluation of all patients with LEMS should include screening tests for thyroid disease, diabetes mellitus, and myasthenia gravis. Specific testing for the other diseases should be performed if there are clinical indications.

Antibodies to the P/Q-type VGCC have been found in the serum of up to 100% of cancer-related LEMS patients and in up to 90% of those with NCD-LEMS. Thus, the presence of these antibodies does not distinguish cancer-related from NCD-LEMS. However, antibodies to the N-type VGCC have been found twice as often in SCLC-LEMS as in NCD-LEMS and thus provide some diagnostic and prognostic information. Antibody patterns that distinguish all cancer-related LEMS from NCD-LEMS may become known in the near future and would have considerable prognostic value. VGCC antibody titers do not correlate with disease severity among individuals but do fall as the disease improves in patients receiving immunosuppression.

Because LEMS may lead to the early detection of SCLC, the prognosis for SCLC in patients with SCLC-LEMS is said to be better than that for SCLC without LEMS. Also possible is that SCLC patients who develop LEMS have a more effective immunologic response to the cancer, thereby improving their survival rate.

Therapies Affecting Prognosis

In patients with cancer-related LEMS, treating the cancer effectively is also the best treatment of LEMS. When the cancer responds to treatment, the LEMS-induced weakness usually abates as well. The degree of persistent weakness and dysfunction

12 months after completion of cancer therapy gives a good indication of the expected long-term response. If weakness worsens later, recurrence of cancer should be suspected.

When LEMS has been symptomatic for at least 2 years and no underlying cancer has been demonstrated, it is likely LEMS arose as an autoimmune process. At that point, the prognosis is determined by the severity of dysfunction and the presence and severity of other autoimmune conditions. Although exceptions occur, weakness does not affect severely the vital muscles in most LEMS patients. Maximum severity usually becomes established within several months of symptom onset in NCD-LEMS patients. Without treatment, the weakness and dysfunction from LEMS usually do not vary significantly thereafter, except during periods of exacerbation induced by intercurrent illness.

Symptomatic treatment of LEMS includes the use of cholinesterase inhibitors, guanidine, or aminopyridines. Cholinesterase inhibitors improve strength in some patients with LEMS and frequently relieve the mouth dryness that is a distressing symptom in many patients. Guanidine hydrochloride increases the release of ACh and produces temporary improvement in strength in many LEMS patients. Pyridostigmine enhances the therapeutic response to guanidine and permits use of a lower dose. However, guanidine frequently produces severe side effects, including bone marrow depression, renal tubular acidosis, chronic interstitial nephritis, cardiac arrhythmia, hepatic toxicity, pancreatic dysfunction, peripheral paresthesias, ataxia, confusion, and mood alterations. Deaths attributable to the drug have been reported.

Aminopyridines also improve neuromuscular transmission by facilitating the release of ACh from the motor nerve terminal. 3,4-Diaminopyridine (DAP) produces improvement in strength and autonomic function in most LEMS patients. The effects of DAP are augmented by concurrent administration of pyridostigmine. Side effects usually are negligible, consisting solely of transitory perioral and digital paresthesias after higher doses in most patients. However, seizures may occur in patients taking high doses of the agent. Although it promises to be a safe and effective treatment of LEMS, DAP is not currently available for clinical use in the United States.

Immunosuppression produces sustained improvement in many LEMS patients, but (in my experience) most continue to have significant dysfunction

despite aggressive immunotherapy. Patients with underlying cancer run the theoretic risk that immunotherapy may reduce immunologic suppression of tumor activity and may facilitate tumor growth. This outcome has not been proved, but the possibility must be considered in deciding whether to use immunosuppression in LEMS patients who are known or suspected to have cancer. Decisions about immunotherapy also must consider the severity of weakness, the degree and duration of response to previous treatments, and the side effects and expense of immunosuppression.

When weakness is severe, plasma exchange (PEX) or high-dose intravenous immunoglobulin (IVIG) may be used to induce rapid, albeit transitory, improvement. Usually, repeated treatments with PEX or IVIG are necessary to maintain the response. Immunosuppressant medications may be used, either with or without PEX or IVIG, to induce more sustained improvement. Prednisone, azathioprine, and cyclosporine are the immunosuppressants used most frequently, given alone or in combination.

Short-Term Prognosis

The course, progression, and severity of weakness in LEMS are determined largely by the presence of underlying malignancy or associated autoimmune disease. The weakness of LEMS rarely is life-threatening but usually is disabling unless effective treatment is applied. Unless there is an underlying cancer or severe autoimmune disease, the symptoms typically progress insidiously over several months and remain relatively constant thereafter. Frequently, cholinesterase inhibitors give relief from dry mouth and occasionally produce useful improvement in strength. Guanidine or DAP produces dramatic symptomatic improvement in some patients, and the latter may provide sustained relief from weakness without significant toxicity. Immunosuppression relieves symptoms in many patients, rarely leads to normal function, and carries significant costs and risks of side effects.

Long-Term Prognosis

The long-term prognosis also is determined by the presence of underlying malignancy or associated autoimmune disease. Effective treatment of underlying cancer leads to sustained improvement or even complete remission of weakness in many patients. The long-term prognosis in these patients is determined by the recurrence rate for the cancer. Judiciously selected treatment with combinations of symptomatic agents and immunosuppression can improve function significantly in many LEMS patients, but most will continue to have some disability despite these therapeutic measures.

Additional Reading

Chalk CH, Murray NM, Newsom-Davis J, et al. Response of the Lambert-Eaton myasthenic syndrome to treatment of associated small-cell lung carcinoma. Neurology 1990;40:1552–1556.

Elrington G, Newsom-Davis J. Clinical Presentation and Current Immunology of the Lambert-Eaton Myasthenic Syndrome. In RP Lisak (ed), Handbook of Myasthenia Gravis and Myasthenic Syndromes. New York: Marcel Dekker, 1994;81–102.

Gutmann L, Crosby TW, Takamori M, Martin JD. The Eaton-Lambert syndrome and autoimmune disorders. Am J Med 1972;53:354–356.

Gutmann L, Phillips LH, Gutmann L. Trends in the association of Lambert-Eaton myasthenic syndrome with carcinoma. Neurology 1992;42:848–850.

Lambert EH, Eaton LM, Rooke ED. Defect of neuromuscular conduction associated with malignant neoplasms. Am J Physiol 1956;187:612–613.

Lennon VA, Kryzer TJ, Griesmann GE, et al. Calcium-channel antibodies in the Lambert-Eaton syndrome and other paraneoplastic syndromes. N Engl J Med 1995;332:1467–1474.

Lundh H, Nilsson O, Rosen I, Johansson S. Practical aspects of 3,4-diaminopyridine treatment of the Lambert-Eaton myasthenic syndrome. Acta Neurol Scand 1993;88:136–140.

McEvoy KM, Windebank AJ, Daube JR, Low PA. 3,4-Diaminopyridine in the treatment of Lambert-Eaton myasthenic syndrome. N Engl J Med 1989;321:1567–1571.

O'Neill JH, Murray NM, Newsom-Davis J. The Lambert-Eaton myasthenic syndrome. A review of 50 cases. Brain 1988;111:577–596.

Sanders DB. Lambert-Eaton myasthenic syndrome: clinical diagnosis, immune-mediated mechanisms, and update on therapy. Ann Neurol 1995;37(suppl 1):S63–S73.

Part XII
Metabolic and Toxic Disorders

Chapter 67

Vitamin B₁₂ Deficiency

Laurence J. Kinsella

Vitamin B_{12}, or cobalamin, deficiency most commonly is the result of pernicious anemia, an autoimmune disorder in which polyclonal antibodies are directed against intrinsic factor, a binding protein—secreted by gastric parietal cells—that facilitates B_{12} absorption. Cobalamin is required by two mammalian enzyme systems: (1) the conversion of homocysteine to methionine and S-adenosylmethionine, which is essential for the methylation of myelin proteins and phospholipids; and (2) the conversion of methylmalonate to succinate.

The mechanism of neurologic dysfunction in B_{12} deficiency is uncertain, but the inability to methylate myelin proteins and phospholipids may result in abnormal nerve conduction. Deficient B_{12} also leads to an accumulation of methylmalonyl coenzyme A, which in turn competes with acetyl coenzyme A for the production of fatty acids, a process that leads to the production of "odd-chain" fatty acids. The incorporation of odd-chain fatty acids into the myelin sheath may result in abnormal impulse propagation.

The disease leads to progressive dysfunction of the spinal cord, cerebral hemispheres, peripheral nerves, and (less commonly) the optic nerves. A bimodal incidence affects young women ages 20 to 40 years and men and women older than 65 years. In the United States, the incidence rises with increasing age.

Natural History

Patients develop paresthesias in the feet, vibratory and position sense abnormalities, ataxia, spasticity, and neuropathic signs of absent ankle reflexes and diminished cutaneous sensation. Patients also may develop cognitive deficits, psychosis, and affective disorders. Optic neuropathy occurs rarely. Subacute combined degeneration is the pathologic finding of demyelination of the posterior and lateral columns within the spinal cord. Myeloneuropathy indicates the coexistence of subacute combined degeneration and peripheral neuropathy. If untreated, the disease progresses to severe spastic weakness, neuropathy, ataxia, dementia, megaloblastic anemia, and death due to cardiovascular collapse or autonomic failure.

The natural history can be divided into the pre–cobalamin supplementation era and the post–cobalamin supplementation era. Before the 1921 discovery by Minot and Murphy of the curative effects of large amounts of cooked liver fed to patients with pernicious anemia, the disease had a mortality rate in excess of 90%. Ungley reviewed 31 patients admitted to hospital before the introduction of liver therapy and found that 28 died and 3 worsened 2 years after diagnosis. Since the advent of intramuscular crystalline B_{12} and oral supplements, mortality virtually has been eliminated, and progressive disability may be arrested or reversed.

Pernicious anemia accounts for approximately 80% of all patients with B_{12} deficiency. The next most likely cause is malabsorption due to a variety of causes, including Crohn's disease, ulcerative colitis, *Diphyllobothrium latum* infestation, ileal resection, and food-cobalamin malabsorption.

Food-cobalamin malabsorption results from atrophic gastritis and achlorhydria, an inability to

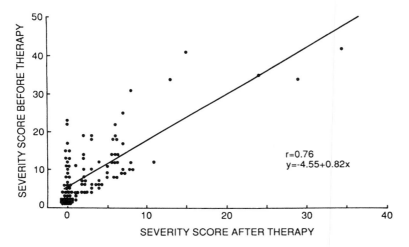

Figure 67-1. Relationship between severity score before and after treatment with cyanocobalamin in 112 episodes of deficiency involving the nervous system. (Reprinted with permission from EB Healton, DG Savage, JCM Brust, et al. Neurologic aspects of cobalamin deficiency. Medicine 1991;70:238.)

secrete the gastric acid necessary to separate vitamin B_{12} from food protein in the stomach despite a normal amount of intrinsic factor. Atrophic gastritis is common in the elderly, and perhaps 2% of B_{12} deficiency may be due to food-cobalamin malabsorption, which gives a normal Schilling's test result.

B_{12} deficiency can occur also in patients with serum binding protein abnormalities (transcobalamin I, II, and III), congenital enzymatic defects, and strict vegetarianism. An acute myeloneuropathy may occur in patients who have borderline stores of B_{12} and receive prolonged nitrous oxide anesthesia.

The normal body stores of cobalamin are 3,000 to 5,000 µg, stored mostly in the liver. Daily turnover is approximately 2 µg. Many months or years may be required before B_{12} deficiency develops in patients with malabsorption or strict vegetarianism. Perhaps for this reason, most patients do not develop neuropsychiatric symptoms until the seventh decade.

Factors Affecting Prognosis

The duration and severity of signs and symptoms at the time of diagnosis are the most important determinants of prognosis. When gait is impaired for less than 3 months, 56% of patients recover fully with cobalamin replacement, as opposed to 24% with gait impairment for longer than 2 years. In Healton's series, in only 2 of 10 patients did the most severe symptoms (spasticity, ataxia, incontinence, confusion, profound sensory loss) resolve completely after B_{12} replacement (Fig. 67-1). Paradoxically, anemia

and macrocytosis are related inversely to severity, and 20% of symptomatic patients have no hematologic abnormalities. Therefore, neurologic complications may progress to an advanced stage before a significant anemia develops.

The distribution of neurologic complaints also affects prognosis. Mild cognitive deficits, paresthesia, and ataxia are most responsive to cobalamin supplementation. Spinal cord dysfunction is less responsive but may improve after many months of treatment. Vibratory and cutaneous sensory impairment are the most resistant. The most responsive aspect of the disorder is the megaloblastic anemia.

Evaluation for Prognosis

The evaluation for prognosis requires an assessment of the duration and severity of the patient's physical findings. Clinical evidence of advanced and prolonged spinal cord dysfunction, including hyperreflexia, extensor plantar responses, spasticity, and profound loss of position sense, vibratory sensation, and cutaneous sensation, implies a worse prognosis after treatment.

Nerve conduction studies, electromyography, and somatosensory evoked potentials can help to identify the degree of nerve and spinal cord involvement and, thus, to enhance determination of prognosis. Magnetic resonance imaging of the brain and spinal cord occasionally demonstrates periventricular white-matter lesions and focal demyelination of the posterior columns.

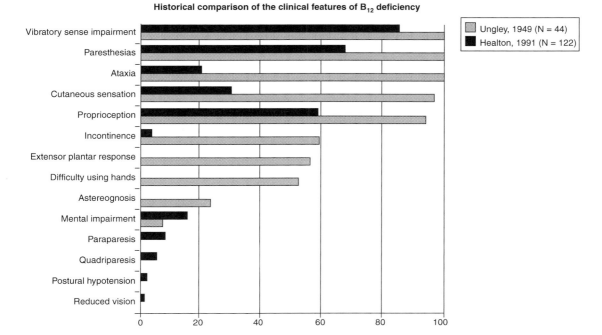

Figure 67-2. Historical comparison of the presenting clinical features of vitamin B$_{12}$ deficiency from 1949 to 1991. The classic features of spasticity and ataxia are less frequent in current practice. (Data from EB Healton, DG Savage, JCM Brust, et al. Neurologic aspects of cobalamin deficiency. Medicine 1991;70:229–245; and from CC Ungley. Subacute combined degeneration of the cord: I. Response to liver extracts. II. Trials with B$_{12}$. Brain 1949;72:382–427.)

Therapies Affecting Prognosis

The introduction of liver extract and, later, crystalline cyanocobalamin, has had the greatest impact on prognosis. In 1991, Healton found that 47% of patients who experienced cobalamin deficiency and who were followed for a mean of 37.6 months responded completely to parenteral B$_{12}$; 53% had a partial response; and 6% had no response. In 1949, Ungley found that 46% of patients improved after parenteral liver extract or B$_{12}$, ranging from 56% of those with impaired gait for less than 3 months to 26% for those whose difficulty in walking had lasted longer than 2 years. Most experienced peak improvement by 6 months. None of Ungley's patients experienced complete recovery, an outcome possibly owing to the greater severity and duration of deficits as compared to the modern series (Fig. 67-2).

Ungley further subdivided response to therapy according to physical findings (Fig. 67-3). The features least likely to improve were vibratory sensation, extensor plantar responses, and cutaneous sensation in the hands.

Short-Term Prognosis

Paresthesias often improve within several weeks, whereas improvement for spinal cord dysfunction may require several months. Some 2% of patients experience an acute worsening of paresthesias immediately after B$_{12}$ supplementation, but this does not impair the long-term response to therapy. Folate supplementation may reverse the hematologic abnormalities but will not prevent neurologic deterioration.

Long-Term Prognosis

With early disease recognition, patients may resume a normal lifestyle with limited impairment of gait or cognition. Spasticity due to spinal cord dysfunction may continue to improve over many months to years.

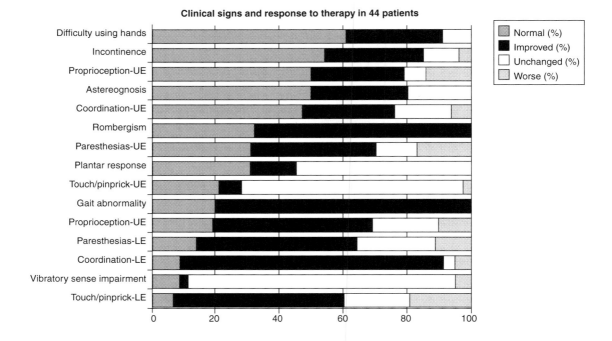

Figure 67-3. The clinical response of certain clinical features of vitamin B_{12} deficiency. Vibratory abnormalities, cutaneous sensation, and extensor plantar responses were least likely to respond to supplementation. (UE = upper extremity; LE = lower extremity.) (Adapted from CC Ungley. Subacute combined degeneration of the cord: I. Response to liver extracts. II. Trials with B_{12}. Brain 1949;72:382–427.)

Some 10 to 20% of patients may relapse, owing to noncompliance with long-term supplementation. These patients often develop identical symptoms that respond equally well to repeat treatment.

Additional Reading

Green R, Kinsella LJ. Current concepts in the diagnosis of cobalamin deficiency. Neurology 1995;45:1435–1440.

Healton EB, Savage DG, Brust JCM, et al. Neurologic aspects of cobalamin deficiency. Medicine 1991;70: 229–245.

Savage DG, Lindenbaum J. Neurological complications of acquired cobalamin deficiency: clinical aspects. Bailliere's Clin Haematol 1995;8:657–678.

Ungley CC. Subacute combined degeneration of the cord: I. Response to liver extracts. II. Trials with B_{12}. Brain 1949;72:382–427.

Chapter 68

Alcohol Withdrawal and Related Nutritional Syndromes

Marvin P. Rozear

Considered in this chapter are the alcohol abstinence or withdrawal syndromes (including delirium tremens and withdrawal seizures) and alcohol-related withdrawal and nutritional diseases, including Wernicke's encephalopathy and Korsakoff's psychosis, alcoholic cerebellar degeneration, and alcoholic peripheral neuropathy. Other rare diseases or those of less certain relationship to alcohol are not included.

Natural History

The clinical features of alcohol (ethanol) intoxication are well known. Within a few hours of cessation of alcohol intake, spree drinkers and steady drinkers who suddenly cease drinking develop tremulousness ("shakes" or "jitters"); agitation, insomnia, irritability, and excessive startle; and vomiting. The tremor is similar to an exaggerated essential tremor. These symptoms and signs peak at some 24 to 36 hours, then gradually diminish and disappear over 7 to 10 days. The prognosis in acute alcoholic tremulousness is excellent. Frequently, however, the patient resumes drinking, which both relieves the acute discomfort and prolongs the period of intoxication, which will have to be terminated sooner or later.

Approximately 25% of patients who experience tremulousness develop alteration of perception, ranging from mild illusions (with misinterpretation of stimuli) to overt hallucinations that, though more often visual, can involve any sensory modality.

Alcoholic auditory hallucinosis (with hallucinations evincing frequently paranoid overtones and experienced only in the auditory sphere) may have a different pathophysiology, possibly arising from a subclinical or coexistent thought disorder. The prognosis is good in this situation, in which no signs of systemic derangement are evident.

In 5 to 10% of withdrawing patients (obviously in the absence of firm statistics in this area), delusions and hallucinations increase; confusion, including disorientation, develops along with more severe agitation and tremor; and signs of sympathetic nervous system overactivity (diaphoresis, fever, tachycardia, blood pressure fluctuations, and dilated pupils) appear. A diagnosis of delirium tremens then can be made, the duration of which in uncomplicated cases is 4 days or less, although exceptional patients have experienced protracted or relapsing delirium for as long as 4 weeks. Exhausted by the excessive activity, patients eventually fall into a deep sleep, from which they usually awake amnesic for the episode. The prognosis for delirium tremens is less favorable than that for uncomplicated alcoholic hallucinosis, with mortality rates of 15% or more. Death frequently is caused by infection, dehydration and circulatory collapse, accidental injury or, especially in older individuals, myocardial infarction. Often, pinpointing the precise cause of death is difficult.

Alcohol withdrawal seizures occurring in this setting usually precede the onset of delirium. The seizures are generalized in type; any focal features of the seizures compel investigation of the patient for pathology other than, or in addition to, the withdrawal state. Results of such investigations not infrequently have adduced lesions (e.g., subdural or intracerebral masses) that required surgical attention. The peak incidence of these seizures, which are brief, is between 12 and 24 hours after cessation of drinking; they can occur with a delay as long as a week (though statistics about such time frames also are less than crisp). Most seizures (usually one to six) transpire over a period of 6 hours from their inception. A significant role for hypomagnesemia in this syndrome has been suggested, based mainly on a temporal association. Approximately 30% of patients experiencing alcohol withdrawal seizures also develop delirium tremens. Except for the small percentage of such patients whose seizures are in fact status epilepticus, the mortality rate in this group probably lies in the 15 to 20% range. Status epilepticus is a medical emergency with a greater overall mortality.

Chronic alcoholics frequently experience nutritional deficiencies, notably thiamine (vitamin B_1) deficiency, which may result in Wernicke's encephalopathy. These patients present with acutely altered mental status, ophthalmoplegia, and ataxia. In a majority, the syndrome is initiated by ataxia, then ophthalmoplegia, and followed by confusion. The mental status changes usually amount to a global confusional state without decreased levels of consciousness. Nystagmus is seen in almost 90% of patients; lateral rectus palsy in more than 50%; other ophthalmoplegias are less common.

Patients also frequently show results of other toxic effects of alcohol on the nervous system: A majority have neuropathy. Orthostatic hypotension may be due to dehydration and electrolyte disturbance or may be caused directly by the Wernicke's disorder. Pathology, including hemorrhage, endothelial proliferation, and demyelination in the cerebellar vermis and periventricular gray regions, is linked somehow to thiamine's role as a cofactor for several enzymes involved in neuronal metabolism. Similar lesions are found in Leigh's disease, a mitochondrial cytopathy with derangements of similar energy pathways. Pinpointing the natural history of Wernicke's encephalopathy is difficult, as the treatment is so simple and cheap and untreated cases are rare.

However, as many as 75% of treated patients recovering from Wernicke's encephalopathy experience a severe amnesic syndrome—Korsakoff's psychosis. Typically, such patients show inappro-

priate lack of concern for their deficits and tend to confabulate. Generally, they are able to access remotely stored or "crystallized" material but do not store new memories and, although they may be gregarious, glib, and entertaining, are unable to function independently. Lesions in the dorsomedial thalamus, part of the limbic system, in addition to the residuals of pathology in areas damaged by the Wernicke's disorder, are believed to be responsible for the memory loss. Probably related is a generally acknowledged increased incidence of diffuse cortical atrophy seen in the computed tomography and magnetic resonance imaging scans of chronic alcoholics, with gyral shrinkage and compensatory sulcal and ventricular enlargement.

Some alcoholics develop progressive, irreversible gait ataxia. The ataxia involves trunk and legs, less so the arms, and nystagmus is not seen. Pathologically, alcoholic cerebellar degeneration demonstrates selective atrophy due to loss of cells, especially Purkinje cells, of the anterior vermis and anterior lobes of the cerebellum. The clinical features resemble the ataxia seen in Wernicke's encephalopathy, except that in the former, the ataxia progresses gradually over weeks or months, whereas in the latter, ataxia tends to appear more suddenly and may be reversible, with resolution of the acute attack.

A well-known problem among chronic drinkers is alcoholic peripheral neuropathy. Binge drinkers apparently are affected less severely because they experience less severe nutritional deficiencies. In this predominantly distal, sensory axonopathy, numbness (which is frequently painful, leading to "burning feet syndrome") is caused by degeneration in the peripheral nerves, more severe in axons than in myelin. Motor nerves can be involved and, in more severe cases, autonomic and even cranial nerves can be affected. Neuropathy is equally common among male and female alcoholics and has been reported in more than 90% of alcoholics admitted to a large city hospital. Patients experience gradually progressive sensory disturbances, followed by weakness involving first the feet, then the legs, and later the fingers and hands. Patients frequently show other effects of alcohol and malnutrition on the nervous system (e.g., features of Wernicke's encephalopathy) and body in general (e.g., liver, skin). Similarity of alcoholic peripheral neuropathy to the neuropathy of beriberi and the fact that it can be prevented even in persistent heavy drinkers if they simply maintain nutrition (especially thiamine), leads to the (still argued) conclusion that nutritional factors are more important than are toxic factors in this disease. Multiple factors (including several vitamin deficiencies) no doubt are responsible for this process.

Factors Affecting Prognosis

The two most important factors in all the syndromes described here are (1) whether the patient is able to discontinue alcohol abuse or will continue drinking and (2) whether the patient can achieve an adequate and prolonged source of nutrition, including multivitamins. Unfavorable answers to both questions suggest a tendency for recurrence of acute attacks (frequently requiring extensive and expensive medical interventions) and progressive deterioration of cognitive, cerebellar, and peripheral nerve function, leading eventually to total disability and (frequently) institutionalization.

Evaluation for Prognosis

Prime considerations in this context are the severity of deficits at the time of evaluation and the willingness of the patient to abstain. Equally significant is the consideration of agencies and facilities to educate and support the patient in abstinence and rehabilitation. A general physical and psychosocial evaluation is essential to assess the patient's general medical condition, level of nutrition (especially in terms of liver function), and ability and desire to participate in rehabilitation. Besides a careful neurologic examination, which can provide precise data on current functioning of the patient's cognition, memory, and cerebellar and peripheral nerve function, laboratory and radiographic testing may expand the evaluation. As regards higher cortical functioning, imaging studies can both indicate the extent of cerebral atrophy, presumably largely irreversible, and screen for other coexistent pathologies that may be amenable to treatment, such as extracerebral collections, hydrocephalus, and the like.

Psychodiagnostic evaluation will provide quantitative estimates of "organic" deficits in cognitive and memory functioning and also may reveal factors that could be manipulated to achieve a more favorable outcome, such as depression or other "treatable" psychiatric disease. As regards cerebellar function, imaging studies can give estimates of the degree of vermian atrophy that, if severe, would correlate with irreversibility of the process and a poor prognosis. Peripheral nerve function can be evaluated by nerve conduction studies and electromyography. Early in the course of the predominantly sensory axonopathy, presumably when pathologic changes are relatively reversible, these electrical studies may be normal. However, with progressive (and frequently irreversible) peripheral nerve damage, nerve conduction studies show reduced amplitude, then absence of evoked sensory responses, at first with modest reduction in conduction velocities. As the damage progresses and myelin is affected secondarily, more slowing of conduction is noted, and abnormalities of motor conduction are found along with electromyographic manifestations of denervation of distal, then progressively proximal lower-extremity muscles and, eventually, upper-extremity nerves and muscles. Such denervation occurs relatively late, mainly in advanced cases, is largely irreversible, and connotes a poor prognosis.

Therapies Affecting Prognosis

Scientific data regarding therapy are lacking. However, neurologists generally maintain that if the patient can be persuaded to abstain and to maintain satisfactory nutrition while the symptoms and signs (and presumably, pathologic changes) are relatively early, many of the deficits can be reversed, leading to good recovery.

Treatment of acute alcohol tremulousness with or without hallucinations consists mainly of sedation, reassurance, and measures to begin rehabilitation. If the patient develops delirium tremens, more intensive therapy is required with fluid, electrolyte, vitamin, and nutritional replacement; search for and treatment of associated infections, pancreatitis, liver dysfunction, gastrointestinal bleeding, and the like; and sedation with paraldehyde, barbiturates, benzodiazepines, phenothiazines, and other tranquilizers. Despite vigorous measures and glowing claims of efficacy, the mortality in delirium tremens has not changed much in the last century.

Treatment of alcohol withdrawal seizures is controversial. One school contends that only nonspecific, supportive measures are necessary and indicated, as the seizures are brief and the number of seizures and period of seizure activity is limited. In fact, in such a situation, although proving drug efficacy is difficult, many neurologists recommend administration of phenytoin, phenobarbital, or lorazepam for a brief course to prevent the rare but well-known and dangerous development of status epilepticus (if for no other reason). Of course, if the patient has focal seizures or some other indication of origin of seizures for some reason other than simply alcohol withdrawal, treatment is mandatory in conjunction with investigative efforts to discover an etiology. Long-term anticonvulsant administration has no place in the treatment or prevention of recurrent, uncomplicated alcohol withdrawal seizures and, in some instances, has been associated with increased mortality.

Treatment of the acute phase of Wernicke's encephalopathy is more rewarding. The ocular manifestations vanish, frequently within a few hours of the administration of thiamine, 50 mg intravenously, the vitamin being continued intramuscularly or orally as tolerated for the duration of hospitalization, along with other nutritional and vitamin replacement. Mortality rate (usually because of comorbidity) is near 15%. Virtually 100% of ophthalmoplegias clear within 48 hours of initiation of such vigorous therapy, though in perhaps one-half of patients, horizontal nystagmus persists. Ataxia clears more slowly, usually over 1 to 4 weeks, and is complete in only approximately 50% of patients. Clearing of mental status changes is even less impressive. Some 10% of patients show improved cognitive and memory function within 2 weeks, but most experience persistent deficits, merging gradually into what becomes, in effect, a Korsakoff's psychosis. Once this more chronic status is reached, prognosis is poor, significant improvement being seen in fewer than 25% of patients. The lesions responsible apparently are irreversible, and thiamine and other vitamins do not seem to improve patient functioning, though most neurologists recommend that the patients continue use of these supplements.

Unlike the acute ataxia associated with Wernicke's encephalopathy, the gait disturbance associated with alcoholic cerebellar degeneration, once established, is not benefited by nutritional or vitamin supplementation. Acute episodes of peripheral neuropathy associated with acute toxic exposure may be benefited by intensive nutritional and vitamin replacement and supplementation, but results are modest, and most relief is achieved through measures to control pain, prevent contractures and skin breakdown, and other nonspecific efforts.

Short-Term Prognosis

In all the diseases caused by the ravages of alcoholism, the short-term prognosis for acute illness generally is favorable, if the patient can be separated from the toxin, can be given nutritional, vitamin, fluid, and electrolyte support, and can be investigated and treated for comorbidity (bleeding, infections, liver failure, etc.). However, mortality from the more serious complications (delirium tremens without and with withdrawal seizures, and Wernicke's encephalopathy) remains near 15%.

Long-Term Prognosis

After stabilization of the patient and treatment of the mentioned acute episodes, assuming the absence of already irreversible, disabling damage to higher cerebral functions, cerebellum, or peripheral nerves, the issue becomes one of rehabilitation, the core point of which is abstinence. Volumes have been written about this subject, and the plans, programs, and centers—with treatments ranging from religious to psychological to mystic to chemical—are boundless. Across the board, most consistent results are reported by Alcoholics Anonymous, an organization that indicates that of patients who make a serious effort to abstain, some one-half are successful. Those who continue to drink experience relentlessly progressive neurologic disability.

Additional Reading

Greenberg DA. Ethanol and sedatives. Neurol Clin 1993; 11:523–534.

Victor M. Neurologic Disorders Due to Alcoholism and Malnutrition. In AB Baker (ed), Clinical Neurology (vol 4). Philadelphia: Harper & Row, 1983;1–83.

Victor M, Adams RD, Collins GH. The Wernicke-Korsakoff Syndrome: A Clinical and Pathological Study of 245 Patients, 82 with Post-Mortem Examinations. Philadelphia: FA Davis, 1971.

Chapter 69

Neuroleptic Malignant Syndrome

Joseph H. Friedman

Neuroleptic malignant syndrome (NMS) is an iatrogenic syndrome defined by variable clinical criteria. As a result of a high degree of overlap with several other disorders, multiple definitions have been proposed. The lack of agreement in the literature and the frequent uncertainty of the diagnoses introduce significant problems in deriving generalizations about prognosis. Also likely is that the published literature is biased toward reporting the more severe cases, thus skewing the prognosis.

NMS first was described in 1960 but was not recognized as being more than a rare idiosyncratic drug reaction until 1980, when increasing numbers of articles about the disorder began to appear. Diagnostic and research criteria appear in *Diagnostic and Statistical Manual (of Mental Disorders), 4th edition*, wherein NMS is defined as a syndrome induced by neuroleptic (dopamine-blocking) medication in which there is severe muscle rigidity and hyperthermia associated with two or more of the following: diaphoresis, dysphagia, tremor, incontinence, change in consciousness, mutism, tachycardia, elevated or labile blood pressure, leukocytosis, or elevated creatine kinase levels. Several other definitions have been proposed, but most include hyperthermia, altered level of consciousness (delirium or decreased alertness), and a severe extrapyramidal syndrome, usually rigidity.

The problem in diagnosing the syndrome is the interrelationship among many of the minor criteria. Frequently, fever is associated with tachycardia, diaphoresis, and tachypnea. In the elderly and neurologically impaired, fever will frequently cause delirium or stupor and will exacerbate pre-existing extrapyramidal syndromes. Thus, the major differential diagnostic problem is distinguishing NMS from infection in a neuroleptic-treated patient. The concurrence of NMS and infection blurs the diagnosis even more. In the only report looking at diagnostic accuracy, 10 of 34 suspected NMS cases actually had serious medical causes for the syndrome rather than NMS.

Natural History

Although NMS usually begins within 3 to 9 days after initiation of a neuroleptic drug, it may occur years after a stable dose of drugs or as early as the day the drug was begun. Half the patients developed NMS within 1 week of a medication change, and only 3% developed it after 3 months on a stable drug schedule. It may develop in a fulminant fashion or may evolve over days. In a large review of the literature, 43% of patients developed a mental change as the first symptom. In 39%, rigidity was the first change. Fever or autonomic dysfunction was a less common initial manifestation. In 70% of cases, mental status changes were followed by rigidity, then hyperthermia and autonomic dysfunction. This sequence of events relies on one particular interpretation of the literature, whereas other interpretations probably are equally valid.

Once the offending agent is discontinued, the mean duration of NMS is 13 days for oral medication and 26 days for depot neuroleptic, with all reported cases resolving by 30 days. Ten percent of cases resolved without stopping the neuroleptic.

Factors Affecting Prognosis

The only drug factor that has been found uniformly to affect prognosis is the use of depot neuroleptic, which prolongs the duration of the syndrome. The dose of neuroleptic does not appear to affect mortality or duration of the disorder. Agreement has not been reached as to whether the concurrent use of lithium, which is not a neuroleptic, either predisposes to the disorder or worsens outcome. The largest number of cases have been associated with the use of haloperidol, but the mortality rate is somewhat less with this neuroleptic.

Exact mortality figures cannot be provided for each major medical aspect of the syndrome, but the degree of temperature elevation, myoglobinuria, respiratory dysfunction, and autonomic instability are of major importance. Maximum core temperature higher than 41°C is associated with a mortality of 34%. Myoglobinuria is a risk factor for renal failure. Renal failure, rather than muscle necrosis per se, is a risk factor for mortality but has not been quantitated. Frequency of cardiovascular collapse due to autonomic instability or persistent tachycardia also cannot be tabulated from collected reports. In one large review, cardiorespiratory arrest was the leading cause of death, followed by pneumonia and pulmonary embolism.

Although not quantifiable, rigidity is undoubtedly a major risk factor for morbidity and mortality. It is associated with dysphagia and the risk of aspiration, fever, and myoglobinuria leading to renal failure.

Evaluation for Prognosis

Probably the most important test for early prognosis is the creatine kinase level. This test provides an indication of the extent of muscle damage and an indirect measure for the risk of renal failure. Another risk factor for death is autonomic dysfunction. Though not directly measurable, the extent of blood pressure lability, the variability of heart rate, and the height of the fever have negative impacts on outcome.

Therapies Affecting Prognosis

As no study has been performed, no convincing data can corroborate that therapy, other than good supportive medical care, alters outcome in NMS. The decline in mortality recorded since the 1960s has been ascribed variously to earlier recognition leading to earlier and better care, recognition of milder cases with a more benign natural history, and treatment with one of several interventions.

Dantrolene, amantadine, bromocriptine, and electroconvulsive therapy have been reported to improve outcome. In one review, supportive care only or benzodiazepines plus supportive care resulted in a death rate of 28%, whereas dantrolene-treated patients experienced a mortality rate of only 6%. As regards only treatment benefits rather than mortality, bromocriptine was helpful in 12 of 13 cases, dantrolene in 29 of 34, and amantadine in 9 of 10. Evaluating electroconvulsive therapy has been more difficult.

The use of paralyzing agents in parallel with bromocriptine and dantrolene in cases of severe rigidity and myoglobinuria has not been reported. However, this approach could alter the outcome of severe cases with extreme rigidity, hyperthermia, and muscle necrosis leading to renal failure.

Short-Term Prognosis

Two separate questions attend the short-term prognosis. One is the medical outcome, and the other is the psychiatric outcome (i.e., whether an antipsychotic can be restarted). The 1980 mortality rate initially was estimated as 20%, but later reports have documented much lower (although highly variable) estimates for mortality. Experience since 1980 suggests that mortality may be diminishing, an outcome ascribed to better recognition and better treatment. One review noted a 76% mortality before 1970, 23% between 1970 and 1980, and 14% from 1980 to 1987. A second review noted a drop from 25% mortality before 1984 to 11.6% from 1984 to 1987. Estimates of mortality vary from 4 to 30%.

Mortality usually is due to a combination of pneumonia, renal failure secondary to myoglobinuria, and autonomic lability. Observed risk factors for death include organic brain disorders (including drug addiction, retardation, cerebral palsy, dementia), with a risk of death of 38%, and myoglobinuria and renal failure, with a mortality risk of 50%. Pneumonia was considered the cause of death in 25% of the fatal cases in one review.

Recurrence rate in restarting a neuroleptic within the first few weeks of an episode of NMS is estimated at 20 to 75%. However, no evidence has accrued to determine whether risk is lowered by starting a drug in a chemical class different from that which caused the syndrome.

Long-Term Prognosis

Very little data exist on the subject of long-term outcome of patients who have experienced an episode of NMS. Clearly, if the patient developed a permanent complication of the NMS (e.g., brain injury from hypoxia or heat stroke) or irreversible renal failure, these complications will be persistent. Isolated reports of a cerebellar syndrome from heat stroke, a peripheral neuropathy, and persistent amnesia have been published. Most patients who survive appear to be clinically unchanged by the experience, but most patients on neuroleptics have some degree of mental impairment at baseline and usually have not been tested formally before the NMS incident, rendering interpretation of follow-up neuropsychometric tests questionable. Some 3.3 to 21.0% of NMS survivors are reported to have permanent neurologic sequelae, but this finding most likely is an overestimate.

The recurrence rate of NMS on repeated neuroleptic treatment is another important question. The largest study of long-term follow-up involving only 20 patients found no recurrence among the 11 who resumed neuroleptic therapy, accruing a total of 16 years of drug treatment. A long-term study of only three patients rechallenged with a neuroleptic reported that one of the three had a repeat episode of NMS after the first episode. Most authorities suggest using a neuroleptic from a different chemical class when reinitiating antipsychotic therapy, but again, with little evidence to support this measure.

Additional Reading

Addonizio G, Susman VL, Roth SD. Neuroleptic malignant syndrome: review and analysis of 115 cases. Biol Psychiatry 1987;22:1004–1020.

Bristow MF, Kohen D. How "malignant" is the neuroleptic malignant syndrome? BMJ 1993;307:1223–1224.

Buckley PF, Hutchinson M. Neuroleptic malignant syndrome. J Neurol Neurosurg Psychiatry 1995;58:271–273.

Caroff S. The neuroleptic malignant syndrome. J Clin Psychiatry 1980;41:79–83.

Kellam AMP. The neuroleptic malignant syndrome, so-called. A survey of the world literature. Br J Psychiatry 1987;150:752–759.

Levenson JL, Fisher JG. Long-term outcome after neuroleptic malignant syndrome. J Clin Psychiatry 1988;49:154–156.

Pope HG, Aizley HG, Keck PE Jr, McElroy SL. Neuroleptic malignant syndrome: long-term follow-up of 20 cases. J Clin Psychiatry 1991;52:208–212.

Sewell DD, Jeste DV. Distinguishing neuroleptic malignant syndrome from NMS-like acute medical illnesses: a study of 34 cases. J Neuropsychiatry Clin Neurosci 1992;4:265–269.

Shalev A, Hermesh H, Munitz H. Mortality from neuroleptic malignant syndrome. J Clin Psychiatry 1989;50:18–25.

Velamoor VR, Norman RMG, Caroff SN, et al. Progression of symptoms in neuroleptic malignant syndrome. J Nerv Ment Dis 1994;182:168–173.

Part XIII

Congenital and Developmental Disorders

Chapter 70

Genetic Neurometabolic Disease

Generoso G. Gascon and Pinar T. Ozand

Genetic neurometabolic disease is defined as inborn errors of metabolism that prominently affect the nervous system. They present primarily in childhood as progressive encephalopathies, with or without long-tract or extrapyramidal signs or seizures, depending on which regions of the brain—white matter, cortical, or subcortical gray matter—are affected earliest. Juvenile and adult-onset variants exist and usually present as dementia. This chapter discusses prognosis in the aminoacidurias, organic acidurias, urea cycle disorders, lysosomal storage diseases, peroxisomal disorders, and mitochondrial disorders. Excellent references are available, to which the reader is referred (Scriver, McKusick, Lyon, and Adams), as this brief chapter cannot review comprehensively all individual diseases in these categories. Because all these diseases are rare, only certain ones provide substantial longitudinal experience to derive clinical prognosis, such as phenylketonuria (PKU), Tay-Sachs disease, adrenoleukodystrophy, and the biotin-responsive encephalopathies. In others (particularly peroxisomal and mitochondrial disorders), discoveries resulting from molecular neurobiology are likely to alter prognoses significantly in the near future.

Natural History

Aminoacidurias usually present in infancy as developmental retardation (e.g., PKU), though several have unique presentations (e.g., biopterin-dependent PKU) and other associated multisystem findings (e.g., homocystinuria) and result in mental retardation if untreated.

Organic acidurias may present in infancy as subacute to chronic encephalopathies with dystonia (e.g., glutaric aciduria type 1). However, in common with aminoacidurias, such as maple syrup urine disease, they may have a devastating neonatal onset as an acute encephalopathy (e.g., propionic aciduria, methylmalonic aciduria), with metabolic acidosis, with or without ketosis, lactic acidosis, or hyperammonemia, particularly when first feedings occur. If the disease is untreated, these babies die.

Lysosomal storage diseases present in infancy with mental retardation and with combinations of dysmorphic facial features (mucopolysaccharidoses [MPS]), hepatosplenomegaly (Niemann-Pick disease, Gaucher's disease, MPS), or cardiomegaly (glycogen storage diseases). They result chronically in severe to profound mental retardation. Peroxisomal disorders have varying presentations over time with varying prognoses: Zellweger's syndrome, presenting at birth, results in death; adrenoleukodystrophy (ALD) presents in midchildhood and causes chronic progressive encephalopathy and death; adrenomyeloneuropathy (AMN) presents in adolescence or adulthood, with chronic peripheral disability. Mitochondrial disorders present as either disorders of oxidative phosphorylation or disorders of fatty oxidation. Presentations are myriad, from subacute to chronic encephalopathies, with seizures, extrapyramidal signs, or stroke-like episodes, to skeletal and cardiac myopathies, to acute encephalopathies due to

Table 70-1. Degree of Absence of Enzyme Related to Prognosis

Near-Complete Absence: Severe Outcome	Partial Absence: Milder Outcome
Hurler's disease	Hurler-Scheie disease
Hunter's disease, severe	Hunter's disease, mild
Glycogen storage disease type 2, early infantile onset	Glycogen storage disease type 2, late juvenile onset
Sialidosis type 2 (infantile)	Sialidosis type 1 (juvenile)
Niemann-Pick disease type A (severe neuronopathic)	Niemann-Pick disease type B (childhood to adolescent onset)
Gaucher's disease type 1 (infancy to young adulthood)	Gaucher's disease type 2 (neuronopathic)
Krabbe's disease, infantile	Krabbe's disease, juvenile
MLD, infantile onset	MLD, juvenile or adult onset
MSD, early infantile	MSD, juvenile (Japanese)
GM_1 gangliosidosis, early infantile	GM_1 gangliosidosis, chronic late onset (20–30 yrs)
Galactosialidosis, early infantile (lethal)	Galactosialidosis, late variant with normal intelligence
GM_2 gangliosidosis, early infantile (Tay-Sachs disease, Sandhoff disease)	Juvenile Tay-Sachs or Sandhoff disease
MSUD,[a] classic severe	MSUD, intermittent, intermediate severity
GAT 1,[b] infantile onset	GAT 1, childhood or adult onset forms
GAT 2,[b] neonatal onset	GAT 2, childhood onset phenotype
3 MGA,[b] neonatal form	3-MGA, Behr's disease
Classic neonatal onset of CPS, OTC, ASA-L[c]	Late-onset, partial deficiency phenotypes
PDH deficiency, neonatal onset[d]	PDH deficiency, late-onset variants
COX deficiency, neonatal[d]	COX deficiency, infantile, later onset

[a]Aminoacidurias.
[b]Organic acidurias.
[c]Urea cycle disorders.
[d]Mitochondrial disorders.
MLD = metachromatic leukodystrophy; MSD = multiple sulfatase deficiency; MSUD = maple syrup urine disease; GAT = glutaric aciduria; 3 MGA = 3-methylglutaconic aciduria; CPS = carbamyl phosphate synthetase; OTC = ornithine transcarbamylase; ASA-L = arginosuccinatelyase; PDH = pyruvate dehydrogenase; COX = cytochrome C oxidase.

hypoglycemia, to migraine syndromes. Outcomes range from sudden death (sudden infant death syndrome in medium-chain acyl–coenzyme A [acyl-CoA] dehydrogenase deficiency), chronic

encephalopathy, cardiomyopathy and heart failure, to asymptomatic outcome, depending on the degree to which various organ systems are affected.

Factors Affecting Prognosis

Age at Onset and Degree of Enzyme Absence

Generally, the younger the onset, the worse the prognosis, particularly in those diseases in which the crucial enzyme deficiency is quantitatively less than in later-onset cases (e.g., infantile onset versus adult onset of metachromatic leukodystrophy). However, this factor interacts with the availability of specific therapy, early diagnosis, and birth order. If therapy is available, with later onset the physician has more time to organize management, as therapy generally is more effective given early in a disease, or presymptomatically (e.g., younger brother of a confirmed ALD patient). For example, in the peroxisomal disorders, total absence of peroxisomes (Zellweger's syndrome) presenting in the neonate is untreatable, whereas early bone marrow transplantation in ALD, a single peroxisomal enzyme deficiency disease presenting in childhood, can result in prevention of symptom expression or in stabilization of neurologic findings.

If a disease begins in utero, the newborn already is affected, and prognosis ultimately is fatal. Examples are hydrops fetalis causing GM_1 gangliosidosis, galactosialidosis, beta-glucuronidase deficiency, sialidosis type II, Gaucher's disease type II with ichthyosis, and severe forms of medium-chain acyl-CoA dehydrogenase deficiency. Partial enzyme deficiencies cause less severe disease (Table 70-1).

Birth Order

The first child affected in a family, particularly with an autosomal recessive disease, has the worst prognosis, as the diagnosis, if made at all, is made late. Once the diagnosis is made, subsequent siblings can be screened selectively (e.g., all male family members in X-linked recessive diseases, all siblings in autosomal recessive diseases) and treated early.

Prenatal Identification

When a genetic neurometabolic disease is fatal, submits to no treatment, and presents in early infancy, prenatal diagnosis may produce several options that influence prognosis, including offering the parents a choice for terminating pregnancy, putting obstetricians and neonatologists on alert for immediate neonatal diagnosis and treatment, and possibly offering intrauterine, prenatal treatment. The overall incidence of Tay-Sachs disease has fallen remarkably because of prenatal diagnosis. Glutaric aciduria type 1, presenting with macrocephaly and the open opercular sign at birth, if identified with neonatal screening, can be treated prenatally by giving carnitine and riboflavin to the mother. In Menkes' disease diagnosed prenatally, babies usually are delivered at some 32 weeks of gestation so that copper-histidinase injections can be given before the blood-brain barrier matures.

Neonatal Screening

The availability of routine neonatal screening laboratory tests certainly has affected the prognosis of the more common neurometabolic diseases. Classic PKU diagnosed in the newborn period with early institution of dietary restriction has resulted in remarkably improved long-term cognitive functioning. Ideally, screening should be performed for all treatable amino acid and organic acid disorders, but cost-effectiveness is an issue.

Selective screening has been successful in high-risk families or in certain regions of the world with high incidence related to the level of consanguinity in the population. The best method is that based on tandem mass spectroscopy. If the disease is not of a severe phenotype, such as methylmalonic aciduria, acute metabolic decompensation will be minimal, because of early dietary restrictions and the use of intravenous carnitine or arginine. Even in diseases with severe phenotypes, such as propionic acidemia and maple syrup urine disease, 80% will be treated successfully. At the King Faisal Specialist Hospital and Research Centre in Riyadh, Saudi Arabia, more than 300 patients with inborn errors of metabolism have been identified at birth in the last 5 years; not one with methylmalonic aciduria has died or had neurologic residua.

Other diseases diagnosable by tandem mass spectroscopy are the bile acid metabolic errors. Two important diseases not diagnosable by tandem mass spectroscopy but by other procedures are galactosemia and biotinidase deficiency. The latter is significant because it presents as a chronic progressive cerebral palsy, but the upper motor neuron signs and encephalopathy are treatable and reversible by high-dose biotin therapy.

Therapies Affecting Prognosis

The probability of neurologic dysfunction being reversible is inversely proportional to treatment latency (i.e., the probability of reversibility is greater if the time from disease onset to treatment is shorter).

Genetic counseling, though not specifically a treatment, well may have the most import in lowering the incidence of these diseases. The availability of substrate measurements, enzyme analysis, and more specific molecular diagnosis has led to a new kind of genetic counseling that can proceed beyond the starting point of pedigree analysis and the probabilities of mendelian or maternal inheritance to offer families management choices. These choices include abortion, presymptomatic sibling diagnosis, familial studies for heterozygote identification, and presymptomatic or even prenatal treatment. However, this counseling still must be conveyed sensitively, with appreciation of a family's moral beliefs and cultural sensibilities.

Coping with those diseases requiring restricted diets is difficult for parents, and compliance with therapy can become a major issue. Chronic vomiting and anorexia are not uncommon in organic acidemias. Infants with a genetic neurometabolic disease are fragile, and minor infections, because of immune compromise, and fasting easily precipitate acute metabolic crises. The degree to which parents can comply with the requirements of diet administration often depends on the easy availability of a support team: metabolic dietitian, physician, social worker, and home health care nurse.

The following socioeconomic and cultural factors influence prognosis, because they influence compliance and whether treatment is made available in a timely fashion.

1. Availability of diets and unusual treatments, such as intravenous carnitine, intravenous

Table 70-2. Prognosis of Selected Aminoacidurias

Disease	Fatal	Treatable (with Sequelae)	Treatable (without Sequelae)	Major Complication	Progressive
PKU, classic	No	—	Yes	MR	Static, if treated
PKU, biopterin	SIDS, if late diagnosis	Yes, if late diagnosis	Yes, if early diagnosis	Quadriplegia	Not if treated early
Tyrosinemia type 1	In severe phenotypes	—	Yes, if NTBC-liver transplant	Brain edema, acute porphyria, hepatomas	Yes
Tyrosinemia type 2	No	—	Yes	Mild MR	No
Homocystinuria, classic	—	Yes	Yes, if pyridoxine-responsive	Brain infarcts, MR, cataracts	Yes
MSUD, classic	In severe phenotype	Yes	Yes	Cerebellar ataxia, MR	Yes
MSUD, intermittent	—	Yes	Yes	Cerebellar ataxia, MR	Slowly
Nonketotic hyperglycinemia	If late diagnosis	Yes	—	Central hypotonia, or spasticity, MR	Yes
Hyperprolinemia	—	—	—	MR	Yes

PKU = phenylketonuria; SIDS = sudden infant death syndrome; NTBC = 2(nitro-4-trifluoromethylbenzoyl)-1,3-cyclohexandione; MR = mental retardation; MSUD = maple syrup urine disease.

arginine, hemodialysis facilities in acute-care centers.

2. Cost of diets and medications.
3. Availability of immediate diagnosis (pH, blood gases, ammonia, lactic acid, pyruvate, ketones, glucose; high-pressure liquid chromatography, gas chromatography-mass spectroscopy, tandem mass spectroscopy). Delayed diagnosis in an acute-care setting risks death or brain damage.
4. Healthy home setting (infection- and toxin-free).
5. Awareness by primary care physicians of signs of neurometabolic disease for prompt referral to a tertiary care center.
6. Parental and family education, particularly true if socioeconomic circumstances, ethnic dietary preferences, or alternative therapies (herbs, prayer, cautery, acupuncture, chiropractic) impede compliance with prescribed treatment.

Short- and Long-Term Prognosis

Assuming early diagnosis and treatment and assuming the most favorable of the prognostic factors discussed, one can make some generalities about overall prognosis. In the amino and organic acidemias, favorable phenotypes do well; severe phenotypes die. A notable exception is propionic acidemia; even under the best care, only 10 to 20% survive with minimal mental retardation and hypotonia.

In the long term, all storage diseases and peroxisomal disorders are lethal (the possible exception being AMN). Mitochondrial disorders generally are lethal, particularly if encephalopathy prominently involves the brain stem (Leigh's syndrome) or if cardiomyopathy exists. Several summary tables are provided (Tables 70-2 through 70-8).

Table 70-3. Prognosis of Selected Organic Acidurias

Disease	Fatal	Treatable (with Sequelae)	Treatable (without Sequelae)	Major Complication	Progressive
Isovaleric	—	—	Yes	—	No
Propionic	Can be	Yes	Rarely	MR	Yes
Methylmalonic	Rarely	—	Yes	—	Sometimes
HMG CoA lyase	Rarely	—	Yes	—	No
Biotinidase	—	If late diagnosis	Yes	Deafness	Chronically
Beta-ketothiolase	—	—	Yes	Motor clumsiness	No
Ethylmalonic	Always	—	—	Spastic quadriplegia	Rapidly
Glutaric aciduria 1	Rarely, SIDS	—	Yes, if diagnosis at birth	Chorea, dystonia, athetosis	Yes
Glutaric aciduria 2	Neonatal onset	Yes, infantile, late onset	Yes, infantile, late onset	Myopathy, cardio-myopathy	Yes
Canavan's disease (acetyl aspartic aciduria)	Always, in teen years	—	—	Neurovegetative state	Yes

MR = mental retardation; HMG CoA = hydroxymethylglutaryl coenzyme A; SIDS = sudden infant death syndrome.

Table 70-4. Prognosis of Selected Lysosomal Storage Diseases

Disease	Fatal	Treatable (with Sequelae)	Treatable (without Sequelae)	Major Complication	Progressive
GM$_2$ gangliosidosis, (Tay-Sachs, Sandhoff diseases)	Yes	—	—	Anterior horn cell disease, late onset phenotypes	Yes
GM$_1$ gangliosidosis	Yes	—	—	Neurovegetative state	Yes
Galactosialidosis	Yes, severe variants	Yes, mild variants	—	Cardiac disease	Chronically
Sialidosis 1 (cherry-red spot, myoclonus)	—	Yes	—	Action myoclonus, blindness	Chronically
Niemann-Pick disease types A and B	Yes	—	—	Pulmonary infiltrates	Yes
Niemann-Pick disease type C	Yes	—	—	Ataxia, dementia, liver disease	Yes
Gaucher's disease type 1	No, if BMT and alglucerase injection (Ceredase)	Yes	Yes	Thrombocytopenia, anemia	Yes
Gaucher's disease type 2 (infantile onset)	Yes	—	—	Trismus, opisthotonus, strabismus	Yes
Mucopolysaccharidoses, severe types	Yes	—	—	Cardiac, MR	Yes
Mucopolysaccharidoses, mild types	—	Yes, with good orthopedic care	—	Skeletal deformities, cardiac, MR	Yes
Mucolipidoses	Yes	—	—	Cardiac, MR	Yes
Pompe's disease, infantile	Yes	—	—	Cardiac	Yes
Pompe's disease, juvenile	Yes, but late	Yes, in mild cases	—	—	Yes
Fabry's disease	Yes, delayed with transplantation	Yes	—	Kidney	Yes
Krabbe's disease	Yes	—	—	Dementia, spastic quad	Yes
Metachromatic leukodystrophy	Yes, unless early BMT	Yes	—	Dementia, spastic quad	Yes

BMT = bone marrow transplant; MR = mental retardation; spastic quad = spastic quadriparesis.

Table 70-5. Prognosis of Selected Peroxisomal Disorders

Disease	Fatal	Treatable (with Sequelae)	Treatable (without Sequelae)	Major Complication	Progressive
X-linked ALD	Yes, unless early BMT	Yes	—	Dementia, blindness, seizures	Yes
Neonatal ALD	Yes	—	—	Seizures, spastic quad	Yes
Zellweger's syndrome	Yes	—	—	Seizures, spastic quad	Yes
Pipecolic aciduria (Zellweger-like syndrome)	Yes	—	—	Neurovegetative state	Yes
X-linked AMN	No	Yes	—	Peripheral neuropathy, paraplegia	Yes
Refsum's disease	No	Yes	—	Peripheral neuropathy, deafness	Yes

ALD = adrenoleukodystrophy; BMT = bone marrow transplant; spastic quad = spastic quadriparesis; AMN = adrenomyeloneuropathy.

Table 70-6. Prognosis in Selected Mitochondrial Diseases: Phosphorylative Oxidation Disorders

Disease	Fatal	Treatable (with Sequelae)	Treatable (without Sequelae)	Major Complication	Progressive
Leigh's disease	Yes	Yes	—	—	Yes, subacutely
Congenital lactic acidosis	Yes (neonatal)	—	—	—	—
MERRF	—	Yes	—	Myoclonic epilepsy, ataxia, dementia	Chronic, slowly
MELAS	—	Yes	—	Strokes, myopathy	Chronic, intermittent
Kearns-Sayre syndrome, CPEO	Possible, heart block	—	—	Cardiac conduction defect	Chronic
LHON	No	—	—	Blindness	Chronic
Malignant migraine	No	—	—	Stroke	Unknown
NARP	No	—	—	Neuropathy, ataxia, blindness	Chronically
Mitochondrial myopathies	Usually not	—	—	Weakness	Chronic, variable

MERRF = myoclonic epilepsy, ragged red fiber syndrome; MELAS = mitochondrial encephalopathy, lactic acidosis, and stroke-like episodes; CPEO = chronic progressive external ophthalmoplegia; LHON = Leber's hereditary optic neuropathy; NARP = neuropathy, ataxia, retinitis pigmentosa syndrome.

Table 70-7. Prognosis of Selected Mitochondrial Diseases: Fatty Acid Oxidation Disorders

Disease	Fatal	Treatable (with Sequelae)	Treatable (without Sequelae)	Major Complication	Progressive
SCAD	Yes	—	—	Cardiomyopathy	—
MCAD	SIDS in 20% of first episodes	—	Yes	Residuals of chronic hypoglycemia	Intermittent
LCAD	Yes, SIDS	—	—	Cardiac arrhythmias	—
LCHAD	Yes, SIDS	—	—	Retinitis, neuropathy	—
Carnitine-acyl carnitine translocase	Yes	—	—	Cardiomyopathy	—
CPT II deficiency	Yes, neonatal	—	Yes (adult form)	Myoglobinuria, renal failure (adult form)	Intermittent

SCAD = short-chain acyl–coenzyme A (CoA) dehydrogenase deficiency; MCAD = medium-chain acyl-CoA dehydrogenase deficiency; SIDS = sudden infant death syndrome; LCAD = long-chain acyl-CoA dehydrogenase deficiency; LCHAD = long-chain hydroxyl-CoA dehydrogenase (or trifunctional enzyme) deficiency; CPT = carnitine palmitoyl transferase.

Table 70-8. Prognosis of Urea Cycle Disorders and Selected Miscellaneous Disorders

Disease	Fatal	Treatable (with Sequelae)	Treatable (without Sequelae)	Major Complication	Progressive
CPS and OTC deficiencies	Yes, usually	Yes	—	MR, spastic quadriplegia	Yes
Argininosuccinic aciduria, citrullinemia	Yes, if diagnosed late	Yes	Yes, if treated promptly	MR, spastic quadriplegia	—
Galactosemia	—	—	Yes	MR, cataracts	—
Methylene tetrahydrofolate reductase deficiency	Yes, unless diagnosed and treated early	Yes	—	Brain atrophy, microophthalmia, central apnea	Yes
Menkes' disease	Yes, unless treated very early	Yes	—	Seizures, dementia, bladder and blood vessel rupture	Yes

CPS = carbamyl phosphate synthetase; OTC = ornithine transcarbamylase; MR = mental retardation.

Additional Reading

Desnick RG. Treatment of Genetic Disorders. New York: Churchill-Livingstone, 1991.

Gascon GG, Ozand PT. Aminoacidopathies and Other Neurometabolic Diseases. In C Goetz, E Pappes (eds), Textbook of Clinical Neurology. Philadelphia: Saunders (in press).

Lyon G, Adams RD, Kolodny EH. Neurology of Hereditary Metabolic Diseases of Children (2nd ed). New York: McGraw-Hill, 1996.

Ozand PT, Gascon GG. Organic acidurias: a review (pt 1). J Child Neurol 1991;6:196–219.

Ozand PT, Gascon GG. Organic acidurias: a review (pt 2). J Child Neurol 1991;6:288–303.

Scriver CR, Beaudet AL, Sly WS, Valle D (eds), The Metabolic and Molecular Bases of Inherited Metabolic Disease (7th ed). New York: McGraw-Hill, 1995.

Chapter 71

Chiari Malformation

William D. Graf and Harvey B. Sarnat

The Chiari malformations are a group of central nervous system (CNS) anomalies classified by three types of hindbrain displacement below the foramen magnum. The Chiari I malformation refers to caudal extension of the cerebellar tonsils alone; the Chiari II (previously known as the *Arnold-Chiari malformation*) refers to an elongated, small hindbrain and caudal displacement of the medulla oblongata, fourth ventricle, and the inferior cerebellar vermis through an enlarged foramen magnum into the cervical spinal canal; and the Chiari III malformation designates caudal displacement of the cerebellum and brain stem in association with occipital encephalocele. The type IV malformation described by Chiari denotes global cerebellar hypoplasia without displacement of posterior fossa contents and now is considered a distinct and unrelated condition. This chapter emphasizes prognosis in the Chiari II malformation.

Basic theories regarding the pathogenesis of the Chiari malformations emphasize mechanical causes: The traction theory is based on tethering of the spinal cord, the crowding theory stresses a small posterior fossa, and the pulsion theory proposes rostral hydrodynamic forces as the cause of hindbrain caudal displacement. Molecular theories speculate on the role of primary embryologic defects in hindbrain segmentation regulated by homeotic genes or other signaling molecules. In addition to the manifestation of abnormal hindbrain structure, most individuals with the type II malformation show evidence of other developmental defects. Common findings include a disorder of cortical neuroblast migration (92%), polymicrogyria (55%), cerebellar dysplasia (72%), primary dysgenesis of the medulla (e.g., variable severity of cranial nerve nuclei hypoplasia, poorly formed inferior olives, displaced long tracts; 20%), fusion of the thalami (16%), agenesis of the corpus callosum (12%), and complete or partial agenesis of the olfactory tract and bulb (8%).

The Chiari II malformation almost always is present in persons with myelomeningocele and only rarely in the absence of myelomeningocele. Occasionally, in persons with low-lumbar or sacral-level myelomeningocele, the malformation does not manifest clinically or on imaging studies. Overall, approximately 90% of infants with myelomeningocele develop hydrocephalus secondary to the posterior fossa malformation.

Natural History

Until the first half of the twentieth century, most infants with the Chiari II malformation and myelomeningocele died of ventriculomeningitis or hydrocephalus. After the onset of the antibiotic era, delay of surgery for closure of the myelomeningocele lesion still was recommended for 3 to 18 months, and hydrocephalus was a contraindication for surgery. Until the late 1960s, most published series described a selection process of various indications and contraindications for treatment of infants. General improvement in nursing care, better nutrition, and lack of adherence to a complete nontreatment protocol led to palliative use of antibiotics and survival rates of up to 70% of infants without surgery. Most survivors of nonsurgery protocols were left with neurologic impairments more severe than those in patients who were treated aggressively.

Initial surgeries to treat hydrocephalus, such as plexectomy for communicating hydrocephalus and third ventriculostomy for obstructive hydrocephalus, were associated with considerable perioperative mortality and morbidity. Early large-diameter, rigid, tubular cerebrospinal fluid shunt systems (developed in the late 1940s) failed for multiple reasons. Technical advances in shunt materials, valve-regulated systems, reservoirs, antisiphon devices, and flexible distal tubing now allow a prognosis of 90% or better for survival with low morbidity.

Factors Affecting Prognosis

Progressive Brain Stem and Cerebellar Dysfunction

Clinical symptoms and signs of lower brain stem dysfunction are life-threatening complications related to the Chiari II malformation. Published series indicate that the frequency of lower brain stem dysfunction ranges between 5 and 30%. When the dysfunction is present, the mortality is as high as 12 to 75%, with or without surgical intervention. Its occurrence is not related to the level of the myelomeningocele lesion, the severity of initial hydrocephalus, findings on magnetic resonance imaging (MRI) scan, or the prognosis estimated at the time of birth. Patients usually present with stridor, respiratory distress, dysphagia, central apnea, and bradycardia, or breath holding. Infants who become symptomatic before 2 to 3 months of age typically show more rapid deterioration than do older children and adults, whose symptoms often progress insidiously. In the survivors of this lower brain stem syndrome, some individuals regain CNS function, and others have persistent vocal cord paralysis, sleep apnea, aspiration, and impaired respiration.

Cervical Spinal Cord Dysfunction

Signs and symptoms that localize to the cervical spinal cord occur more typically in older children and adolescents. Patients may present with arm weakness, decreased coordination, sensory changes in the hands, atrophy, or spasticity. The cause may be related to intrinsic brain stem dysgenesis or to hydromyelia, syringomyelia, and syringobulbia.

Hydrocephalus

In infants with the Chiari II malformation, approximately 85% develop ventriculomegaly, parenchymal compression, and increased occipitofrontal circumference by the early postnatal period. Approximately one-third of these affected individuals have already developed these signs during the prenatal period.

Visual Impairment

Various oculomotor impairments are associated with the Chiari malformations, including strabismus and spontaneous nystagmus, convergence defects, ocular motility defects, and oscillopsia. Severity and prognosis are related to such general causes as hydrocephalus and abnormal visual pathways, cerebellar displacement, upper– and lower–brain stem compression, and cranial nerve nuclei hypoplasia. Adaptive mechanisms are variable. Severe and prolonged untreated hydrocephalus rarely may cause stretch and pressure atrophy of the optic radiations (geniculocalcarine tract) and may contribute to cerebral visual impairment.

Neuropsychiatric Complications

Measuring intelligence in this population is difficult owing to the history of selective treatment patterns in many institutions and to a number of confounders in individual cases, such as denial of immediate perinatal care, severe prenatal hydrocephalus, cerebral visual impairment, and meningitis. The majority of persons with the Chiari II malformation and shunted uncomplicated hydrocephalus will reveal normal cognition on psychometric testing. A lower mean IQ (approximately 75) prevails in persons with associated thoracic-level myelomeningocele as compared to persons with sacral lesions (mean IQ, 100). Verbal subtest scores usually are higher than are subtest scores that measure nonverbal reasoning skills and visuospatial perception. In persons with higher-level myelomeningocele, the "cocktail party personality" is a characteristic finding, with superficial, hyperverbal behavior but significant cognitive deficiency.

Seizures

Most series estimate the incidence of seizures in persons with Chiari malformations to be 10 to 20%. Seizures are more likely to occur in persons with complicated hydrocephalus, a history of meningitis, or significant CNS dysgenesis with neuronal migration defects. Usually, seizures can be controlled with antiepileptic drugs, and remission of epilepsy is common.

Evaluation for Prognosis

The diagnosis of Chiari malformation should be suspected in a patient with a clinical history or objective findings of lipomyelomeningocele (Chiari I), myelomeningocele (Chiari II), exertional headache, oculomotor impairment, stridor, central apnea, unexplained respiratory distress, sensory and motor deficits in the hands or arms, progressive hydrocephalus, or increased intracranial pressure. Each imaging technique currently used in clinical practice is useful in management: Cranial ultrasonography, usually the first study performed on the newborn infant to monitor progressive ventriculomegaly serially; computed tomography, readily accessible and used to detect hemorrhage, edema, and infarction and to monitor ventricle size after shunt placement; and MRI, the technique that best defines both posterior fossa and cerebral neuropathology. Sagittal views are particularly useful in determining the caudal extent of the hindbrain displacement and hydromyelia or syringomyelia. Neuroanatomic findings may not accurately correlate with individual prognosis.

Therapies Affecting Prognosis

Hydrocephalus

Ultimately, shunt placement is required in 90% of individuals, and lifelong monitoring of shunt function is necessary. Mortality and morbidity for hydrocephalus are related closely to the overall prognosis of the Chiari II malformation. Shunt revision rates should be no higher than one to two per initial ventriculoperitoneal shunt in most institutions. With modern surgical techniques and the standard use of perioperative antibiotic prophylaxis, shunt infection rates have decreased to approximately 2% in most children's hospitals. Good prognosis depends most on the vigilance of parents and caregivers to recognize early signs of shunt infection, increased intracranial pressure, or shunt obstruction symptoms. Parents and caregivers *must* receive detailed instruction by their treating physicians and have emergency access to neurosurgeons.

In patients with hydromyelia, syringomyelia, and syringobulbia, placement of a shunt from the fourth ventricle or syrinx to the subarachnoid space is indicated for a syrinx-cord ratio of more than 35%.

Progressive Brain Stem and Cerebellar Dysfunction

Brain stem compression frequently is associated with increased intracranial pressure secondary to untreated hydrocephalus or ventriculoperitoneal shunt malfunction. Placement or revision of a shunt leads to reversal of the brain stem dysfunction in many cases. Suboccipital craniectomy, cervical laminectomy, and dural decompression are associated with reversal of brain stem compression signs in some patients. Instability of the cervical spine is a common postoperative complication. No controlled, prospective treatment trials have been performed.

Short-Term Prognosis

Chiari II malformations are associated with a spectrum of severity resulting in a wide range of outcomes: Progressive brain stem dysfunction is the most common cause of death in infancy and early childhood. In the 5 to 30% of patients who develop brain stem dysfunction, high morbidity and mortality are correlated with young age of onset (<3 months), severity of neurologic status at presentation (e.g., myeloschisis, spasticity), multiple shunt revisions, severe hydrocephalus at birth, level of motor paralysis (above L1), and the persistence of postoperative vocal cord paralysis.

Long-Term Prognosis

Estimates of long-term prognosis are complicated by the history of selective nontreatment of certain infants until the 1970s. Conversely, such aggressive surgical interventions as posterior fossa decompression in infants with progressive brain stem dysfunction and postoperative tracheostomy in those with bad outcome may prolong survival but significantly increase pulmonary morbidity.

The majority of persons affected by Chiari malformations without progressive brain stem dysfunction will complete high school and become independent adults vitally concerned about their current and future health. However, studies in adults with the Chiari II malformation and myelomeningocele clearly indicate that continued health deterioration persists and new medical problems emerge. Neurologic signs of intermittent shunt dysfunction, spinal cord atrophy, syringomyelia, and tethered cord occur in addition to many vague neurologic symptoms that may indicate these diagnoses. Patients with associated myelomeningocele experience deterioration of ambulation, back pain, contractures, and progressive musculoskeletal weakness. Joint pain occurs in perhaps 50% and is a major health problem for some patients. Persistent complications of paraplegia in adulthood include decubitus (25%), urinary incontinence resulting in socially unacceptable odor or leakage (40%), chronic urinary tract infection regardless of the method of collection (40%), and prostatitis or epididymitis in men who use clean intermittent catheterization (25%). Psychologically, 40% of surveyed adults report depression requiring treatment, and 9% admitted suicide attempts, most commonly in the young adult years. Furthermore, surveyed young adults affected by Chiari malformations perceive the health professions as having limited knowledge and interest in their ongoing symptoms and health problems.

Additional Reading

Dahl M, Ahlsten G, Carlson H. Neurological dysfunction above cele level in children with spina bifida cystica: a prospective study to three years. Dev Med Child Neurol 1995;37:30–40.

Gilbert JN, Jones KL, Rorke LB, et al. Central nervous system anomalies associated with meningomyelocele, hydrocephalus, and the Arnold-Chiari malformation: reappraisal of theories regarding the pathogenesis of posterior neural tube closure defects. Neurosurgery 1986; 18:559–564.

Griebel ML, Oakes WJ, Worley G. The Chiari Malformation Associated with Myelomeningocele. In HL Rekate (ed), Comprehensive Management of Spina Bifida. Boca Raton, FL: CRC Press, 1991;67–92.

Hays RM, Jordan RA, McLaughlin JF, et al. Central ventilatory dysfunction in myelodysplasia: an independent determinant of survival. Dev Med Child Neurol 1989;31: 366–370.

Lennerstrand G, Gallo JE, Samuelsson L. Neuro-ophthalmological findings in relation to CNS lesions in patients with myelomeningocele. Dev Med Child Neurol 1990; 32:423–431.

Marin-Padilla M, Marin-Padilla MT. Morphogenesis of experimentally induced Arnold-Chiari malformation. J Neurol Sci 1981;50:29–55.

McGinnis W, Krumlauf R. Homeobox genes and axial patterning. Cell 1992;68:283–302.

Pollack IF, Pang D, Albright AL, Krieger D. Outcome following hindbrain decompression of symptomatic Chiari malformations in children previously treated with myelomeningocele closure and shunts. J Neurosurg 1992;77:881–888.

Shurtleff DB. Selection Process for the Care of Congenitally Malformed Infants. In DB Shurtleff DB (ed), Myelodysplasia and Exstrophies: Significance, Prevention, and Treatment. Orlando, FL: Grune & Stratton, 1986;89–115.

Tew B. The Effects of Spina Bifida and Hydrocephalus Upon Learning and Behavior. In CM Bannister, B Tew (eds), Current Concepts in Spina Bifida and Hydrocephalus. London: Mac Keith Press, 1991;158–179.

Chapter 72

Myelomeningocele

William D. Graf and Harvey B. Sarnat

Myelomeningocele is the most common form of neural tube defect (NTD), a heterogeneous group of complex developmental malformations that involve errors in primary neurulation. Virtually all persons with myelomeningocele also have an anomaly of the hindbrain and the upper cervical spinal cord known as the *Chiari II malformation*. Usually, this malformation is accompanied by hydrocephalus. Most of the neurologic impairments that affect the prognosis of patients with myelomeningocele are related to primary spinal cord dysraphism and the Chiari II malformation. Other problems frequently observed in patients affected by myelomeningocele, such as growth retardation, wound healing problems, and latex allergies, may be related to genetic and metabolic differences underlying the condition.

Because multiple factors contribute to their genesis, NTDs are an ecogenetic model of developmental disorders. Genetic predisposition, certain environmental risk factors, and teratogens (especially the antiepileptic drug valproic acid) are associated with higher occurrences of myelomeningocele and other NTDs. Significant associations between myelomeningocele and lower socioeconomic status, diabetes mellitus, maternal hyperthermia in early pregnancy, and dietary deficiencies have been shown.

Natural History

Until the late 1950s, few infants with myelomeningocele were treated actively, and most died. In the 1960s, early surgical closure of the spinal lesion in the neonatal period allowed extended survival; however, the long-term disabilities of survivors became apparent. During the 1970s, a period of selective nontreatment for surgery of the most severe cases led to serious ethical and legal issues. Since that time, the vast majority of infants with myelomeningocele have had early back closure and ventriculoperitoneal shunt placement for management of hydrocephalus. In the 1980s, methods were developed for antenatal diagnostic screening tests (maternal serum alpha-fetoprotein and ultrasonography) that were complemented by amniocentesis when screening tests were positive, allowing informed parents the choice of abortion of an abnormal fetus or an atraumatic form of delivery. More recently, prospective controlled randomized trials demonstrated that periconceptional folic acid supplementation resulted in prevention of some NTDs. The biological mechanism of this vitamin remains unknown.

The total prevalence of myelomeningocele in Europe and North America has declined from the early 1970s to an apparent plateau in the 1990s. The availability of prenatal screening with selective termination of pregnancy has had the largest impact on the prevalence of NTDs. Despite these trends, the defects remain an important group of severe congenital anomalies. Approximately 1,500 infants annually are born with myelomeningocele in the United States.

In this country, folic acid fortification of all enriched foods began in 1998. This action should achieve a daily supplement of some 100 to 400 µg

Table 72-1. Approximate Functional Neuromuscular Prognosis in Myelomeningocele for Each Anatomic Level of the Embryologic Lesion

Level of Paralysis	Expected Motor Function	Expected Mobility
Thoracic	Complete paraplegia of legs and hips T5–T10: paralysis of abdominal muscles, poor sitting posture, and decreased respiratory function T12: good trunk musculature and sitting posture	Nonambulatory; 50% with significant MR affecting independence; full wheelchair dependency
High lumbar (L1–L2)	L1: weak hip flexion L2: mild hip adduction; possibly at risk for unopposed hip muscle flexion contractures	Nonfunctionally ambulatory (use of KAFO or RGO usually only in therapy); wheelchair-dependent; 50% MR
Midlumbar (L3)	Strong hip flexion and adduction, some knee extension	In household, ambulatory with KAFO and forearm crutches; wheelchair for community use; 15% MR
Midlumbar (L4)	Strong knee extension and ankle dorsiflexion, some knee flexion; possibly at risk for calcaneal foot deformities from unopposed anterior tibialis muscle	In community, ambulatory with AFO and forearm crutches; wheelchair possibly useful for longer distances in childhood, increased wheelchair dependency in adulthood
Low lumbar (L5)	Fair antigravity knee flexion with weak hip extension using hamstrings, weak hip abduction, weak plantar flexion with inversion; calcaneus foot deformities secondary to muscle imbalance	In community, ambulatory with AFO; forearm crutches or wheelchair possibly useful for longer distances; 15% MR
High sacral (S1)	Mild gluteus maximus strength, fair plantar flexion and toe strength; usually mild foot deformities	Mild disability; possible difficulty in climbing stairs; usual walking without orthoses; 15% MR
Low sacral (S2–S5)	Fair to good hip flexion (gluteal muscles) and plantar flexion of foot	Essentially normal gait, possibly some weakness in running or jumping

MR = mental retardation (IQ ≤70); KAFO = knee-ankle-foot orthoses; RGO = reciprocating-gait orthoses; AFO = ankle-foot orthoses.

folic acid for the average pregnant woman, significantly less than the folic acid doses of 0.8 mg and 4.0 mg used in the trials of periconceptional vitamin supplementation.

Factors Affecting Prognosis

Associated Malformations

More than one-half of spontaneously aborted embryos with NTDs have chromosomal anomalies. Approximately 10 to 20% of fetuses with myelomeningocele diagnosed in utero have chromosomal anomalies or other dysgenesis syndromes. The occurrence of triploidy and trisomy (especially 13 and 18) is highest in mothers younger than 20 and older than 35. Myelomeningocele occurs with an increased frequency in patients with family histories of schisis anomalies, such as cleft lip and palate, or together with other rare genetic (e.g., chromosome 22q11 deletion) or teratologic (e.g., fetal valproate) syndromes. The prognosis for

long-term survival is reduced significantly for these syndromes with severe developmental anomalies of the heart, urinary tract, and gastrointestinal tract.

Neuroanatomic Level of the Congenital Dysraphic Lesion

The primary embryologic defect results in denervation at the level of the spinal nerve root, with variable leg paralysis, loss of leg sensation, and functional loss of anal sphincter and urinary control. The level of motor function assessed in the perinatal period is an important indication of overall prognosis for complete or incomplete paraplegia, likelihood of spinal deformities, cognitive development, and expected mobility (Table 72-1). Common secondary musculoskeletal deformities may be congenital because of spinal anomalies and intrauterine positioning or may be acquired because of muscle imbalances, abnormal posture, joint contractures, spasticity, or fractures. Kyphosis and scoliosis occur in the great majority of persons with thoracic and high-lumbar myelomeningocele and are the orthopedic complications most likely to affect prognosis adversely. Spinal deformities are progressive with age and result in pain, decreased posture, additional impairment of mobility, and restrictive pulmonary function.

Complications of Neuropathic Bladder

Persons with myelomeningocele may have a combination of upper and lower motor neuron type neurogenic bladder dysfunction. Both hypertonic (spastic) and hypotonic (flaccid) bladder musculature in combination with sphincter dysfunction can lead to urinary reflux, hydronephrosis, and other upper urinary tract deterioration. Continuous surveillance of the urinary tract is essential to prevent, diagnose, and treat vesicoureteral reflex, urinary tract infections and pyelonephritis and to prevent subsequent renal injury.

Neurogenic Bowel

Ninety-five percent of persons with myelomeningocele have bowel dysautonomia and anal sphincter dysfunction. Depending on the type of denervation, either a hypertonic (spastic) or hypotonic (flaccid) anus can be present, with either obstruction or incontinence of stool. The majority of children can master a bowel training program by school age and can attain "social continence."

Progressive Neurologic Dysfunction

A decline in motor and sensory function, change in bowel and bladder function, lower-back pain, or spasticity commonly are observed in patients with myelomeningocele. The tethered cord syndrome, diastematomyelia, hydrocephalus, and syringomyelia are preventable or reversible causes of progressive neurologic dysfunction if diagnosis and treatment are immediate. Other causes of progressive neurologic deterioration, such as syringobulbia and spinal cord hypoplasia, often are associated with irreversible loss of function and spasticity.

Continuity of Medical Care

Because of the complexity and multidisciplinary aspects of myelomeningocele, care from teams composed of medical, surgical, nursing, nutrition, and psychology personnel, social workers, and therapists is essential in identifying the subtle needs of the patient and the family. The expected neurologic function is based on the perinatal examination, the longitudinal record of growth and development, and the individual problem list. Reversible growth failure, early onset of puberty, and acquired loss of function may be missed in the absence of pertinent medical records and continuous care from the same team of providers.

Other Factors Related to Increased Morbidity and Mortality

Skin breakdown and decubitus ulcers can be a serious complication of prolonged pressure on insensitive areas. Severe neurogenic vascular insufficiency in some persons with higher-level myelomeningocele may lead to edema, skin breakdown, osteomyelitis, and amputation. Latex allergy, recognized since the early 1990s as present in 15 to 50% of persons with myelomeningocele, is a significant risk factor for anaphylaxis and sudden death.

Evaluation for Prognosis

The first visit of a patient with myelomeningocele should include a thorough medical and surgical history, physical and neurologic examination, and assessment of functional abilities. If the initial neurologic examination is performed at birth, the prognosis for partial or complete functional deficits at the affected neuroanatomic level can be estimated (see Table 72-1). A description of the neural elements within the meningeal sac during the surgical closure of the lesion is a useful record and should be available for later reference. The prognosis for severe cognitive impairment is increased in the presence of marked congenital thinning of the cerebral cortex. A computed tomography scan or magnetic resonance imaging (MRI) scan of the head should be obtained after the initial ventriculoperitoneal shunt placement for the treatment of congenital hydrocephalus. An MRI scan of the spine may reveal upper cervical cord compression, syringomyelia, subarachnoid cysts, spinal cord atrophy, or diastematomyelia. A renal ultrasonographic reading should be obtained shortly after birth to assess for renal anomalies or hydronephrosis. Cytogenetic studies and echocardiography should be obtained if clinically indicated.

Therapies Affecting Prognosis

Progressive spine deformities are managed best prospectively by pediatric orthopedists and neurosurgeons in a multidisciplinary care setting. Tethered spinal cord should be considered in persons with low-lumbar or sacral myelomeningocele and scoliosis, pain, and loss of motor or sensory function. In patients with high-lumbar and thoracic lesions, aggressive surgical treatment with rigid spinal instrumentation and fusion leads to permanent correction. Spinal fusion should be postponed until after the onset of puberty to avoid shortening of the torso.

Short-Term Prognosis

Survival of infants and young children with myelomeningocele has increased significantly since the 1960s, but less progress has been made in long-term survival. Whereas persons with sacral level lesions can expect a prognosis of mild disability, the quality of life for those who survive with thoracolumbar myelomeningocele typically is associated with moderate to severe impairment, lifelong disability, dozens of surgical interventions, and enormous financial expenditures.

Long-Term Prognosis

Surgical and medical management has improved childhood survival only modestly since the 1970s. Long-term follow-up of patients reported in three large series suggests a low, delayed mortality extending beyond the period of the studies. For all patients, only a 70% survival rate to young adulthood is estimated.

The prognosis for independent living is significantly lower for adults with thoracic and high-lumbar myelomeningocele who are more likely to have cognitive deficiencies and major disabilities in mobility, transfers, and self-care. These patients usually require a supervised living situation throughout adulthood and rarely obtain competitive employment. Approximately one-half of persons with midlumbar myelomeningocele will achieve independent living as adults. At least 80% of individuals with low-lumbar and sacral-level myelomeningocele will achieve independent living, but full employment rates are below the average rates of the general population.

Additional Reading

Bamforth SJ, Baird PA. Spina bifida and hydrocephalus: a population study over a 35-year period. Am J Hum Genet 1989;44:225–232.

Birth Defects and Genetic Diseases Branch and Developmental Disabilities 877 Branch DoBDaDD, Center for Environmental Health and Injury Control, CDC. Economic Burden of Spina Bifida—United States, 1980–1990. MMWR Morb Mortal Wkly Rep 1989;38:264–267.

Centers for Disease Control. Spina bifida incidence at birth—United States, 1983–1990. MMWR Morb Mortal Wkly Rep 1992; 41:497–500.

Centers for Disease Control. Recommendations for the use of folic acid to reduce the number of cases of spina bifida and other neural tube defects. MMWR Morb Mortal Wkly Rep 1992;41:1–8.

Elwood JM, Little J, Elwood JH. Epidemiology and Control of Neural Tube Defects. In JM Elwood, J Little, JH Elwood (eds), Monographs in Epidemiology and Biostatistics (vol 20). Oxford, NY: Oxford University Press, 1992.

Hunt GM, Poulton A. Open spina bifida: a complete cohort reviewed 25 years after closure. Dev Med Child Neurol 1995;37:19–29.

Luthy DA, Wardinsky T, Shurtleff DB, et al. Cesarean section before the onset of labor and subsequent motor function in infants with myelomeningocele diagnosed antenatally. N Engl J Med 1991;324:662–666.

McLaughlin JF, Shurtleff DB, Lamers JY, et al. Influence of prognosis on decisions regarding the care of newborns with myelodysplasia. N Engl J Med 1985;312:1589–1594.

Murphy M, Seagroatt V, Hey K, et al. Neural tube defects 1974–94—down but not out. Arch Dis Child 1996;75: F133–F134.

Shurtleff DB. Myelodysplasia and Exstrophies: Significance, Prevention, and Treatment. Orlando, FL: Grune & Stratton, 1986.

Chapter 73

Mental Retardation

Allen C. Crocker

The term *mental retardation* is a human behavioral descriptor, helpful in many clinical ways but subject to serious misuse and distortion. The widely used 1992 American Association on Mental Retardation definition states that

> mental retardation refers to substantial limitations in present functioning. It is characterized by significantly subaverage intellectual functioning, existing concurrently with related limitations in two or more of the following applicable adaptive skill areas: communication, self-care, home living, social skills, community use, self-direction, health and safety, functional academics, leisure, and work. Mental retardation manifests itself before age 18.

The Association goes on to caution that the definition must be applied in an ecologic context, with attention to diversity and acknowledgment that important additional adaptive and personal capabilities may coexist.

The diagnosis of mental retardation requires specific measurement, with attention paid to multiple dimensions. Persons so identified constitute approximately 1.5% of the population. Their status represents both part of a continuum with that of average individuals and, in other instances, a result of very special personal aberrations. Because of their special characteristics, individuals with mental retardation have often taken on aspects of a cultural minority, albeit loosely conceived; since the 1970s there has finally been a more substantial incorporation of persons with mental retardation into the societal mainstream. Perhaps 85% of those involved have "mild" mental retardation, with IQs in the 50 to 70 range, 10% are affected moderately, and only 5% have severe or profound limitations.

Natural History

Discussion of the life course of (and prognosis for) persons with mental retardation is a somewhat arbitrary exercise because of the enormously wide range of causes that underlie this personal situation. One often hears that mental retardation represents more than 300 etiologies; this statistic is meaningless (and grossly incomplete). More relevant is acknowledgment that any process that affects brain development or function, either congenital or acquired, can produce the condition of mental retardation. For the purposes of this chapter, the following six major categories of circumstances are identified:

1. Hereditary disorders, including an entire spectrum of single gene or polygenic syndromes
2. Early alterations in conception or embryonic development, encompassing chromosomal aberrations or early congenital anomaly syndromes
3. Pregnancy and perinatal problems, such as placental difficulties, preterm birth, or obstetric complications
4. Acquired childhood diseases, such as head injury, infection of the nervous system, intoxications, and the like
5. Environmental problems and certain unexplained behavioral syndromes, including psychosocial deprivation
6. Unknown, unclear, or multiple origins

In clinical experience, the relative prominence of these diverse causes varies greatly. Psychosocial deprivation is a common background for mild mental retardation; chromosomal changes, embryodys-genesis, or notable preterm birth likely will be associated with organic brain changes and more serious functional limitations.

The natural histories of persons with these heterogeneous disorders are obviously of several sorts. The most common course for people with significant mental retardation is relative stability, wherein the variant developmental programming appears to have been established early and then continues at its own rate and schedule throughout life. This course is true, for example, of most chromosomal disorders or congenital anomaly syndromes. Some of the hereditary syndromes, however, start off with minor differences but then experience progressive change (and even fatal outcome). The inborn errors of metabolism may show this configuration. Acquired disorders, such as brain injury, will have a deflection in course and later partial recovery. Young persons with irregular environmental trauma can be subject to varying periods of better or lesser progress as their lives proceed.

Factors Affecting Prognosis

Prognosis can have deeply rooted biological or circumstantial qualifiers. Many persons with mental retardation encounter other issues that ultimately can determine their health and survival. These events constitute the phenomenology of secondary conditions. The pathologic processes or impairments in one or another fashion derive sequentially from the disability picture of a given individual. In the course of syndromes involving mental retardation, the following six kinds of troubles eventually may become important:

- A complication, deriving directly from syndromic vulnerability, such as decubitus ulcers in a person with limited mobility, or subluxation of the cervical spine in a person with Down syndrome
- A contingency, or indirect event, such as pulmonary fibrosis in someone who is having gastroesophageal reflux and aspiration, or renal failure in a person with a neural tube defect syndrome
- An unexpected progression, such as acquired hypothyroidism in Down syndrome or loss of ambulation in severe cerebral palsy

- A comorbidity (e.g., a seizure disorder)
- Other health concerns, possibly masked or confounded by the mental retardation (a concern that could include late detection of malignancy)
- Effects of aging, including those that become additive to the mental limitations, such as memory loss

Acknowledgment of the importance of the development of secondary conditions as impingements on quality of life or as threats to survival has evolved slowly. Management plans and quality assurance programs are now much more attentive.

Therapies Affecting Prognosis

The atmosphere for accurate and resourceful health care for persons with the various mental retardation syndromes has undergone a very favorable enhancement since the 1980s. This improvement has been assisted by a substantially improved knowledge base (etiology, biology, course) but even more by a vigorous consumer movement. Parent and family organizations feature health care discussions in their conferences and publications and are demanding more partnership from involved professionals. One inspired publisher (Woodbine House) has creditable texts for parents on care in Down syndrome, spina bifida, epilepsy, cerebral palsy, and six other syndromes. Family members exchange guides to health care by electronic communication and telephone networks in an extraordinarily lively fashion. Professionals find themselves in new and important alliances.

A significant characteristic of the human service field as it reaches to persons with mental retardation and related developmental disabilities is the earnest concern with health maintenance. Currently, active committees on "health promotion" are found in such organizations as The Arc (formerly Association for Retardation Citizens) and the American Association on Mental Retardation. The Down Syndrome Medical Interest Group publishes a preventive medicine checklist for lifelong monitoring of health progress. *HEALTHWATCH* guides are available for a number of the major syndromes. Much concern is being expressed for greater attention to syndrome objectives in the *Healthy People 2010* compendium from the Public Health Service. All these efforts focus on the challenge of preventing secondary conditions.

Certain therapies have made especially valuable contributions to care of persons with mental retardation syndromes and have very real prognostic implications. The single most dramatic example is the definitive repair of major congenital heart lesions in youngsters with Down syndrome, thereby averting fatality. The campaign began seriously some 40 years ago and now is largely secured. Also dramatic has been the provision—via bone marrow transplant—of missing enzyme to children with Hurler's syndrome and certain other inborn errors of metabolism, still an arduous procedure but tantalizing when successful. The thoughtful use of advanced assistive technology devices for disabled persons (mobility, language) ultimately will affect the prognosis for these patients in several ways.

Short-Term Prognosis

Several representative syndromes within the territory of mental retardation can serve to illustrate the varying courses and outcomes. Persons with Down syndrome now are living almost entirely within community settings and are vigorous local citizens. They are broadly recognized and have well-documented clinical issues, and the condition carries a relatively high prevalence (birth incidence, 1 per 1,000; "the most common clinical cause of mental retardation," according to the National Down Syndrome Congress). Growth is somewhat limited, and obesity is a risk. Usually, retardation is in the mild to moderate range. Personal success is much influenced by the quality and quantity of verbal language.

Young people with the various mucopolysaccharidosis syndromes (Hurler's, Hunter's, Sanfilippo's, and others) experience an increasing intrusion on health and activity as the years pass, with joint restriction, airway obstruction, and progressive neuronal loss and gliosis. Their most favorable developmental status is in early to middle childhood.

Girls with Rett syndrome experience a mysterious central nervous system disorder of low incidence. It is expressed only in female subjects. Such patients first have an inexplicable progressive loss of function and then a stable, long-lasting, severely retarded state.

In many other mental retardation situations, the medical and nursing elements are not so notable, but thoughtful health maintenance programs remain a major strategy. Habilitative therapies (physical, occupational, speech, creative arts, therapeutic equitation) bring critical learning and support. Community medical offices are developing increasing familiarity with wellness efforts, and public and private agencies are committed in varying degrees.

Long-Term Prognosis

Nowhere in this field has the shift in survival been more striking than in persons with Down syndrome. Life expectancy was 9 years in 1929 and 21 years in 1947. In the latter period, fewer than 50% of infants survived the first year. Now the more than 40% of children who have Down syndrome with important congenital heart lesions are receiving reparative cardiovascular surgery, and many other health care elements are treated more effectively. Current life expectancy is near 58 years. Ironically, the major concern now for failure and mortality is a result of aging: the occurrence of premature senescence in an Alzheimer-like pattern. This condition typically appears in the sixth decade, affects a significant percentage of persons, and is assumed to have a direct gene-overdose origin from the trisomy of chromosome 21.

For young persons with the prototypic mucopolysaccharidoses, death characteristically follows progressive cardiac and pulmonary failure. A small but growing cohort of children and youth are appearing who have received successful bone marrow transplants. For them, the diseases appear to be standing still, and the prognosis is completely unknown.

In other mental retardation situations with less singular or discrete somatic liabilities, the outlook for life expectancy generally is correlated with the complexity of disability expression (and the functional limitations). Life expectancy is normal or near normal in the mild range of mental retardation. One finds enhanced usage patterns for medical care with increasing disability, a phenomenon noticed by those enrolling patients in managed care plans. Some of the survival implications of these health concerns probably can be overcome, and a reasonable assumption is that a more systematic commitment to health care in the community will continue to increase life expectancy. At the most serious end of the scale, Eyman and associates have carried out a monumental analysis of mortality. Drawing on California state systems data from nearly 100,000 clients with mental retardation and related developmental disabilities, these investigators clustered some 7,000 who had the greatest limitations. Those who were immobile and required tube feeding had 4 to 5 additional years of life expectancy, those immobile but able to eat with personal assistance had an expectancy of approximately 8 years, those with some mobility (but who were not ambulatory), not toilet-trained, and who were using personal assistance for eating would have an average of 23 additional years. Infection and accompanying troubles with pulmonary ventilation were the primary issues.

Additional Reading

Crocker AC. The causes of mental retardation. Pediatr Ann 1989;18:623–636.

Eyman RK, Borthwick-Duffy SA. Trends in Mortality Rates and Predictors of Mortality. In MM Seltzer, MW Krauss, MP Janicki (eds), Life Course Perspectives on Adulthood and Old Age. Washington, DC: American Association on Mental Retardation, 1994;93–105.

Eyman RK, Grossman HJ, Chaney RH, Call TL. The life expectancy of profoundly handicapped people with mental retardation. N Engl J Med 1990;323:584–589.

Eyman RK, Grossman HJ, Tarjan G, Miller CR. Life Expectancy and Mental Retardation. Washington, DC: American Association on Mental Retardation, 1987.

Lai F. Alzheimer Disease. In SM Pueschel, JK Pueschel (eds), Biomedical Concerns in Persons with Down Syndrome. Baltimore: Paul H. Brookes, 1992;175–196.

Luckasson R, Coulter DL, Polloway EA, et al. Mental Retardation: Definition, Classification, and Systems of Supports. Washington, DC: American Association on Mental Retardation, 1992.

Rubin IL, Crocker AC. Developmental Disabilities: Delivery of Medical Care for Children and Adults. Philadelphia: Lea & Febiger, 1989.

Sadovnick AD, Baird PA. Life Expectancy. In SM Pueschel, JK Pueschel (eds), Biomedical Concerns in Persons with Down Syndrome. Baltimore: Paul H. Brookes, 1992;47–57.

Eberly S, Van Dyke DC, Mattheis P, et al. Medical and Surgical Care for Children with Down Syndrome: A Guide for Parents. Bethesda, MD: Woodbine House, 1995.

Chapter 74

Cerebral Palsy

Beth A. Rosen and Israel F. Abroms

Cerebral palsy is a nonprogressive, early-onset brain disorder characterized by abnormal control of movement and posture. The causes include cerebral malformation, intrauterine infection, prematurity, birth asphyxia, meningitis, and trauma. The unifying feature is either failure of normal brain development or injury to the developing brain. With improvements in imaging techniques and other diagnostic testing, the term *cerebral palsy* has little use as a medical diagnosis but is useful to describe a group of individuals with similar educational and rehabilitation needs. As the nervous system matures, the clinical manifestations of cerebral palsy may change, but no structural changes occur in the brain.

Cerebral palsy can be divided into three major types: spastic, extrapyramidal, and mixed. Spastic cerebral palsy (>80%) is the most common and is characterized by hypertonia of the clasp-knife type, hyperreflexia, and extensor plantar responses. Extrapyramidal cerebral palsy, occurring in 9 to 22% of cases, involves deficits in movement and posture, including dystonia, athetosis, and ataxia. A third group called *mixed cerebral palsy* (also estimated at 9 to 22%) has features of both types.

Spastic cerebral palsy can be divided further by pattern of the limbs involved. Spastic hemiplegia (25 to 40%) involves one side of the body, usually the arm greater than the leg. Spastic quadriplegia (9 to 43%) involves all four extremities, with the legs usually affected to an extent greater than the arms. Spastic diplegia (10 to 33%), the most common type seen in premature infants, involves the lower extremities, though the upper extremities almost always are involved to some degree.

Natural History

Maternal and prenatal factors appear to play an important role in the etiology of cerebral palsy. Large population studies do not support the popular belief that birth asphyxia is the major cause. Only 20% of patients have a history of birth asphyxia and, in a large percentage of those, other known risk factors are present. The strongest association with the development of cerebral palsy has been low birth weight (<2,000 g) of both full-term and premature infants and congenital anomalies in infants. Maternal mental retardation, twin gestation, and breech presentation have been cited also as risk factors. Despite improvements in obstetric and neonatal care, the incidence of cerebral palsy has not decreased in any birth-weight group, and the etiology in many cases remains unknown.

The diagnosis of cerebral palsy usually is made after delay in the attainment of normal developmental milestones, such as head control, rolling over, sitting, and crawling. However, signs and symptoms may be present even in the perinatal period. Associated with the subsequent development of cerebral palsy are the following: Apgar score of 3 or less at 10 minutes, seizures in the first 48 hours of life, diminished or delayed cry, and apneic spells. On examination, infants with cerebral palsy usually have tone abnormalities, most often hypotonia evolving into hypertonia, and persistence of primitive reflexes (such as the Moro embrace reflex and the asymmetric tonic neck reflex), and fail to develop such normal protective and righting reflexes as the parachute response. Obligatory hand fisting and failure to develop hand usage may be present. Established handedness before 12 to 15 months may indicate a hemiplegia on the opposite side. Deep-tendon reflexes may be brisk, with cross adductor reflexes and Babinski's signs.

As individuals with cerebral palsy proceed through childhood, all but the most severely affected will attain some developmental milestones. Estimates maintain that between 55 and 80% ultimately will walk, with a lower percentage able to ambulate independently outside of the home. At present, no cure exists for the tone abnormalities of cerebral palsy (i.e., spasticity) and, despite therapy, many individuals will develop progressive orthopedic problems, especially contractures. Total lifelong care will be required for approximately 25% of those with spastic quadriparesis.

Though by definition cerebral palsy is a disorder of the motor system, most individuals also have other neurologic disabilities. Mental retardation occurs in at least 50% of patients, and those with normal intelligence often have learning disabilities. One-third to one-half have a seizure disorder, with the highest incidence in those with spastic hemiplegia or mental retardation. Abnormalities of the visual system, especially strabismus, are common. A high incidence of speech and language disorders, feeding difficulties, and behavior disorders is seen.

Factors Affecting Prognosis

Multiple factors can affect prognosis in cerebral palsy, including etiology, type of cerebral palsy, pattern of limb involvement, intelligence, associated disabilities, and such psychosocial factors as family support and motivation. Among individuals with spastic cerebral palsy (the most common form), an important factor is pattern of limb involvement. For example, nearly all patients with hemiplegia ambulate before their third birthday. The percentage is considerably lower for children who have spastic diplegia and spastic quadriplegia. A reasonable estimate would be that at least 50% of those with spastic diplegia eventually walk,

whereas the number drops to 25 to 33% of those with spastic quadriplegia.

Factors related to the neurodevelopmental examination also can affect prognosis. Again, using the example of ambulation, two factors that have been identified as important clinical predictors include the age of achievement of sitting and the loss of primitive reflexes. The majority of children who achieve sitting by age 2 years become functionally ambulatory, and most children who do not sit unsupported by age 4 years will not walk. The persistence of primitive reflexes (including the Moro embrace reflex and the asymmetric tonic neck reflex) beyond age 18 to 24 months signifies a poor prognosis for ambulation, especially if these reflexes are obligatory. Most functional walkers will have lost these reflexes by age 12 months.

In all types of cerebral palsy, associated disabilities negatively affect prognosis. Most notable of such disabilities are intellectual deficits, seizure disorders, and severe visual impairment.

Evaluation of Prognosis

Prognosis in cerebral palsy is determined largely on clinical grounds. Such neuroimaging studies as computed tomography and magnetic resonance imaging are useful in determining etiology and the extent of the lesion. Both of these findings may be useful to some degree in predicting outcome but should never be used as absolute indicators of prognosis. Neurophysiologic studies are not useful. Even the most severely involved individuals may have normal electroencephalograms. Metabolic studies may be useful to rule out a degenerative neurologic disorder when indicated.

Therapies Affecting Prognosis

Currently, no treatment is available to repair the abnormal development or damage to the brain that leads to cerebral palsy. Physical and occupational therapy, special education, and orthopedic intervention have been mainstays of treatment. Services frequently begin in state-funded early intervention programs as soon as the diagnosis is established. The goals of physical and occupational therapy programs include maximizing movement and function and the prevention of deformities. Neurodevelopmental therapy for children with cerebral palsy is a commonly used modality that attempts to correct abnormal postures and reflexes and to enhance normal movement patterns. However, despite their widespread use and acceptance, no clear evidence substantiates that therapy programs improve ultimate prognosis for any selected outcome.

Adjunctive therapies include the use of orthotics, casting, and adaptive equipment. Walkers, wheelchairs, specialized seats and standers, modified utensils, and sophisticated communication devices clearly have improved the quality of life for many individuals with cerebral palsy. Less clear is whether they modify overall prognosis.

Several medications have been advocated to improve prognosis in cerebral palsy by reducing spasticity. When taken orally, the most commonly used medications, (baclofen, diazepam, and dantrolene sodium) may have the unacceptable side effect of sedation. Localized nerve blocks that cause partial denervation of a specific nerve and decrease spasticity in a target muscle can improve range of motion and allow more use of orthotics. However, the nerve block wears off after 4 to 6 months, and uncertain is whether the benefits gained during the window of decreased spasticity provide any long-term benefit.

Two new treatments to reduce spasticity have been introduced. One, intrathecal baclofen, allows this medication to be delivered directly into the cerebral spinal fluid using a programmable pump. By reducing the necessary dosage as compared to the oral dose, the side effect of sedation is minimized. In addition, dosage can be customized for each patient. Botulinum toxin A, a naturally occurring poison that acts at the neuromuscular junction, can be injected directly into the muscle to reduce spasticity. Its advantages over nerve block are easier administration and repeat dosing, though the development of resistance raises some concern. Though both new treatments are exciting and appear to confer short-term benefits, a positive effect on long-term prognosis remains to be proved.

Finally, surgery continues to play an important role in the treatment of cerebral palsy. Orthopedic surgery is used to lengthen and release tight muscles and to relieve contractures. This modality may lead to improved standing and ambulation and, in more severely affected individuals, may allow better positioning and hygiene. However, surgery cannot always prevent long-term deformities common in patients with spastic cerebral palsy.

A neurosurgical procedure called *selective dorsal rhizotomy* involves the isolation and sectioning of selected posterior spinal roots from the second lumbar nerve to the first sacral nerve. Intraoperative electrical stimulation of the nerves is performed, and those that appear to contribute most to spasticity are cut. Proponents of the procedure claim that lower-extremity spasticity and gait are improved, and gains in upper-extremity and cognitive function have been cited. Whether the improvements seen in patients are a result of the surgery or part of the natural history of the disorder remains controversial.

As in any condition for which there is no cure, a variety of alternative therapies are available. Many are time-consuming and expensive, but none have shown any definite benefit in improving prognosis.

Short-Term Prognosis

For those children who survive the neonatal period, the short-term prognosis is good. Improvements in health maintenance and nutritional support allow most children to live at home with their families and to attend a school program, often in special education. Psychosocial factors play an important role in a family's ability to adapt to a child with a significant disability.

Long-Term Prognosis

Life expectancy for individuals with cerebral palsy does not appear to be diminished greatly in comparison to that of the general population. Two studies cited 20-year survival rates of approximately 90%. Only among a subgroup of those with severe spastic quadriparesis, characterized by mental retardation and immobility, was the survival rate substantially lower, ranging between 40 and 60% by age 20 years.

Less well understood is long-term prognosis as it relates to the ability to function in society. Employment is one outcome measure that has been studied. Several factors, including the type of cerebral palsy, the degree of disability, and especially the level of intelligence, clearly are important. Those with spastic diplegia and spastic hemiplegia are most likely to become employed, and those with spastic quadriparesis are the least likely. Useful hand function and intelligible speech have a positive correlation, as does the ability to live independently. Individuals who have completed 12 years of schooling and have normal or borderline intelligence have the highest rate of employment.

Cerebral palsy is a disorder for which no cure exists. All affected individuals have some degree of disability—ranging from mild to severe—that has an impact on their developmental and functional potential. Though many treatments are available, none have been proved with any certainty to alter prognosis significantly. With data suggesting that life expectancy may approach normal for many individuals with cerebral palsy, programs must be designed to maximize function and quality of life for both children and adults while researchers continue to search for more effective treatments.

Additional Reading

Evans PM, Evans SJW, Alberman E. Cerebral palsy: why we must plan for survival. Arch Dis Child 1990;65: 1329–1333.

Hutton JL, Cooke T, Pharoah POD. Life expectancy in children with cerebral palsy. Br Med J 1995;309:431–435.

Molnar GE, Gordon SU. Cerebral palsy: predictive value of selected clinical signs for early prognostication of motor function. Arch Phys Med Rehabil 1976;57:153–158.

Nelson KB. Cerebral Palsy. In Swaiman KF (ed), Pediatric Neurology. St. Louis: Mosby, 1994;471–477.

O'Grady RS, Crain LS, Kohn J. The prediction of long term functional outcomes of children with cerebral palsy. Dev Med Child Neurol 1995;37:997–1005.

Palmer FB, Shapiro BK, Wachtel RC, et al. The effects of physical therapy on cerebral palsy: a controlled trial in infants with spastic diplegia. N Engl J Med 1988;318: 803–808.

Chapter 75

Wilson's Disease

James R. White and James M. Gilchrist

Wilson's disease is a rare, autosomal recessive disorder of copper metabolism associated with a gene mutation on chromosome 13. An unknown molecular defect impairs excretion of copper by the liver, causing accumulation of this metal in the liver, brain, and other organs. The copper deposition causes a wide range of clinical signs and symptoms, the most common of which are due to neurologic or hepatic dysfunction. Before the 1950s, Wilson's disease always was fatal, death occurring usually within 2 to 3 years of the onset of neurologic symptoms. In 1948, Cumings established the relationship between the abnormal deposits of copper and the lesions associated with Wilson's disease. A few years after this discovery, copper-chelating agents were found to be effective treatment.

Natural History

Most studies indicate that the average symptom onset age is the second decade. Rare patients will develop the illness before age 4 years or after age 50 years. Patients presenting with hepatic symptoms generally have an earlier onset age than do those presenting with neurologic deficits that usually present late in the second decade or early third decade of life.

The presenting symptoms and signs of Wilson's disease are highly variable. Approximately 40 to 60% of patients present with a neurologic illness. The most common neurologic signs include dysarthria, tremor, writing difficulties, dystonia, and ataxia. At the time when neurologic disease becomes manifest, a Kayser-Fleischer ring, due to deposition of copper in Descemet's membrane in the cornea, is seen in virtually every case. Hepatic disease (e.g., fatty liver infiltration, cirrhosis, and acute fulminant hepatic necrosis) also occurs. Patients also may develop hemolytic anemia and various renal abnormalities.

Deiss and coworkers suggested a five-stage model of the natural history of Wilson's disease (Fig. 75-1). During the first years of life, patients remain asymptomatic as progressive hepatic copper accumulation occurs (stage I). Then copper is released from the liver once hepatic binding sites are saturated. This finding is supported by evidence that the concentration of copper in the liver of asymptomatic patients is significantly greater than that in the liver of neurologically impaired patients. Approximately 60% of patients are asymptomatic during this stage (stage II) of hepatic copper release. Others may develop hemolytic anemia (stage IIA). Some patients may not release the copper as readily, and necrosis of liver cells and hepatic failure ensues (stage IIB). These nonneurologic manifestations of Wilson's disease present most commonly early in the second decade of life. The patients who survive enter the stage of cerebral copper accumulation (stage III). Once the concentration of copper reaches a critical level in the brain, neurologic disease develops (stage IV). Unless treatment is initiated (stage V), all patients will develop a progressive, and eventually fatal, neurologic disease.

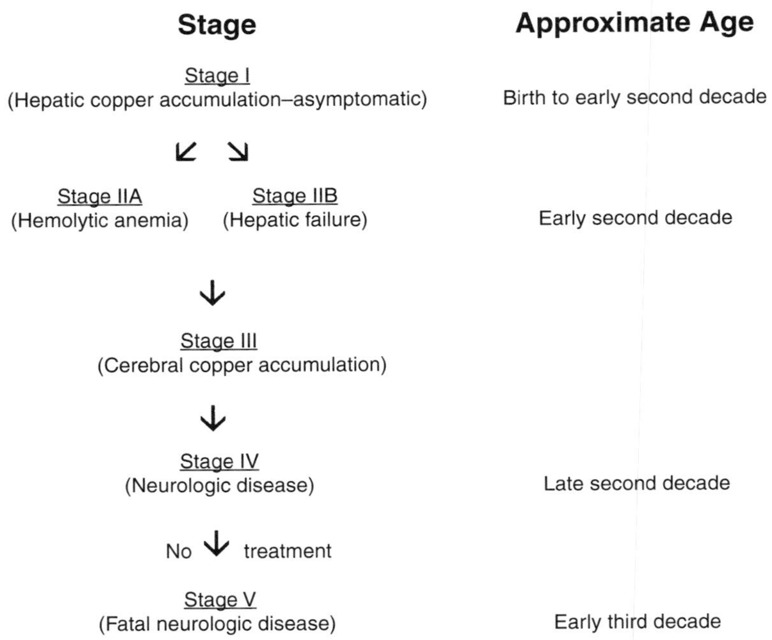

Stage	**Approximate Age**

Figure 75-1. A model for the natural history of Wilson's disease.

Stage I
(Hepatic copper accumulation–asymptomatic)   Birth to early second decade

↙   ↘

Stage IIA   Stage IIB
(Hemolytic anemia)   (Hepatic failure)   Early second decade

↓

Stage III
(Cerebral copper accumulation)

↓

Stage IV
(Neurologic disease)   Late second decade

No ↓ treatment

Stage V
(Fatal neurologic disease)   Early third decade

Factors Affecting Prognosis

Patients who are asymptomatic at the time of diagnosis have the best prognosis. In general, neurologic deficit at presentation carries a worse prognosis than does presentation with other manifestations of the disease. Patients with a neurologic disorder demonstrating marked involuntary movements, such as chorea and pseudosclerosis (dysarthria and flapping tremor), long have been thought to have a more favorable prognosis than do patients with parkinsonism or dystonia. A study by Walshe and colleagues supports this observation. The best prognosis is seen in patients presenting with pseudosclerosis; they have an 82% chance of good response to treatment (defined as becoming symptom-free or characterized by only minor neurologic deficit). Those with a choreic syndrome have a 75% chance of good response, whereas patients with parkinsonism or dystonia have a relatively reduced chance of good response (being 63% and 53%, respectively).

Overall, patients presenting with hepatic disease have a good prognosis. However, those with end-stage liver disease tend to have poor outcomes secondary to fulminant hepatic failure or complications of cirrhosis, such as massive bleeding. It is important to note that some patients' first manifestation of Wilson's disease is fulminant hepatic necrosis, a condition with high mortality.

Evaluation for Prognosis

Though establishing the diagnosis of Wilson's disease unequivocally is of the utmost importance, especially given the toxic and lifelong treatment, no test accurately predicts prognosis in individual patients. The biochemical abnormalities in Wilson's disease include a low serum copper, a low ceruloplasmin, a high serum free copper, an increased urinary output of the metal, and high concentration of copper on liver biopsy. Several studies have examined these parameters, and no correlation with disease progress could be made. An asymptomatic patient may have more severe derangements in these parameters than does a patient who dies from the disease.

As mentioned in the previous section, fulminant hepatic failure is an important cause of death in Wilson's disease. Nazer and associates used certain ranges of prothrombin time, aspartate transaminase, and bilirubin concentration to formulate a numeric prognostic index. By use of this prognostic index retrospectively, 17 survivors were differentiated from 18 patients who died of liver disease. Other investigators found this prognostic index to have poor predictive value, however.

Therapies Affecting Prognosis

Before the use of copper-chelating agents, Wilson's disease universally was fatal. Currently, most physicians use the chelating agent D-penicillamine for Wilson's disease, especially for patients with neurologic presentation. Unless serious toxicity develops, this medication is continued for the duration of life. Approximately 10 to 20% of patients with neurologic disease experience clinical worsening during the first weeks or months after starting D-penicillamine. One study observed that half of those who worsened did not recover to their pre-penicillamine baseline. This phenomena is not seen in asymptomatic or other nonneurologic presentations of Wilson's disease. Most patients who are started on D-penicillamine before irreversible neurologic deficit have good recovery. However, predicting irreversible disease in a given patient is not possible. Poor compliance with the medication has been demonstrated to worsen patients' prognosis.

Side effects of the medications used in the treatment of Wilson's disease can complicate treatment and can affect prognosis adversely. Penicillamine toxicity occurs in some 20% of treated patients. The most common reaction to penicillamine is an urticarial rash. The late immune reactions, such as immune complex nephropathy and systemic lupus erythematosus (SLE), can have significant morbidity. Also, SLE can be reactivated by most of the medications used in the treatment of Wilson's disease. Other adverse reactions include polyneuropathy, myasthenia gravis, leukopenia, Goodpasture's syndrome, epidermolysis bullosa, and oral ulceration.

Approximately 5 to 7% of patients cannot tolerate D-penicillamine. Usually, such patients are treated with trientine, another copper-chelating agent. It has less of a cupruretic effect than does penicillamine, but its clinical effectiveness is similar. No controlled trial has compared the two medications. The side effects of trientine include reactivation of penicillamine-induced SLE and sideroblastic anemia.

Zinc, which blocks the intestinal absorption of copper, is another useful medication. Some authors suggest that it is the treatment of choice for maintenance therapy, treatment of the presymptomatic patient, and treatment of the pregnant patient because of its relatively low toxicity. Zinc can produce iron deficiency anemia and significant epigastric pain, nausea, and vomiting.

Less experience with ammonium tetrathiomolybdate is available. The agent forms a complex with copper and protein, blocks intestinal absorption of copper, and renders serum copper nontoxic. A study of 17 patients with neurologic symptoms treated with ammonium tetrathiomolybdate suggests it is a safe and effective medication. Patients do not appear to be at risk for early neurologic deterioration with this medication, in contrast to D-penicillamine. Bone marrow suppression is one important side effect of tetrathiomolybdate.

Although delay in starting treatment of Wilson's disease has risk, no clear correlation connects delay in therapy with prognosis. For example, one study observed the paradoxical effect of better response to treatment in patients whose diagnosis was delayed by 7 months or longer as compared to patients with a 1- to 6-month delay. Nevertheless, therapy should not be delayed in patients with Wilson's disease. At some point, accumulated copper causes irreversible neuronal damage, though currently no method can predict the point at which this threshold is reached. Furthermore, patients can die from fulminant hepatic failure early in the course of the disease.

Another important treatment of Wilson's disease is liver transplantation. This procedure is reserved for patients who have end-stage liver disease and are at high mortal risk. If the liver transplantation is successful, the patient's biochemical abnormalities normalize, and the Wilson's disease appears to be cured. Few descriptions of the effect of liver transplantation on neurologic symptoms exist. In the reported cases, some appear to have improvement of their neurologic deficit, though cases of severe neurologic impairment may not benefit.

Short-Term Prognosis

The most significant negative prognostic factor in the early stages of Wilson's disease is the development of hepatic failure, which causes significant morbidity and mortality. Generally, neurologic symptoms slowly improve over time with appropriate treatment. Up to several months might pass after initiation of treatment before improvement is noted, especially in neurologic Wilson's. A significant number of patients with neurologic disease initially worsen in the weeks to months after starting D-penicillamine.

Long-Term Prognosis

Overall, of those patients with appropriately treated neurologic Wilson's disease, approximately 40% will have an excellent response and become symptom-free. Twenty-five percent can be expected to have a good response, with only minor neurologic deficit. The remaining one-third will have a poor response, with severe neurologic deficit or death. Long-term prognosis for survival does not appear to be reduced in patients with treated Wilson's disease (neurologic and nonneurologic) as compared to gender- and age-matched controls. Untreated Wilson's disease is fatal.

Additional Reading

Brewer GJ, Terry CA, Aisen AM, Hill G. Worsening of neurologic syndrome in patients with Wilson's disease with initial penicillamine therapy. Arch Neurol 1987;44:490–493.

Deiss A, Lynch RE, Lee GR, Cartwright GE. Long-term therapy of Wilson's disease. Ann Intern Med 1971;75:57–65.

Nazer H, Ede RJ, Mowat AP, Williams R. Wilson's disease: clinical presentation and use of prognostic index. Gut 1986;27:1377–1381.

Sternlieb I. Perspectives on Wilson's disease. Hepatology 1990;12:1234–1239.

Stremmel W, Meyerrose KW, Niederau C, et al. Wilson disease: clinical presentation, treatment, and survival. Ann Intern Med 1991;115:720–726.

Walshe JM, Yealland M. Chelation treatment of neurological Wilson's disease. Q J Med 1993;86:197–204.

Walshe JM, Yealland M. Wilson's disease: the problem of delayed diagnosis. J Neurol Neurosurg Psychiatry 1992; 55:692–696.

Part XIV
Miscellaneous Disorders

Chapter 76

Neurosarcoidosis

Thomas F. Scott

Sarcoidosis is an idiopathic inflammatory disorder characterized by granulomatous inflammation involving multiple organs. Pulmonary involvement is seen in most cases, and much less commonly involved organs and tissues include abdominal viscera, skin, bones, orbital tissues, and muscle. In some 5% of cases, the nervous system is involved.

Natural History

The natural history of neurosarcoidosis depends on the organ systems involved and the response to therapy. Death due to sarcoidosis results generally from pulmonary or cardiac involvement, but death from neurologic involvement has been reported in several cases (though rare overall). Much that is known about neurosarcoidosis is presented in isolated case reports and small case series, though a few series of more then 30 patients are available. Long-term studies of patients with neurosarcoidosis are rare.

Neurosarcoidosis may be an autoimmune illness, but the neuroimmunology of the disease is poorly understood. Like most autoimmune illnesses, neurosarcoidosis may entail relapsing-remitting symptoms. However, most patients (perhaps 70%) will not relapse after initial treatment, and the maximum severity of illness for these patients tends to occur around the time of diagnosis or initial presentation. Improvement after treatment (initially with steroids) generally occurs over weeks to months. The natural history of untreated neurosarcoidosis is unknown.

Patients who experience relapse tend to have multiple relapses or disease that is difficult to control. Relapses have a strong tendency to affect the same area of the nervous system as did the initial attack. Patients who have disabling symptoms and do not respond well to initial treatment tend to have disease that is more difficult to control. If the initial attack involves very sensitive areas of the nervous system (e.g., the spinal cord or brain stem) and initial deficits are severe, patients may have static but severe neurologic deficits causing significant disability.

Factors Affecting Prognosis

As in other autoimmune disease, the course of neurosarcoidosis may be punctuated by multiple relapses. An initial relapse tends to portend further relapses, making an initial relapse a poor prognostic sign. Usually, multiple relapses are associated with increasing disability. As with the initial attack of neurosarcoidosis, prognosis after relapse appears to be influenced by treatment (controlled studies of which are not available). Response to steroids seems evident in most cases but, in patients in whom steroid therapy fails or is intolerable, such immunosuppressives as azathioprine, cyclosporine, and methotrexate have a fairly well-defined role as rescue therapy and most likely influence prognosis. In desperate situations, radiotherapy has been used successfully.

Neurosarcoidosis can involve either the peripheral nerves or the central nervous system. Patients with peripheral neuropathy or Bell's palsy as the sole manifestation of neurosarcoidosis tend to pursue a benign monophasic course. In my experience, involvement of both the peripheral and central nervous systems is rare.

I (and others) would propose several clinical factors as important in determining prognosis; however, patient numbers have been insufficient to make speculation more secure. Stern and coworkers have noticed that several of their patients with seizures had a poor neurologic outcome. In my experience and in several anecdotal reports, optic neuropathy due to neurosarcoidosis often is refractory and requires more aggressive treatment.

My institution has experienced a single death owing to hydrocephalus and brain edema in a patient with fulminant meningitis resulting from (apparently noninfectious) neurosarcoidosis. Others (rarely) have reported similarly malignant cases, though successful treatment also has been reported. Sarcoidosis involving the spinal cord may be particularly disabling. As is seen with multiple sclerosis, once a severe myelopathy is established for a period of months, significant recovery is rare.

Many reports agree with my experience that intracranial mass lesions often respond well to treatment with steroids, though treatment failures occur. Some patients retain large enhancing intracranial lesions by magnetic resonance imaging (MRI) and yet do well clinically. This outcome is due likely to a slow transformation of active inflammation into a chronic, vascularized, fibrotic scar. Stress (mental or physical) does not appear to be a factor in progression or relapse of neurosarcoidosis.

In my experience, lack of initial improvement of laboratory parameters does not correlate with prognosis. Serum and cerebrospinal fluid (CSF) angiotensin-converting enzyme level, total spinal fluid protein, and CSF immunoglobulin G (IgG) index may correlate with disease activity in some cases, but no prognostic significance has been derived from the limited studies available in this area.

Evaluation for Prognosis

MRI scanning with gadolinium is important for the initial evaluation of most patients with central nervous system sarcoidosis, but repeat MRI scanning may be necessary only when a clinical response to treatment is lacking. CSF analysis is useful for diagnosis, and elevation of opening pressure may correlate with a worse prognosis in patients with aseptic meningitis if the high pressure is related to hydrocephalus. Papilledema or other findings indicating increased intracranial pressure likely are indicative of a worse prognosis.

A patient suspected of having peripheral neuropathy or myopathy should undergo electromyography (EMG) and nerve conduction studies. Some patients with pulmonary sarcoidosis seem in a state of chronic fatigue, complain of poor endurance, but have no objective or EMG evidence of myopathy. Patients with symptomatic EMG or biopsy-proved myopathy may experience either a monophasic, chronic relapsing or a severe, progressive course.

Therapies Affecting Prognosis

In the absence of controlled studies of steroid treatment in neurosarcoidosis, common practice is to treat all symptoms of recent onset with moderate- or high-dose steroids, usually tapered over a period of months. Rapid response to therapy seems a good prognostic sign, and ultimately two-thirds of patients will have an easily treated monophasic illness. In neurosarcoidosis affecting peripheral nerves, failure of steroids to improve symptoms is exceedingly rare and, in a few reported cases, therapy was withheld, and patients progressed. Many reports cite both successful steroid treatment of intracranial lesions and some treatment failures. Sarcoidosis of the spinal cord also should be treated initially with steroids. Such immunosuppressives as azathioprine, cyclophosphamide, methotrexate, and cyclosporine have produced steroid-sparing effects in patients requiring long-term immunosuppression. Cranial irradiation has been used successfully in cases refractory to either steroids or immunosuppression.

Short-Term Prognosis

The majority of patients with neurosarcoidosis respond within weeks or months to steroid treatment alone and may be weaned from steroids without serious consequences. Many patients have mild disease that can be controlled easily.

Long-Term Prognosis

Although patients may be left with significant long-term disability from an initial neurosarcoidosis attack, most patients experience improvement after their initial bout and remain relapse-free. In perhaps 50% of patients with more severe illness characterized by multiple relapses or slow progression, disease can be controlled eventually with aggressive immunosuppressive therapy. Patients with insidious onset of severe disabilities rarely recover.

Death rarely results from neurosarcoidosis but not uncommonly results from pulmonary sarcoidosis. Pulmonary sarcoidosis may be less steroid responsive, as a controlled study of steroid treatment failed to provide more than temporary symptomatic improvement in this setting.

Additional Reading

Agbogu BN, Stern BJ, Sewell C, Yang G. Therapeutic considerations in patients with refractory neurosarcoidosis. Arch Neurol 1995;52:875–879.

Delaney P. Neurologic manifestations of sarcoidosis: review of the literature, with a report of 23 cases. Ann Intern Med 1977;87:336–346.

Herring AB, Urich H. Sarcoidosis of the central nervous system. J Neurol Sci 1969;9:405–422.

Krumholz A, Stern BJ, Stern EG. Clinical implications of seizures in neurosarcoidosis. Arch Neurol 1991;48:842–844.

Matthews WBE. Sarcoidosis of the nervous system. J Neurol Neurosurg Psychiatry 1965;28:23–29.

Scott TF. Neurosarcoidosis: progress and clinical aspects. Neurology 1993;43:8–12.

Stern BJ, Krumholz A, Johns C, et al. Sarcoidosis and its neurological manifestations. Arch Neurol 1985;42:909–917.

Wiederholt WC, Siekert RG. Neurological manifestations of sarcoidosis. Neurology 1965;15:1147–1154.

Chapter 77

Idiopathic Intracranial Hypertension (Pseudotumor Cerebri)

Valerie Biousse and Nancy J. Newman

Idiopathic intracranial hypertension (IIH), also called *pseudotumor cerebri*, is defined as increased intracranial pressure—without underlying intracranial mass lesions, hydrocephalus, or venous sinus thrombosis—and normal cerebrospinal fluid composition (Table 77-1). The symptoms of IIH are those of raised intracranial pressure without any neurologic localizing signs (Table 77-2). By definition, raised intracranial pressure related to such entities as cerebral venous thrombosis or chronic meningitis is not classified as IIH and should be considered in alternative diagnoses. The syndrome of IIH is more frequent in women of reproductive age, especially those with recent weight gain. However, multiple conditions and diseases have been reported to be associated with IIH, most with only anecdotal supporting evidence (Table 77-3).

Natural History

The natural history of IIH is highly unpredictable. The disease is spontaneously remitting and relapsing. Recurrences can occur as long as 14 years after the last manifestations. The symptoms and signs are variable, from the patient with severe headache but no recognized papilledema to the asymptomatic patient with chronic atrophic papilledema and insidious, severely constricting visual field loss. Predicting the evolution of IIH for a specific patient is impossible.

Headache can vary in severity, even in the same patient over time. Although individuals may have headaches that consistently herald the return of raised intracranial pressure, resolution of headache does not always mean that IIH has remitted. These patients still may be at risk for persistent papilledema and vision loss.

The most significant sequel of IIH is permanent loss of vision caused by prolonged papilledema and secondary optic atrophy. Up to 50% of IIH patients have been reported with visual field or visual acuity deficits, with severe, legally blinding deficits in up to 25%. Vision impairment may occur early or late in the course of the disease. Although usually insidiously progressive, vision loss occasionally may present suddenly, often associated with superimposed ischemic optic neuropathy. Initially, most of the patients have only minor abnormalities of their visual fields, particularly enlargement of the physiologic blind spots. With time, however, patients may experience progressive constriction of the visual fields, characterized by inferior nasal defects and arcuate defects, with relative sparing of central visual acuity until late in the course of the disease. Therefore, by the time patients start to complain about their vision, attempts to save it often are too late. The interval from onset to remission varies with patients and their treatment, ranging from a few days to many months.

Factors Affecting Prognosis

Transient visual obscurations have been associated with vision loss and have been used by some as an indication for surgical treatment; however, multiple

Table 77-1. Modified Dandy's Criteria for the Diagnosis of Idiopathic Intracranial Hypertension

1. Signs and symptoms of raised intracranial pressure
2. No localizing neurologic signs, in an alert patient, other than abducens nerve paresis
3. Normal neuroimaging studies, except for small ventriculi or empty sellae (neuroimaging should include a good quality magnetic resonance imaging or magnetic resonance venography to rule out cerebral venous thrombosis)
4. Documented increased opening pressure (250 mm of water or more) but normal cerebrospinal fluid composition
5. Primary structural or systemic causes of elevated intracranial venous sinus pressure excluded (e.g., chronic meningitis or cerebral venous thrombosis)

Table 77-2. Demographics, Symptoms, and Signs in Idiopathic Intracranial Hypertension

Demographics
  Female (65–95%)
  Age peak (21–34 yrs)
  Obesity (44–94%)
Symptoms
  Headache (75–99%)
  Visual symptoms (transient visual obscurations; visual loss: 30–68%)
  Diplopia (20–38%)
  Tinnitus (often pulsatile: 0–80%)
  Distal paresthesias
Signs
  Papilledema (98–100%)
  Sixth nerve palsy (14–35%)
  Visual field defects (3–51%)
  Decreased visual acuity (2–25%)

Table 77-3. Conditions and Diseases Having a Suggested Association with Idiopathic Intracranial Hypertension

Conditions
  Female gender
  Reproductive age group
  Obesity and recent weight gain
Endocrine diseases
  Hypothyroidism
  Addison's disease
  Cushing's disease
  Hypoparathyroidism
Miscellaneous diseases
  Iron-deficiency anemia
  Chronic renal failure
  Systemic lupus erythematosus
  Dural arteriovenous malformations
Medications
  Multivitamins (vitamin A)   Cimetidine
  Isoretinoid   Lithium carbonate
  Tetracycline   Steroids and steroid
  Nalidixic acid   withdrawal
  Nitrofurantoin   Anabolic steroids
  Sulfa antibiotics   Norplant implants
  Amiodarone   Tamoxifen
  Danazol   Cyclosporine
  Diphenylhydantoin

studies have shown that this symptom is not associated with poor visual outcome. Furthermore, the presence of transient visual obscurations does not correlate with the degree of intracranial hypertension or the extent of papilledema. As optic disk edema is the cause of vision loss in IIH, some have suggested that the severity of vision loss could be predicted from the severity of papilledema. However, this too is not a reliable indicator of disease progression, as chronic compression of the optic nerve by edema results in axonal loss and optic atrophy and, therefore, subsequent decrease in the amount of papilledema (which is to say, "Dead axons can't swell").

Numerous studies have emphasized the association of IIH with a variety of conditions and medications (see Table 77-3), but not clear is whether these associated factors affect the prognosis of IIH. In a retrospective study, Corbett and coworkers found systemic hypertension to be the only statistically significant risk factor for poor vision outcome; systemic corticosteroid administration and raised intraocular pressure were presumed to be additional risk factors. These investigators noted also that if visual function already was affected severely at the time of presentation, return of visual function was unlikely. Digre and colleagues (see Radhakrishnan and coworkers) showed that black men were particularly at risk for severe visual impairment. In a prospective study, Wall and associates reported recent weight gain as the only factor significantly associated with worsening of vision. Finally, Radhakrishnan and coworkers found that the only factor related to poor visual outcome was the duration of IIH-related symptoms before diagnosis.

Figure 77-1. Automated perimetry (Humphrey 30-2) in a patient with idiopathic intracranial hypertension. The right eye is on the right and the left eye is on the left. Dark areas are areas of visual field loss. A. Substantial visual field loss is noted on presentation, left eye worse than right. B. At 1-month follow-up, note worsening visual field loss in both eyes. C. After optic nerve sheath decompression in the left eye, note visual field improvement in both eyes. (Reprinted with permission from V Biousse, NJ Newman. Management of optic nerve disorders: II. Idiopathic intracranial hypertension. Drugs Today 1997;33:21.)

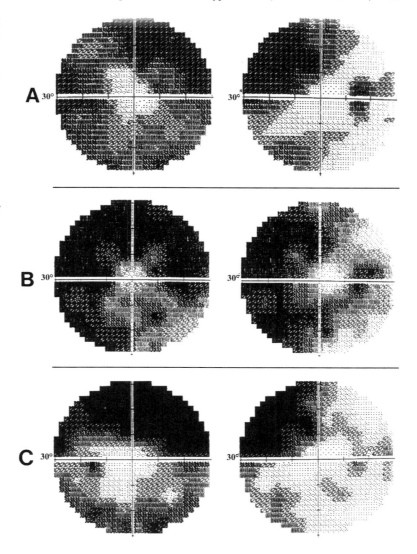

Evaluation for Prognosis

The only permanent morbidity from IIH is loss of vision. Therefore, the evaluation for prognosis is the detection of the presence and progression of vision loss. It has been shown that visual acuity and visual evoked potentials are insensitive to the vision loss resulting from IIH. As progression can be insidious and unpredictable, careful follow-up with serial vision field testing is mandatory. Many authors have proposed measurement of blind spot enlargement to follow these patients. However, refraction often eliminates this defect, so blind spot enlargement should not be considered as significant vision loss unless it encroaches fixation. Furthermore, as the size of a blind spot is so dependent on refraction, it should not be used to follow the course of therapy. Visual field testing with quantitative, automated perimetry of the central 30 degrees of vision is the most sensitive test (Fig. 77-1). Serial fundus photography may prove useful in gauging the effects of therapy and in the resolution or recurrence of papilledema.

Therapies Affecting Prognosis

The spontaneous remission rate for IIH is high, and this finding renders difficult the evaluation of any treatment regimen. Furthermore, no prospective randomized study comparing various treatments in IIH patients has been performed. Management of the disorder focuses on the early detection and prevention of vision loss. Therefore, in the patient with severe or progressive vision loss, prompt and invasive intervention may be required. As vision loss occurs as a complication of chronic papilledema from raised intracranial pressure, all treatment regimens aim to lower the intracranial pressure and to improve prognosis of IIH. Correction of predisposing factors, such as withdrawal of a potentially offending medication and weight reduction, probably are useful in limiting the duration of the disease and in preventing recurrences.

Repeated lumbar punctures (LPs) have been used to treat IIH. Indeed, the LP performed at the time of diagnosis often is the first treatment for IIH, as most patients report an immediate resolution of symptoms. Occasionally, complete resolution of IIH occurs after the first or second LP. However, the use of this treatment is tempered by tolerance and by the risk in some patients of visual loss rather than improvement after serial LPs.

Medical therapy includes the carbonic anhydrase inhibitor acetazolamide, which is effective and safe in reducing intracranial hypertension. Steroids also may be effective in the treatment of IIH. However, recurrence rates of IIH are high after steroid withdrawal, and chronic steroid use in an obese population is to be avoided.

Surgical intervention is required for significant optic nerve dysfunction despite maximum medical therapy. The two primary surgical options for IIH patients are optic nerve sheath decompression and placement of a lumboperitoneal shunt. Decompression of the optic nerve—by making a window or multiple slits in its dural sheath from a transconjunctival medial or lateral approach—is effective for reversing vision loss and protecting the optic nerve from further IIH damage. In addition to immediate decompression of the optic nerve, this fenestration likely results in long-term filtration of cerebrospinal fluid. Indeed, more than 50% of patients show improvement in headache and contralateral visual function after unilateral surgery. However, the results may not be permanent, with a failure rate of 32% within 3 years. In addition, this procedure is not without risk. Minor transient complications include Adie's tonic pupil and diplopia. More serious complications include orbital hemorrhage and vascular occlusions in up to 11% of cases. Lumboperitoneal shunting once was considered the optimum surgical treatment of IIH but was abandoned by many physicians in favor of optic nerve sheath decompression. Many complications have been reported after lumboperitoneal shunting, mainly shunt failure from obstruction or disconnection, (requiring revisions in approximately 50% of patients), secondary intracranial hypotension with low-pressure headache, abdominal pain, subdural hematoma, and infection. In addition, this procedure failed to prevent progressive vision loss in some patients with IIH. Nevertheless, one study suggested that lumboperitoneal shunt was a safe procedure without any major complications (other than obstruction of the shunt) and was effective in alleviating the signs and symptoms of IIH and in preventing visual complications.

Short-Term Prognosis

Generally, the course of IIH is limited to several months or a few years. The first months are crucial, as the pattern of visual involvement typically is dictated at presentation, and early intervention may prevent progressive deterioration.

Long-Term Prognosis

Depending on the series, a variable percentage of patients (up to 37%) are shown to have recurrences after months or years of follow-up. Usually, the recurrences are no worse than was the initial presentation, and no trend toward a worse visual outcome has been noted in patients with recurrences. Except for visual deficits, no trend toward development of any other problem is evident. However, substantial and permanent visual compromise can result from untreated disease.

Additional Reading

Ahlskog JE, O'Neill BP. Pseudotumor cerebri. Ann Intern Med 1982;97:249–256.
Biousse V, Newman NJ. Management of optic nerve disorders: II. Idiopathic intracranial hypertension. Drugs Today 1997;33:19–24.

Corbett JJ, Savino PJ, Thomson HS, et al. Visual loss in pseudotumor cerebri: follow-up of 57 patients from 5 to 41 years and a profile of 14 patients with permanent severe visual loss. Arch Neurol 1982;39:461–474.

Corbett JJ, Thomson HS. The rational management of idiopathic intracranial hypertension. Arch Neurol 1989;46: 1049–1051.

Eggenberger ER, Miller NR, Vitale S. Lumboperitoneal shunt for the treatment of pseudotumor cerebri. Neurology 1996;46:1524–1530.

Radhakrishnan K, Ahlskog JE, Garrity JA, Kurland LT. Idiopathic intracranial hypertension. Mayo Clin Proc 1994;69:169–180.

Spoor TC, McHenry JG. Long term effectiveness of optic nerve sheath decompression for pseudotumor cerebri. Arch Ophthalmol 1993;111:632–635.

Wall M, George D. Idiopathic intracranial hypertension. A prospective study of 50 patients. Brain 1991;114:155–180.

Wall M. Idiopathic intracranial hypertension. Neurol Clin 1991;9:73–95.

Chapter 78
Trigeminal Neuralgia

Gary Johnson

Trigeminal neuralgia is characterized by paroxysmal shooting, jabbing, burning, or electriclike facial pain in the territory of the trigeminal nerve. The paroxysms are primarily unilateral and occur sporadically or clustered in bursts. They can be spontaneous or initiated by movements of the face or by sensory stimulation in defined "trigger zones." The disorder tends to have exacerbations and remissions. Although the pain varies in intensity, frequently it is severe and characteristically unresponsive to analgesics. A favorable response to anticonvulsants, though not diagnostic, is characteristic of trigeminal neuralgia.

Natural History

The peak onset of the disorder is in the sixth to seventh decades. Women are affected one and a half times more often than are men. The maxillary and mandibular divisions of the trigeminal nerve are affected most often. The ophthalmic division is affected infrequently, occurring in isolation in only 4% of incidents. The right side of the face is affected almost twice as often as is the left. Bilateral trigeminal neuralgia occurs in perhaps 3% of cases.

Both the episodes of pain and the periods of remission vary widely and are unpredictable and may persist for days to years. In one series, 50% of patients described had one or more spontaneous remissions of 6 months or longer, and 25% described remissions of 12 months or more. In general over time, the intensity, duration, and frequency of the pain episodes increase progressively.

Some authors report that patients may not report the typical description of pain at presentation but rather will describe a dull, longer-lasting, toothache-like pain that can develop over months to years into true trigeminal neuralgia involving the same distribution. This type of pain, called *pre–trigeminal neuralgia*, often is paroxysmal and responsive to anticonvulsants.

The association of multiple sclerosis and trigeminal neuralgia is well described but insufficient information precludes directly linking the two disorders. Between 1.7 and 8% of patients with trigeminal neuralgia are reported to have multiple sclerosis.

Factors Affecting Prognosis

Patients with pain that corresponds to the typical description of trigeminal neuralgia have the best medical and surgical outcomes. Some patients describe a superimposed pain consistent with atypical facial pain. Patients with mixed facial pain may be refractory to medical therapy and have a higher recurrence rate with some surgical therapies, such as microvascular decompression and retrogasserian glycerol rhizotomy.

A number of studies have suggested that trigeminal neuralgia has an earlier age of onset in patients with multiple sclerosis. Multiple sclerosis patients have a higher rate of recurrence, and managing them with anticonvulsants is more difficult, owing to a lack of tolerance to the medications. No correlation seems to exist between the course of the trigeminal neuralgia in patients with multiple sclerosis and the course of the exacerbations and remissions in multiple sclerosis. Additionally, in multiple sclerosis patients treated for trigeminal neuralgia with percutaneous radiofrequency rhizotomy, the recurrence rate of facial pain is comparable to the recurrence rate of those who did not have multiple sclerosis. Patients with multiple sclerosis have bilateral trigeminal neuralgia more commonly than do patients with only unilateral trigeminal neuralgia.

A number of studies have suggested that patients with sensory loss in association with trigeminal neuralgia have a higher recurrence rate. The data supporting this contention are confusing, as some of the patients described had previous destructive surgeries or atypical features, both of which are associated with a higher rate of recurrence.

Evaluation for Prognosis

Magnetic resonance imaging (MRI) is useful in excluding tumors, aneurysms, demyelination, and aberrant blood vessels as a cause of trigeminal neuralgia but has limited prognostic benefit. MRI scans may show a neurovascular contact at the root entry zone of the trigeminal nerve, but this finding is not an indication for microvascular decompression, because more than 25% of asymptomatic controls also show such nerve-vessel contacts. In Jannetta's series of patients treated with microvascular decompression, the response to surgery in the 2% of patients with tumors was roughly equivalent to the response in the majority of patients in whom vascular lesions were noted. Therefore, the determination of a vascular lesion or tumor by MRI does not confer a specific outcome related to microvascular decompression. However, patients with abnormalities associated with multiple sclerosis tend not to be candidates for microvascular decompression.

Therapies Affecting Prognosis

Carbamazepine is the most effective medication for trigeminal neuralgia. Its efficacy relates to the suppression of impulse conduction through increased segmental inhibition. Approximately 70 to 80% of patients treated with carbamazepine respond well, with 94% gaining relief in 48 hours. However, only some 50% of patients continue to respond after 5 to 16 years of treatment.

Phenytoin is effective in 50 to 70% of patients after 2 weeks of therapy. In one study, all phenytoin-treated patients who benefited from treatment experienced improvement within 24 to 48 hours, occasionally after the first dose. Intravenous phenytoin is particularly helpful in patients who are in severe pain and cannot take oral medications. Few long-term reports can confirm the efficacy of phenytoin, but fewer than 30% of patients respond after 2 years of treatment. No studies have compared phenytoin and carbamazepine rigorously.

Baclofen is not as effective as carbamazepine on the basis of a double-blind placebo-controlled trial and of a larger, open-label trial. During a 12-month follow-up period, 7 of 10 patients were pain-free or almost pain-free on 60 to 80 mg of baclofen per day. Baclofen has been shown to be effective in conjunction with phenytoin and particularly effective in combination with carbamazepine. Clonazepam has good results, but most patients are limited by sedation. Anecdotal evidence suggests that lamotrigine may have antineuralgic properties.

Surgical therapy is reserved for patients who have typical trigeminal neuralgia with a less-than-satisfactory response to medications. A wide range of effective surgical techniques target different points along the course of the trigeminal nerve. Peripheral techniques aim to produce selective trauma to the branches of the trigeminal nerve, thereby preventing the conduction of painful stimuli. Surgery at the level of the gasserian ganglion is directed at the trigeminal root, primarily affecting A-delta and C fibers. With the exception of rhizotomy, the aim of posterior fossa surgery is restoring functional anatomy. In general, the more peripheral procedures have higher rates of recurrence, are more likely to have significant sensory loss, but have much less morbidity and mortality.

The most peripheral techniques, such as cryotherapy, neurectomy, or phenol or alcohol injections, have similar efficacy and recurrence rates. The success rates range from 50 to 100%. Most patients have immediate relief, but recurrence rates are measured in months rather than years. Local complications, persistent sensory loss, and possible anesthesia dolorosa are common. These therapies rarely are indicated but may be used in some medically complicated or elderly patients.

Surgical therapies at the gasserian ganglion currently are the procedures used most commonly for treatment of trigeminal neuralgia. Percutaneous radiofrequency rhizotomy of the gasserian ganglion is effective in 70 to 80% of patients. The recurrence rates quoted in the literature range from 4 to 65% over variable assessment times and using varied assessment criterion. In some studies, the degree of postoperative sensory loss is linked to the recurrence rate such that patients with no postoperative sensory loss had 100% recurrence rate in 5 years, whereas those with clear postoperative sensory deficits had a 25% recurrence rate in 5 years. Some investigators suggest that the recurrence rate rises sharply in the first year and then gradually trails off. Corneal sensory loss is the major complication of the procedure, with involvement in up to 20% of patients. Disturbing sensory loss occurs in up to 21% of patients, with anesthesia dolorosa in 1 to 5%.

Percutaneous glycerol rhizotomy affords pain relief in 50% of patients within 24 hours, with most achieving benefit in 7 to 10 days. The procedure is effective in up to 90% of patients. Although the recurrence rates range from 10 to 72%, in most series the recurrence rate was less than 47%. Recurrences are most frequent within the first 6 months. The mean time to recurrence is 3 years. Similar to radiofrequency rhizotomy of the gasserian ganglion, the best prognostic factor for long-term relief is the degree of postoperative sensory loss (i.e., the more sensory loss, the less chance of recurrence). On the other hand, sensory loss is the most important complication, with mild loss of light touch in 26 to 71% of patients. Painful paresthesias or anesthesia dolorosa occurs in up to 2% of patients.

The initial success rate of percutaneous microcompression of the gasserian ganglion is near 80 to 90%. The recurrence rates range between 10 and 25% over a 3- to 7-year period, with the mean time to recurrence at 6.5 months. One of the major complications of this procedure is perioperative hypotension and bradycardia, related to distension of the balloon catheter. As a result, cardiac disease is a contraindication for the procedure. Sensory loss, especially involving the third division of the trigeminal nerve, occurs in the majority of patients. Painful dysesthesia occurs in some 10% of patients, whereas corneal anesthesia and anesthesia dolorosa are exceedingly infrequent.

Microvascular decompression is the posterior fossa technique used most frequently. As with many of the other surgical techniques, no clinical trials can support the comparative efficacy of the procedure. The experience of Jannetta and others is well documented. Some 70% of patients were pain-free and off medications for up to 10 years after the procedure. Recurrences were most likely to occur in the first 2 years after surgery, with the annual rate of recurrence tapering down to 1% in 10 years.

Though their results were argued by some authors, Barker and coworkers found in their series that significant predictors of eventual recurrence were female gender, symptoms of longer than 8 years' duration, venous compression of the trigeminal root entry zone, and lack of immediate postoperative relief of pain. Patients with prior destructive therapies have higher rates of burning or aching pain, likely unmasked by removal of the paroxysmal pain.

The degree of compression is another prognostic variable, though measuring it consistently is difficult. The patients with the least degree of vascular compression of the trigeminal nerve root have the highest recurrence rates. A strong relationship is seen between the skill of the surgeon and the risk of significant morbidity and mortality associated with posterior fossa procedures, such as microvascular decompression. Operative mortality ranges from 0.2 to 1.0%, the highest of all reported mortality rates among the various surgical therapies for trigeminal neuralgia. Initial morbidity may be as high as 60%; however, morbidity lasting for longer than 3 months is seen in fewer than 10 to 30% of patients. Transient hearing loss or other cranial neuropathies occur in slightly more than 20% of patients but are more common in the few patients with tumors. Though mild postoperative sensory loss is seen occasionally in patients, the procedure is not associated with significant sensory loss or anesthesia dolorosa.

The technique for rhizotomy using the posterior fossa approach is similar to that for microvascular decompression. This procedure, though performed infrequently, may be indicated in microvascular decompression cases wherein no compression of the trigeminal nerve root is found at operation. The results described in the literature are comparable to those of microvascular decompression. Some 96 to 99% of patients are pain-free at follow-up of less than 5 years. The result is a trend toward recurrence rates higher than those in microvascular decompression. Mortality and complication rates are similar to those for microvascular decompression, but significant sensory loss is much more common in rhizotomy. Painful facial dysesthesia and anesthesia dolorosa may occur in up to 8% of patients, most frequently occurring after near-complete section of the trigeminal root.

Short-Term Prognosis

The periods of pain from trigeminal neuralgia usually are interspersed with relatively long periods of remission. Medical therapy is the first choice of therapy, and the initial response is excellent in most patients.

Long-Term Prognosis

The ability to control symptoms with medications lessens as the episodes of pain become longer and periods of remission become shorter. Surgery should be considered at this point. The choice of surgical technique depends on the patients' preferences, age, and associated medical conditions. If relapses occur, they can be treated with repeat surgical procedures or medications. The long-term prognosis should be recognized as mainly determined by the quality of the long-term medical and surgical follow-up.

Additional Reading

Barker FG, Jannetta PJ, Bissonette DJ, et al. The long-term outcome of microvascular decompression for trigeminal neuralgia. N Engl J Med 1996;334:1077–1083.

Burchiel KJ, Steege TD, Howe JF, Loeser JD. Comparison of percutaneous radiofrequency gangliolysis and microvascular decompression for the surgical management of tic douloureux. Neurosurgery 1981;9:111–118.

Fromm GH, Sessle BJ (eds). Trigeminal Neuralgia: Current Concepts Regarding Pathogenesis and Treatment. Boston: Butterworth, 1991.

Katusic S, Beard CM, Bergstralh E, Kurland KT. Incidence and clinical features of trigeminal neuralgia. Ann Neurol 1990;27:89–95.

Lichtor T, Mullan JF. A 10-year follow up review of percutaneous microcompression of the trigeminal ganglion. J Neurosurg 1990;72:49–54.

Rovit RL, Murali R, Jannetta PJ. Trigeminal Neuralgia. Baltimore: Williams & Wilkins, 1990.

Steiger HJ. Prognostic factors in the treatment of trigeminal neuralgia. Analysis of a different therapeutic approach. Acta Neurochir (Wien) 1991;113:11–17.

Sweet WH. The treatment of trigeminal neuralgia (tic douloureux). N Engl J Med 1988;315:174–177.

Zakrzewska JM. Trigeminal Neuralgia. London: Saunders, 1995.

Chapter 79

Migraine

David W. Dodick and David J. Capobianco

Headache is one of the most common complaints referred to primary care physicians and neurologists. The vast majority of these headaches represent benign recurrent disorders, such as migraine and tension-type headache. Migraine is a highly prevalent condition in the United States, with estimates exceeding 23 million patients.

Migraine is an episodic headache syndrome that usually is unilateral and associated with nausea, vomiting, photophobia, and phonophobia. Diverse prodromal and neurologic symptoms may be associated with migraine attacks, which reflect the attacks' central pathophysiology. Although a unifying concept of migraine pathogenesis remains elusive, the susceptibility to migraine appears to be inherited, and the migrainous brain is more vulnerable and reactive to changes in the external and internal milieu. This vulnerability is based on defined biochemical differences, whereas the reactivity is augmented through critical brain stem reflexes that produce upstream changes in vascular tone and cerebral blood flow and downstream changes in endogenous pain-modulating pathways.

In 1988, the International Headache Society proposed a new classification of headache. *Migraine without aura* supplanted the term *common migraine*. *Migraine with aura* now refers to what was termed *classic migraine*.

Natural History

Information concerning the natural history of migraine is limited. Cross-sectional epidemiologic studies provide little definitive data concerning the prognosis of migraine. Longitudinal prospective epidemiologic studies, following a representative population over time, are required to generate any meaningful information concerning the natural history of migraine.

Much of the knowledge concerning the natural history of childhood migraine is credited to Bille. In a longitudinal study spanning 30 years, he compared 73 children with migraine to 73 children free of migraine. The children were ages 7 to 15 years at study onset. In the migraine group, the percentage of patients who were migraine-free at 6 and 30 years of follow-up was 34% and 40%, respectively. Thirty percent of the original 73 migraine children experienced migraine continuously throughout childhood. An unfavorable prognosis was demonstrated in girls as compared to boys and in children with visual aura. Alternatively, at the 16-year follow-up, 8 (11%) of the 73 children in the migraine-free cohort had developed migraine. This subgroup, of whom five had a family history of migraine, was exclusively female.

A study of 2,921 Finnish children beginning school at age 7 years found that 41% of the children with migraine either were unchanged or were experiencing more severe migraine at age 14 years, whereas 22% were migraine-free (Sillanpaa 1983). Similar to Bille's observations, boys had a more favorable prognosis when migraine began before school age. These gender differences are in accordance with previous prevalence estimates indicating equal prepubescent male to female ratios (2.5%), whereas adult migraine prevalence is estimated to be 17.8% in women and 5.7% in men.

In a population of 90 migraineurs observed over 15 to 20 years, Whitty and Hockaday have provided the most valuable prospective data on the natural history of adult migraine. The first migraine attack in this group ranged from 16 to 69 years before evaluation. Despite the pitfalls of a selected population with the potential for recall errors, this study highlighted several important points. Although 70% of patients (63 of 90) at follow-up were still having migraine attacks, 70% of this group (44 of 63) experienced improvement, as defined by a reduction in attack frequency or attack severity. Headache persistence was not associated with age at headache onset, age at the time of evaluation, or duration of migraine. The regenerative and enduring capacity to develop migraine was evident in some patients whose headaches later recurred after complete cessation of attacks during early adult life.

Contrary to widely held belief, no consistent change in attacks occurred either after menopause or after specific treatment. Of the 40 patients in whom menopause had occurred by the time of follow-up, 24 of 40 either had unchanged persistence of attacks (18 of 40) or had worsened (6 of 40). Furthermore, of the patients older than 64 years, 50% (9 of 18) still were having migraine attacks. Only 2 of the 27 headache-free patients could attribute migraine cessation to either the onset of menopause or to a course of specific treatment.

A relationship also appears to exist between migraine prevalence and age, with a peak at perhaps age 40 years. In a Selby and Lance study of 500 migraine patients, 92% experienced their first attack within the first four decades, whereas only 2% experienced the first attack after age 50 years. Although the data are limited, the capacity to generate migraine attacks increases with age during the first four decades and continues throughout adult life, even after prolonged attack-free intervals. However, severity appears to attenuate over time, and the likelihood of disappearance increases with advancing age.

Factors Affecting Prognosis

Migraine is associated with several comorbid psychiatric and neurologic conditions that can influence prognosis and treatment. Neurologic comorbidities include stroke and epilepsy. Psychiatric comorbidities include phobias, anxiety, and depression.

One study demonstrated that the relative risk of ischemic stroke was elevated in women who had migraine, although the absolute risk of stroke in the migraine population still was very low (19 per 100,000 woman-years). Curiously, the risk of stroke was slightly higher in women with migraine with aura. The use of oral contraceptives, cigarette smoking, and a family history of cardiovascular disease also increased the risk.

The association between migraine and epilepsy is complex but unequivocal. Epileptic individuals are 2.4 times more likely to develop migraine than are their relatives without epilepsy. Conversely, the prevalence of epilepsy in patients with migraine is approximately 5.9%, a percentage greatly exceeding the prevalence (0.5%) in the general population. This comorbidity may be explained by a state of neuronal hyperexcitability that increases the risk of both disorders.

Migraine also occurs commonly in complex heredofamilial disorders associated with both ischemic stroke and seizures. CADASIL (*c*erebral *a*utosomal *d*ominant *a*rteriopathy, *s*ubcortical *i*nfarcts, and *l*eukoencephalopathy), a hereditary disorder linked to chromosome 19, is composed of several core features, including migraine, strokes, seizures, and cognitive deterioration. Myoclonic epilepsy with ragged red fibers and mitochondrial encephalopathy with lactic acidosis and stroke-like syndromes are mitochondrial disorders that share migraine as a common comorbid feature.

Many studies have examined the comorbidity of primary headache and psychiatric illness. The lifetime prevalence of anxiety, phobia, and depression is significantly greater in migraineurs than in nonmigraine control groups. A fourfold risk of major depression is seen in migraine patients as compared to that seen in their nonmigrainous counterparts.

Comorbid illnesses impose therapeutic restrictions but also provide therapeutic opportunities. For example, tricyclic antidepressants must be used cautiously in patients experiencing both migraine and epilepsy, as they lower seizure threshold. However, divalproex sodium may control both migraine and epilepsy in a patient with both conditions.

Evaluation for Prognosis

The prognostic evaluation for patients with migraine involves securing an accurate diagnosis, educating the patient regarding the pathophysiology and natural history, maintaining a headache diary, and avoiding potential trigger factors. Other issues to discuss include the important role of nonpharmacologic modalities in the treatment of migraine, the appropriate use of abortive and prophylactic medications, and the importance of not using analgesics more often than 2 days per week to avoid medication-induced chronic daily headache (CDH) or transformed migraine. Diagnostic testing (e.g., computed tomography, magnetic resonance imaging, lumbar puncture, and cerebral angiography) is not routinely required.

Therapies Affecting Prognosis

Frequent overuse of symptomatic medications used to treat episodic headache is well recognized. Analgesic-ergotamine overuse appears to be the most common factor leading to "transformed migraine," although such comorbidities as anxiety, depression, abnormal personality profile, and stress may be important contributing factors. *Transformed migraine* refers to an evolutionary form of CDH that arises from episodic migraine and accounts for 75 to 80% of patients with daily or near daily headaches seen at tertiary headache referral centers. In a certain group of patients, migraine may evolve spontaneously into a CDH pattern. Manzoni reported no apparent factors that could be implicated in 22% of a cohort of patients with transformed migraine. This disorder not only exacts an enormous personal toll but is an important public health problem that accounts for a disproportionate share of indirect costs and health care use.

Removal of the offending agent or agents is the first step in the management of this difficult problem. However, despite appropriate management, the condition remains intractable in approximately 30% of these patients. This fact underscores the importance of physician awareness and patient education in avoiding analgesic overuse and the consequent development of CDH. Excessive use of symptomatic medications not only renders standard prophylactic and abortive migraine therapy ineffective but may alter irrevocably the natural history of migraine.

Realistic expectations regarding the prognosis of migraine must be established from the outset. Migraine is a familial disorder with a lifelong potential to develop at any age. Whether prophylactic therapy affects the long-term prognosis of migraine remains unclear. Certainly, appropriate prophylactic treatment in patients with frequent and severe migraine attacks may obviate the need and tendency to increase the use of analgesic compounds, thereby decreasing the incidence of CDH that may affect prognosis permanently.

Short-Term Prognosis

Although the short-term prognosis varies, patient education and appropriate use of nonpharmacologic therapies, migraine-specific agents, and prophylactic medications will pay dividends for both the patient and the treating physician. With the development of novel superselective serotonin receptor agonists, the success rate in terminating an acute attack of migraine is approximately 70 to 80%. However, this advance in acute treatment has not been paralleled by similar progress in migraine prophylaxis. This discrepancy almost certainly reflects the poorly understood mechanisms by which prophylactic medications exert their effect. The efficacy of the four most commonly used migraine prophylactic agents (beta-blockers, calcium-channel blockers, tricyclic antidepressants, and valproate) does not exceed 50% over placebo.

Long-Term Prognosis

At present, a cure for migraine does not exist. Although the majority of patients may continue to experience varying manifestations of migraine, this same majority will enjoy the self-limited nature and tendency for attenuation over time. Whether prophylactic measures affect overall long-term prognosis is unclear but, clearly, appropriate measures initiated early (as discussed in Evaluation for Prognosis) will decrease the likelihood of a CDH disorder. Only anecdotal evidence suggests that a proportion of migraine patients successfully treated with prophylactic agents will remain headache-free, or nearly so, after treatment has been discontinued. Individualizing therapy for those with medical, neurologic, or psychiatric comorbidities is critical. Ongoing research in neuropharmacology and genetics likely will provide more effective means to combat the pervasive problem of migraine.

Additional Reading

Bille B. Migraine in Childhood: A 30 Year Follow-Up. In G Lanzi, U Balottin, A Cerniborn (eds), Headache in Children and Adolescents. Amsterdam: Elsevier, 1989;19–26.

Breslau N, Merikangas K, Bowden CL. Comorbidity of migraine and major affective disorders. Neurology 1994;44(suppl 7):17–22.

Manzoni GC, Miciele G, Granella F, et al. Daily chronic headache: classification and clinical features: observation on 250 patients. Cephalalgia 1987;7(suppl 6):169–170.

Mathew NT. Transformed migraine. Cephalalgia 1993;13 (suppl 12):78–83.

Ottman R, Lipton RB. Comorbidity of migraine and epilepsy. Neurology 1994;44:2105–2110.

Ramadan NN, Schultz LL, Gilkey SJ. Migraine prophylactic drugs: proof of efficacy, utilization and cost. Cephalalgia 1997;17:73–80.

Selby G, Lance JW. Observation on 500 cases of migraine and allied vascular headaches. J Neurol Neurosurg Psychiatry 1960;23:23–32.

Sillanpaa M. Changes in the prevalence of migraine and other headaches during the first seven school years. Headache 1983;23:15–19.

Tzourio C, Tehindrazanarivelo A, Iglesias S, et al. Case-control study of migraine and risk of ischaemic stroke in young women. BMJ 1995;310:830–833.

Whitty CWM, Hockaday JM. Migraine: a follow-up study of 92 patients. BMJ 1968;1:735–736.

Chapter 80

Normal-Pressure Hydrocephalus

Neill R. Graff-Radford

Normal-pressure hydrocephalus (NPH), also called *symptomatic hydrocephalus*, is an entity characterized by hydrocephalus (ventriculomegaly out of proportion to cortical atrophy), difficulty in walking, cognitive impairment, and urinary incontinence. The causes can be classified into primary, secondary (related to subarachnoid hemorrhage, meningitis, head injury, and previous intracranial surgery), and congenital. The latter accounts for 10% of cases in some series and is characterized by a large head size. Neuroimaging in congenital hydrocephalus shows chronic hydrocephalus without periventricular cerebrospinal fluid (CSF) leakage and, sometimes, a cause of the hydrocephalus, such as Arnold-Chiari malformation or aqueductal stenosis. At lumbar puncture, the CSF pressure usually is normal but, with intracranial pressure monitoring, some reports indicate that the more frequently the pressure is more than 20 cm of water, the better the prognosis for surgery.

Natural History

The natural history of NPH is not known. No controlled studies place shunts in one group but not in another group and then follow the groups over time. In following patients with serial videotaping of their gait and with repeat neuropsychological testing before shunt surgery, I have found clear progression over 3 to 12 months in some patients but relative stability in others. In their histories, patients and their families describe deterioration over months to years before seeking medical attention.

Factors Affecting Prognosis

Several factors have been shown to affect prognosis from a shunt surgery point of view. If the NPH is secondary, surgical outcome is more favorable than if the disease is idiopathic or primary. A history of alcohol abuse results in a poor surgical outcome. If the gait difficulty began before or at the same time as the dementia, the surgical prognosis is better. In contrast, if the dementia began before the gait difficulty or if the dementia has been present for 2 or more years, the prognosis is worse.

Patients with an anomia have a worse surgical prognosis. One may speculate that the anomia may be a surrogate marker of a cortical dementia, such as Alzheimer's disease.

Evaluation for Prognosis

In a summary of all the patients reported to have undergone shunt surgery until 1978, Hughes and coworkers reported that some 50% improved. By accounting for factors that may influence prognosis (as mentioned), doctors can improve the chances of a good surgical outcome. The following tests also have been used to improve surgical prognosis.

Cortical Atrophy by Imaging Studies

In patients with hydrocephalus, the absence of sulcal enlargement is a favorable factor in surgical prognosis; however, with combined sulcal enlargement and hydrocephalus, patients still can improve. Borgesen and Gjerris measured the largest sulcus in the high frontal or parietal region and found that if the cortical sulci were less than 1.9 mm, 17 of 17 shunted patients improved; if the sulci were 1.9 to 5 mm, 17 of 20 shunted patients improved; and if the sulci were 5 mm or more, 15 of 27 shunted patients improved.

Magnetic Resonance Detection of Cerebrospinal Fluid Flow Through the Cerebral Aqueduct

In 1991, Bradley and colleagues retrospectively reviewed the magnetic resonance imaging scans of 20 patients who had undergone ventriculoperitoneal shunt surgery for NPH. They rated initial surgical outcome as excellent, good, or poor and correlated this with the extent of flow void in the cerebral aqueduct as a marker of CSF flow through the cerebral aqueduct. (The method of acquiring magnetic resonance images may affect the flow void appearance.) They found a significant correlation ($p < 0.003$) between extent of increased aqueduct flow void and initial surgical outcome. More specifically, 8 of 10 patients with increased CSF flow void scores had an excellent or good response to surgery, whereas only 1 of 9 with a normal flow void score improved with surgery. I believe that this method is promising for predicting surgical prognosis in symptomatic hydrocephalus. Future studies should be prospective, should have better quantitation of flow through the aqueduct, and should have more objective measures of surgical outcome.

Regional Cerebral Blood Flow

Regional cerebral blood flow has been studied in symptomatic hydrocephalus of the elderly. Studies addressing the predictive value of this method for surgical outcome were published by Graff-Radford and associates. Patients with Alzheimer's disease often have decreased cerebral blood flow posteriorly, whereas patients with hydrocephalus have decreased blood flow anteriorly. The authors calculated the ratio of blood flow in the anterior over the posterior cortical regions and found that patients with a higher ratio had less chance of improving

than did those with a lower ratio. This method made possible the correct prediction of 5 of 7 nonimprovers and 22 of 23 improvers. Patients with "an Alzheimer pattern" (i.e., decreased blood flow posteriorly) did poorly, whereas those without this pattern did well.

These studies suggest the possibility that single-photon emission computed tomography scanning may be a useful method for predicting surgical prognosis in patients with symptomatic hydrocephalus. Further work should be done in this area.

Cisternography

My experience with cisternography is limited, but the literature suggests numerous cases of patients who have a positive test (radioisotope seen within the ventricles 48 to 72 hours after being injected in the lumbar area) and do not improve with surgery and numerous cases of patients who have equivocal or negative tests and do improve. In a review of their experience with this test, Black and coworkers found the following: Of 11 patients who had a positive test, 9 improved and 2 did not; of 6 patients who had mixed results, 3 improved and 3 did not; of 6 who had negative results, 4 improved and 2 did not. These authors suggested that a positive test was helpful but that an equivocal or negative test was not. A study by Vanneste and colleagues reported that "cisternography did not improve the accuracy of combined clinical and computerized tomography in patients with presumed normal-pressure hydrocephalus." Specifically, of the 65 patients with communicating hydrocephalus who were shunted, cisternography added no predictive value to clinical and computed tomography evaluation. Seventeen showed a better prediction with cisternography than by clinical and computed tomography evaluation, but 23 showed a worse prediction. I do not recommend cisternography routinely as a diagnostic test for symptomatic hydrocephalus.

Cerebrospinal Fluid Drainage Procedures

Gait improvement after removal of a large quantity of CSF by lumbar puncture (30 to 50 ml, which can be repeated daily for several days if needed) would render the patient a good candidate for shunt surgery. A modification of this technique also has been reported: continuous CSF drainage via a catheter placed in the lumbar CSF space. Shortcomings attend this technique: Patients eventually have responded to shunt surgery but have had no obvious improvement for the first postsurgical week. The drainage test could have given a falsely negative result in these patients. In undergoing this test, the patient may appear improved for the duration of the test (the placebo effect) but may not maintain response, leading to a false-positive result. In addition, meningitis and subdural hematoma are possible complications of continuous CSF drainage procedures.

Cerebrospinal Fluid Pressure Monitoring

Some reports have cited a significant relationship between measures of intracranial CSF pressure monitoring and surgical outcome for symptomatic hydrocephalus. For example, in the Borgesen and Gjerris study and in my study, the greater the percentage of time B waves were present, the greater the chance of a good outcome. Also, in my series, the longer the pressure was greater than 15 mm Hg, the better the chance of successful surgery.

Infusion Tests

Borgesen and Gjerris described the CSF conductance test, in which CSF absorption is measured at different fluid pressures. They reported an accuracy of greater than 90% in predicting short-term prognosis after shunt surgery and some 85% accuracy in predicting long-term prognosis. The concept holds that the greater the pressure needed to obtain an amount of absorption, the better chance of that patient improving with shunt surgery. My study found no significant correlation between CSF conductance and improvement. However, the patients were chosen on the basis of the conductance result, so this was not an independent variable. In addition, most of my patients had idiopathic hydrocephalus, whereas many of Borgesen and Gjerris's patients had secondary hydrocephalus. The conductance test, which relates to CSF absorption, may be a better predictor of outcome in secondary hydrocephalus in which an absorption defect may be causative.

Short-Term Prognosis

Shunt complications, both major and minor, occur in 30 to 40% of patients and include intraoperative complications related to general anesthesia in an elderly population, intracranial hemorrhage from ventricular catheter placement, intra-abdominal injury (rare), and arrhythmias from incorrect ventriculoatrial distal catheter placement. Perioperative complications include infection (3 to 8% of cases), CSF hypotensive headaches, and the development of subdural effusions or hematomas. The latter problem is more likely to occur in patients with marked reduction in ventricular size after shunting and is more common when low-pressure valves are used for treatment of these effusions. Depending on symptoms, conservative or surgical therapy may be indicated. Seizures also may complicate shunt surgery. Long-term complications are related primarily to shunt occlusion or catheter breakage. Infection after the first 2 months is unusual.

Long-Term Prognosis

Surgical outcome often has been measured using a five-point scale. The problem with this device is that some of the points on the scale may overlap, rendering the use of this scale subjective. I used three measures: ratings of serial videotapes of gait, neuropsychological testing, and an index of activities of daily living. Patients were followed with all these scales for only 6 months, a period that does not address long-term prognosis fully; however, at 6 months, some 70% of patients were improved. Retrospective analyses have looked at longer-term data, and the results have varied. Determining prognosis accurately from retrospective chart reviews is particularly difficult. Additional long-term prospective data are needed.

Additional Reading

Black P, Ojemann R, Tzouras A. CSF shunts for dementia, incontinence, and gait disturbance. Clin Neurosurg 1985;32:632–651.

Borgesen S, Gjerris F. The predictive value of conductance to outflow of CSF in normal pressure hydrocephalus. Brain 1982;105:65–86.

Bradley W, Whittemore A, Kortman K, et al. Marked cerebrospinal fluid void: indicator of successful shunt in patients with suspected normal-pressure hydrocephalus. Radiology 1991;178:459–466.

Fisher C. The clinical picture in occult hydrocephalus. Clin Neurosurg 1977;24:270–284.

Graff-Radford NR, Godersky JC. Symptomatic congenital hydrocephalus in the elderly simulating normal pressure hydrocephalus. Neurology 1989;39:1596–1600.

Graff-Radford NR, Godersky JC, Jones M. Variables predicting surgical outcome in symptomatic hydrocephalus in the elderly. Neurology 1989;39:1601–1604.

Haan J, Thormeer R. Predictive value of temporary external lumbar drainage in normal pressure hydrocephalus. Neurosurgery 1988;22:388–391.

Hughes C, Siegel B, Coxe W, et al. Adult idiopathic communicating hydrocephalus with and without shunting. J Neurol Neurosurg Psychiatry 1978;41:961–971.

Petersen R, Mokri B, Laws E. Surgical treatment of idiopathic hydrocephalus in elderly patients. Neurology 1985;35:307–311.

Vanneste J, Augustijn P, Davies G, et al. Normal-pressure hydrocephalus. Arch Neurol 1992;49:366–370.

Vanneste J, Augustijn P, Dirven C, et al. Shunting normal-pressure hydrocephalus: do the benefits outweigh the risks? A multicenter study and literature review. Neurology 1992;42:54–59.

Wikkelso C, Andersson H, Blomstrand C, Lindqvist G. The clinical effect of lumbar puncture in normal pressure hydrocephalus. J Neurol Neurosurg Psychiatry 1982;45:64–69.

Chapter 81

Neurocutaneous Disorders

Frank Lieberman and Allan E. Rubenstein

The application of molecular genetic techniques to the study of patients with neurophakomatoses promises to clarify natural history and clinical management issues. Molecular genetics has contributed a new understanding of the range of phenotypic features of each disorder and the pathophysiologic mechanisms underlying several of the important complications, such as neoplasia. However, much still remains unknown about the natural history of these disorders, and prospective longitudinal studies of patients diagnosed using molecular diagnostic techniques are not yet available. In the absence of such studies, predictions regarding prognosis for patients must be based on clinical reports of populations of patients of various ages and comparison of the incidence and prevalence of specific disease manifestations within the different age groups.

Neurofibromatosis 1

NF-1 is one of the most common neurogenetic disorders, with an incidence of 1 in 30,000 in Western populations. The disorder is inherited in an autosomal dominant fashion. The gene for neurofibromatosis type 1 (NF-1) was located by positional cloning on chromosome 17 and subsequently sequenced. The protein product, neurofibromin, is a member of a family of proteins that function as guanosine triphosphatase–activating proteins (GAPs) for the *ras* oncogene signal transduction pathway. The neurofibromin gene appears to function as a tumor-suppressor gene, and aberrant regulation of

the *ras* signaling pathway has been demonstrated in NF-1–related neoplasms.

Although the gene mutation is highly penetrant, expression of the associated phenotype is highly variable. An unknown number of individuals carrying the mutation for NF-1 may manifest only dermatologic signs or insufficient neurologic symptoms or signs to trigger identification and referral. Nonetheless, experienced clinicians believe clinically relevant generalizations can be shared with patients and their families to guide clinical decision making and family planning. The NF-1 gene mutation is pleiotropic in effects, potentially involving every organ system.

Natural History

Cafe-au-lait spots (CLSs) (defined as hyperpigmented macules >1.5 cm in postpubescent patients and >0.5 cm in prepubertal patients) and freckling are the cardinal skin manifestations of NF-1. By definition, the majority of patients with NF-1 will display six or more CLSs. CLSs usually increase in number as the patient ages and may darken with sun exposure or pregnancy. Freckling in intertrigo areas and the axillae is usually absent at birth, appears in young childhood, and becomes increasingly prominent with age. Although CLSs may be cosmetically significant, they are not premalignant lesions.

Neurofibromas are the pathologic hallmark of NF-1. These benign peripheral nerve neoplasms may arise from any component of the peripheral nervous system; from intradermal nerve fibers to the spinal roots. Neurofibromas may be present as congenital neoplasms, but usually visible cutaneous neurofibromas appear during young childhood and increase both in size and number with age.

Although cutaneous neurofibromata may burden patients, the plexiform neurofibromas (PNFs) are the form of neurofibroma usually responsible for major dysmorphic, mechanical, and neurologic complications of the NF-1 mutation. These tumors are usually congenital. PNFs frequently involve the major nerves and trunks of the brachial or lumbar plexi, and their progressive infiltration and enlargement may cause progressive neurologic deficits, pain, and dysfunction of the affected extremity. When these lesions arise in the cutaneous or proximal branches of the fifth cranial nerve, they may lead to deformation of the orbit and facial structures and visual disturbance. Plexiform neurofibromas tend to enlarge over time, and some investigators report an acceleration of symptomatic progression with puberty and during pregnancy.

Seizure disorders are frequent in the NF-1 population, with an incidence of approximately 5%. There are no data suggesting management of seizure disorders in NF-1 patients should differ from patients without NF-1. Generalized seizures are the most common type. It is unclear whether focal abnormalities seen on computed tomography (CT) or magnetic resonance imaging (MRI) scanning increase the risk of seizures.

Learning disabilities, defined as performance two or more grade levels below chronologically appropriate grade in the presence of normal intelligence, occur in approximately 50% of patients with NF-1. The natural history of learning diabilities in NF-1 patients has not been systematically studied.

Multidisciplinary NF clinical centers incorporate CT, and more recently MRI scanning, into the diagnostic evaluation of patients referred for care. A variety of intracranial signal abnormalities have been identified in addition to the neoplasms discussed in the following paragraphs. Focal areas of increased signal on T2-weighted scans may be identified in cortical or white-matter regions. Usually, these abnormalities do not enhance. The white-matter regions of hyperintensity have been termed *unidentified bright objects* (UBOs). UBOs do not demonstrate mass effect, and the histopathologic nature of these lesions is unknown.

Ophthalmologic manifestations of NF-1 include Lisch nodules, hyper- or hypopigmented macular iris lesions with no functional impact on ocular function, congenital glaucoma, and gliomas of the optic pathways. Lisch nodules are usually not demonstrable at birth, but increase in frequency with age so that they are present in 50% of patients at age 60 years. Congenital glaucoma probably occurs in 0.5 to 1.0% of children with the NF-1 mutation and is an ophthalmologic emergency when it occurs.

Tumors of the optic pathway are a major source of vision loss in patients with NF-1. The tumors may arise in any part of the optic pathway from the optic nerve caudally to the optic radiations. Most commonly, the tumors are diffusely infiltrating pilocytic astrocytomas. Approximately 10% of patients who undergo CT or MRI scanning as part of the evaluation of nervous system involvement will have optic pathway tumors. Although these neoplasms may produce progressive vision loss, in many instances the tumors manifest long periods of clinical and radiologic quiescence. Clinical experience argues against radiation therapy or chemotherapy unless lesions demonstrate clinical or radiologic progression.

Cerebral, brain stem, or cerebellar astrocytomas appear with increased frequency in patients with NF-1. Brain stem and hypothalamic involvement often coexists with optic nerve or chiasmal infiltration. These tumors are most frequently pilocytic astrocytomas. Again, these tumors may remain static for protracted periods of time. Patients with NF-1 experience an increased propensity for developing myelogenous leukemia when treated with chemotherapy regimens that include alkylating agents. Chemotherapy for intracranial tumors should be used only when clinical or radiologic progression, or both, of the neoplasm is clearly demonstrable. Malignant astrocytomas occur more frequently in patients with NF-1, but medulloblastomas and ependymomas are relatively rare. It is unclear whether the biological behavior of malignant brain tumors is different in the setting of NF-1 than in sporadic cases.

Although a dreaded and frequently discussed occurrence in NF-1 patients, the development of nonbrain malignant neoplasms is rare. Pheochromocytomas, most frequently of the adrenal medulla, are reported to occur more frequently in patients with NF-1 than in the general population, but the incidence in large, horizontal, population-based studies is less than 1%. Acute myelogenous leukemia (AML) seems more frequent in the NF-1 population, with the juvenile form of AML, in association with karyotypic abnormalities portending drug resistance and poor prognosis, predominating. The incidence of AML, however, is probably also less than 1%.

The most feared and lethal consequence of plexiform neurofibromas is the development of malignant peripheral nerve sheath tumors (MPNST). These tumors usually, if not always, arise within pre-existing plexiform neurofibromas. Perhaps 4 to 10% of patients harboring a plexiform neurofibroma will develop an MPNST over the course of their lifetime.

Short-Term Prognosis

The majority of children with the NF-1 gene mutation will probably manifest cutaneous, ophthalmologic, or neurologic abnormalities related to NF-1 during late childhood or puberty. Learning disabilities are the most common neurologic manifestation of NF-1, occurring in 50% of patients. Although several authors have proposed a relationship between the number and location of abnormalities on CT or MRI and the presence of cognitive disability, the literature is not consistent and further studies are needed to clarify the prognostic implications of MRI abnormalities for school performance.

The disfigurement related to cutaneous and plexiform neurofibromas may be severe. Attempts to correlate the type of mutation or extent of deletion in the NF-1 gene with the propensity to develop neurofibromata have been mostly unsuccessful. There may be increased risk for development of large numbers of cutaneous neurofibromata in patients with large NF-1 deletions. The natural history of plexiform neurofibromas is especially unclear, and a multi-institutional, prospective study of patients with plexiform neurofibromas of the orbit or major plexi is planned to address this question. Not infrequently, these tumors grow in increments, with quiescent periods of variable length. This has complicated both the surgical management of such lesions and the interpretation of clinical trials of cytotoxic chemotherapeutic drugs or biologic response modifiers.

Optic gliomas rarely become symptomatic after age 8 years; if a patient has reached the age of 8 without significant visual disability, the prognosis for maintenance of vision is good. In the younger child, patients should be treated with radiation therapy or chemotherapy only when there is clear, consistent neuroradiologic or clinical evidence of tumor progression.

Long-Term Prognosis

In general, patients with the NF-1 mutation and no other identifiable risk factors for development of malignancy should be reassured that their risk of developing NF-1–related malignancies is less than 5% over their lifetime. Although molecular genetic differences in tumor suppresser and oncogene function have been identified between MPNST and benign plexiform neurofibroma, there is currently no reliable genetic criteria for predicting which patients, or which benign plexiform neurofibromas, will eventually develop MPNST. The prognosis for patients who have MPNST is similar to that of other soft-tissue sarcomas, with most patients dying of intractable local progression or distant metastasis. The mainstay of therapy for MPNST is surgery and intensive local radiotherapy where possible. Chemotherapy currently adds little to the duration of survival or tumor-free survival in patients with MPNST, and adjuvant chemotherapy should probably be limited to patients participating in clinical trials.

Neurofibromatosis 2

Molecular genetic studies have verified the clinical impression that this disorder is distinct from NF-1. The hallmark of NF-2 is the development of bilateral vestibular schwannomas with associated hearing loss. Genotyping allows clarification of the status of patients who manifest a unilateral vestibular schwannoma and additional features of NF-2. These features include meningiomas; schwannomas of other cranial nerves, spinal nerve roots, or peripheral nerves; and cataract.

The NF-2 gene has been identified on chromosome 22 by positional cloning and the protein product, schwannomin or merlin, has been characterized as a member of the moesin-ezrin-radixin family of proteins. The function of the protein is not completely understood, but analogy with other family members suggests a role in mediating interactions between cytoskeletal elements and the extracellular matrix.

Natural History

In addition to bilateral acoustic neuromas, other neoplasms are frequently present. Multiple meningiomas occur throughout the calvarium. Spinal tumors occur with high frequency, including schwannomas, meningiomas, and ependymomas.

The age of onset of vestibular neuroma is variable, spanning youth to adulthood, with the mean age of onset in the third decade. The diagnosis of single, and certainly multiple, meningiomas in a child or adolescent should suggest the diagnosis of NF-2.

The majority of morbidity is related to neoplasms of the nervous system. Symptoms usually begin in early adulthood. Vestibular schwannomas with associated hearing loss are the presenting problem in approximately 40% of patients, with other central nervous system (CNS) tumors accounting for approximately 20%. Probably all patients with an NF-2 gene mutation will develop vestibular schwannomas at some point during their lifetime.

Cataracts are common in NF-2 patients, but permanent vision loss is relatively rare. Vision loss is related to retinal hamartomas or compressive optic neuropathy from canalicular or perichiasmal meningiomas rather than from cataracts.

Other intraparenchymal tumors do occur, but much more rarely. Astrocytomas and ependymomas probably occur in less than 5% of patients. Pilocytic astrocytomas of the optic nerve, chiasm, or optic tracts, though a frequent neoplasm in patients with NF-1, rarely occur in NF-2. Malignant astrocytic tumors and medulloblastoma are not clearly associated with NF-2.

NF-2 patients may manifest cutaneous abnormalities, which overlap somewhat with the phenotype of NF-1. CLSs are present in almost 50% of patients, but few have six or more. Axillary and groin freckling is not a feature of NF-2. Skin tumors occur in approximately 70% of NF-2 patients. The tumors are of two types: (1) soft, raised, hypertrichotic, and slightly pigmented lesions; and (2) subcutaneous, spherical tumors detected along the path of peripheral nerves. The subcutaneous tumors may be schwannomas or neurofibromas.

Factors Affecting Prognosis

With early detection of neuraxis neoplasms by MRI scanning and neurosurgical or radiotherapeutic intervention at the time of tumor progression or symptom development, the impact of NF-2–related neoplasms on longevity and quality of life should be lessened. Genetic screening allows for presymptomatic diagnosis and confirmation of genotype in patients with sporadic appearance of bilateral schwannoma or unilateral schwannoma and other features of the disease. However, it is not yet possible to predict phenotypic severity based on the nature of the genetic abnormality. Studies of relatively small numbers of patients suggest mutations leading to frameshift and premature protein truncation are associated with a more severe phenotype than missense mutations. Although expression within families may vary to some extent, patients within a kindred usually conform to the same phenotype.

With increasingly refined surgical techniques and radiotherapeutic treatments both indicating substantial hope of hearing preservation when applied to small tumors, early tumor removal from a hearing ear is becoming more common. A multicenter, cooperative study of the natural history of vestibular schwannomas in patients with NF-2 is needed, and such studies are being planned.

Short-Term Prognosis

The natural history of NF-2–associated neoplasms is not well understood. Some generalizations may be cautiously applied to prediction of the impact of the disease on a typical patient.

Unlike, NF-1, most patients with NF-2 are of at least normal intelligence. The incidence of learning disabilities is low. Most patients develop hearing loss long after language acquisition. Women with NF-2 are fertile, and the majority who become pregnant carry the fetus to term delivery without NF-2–related complications.

The vast majority of patients will develop acoustic schwannomas at some point in their lifetime; most can expect unilateral hearing loss to manifest by early adulthood. Approximately half may develop meningiomas at one or more loci within the neuraxis, but these tumors may be asymptomatic. The natural history of NF-2–related schwannomas and meningiomas has not been studied in longitudinal trials. It is assumed the propensity for growth and metastasis is similar to sporadic tumors.

In those patients with intracranial or spinal meningiomas, the possibility of increased tumor growth during pregnancy may be inferred from the same effect of pregnancy on sporadic meningiomas and reports of acoustic schwannomas first presenting during pregnancy, but no systematic study of the effect of pregnancy on schwannomas and meningiomas in NF-2 patients is available.

Long-Term Prognosis

The effect of NF-2 on longevity is variable, but the majority of the patients with NF-2 diagnosed on the basis of bilateral acoustic schwannomas die of causes unrelated to NF-2 and live a normal life span. Patients appear to segregate into either a mildly or severely affected group, with respect to both age of onset of first symptoms and eventual tumor burden. Those patients manifesting the severe phenotype may succumb to the neurologic sequelae of unresectable or disseminated meningiomas or schwannomas.

Tuberous Sclerosis

Tuberous sclerosis (TS) is a dominantly inherited neurogenetic disorder that affects the skin and visceral organs in addition to the nervous system. Like NF-1, TS is associated with neurologic dysfunction and maldevelopment, skin abnormalities, and a propensity for development of neoplasia. TS is associated with an increased incidence of both CNS and visceral tumors. Linkage studies have identified genes on chromosome 9 (TSC1) and 16 (TSC2). The TSC2 gene has been cloned and encodes a GAP-activating-protein associated with the Rap1 signal transduction pathway.

The diagnosis of TS is established when a patient manifests one of the following signs: facial angiofibroma or periungual or subungual fibroma; cortical tubers or subependymal hamartomas; or multiple retinal hamartomas. Secondary diagnosis requires two of the following: infantile spasms, hypomelanotic macules, shagreen patch, single retinal hamartoma, subependymal or cortical calcifications on CT scan, multiple renal tumors, cardiac rhabdomyoma, or an immediate relative with TS.

Natural History

Neurologic symptoms are present in the vast majority of patients. Seizures are present in more than 80% of patients. Mental retardation is the next most frequent symptom (60% of patients). The majority of patients with seizure disorders experience generalized seizures, including infantile spasms (30%) and myoclonic seizures (16%). Early onset, generalized seizures correlate strongly with mental retardation. When seizures begin in the first 2 years of life, mental retardation is almost uniformly present. Conversely, 60% of those with a first seizure between age 2 and 5 years have at least average intelligence, and only 33% of those having a seizure older than age 5 years are mentally retarded.

Age of onset of facial angiofibromas has no correlation with intelligence. Perhaps children with infantile spasms and a hypsarhythmic electroencephalogram exhibit more numerous and more extensive hypopigmented macules, but this has limited independent prognostic import since the correlation between infantile spasms and mental retardation is so high.

The kidneys, heart, and lungs are the most frequently involved viscera in TS. The majority of patients with TS have renal angiomyolipomas, highly vascular growths of smooth muscle, and fatty tissue within the substance of the kidney. The incidence increases with age; most patients have bilateral, multiple masses. Angiomyolipomas are infrequently symptomatic, and progressive renal failure is rare. Angiomyolipomas usually are indolent tumors and treatment should aim at preserving functional renal parenchyma. Renal cysts are frequently seen but usually are asymptomatic. Polycystic kidney disease may be the presenting feature of TS in a minority of cases.

A benign cardiac tumor, rhabdomyoma, is frequently associated with TS. When a pediatric rhabdomyoma is present, approximately half of the patients will have other stigmata of TS. Patients may manifest abnormalities of ventricular function, outflow obstruction, or dysrhythmia. These tumors do not metastasize, but can kill the patient by causing outflow obstruction or intractable cardiac failure. Surgical therapy, often transplantation, is required.

Pulmonary macrocystic disease is lethal but rare. When dyspnea appears in early adulthood, death, from progressive pulmonary dysfunction and cor pulmonale or acute spontaneous pneumothorax, usually follows within several years.

Skeletal lesions are common. Multifocal sclerotic areas may be present in the calvarium, spine, pelvis, hands, and feet. The lesions in the hands and feet are typically cystic with periosteal bone formation. These lesions are usually asymptomatic and are not neoplasms.

Dermatologic manifestations are frequently present even in neonates. Hypomelanotic macules (ash-leaf spots) are frequently present at birth and persist throughout life. They are usually 1 cm or more in length and are most common over the trunk and buttocks. These lesions are most easily seen using a lamp that emits 360 nm wavelength light (Wood's light). When present at birth, these lesions are almost pathognomonic for TS. Infants with mental retardation or seizure disorder should be examined with a Wood's light as part of the diagnostic evaluation. Shagreen patches are connective tissue hamartomas usually located on the dorsal skin surface of the lower back.

Facial angiofibromas (adenoma sebaceum) develop in the majority of patients with TS, but are usually not present at birth or in early infancy. These maculopapular lesions usually appear by age 4 years and may become more prominent and numerous during puberty. When present, facial angiofibromas are a pathognomonic sign of TS. Ungual fibromas are similarly pathognomonic.

The major focus of morbidity is the nervous system, and the major cause of early mortality is the growth of intraparenchymal brain neoplasms. Cortical tubers are hamartomatous lesions usually located in the cortical or subcortical parenchyma. Subependymal nodules, however, are usually subependymal giant cell astrocytomas. These are often slow-growing tumors that deform but do not invade adjacent brain parenchyma. The tumors may produce obstructive hydrocephalus or brain stem compression, depending on location. Patients with TS rarely develop other histologic types of intraparenchymal brain tumor.

Retinal and optic nerve involvement occurs in approximately half the patients with TS. Hamartomas of the retina or optic nerve may be classified into two types: (1) noncalcified, relatively flat, semitransparent lesions superficial to the retinal vessels; and (2) calcified, multinodular, mulberry lesions. The retinal and optic nerve lesions usually do not lead to blindness. The lesions are usually indolent. In the majority of patients, visual function is not compromised, the lesions do not grow, and no treatment is indicated. Retinal hamartomas may be mistaken for true malignant neoplasms, such as retinoblastoma, but only rarely is a retinal hamartoma the sole manifestation of TS when the neurologic and cutaneous examinations are carefully performed.

Short-Term Prognosis

The prognosis for normal intellectual development is difficult to assess in the young child. The occurrence of early onset generalized seizures, including infantile spasms, strongly predicts compromised intelligence. In the absence of a cardiac tumor, survival into young adulthood is common.

Long-Term Prognosis

The physician may be cautiously optimistic in predicting normal intellectual function for those patients who reach age 5 years without a seizure. Although the skin lesions may be cosmetically disfiguring and diagnostically helpful in establishing the diagnosis of TS, none of the lesions have neoplastic potential nor predispose to the development of skin malignancy. The skin manifestations of the disease do not impact on longevity. Vision loss is uncommon. The major cause of early mortality is CNS neoplasms.

von Hippel–Lindau Disease

von Hippel–Lindau Disease (VHD) is an autosomal, dominantly inherited disorder manifested by the development of retinal and cerebellar hemangioblastomas. The kidneys, pancreas, and epididymis may also show cystic changes. Positional cloning has identified the VHD gene on chromosome 3. This tumor suppressor gene is mutated not only in germline and tumor DNA in patients with VHD, but also in a substantial percentage of sporadic renal cell cancers.

Natural History

Retinal hemangioblastomas are the ocular hallmark of VHD, but are often asymptomatic. The lesions are often peripheral and rarely congenital. The median age of detection is young adulthood and visual prognosis is variable. Extravasation of fluid through a disrupted retinal vascular barrier and retinal detachment may compromise vision. Probably 50% of patients with retinal lesions will retain normal vision; blindness is unusual. Hemangioblastomas of the optic disk region or macula pose a greater threat.

Cerebellar hemangioblastoma is one of the most frequent manifestations of VHD and is often the first symptomatic manifestation, appearing in the third or fourth decade, and is a cause of substantial mortality and morbidity in most clinical series. Patients present with the signs and symptoms of a cerebellar mass lesion. Hemangioblastomas may also arise in the medulla or spinal cord and perhaps 10% of patients may have multiple tumors. Cerebellar hemangioblastomas may be cured by complete surgical resection.

A large percentage of patients with VHD develop some renal parenchymal abnormality. The most dangerous lesions are malignant hypernephromas. These tumors develop in approximately 25% of patients and are frequently lethal. Bilateral tumors occur frequently and develop earlier in VHD patients than in sporadic cases, with median age of diagnosis in the fifth decade. The tumors are malignant, and do metastasize, but cerebellar lesions detected in a search for metastasis in patients with hypernephroma may be surgically curable hemangioblastomas and not metastatic hypernephroma.

Polycystic disease may affect various visceral organs, including the kidneys, pancreas, and epididymis. These lesions are frequently asymptomatic and rarely compromise organ function. Pheochromocytomas have been reported in some VHD kindreds and may cluster in these families so that a large percentage of affected individuals will develop adrenal pheochromocytoma. Bilateral pheochromocytomas have been reported in VHD families, and the tumors may be asynchronous. The tumors are usually curable by surgery and rarely metastasize.

Short Term Prognosis

Molecular genetic identification should allow identification of presymptomatic individuals in kindreds known to be carrying the VHD mutation. These children should have an excellent short-term prognosis with normal intelligence, functional vision, and good renal function.

Long Term Prognosis

The major sources of morbidity and mortality are neoplasms associated with the VHD mutation. All patients with cerebellar hemangioblastoma or retinal hemangioblastomas should be tested for the presence of germline VHD mutations, which if present, indicate the need for ongoing surveillance to detect the presence of potentially lethal hypernephroma before metastasis. When presymptomatic screening identifies a patient within a known kindred, ongoing surveillance to detect the appearance of cerebellar or renal neoplasms should lead to effective surgical therapy and prolonged survival.

Additional Reading

Decker HJ, Weidt EJ, Brieger J. The von Hippel–Lindau tumor suppressor gene. A rare and intriguing disease opening new insights into basic mechanisms of pathogenesis. Cancer Genet Cytogenet 1997;93:74–83.

Gomez MR (ed). Neurocutaneous Diseases: A Practical Approach. Boston: Butterworths, 1987.

Gutmann DH, Aylsworth A, Carey JC, et al. The diagnostic evaluation and multidisciplinary management of neurofibromatosis 1 and neurofibromatosis 2. JAMA 1997; 278:51–57.

Korf BR. Neurocutaneous syndromes: neurofibromatosis 1, neurofibromatosis 2, and tuberous sclerosis. Curr Opin Neurol 1997;10:131–136.

Rubinstein AE, Korf BR (eds). Neurofibromatosis: A Handbook for Patients, Families and Health Care Professionals. New York: Thieme-Stratton, 1990.

Index